Manual of Pathologic Grossing

Ashley Illingworth

Manual of Pathologic Grossing

A Deliberative Approach

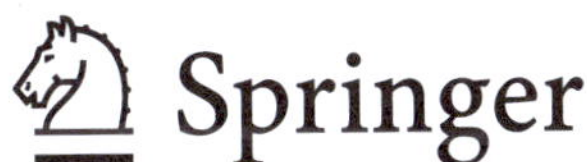 Springer

Ashley Illingworth
Department of Pathology
University of Mississippi Medical Center
Jackson, MS, USA

ISBN 978-3-031-72696-5   ISBN 978-3-031-72694-1   (eBook)
https://doi.org/10.1007/978-3-031-72694-1

This Springer imprint is published by the registered company Springer Nature Switzerland AG
The registered company address is: Gewerbestrasse 11, 6330 Cham, Switzerland

If disposing of this product, please recycle the paper.

To my Iowa family and Mississippi friends,
Thank you for all the love and support throughout my entire
career.
This one's for you!

Ashley

Preface

Throughout many years of experience as a Pathologists' Assistant, I have had two contradictory thoughts. The first: "I've seen so many specimens I could do this in my sleep." The second, which always catches me off guard: "Wow, I've never seen that before." This is why all of us who do this work love what we do. We love to learn. We love to see new things. We love the journey of pathology with all of its twists and turns always being reminded that no two specimens are alike. In fact, each specimen should be approached as if it is totally unique.

I started this textbook as a Word document tabulating the specimens I was grossing on a daily basis. It was a step-by-step tutorial to aid pathology residents learning this essential skill. It was a direct reference for the cases our residents were grossing in the lab at that exact moment. There was no additional information to digest just step 1, step 2, and step 3.

After I made the document available to the department, my coworkers began using my manual instead of existing textbooks. I realized that having a book that gave a deliberative approach focused only on grossing was needed! *The Manual of Pathologic Grossing: A Deliberative Approach* was born! This is a textbook designed to support the pathology assistant, pathology resident, pathologist or medical student. It supplements but will never replace the necessary communication between the grosser and the pathologist. Remember, no two specimens are the same and communicating specimen-specific information is essential.

Experience is the only way to gain confidence in the medical field. I would like to thank the department of pathology at the University of Mississippi Medical Center (UMMC) for allowing me the opportunity to learn and to teach. Specifically, I offer my deepest appreciation to my UMMC colleagues: William Daley, MD, Professor of Pathology who has been my mentor, confidante, and support system; Youssef Al Hmada, MD, Associate Professor of Pathology my advocate and comrade; and Robert T. Brodell, MD, Chair and Tenured Professor of Pathology for the support and encouragement that made this publication possible. Thank you all for helping me, encouraging me, and being with me to see this through. Without you this information would still be in a Word document.

Jackson, MS, USA

Ashley M. Illingworth

Acknowledgments

I would like to give a giant thank you to:

Dr. Robert Brodell for opening the door to this opportunity.

Dr. Ariel Velasques-Evers for all that time spent editing chapters and reviewing them with me. All your efforts are greatly appreciated.

Contents

Pregrossing

Contents

While experience is the best way to learn and gain confidence, there are a few things to know before entering the lab. Always communicate with the pathologist when new situations arise. You do not need to know the answer to everything but you do need to know where to find the answer.

1.1 Transport Medias

There are a multitude of different fixative solutions for different pathologic studies. It is vital to know the difference between each solution as often times, once the tissue is placed in a specific fixative, it cannot be used for any other testing than the purpose of the fixative. Always make sure the vial of fixative is labeled with the patient's information and the name of the solution. The main fixatives used in the surgical pathology lab are as follows:

Formalin Used in standard fixation of surgical specimens. Most laboratories use 10% buffered formalin which is formaldehyde diluted with a phosphate buffer. In general, formalin preserves tissue by stabilizing the proteins. This prevents the tissue from autolyzing.

Zeus or Michel's Transport Media Used for immunohistochemistry (IF) studies for in vitro diagnostic use. The tissue must be received fresh or in saline before being placed in Zeus or Michel's fixative.

A. Illingworth, *Manual of Pathologic Grossing*, https://doi.org/10.1007/978-3-031-72694-1_1

Glutaraldehyde Used for electron microscopy (EM). Tissue should be fresh or in saline before being placed in glutaraldehyde. If tissue is received in formalin and needs electron microscopy studies, communicate with the pathologist signing out the case. It is possible to submit formalin fixed tissue for electron microscopy but it is not the ideal procedure.

Roswell Parker Memorial Institute Medium (RMPI) Used for cytogenetic studies and flow cytometry. It is a nutritive medium that supports cell viability and is therefore not technically a fixative. Tissue must be received fresh or in saline for studies.

Snap Freeze Snap freezing tissue is one of the best ways for long-term preservation. Using liquid nitrogen, place the selected tissue into a labeled vial and close the lid. Place the vial in liquid nitrogen for 45–60 seconds. Snap frozen tissue can then be preserved in a −80 freezer until needed.

1.2   Fixation of Specimens

Proper fixation of all specimens is the key to good sections and histology. Adipose tissue and blood are by far the most difficult types of tissue to achieve good fixation. Remember that formalin penetrates tissue at approximately 1mm per hour and starts fixation from the outside of the specimen, working its way in. Adipose tissue and blood take even longer to fix because of the soft nature of the tissue. Always err on the side of more fixation rather than less and it is acceptable to begin grossing the specimen and then add additional fixation time when the specimen is sliced. Figure 1.1a is unfixed placenta. Notice how hemorrhagic and soft it looks. Figure 1.1b is the same section of placenta after 24 hours of formalin fixation. The time in formalin has allowed the tissue to become more firm which will allow for proper sections.

1.3   The Cassette

Everything in the lab revolves around the cassette. Grossing ends when the cassette closes but what is placed in the cassette and how it is placed in the cassette are incredibly important. Cassettes come in a variety of colors (Fig. 1.2), and each color can designate certain things. However, the colors and designations are laboratory dependent and not universal. Different colors could mean a type of tissue such as green cassettes are for sentinel lymph nodes. Or, different colors can correlate with the number of slides cut in histology such as a white cassette has one slide cut but a pink cassette has three slides cut from the tissue. Some laboratories use a number of different colors, and some only use one color cassette for everything. It all depends on where you work.

So, how do we use the cassette? Obtaining proper orientation in the cassette can be very counterintuitive. The rule is as follows:

The side of the tissue that is placed flat down on the bottom of the cassette is what will show on the slide.

What you need to see on the slide you will not see when you close the cassette lid because it will be placed down in the cassette.

For example: Let's look at this section of small bowel. With the eye, you can see the serosa, submucosa, and mucosa (Fig. 1.3). We also want to see all these layers on the microscopic slide.

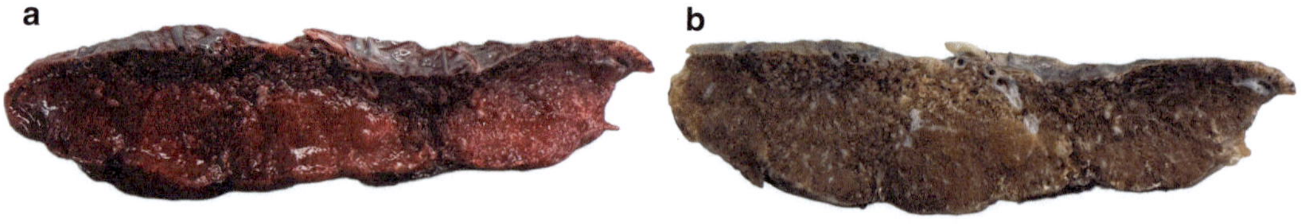

Fig. 1.1 (**a**) Fresh placental tissue with no formalin fixation; (**b**) placental tissue after 24 hr formalin fixation

Fig. 1.2 Cassettes

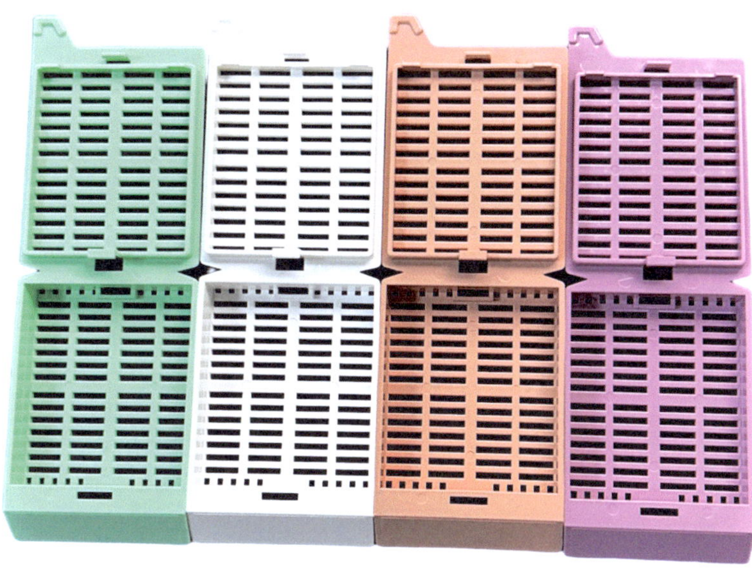

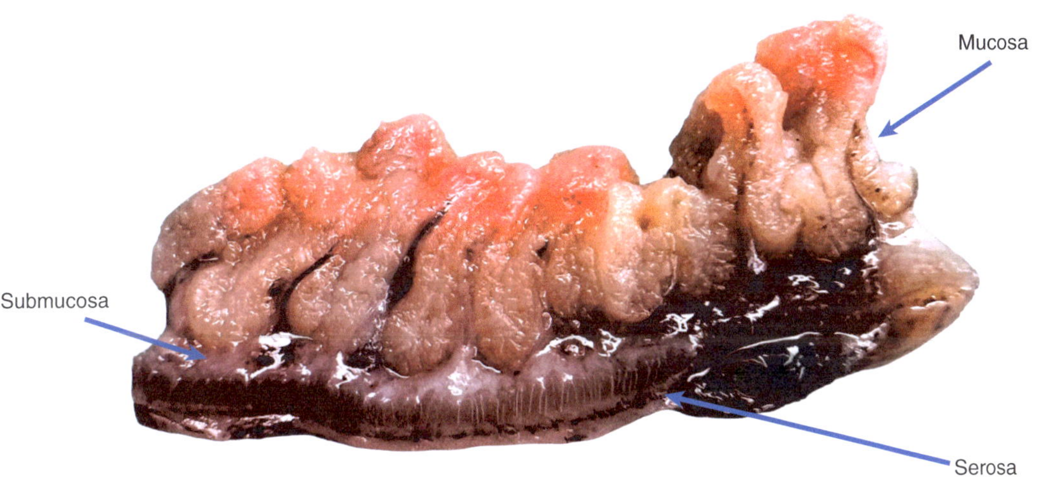

Fig. 1.3 Small bowel longitudinal section

Let's say the blue ink spot on the small bowel fragment is an area of interest (Fig. 1.4). We need to see this area on the slide. How should this section of small bowel be submitted in the cassette?

The blue ink spot on the section of small bowel should be placed flat down in the cassette. (Fig. 1.5). Now the blue ink is not visible.

If the grossing person places the same small bowel section with the serosa flat down in the cassette (Fig. 1.6a), then only serosa will be present on the slide. If the tissue is flipped over and the mucosal surface is placed flat down in the cassette (Fig. 1.6b), then only mucosa will end up on the slide.

Remember, it is imperative that attention be paid to the orientation of the tissue as it is being placed in the cassette. Otherwise, what is placed on the slide could be indecipherable.

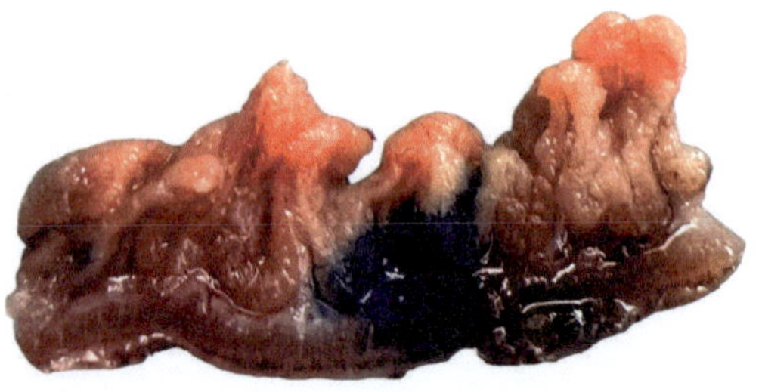

Fig. 1.4 Small bowel with ink designating area of interest

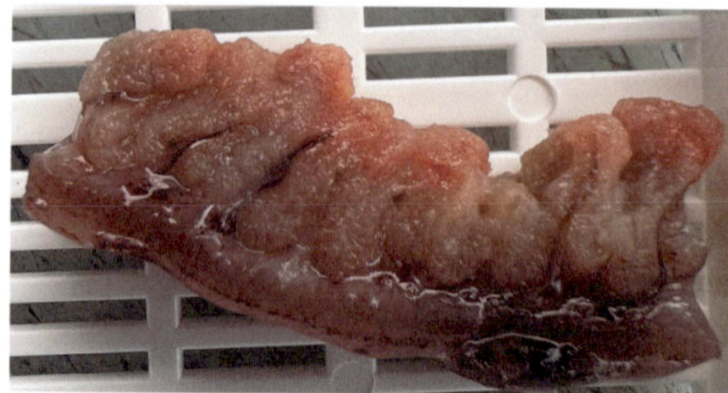

Fig. 1.5 Small bowel cassette submission

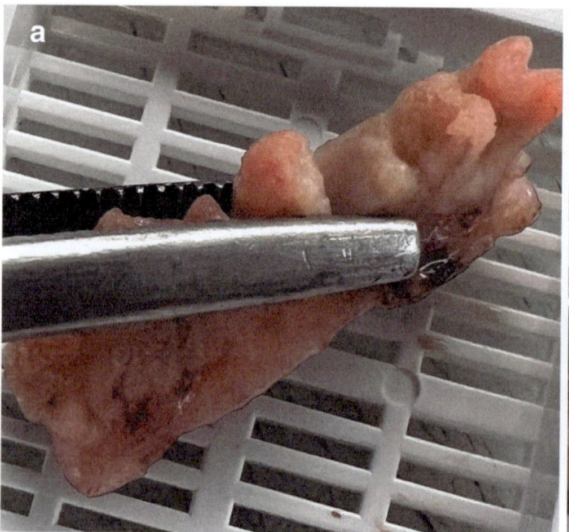

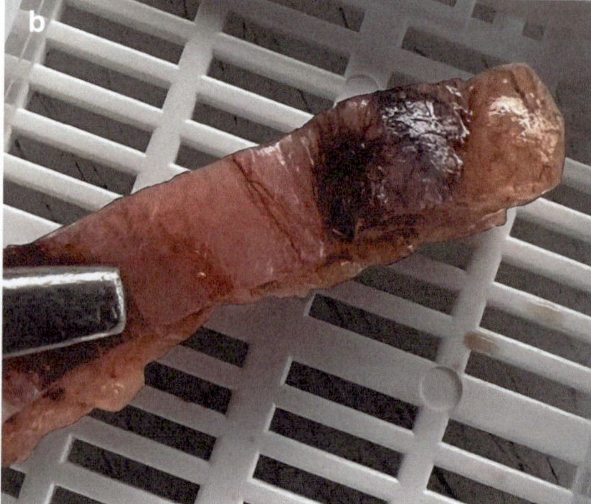

Fig. 1.6 (**a**) Small bowel placed on serosa; (**b**) small bowel placed on mucosa

1.4 Proper Sectioning Technique

There are so many different suggestions concerning proper grossing. However, it is up to you to decide what techniques work best. Two things to always keep in mind:

1. Your sharp instrument works better if it is slightly larger than the specimen or area of the specimen you are cutting. Using a 2-inch scalpel blade on a liver explant will take considerable time to section. However, that 2-inch scalpel blade would work great to remove the hilar vessels of the liver explant.
2. Sections submitted in cassettes need to be thin. Tissue is submitted in the cassette and then embedded in paraffin by histology. Those paraffin-embedded sections are then cut into thin 4–6 micron sections and placed on a glass slide. A histotechnologist needs a small rim of paraffin to surround the tissue section to grab onto while creating the slide. Therefore, it is necessary to submit sections that allow for proper embedding and not over fill the cassette allowing the tissue to touch the edges (Fig. 1.7a). Allow approximately 4–5mm of space between the tissue section and all four edges of the cassette. Also, the tissue needs room in the cassette for infiltration during processing. If the tissue becomes crushed within the cassette (Fig. 1.7b), there is no room for the processing chemicals and paraffin to get inside the cassette. Remember, leave a space between the tissue and the edges of the cassette and lid when closed (Fig. 1.7c)

Fig. 1.7 (**a**) Tissue overfilling fassette; (**b**) tissue too thick; (**c**) appropriate amount of tissue for cassette

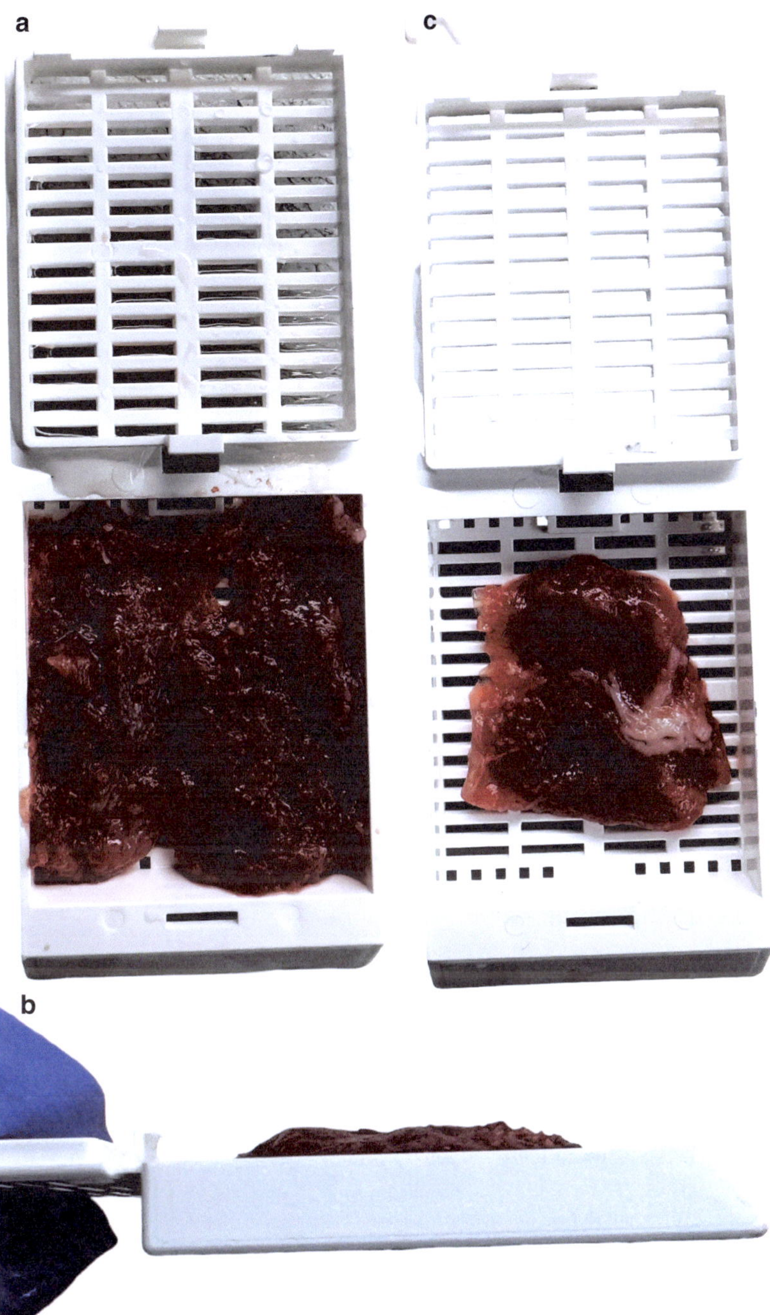

1.5 Use of Decalcifying Solutions

Before decalcifying any tissue, it must first be well fixed in formalin. Proper fixation preserves the cellular structure of the tissue before being introduced to harsh decalcification. Once the tissue is properly fixed, there is a multitude of brand name decalcifying solutions to choose from. These solutions are broken down into three main categories. It is best to discuss decalcifying options with the pathologists before placing any tissue in a decalcifying solution [1].

1. Strong acids: Typically, hydrochloric acid or nitric acid. These are the most rapid action solutions but if the tissue is left in these solutions for an extended period of time it can cause loss of nuclear staining and over soften the tissue. Continually check the tissues when using these decalcifying solutions.
2. Weak acids: Formic acid is widely used as a weak acid decalcifier. These solutions are slower to decalcify but are less likely to hinder nuclear staining.
3. Chelating agents: Ethylenediaminetetraacetic acid (EDTA) is a chelating agent that attaches to and minimizes the calcium ions present in the tissue. Chelating agents work the slowest but are very gentle on the tissue and work the best for ancillary studies such as immunohistochemistry (IHC), fluorescence in situ hybridization (FISH), and polymerase chain reaction (PCR) [1].

Whatever the solution chosen, the tissue should be grossly bendable and able to be cut easily with a blade before submitted the tissue as seen in Fig. 1.8. Once the tissue is ready, thoroughly rinse the tissue in water for a few minutes before placing the tissue in the cassette to remove excess decalcifying solution before processing.

While bone should be properly decalcified before submitting sections, over decalcifying can destroy the tissue, rendering it unacceptable for diagnosis. Notice the difference between these four sections of the same bone. Figure 1.9a is bone with 6 hours of decal time. Figure 1.9b is bone with 24 hours of decal time. Figure 1.9c is 96 hours of decal time, and Fig. 1.9d is bone with 168 hours of decal time. The nuclear structure of the bone begins to dissipate dramatically between 24 hours and 96 hours. At 168 hours, the nuclear structure is almost nonexistent. This is the process that occurs when bone is placed in decalcifying solution and then forgotten. If left too long in decalcifying solution, the section is nearly unreadable.

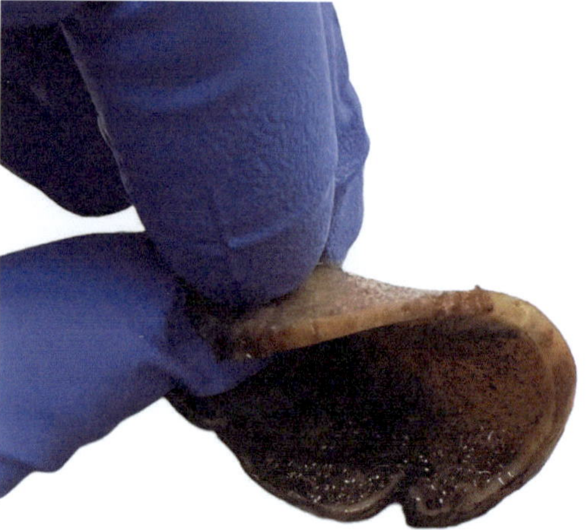

Fig. 1.8 Pliable bone post appropriate decalcification time

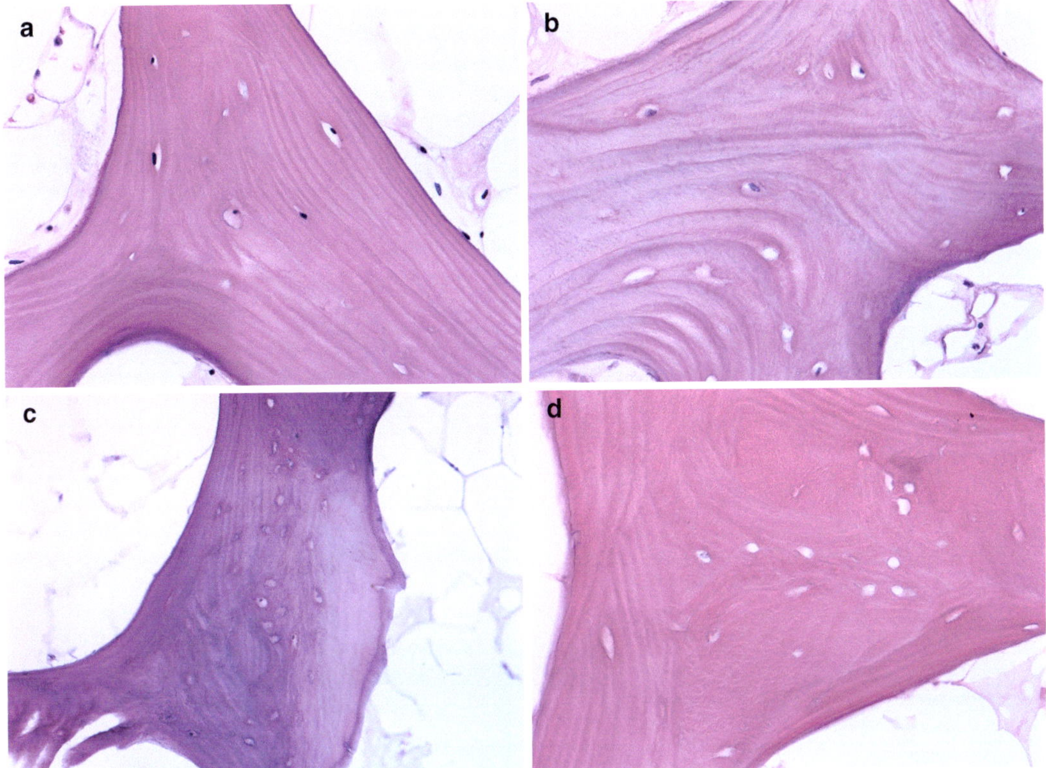

Fig. 1.9 (**a**) Bone decalcified for 6 hours; (**b**) bone decalcified for 24 hours; (**c**) bone decalcified for 96 hours; (**d**) bone decalcified for 168 hour

1.6   Basic Histology Embedding

Knowledge of the process of embedding is extremely important to the grossing person. Orientation of tissue and use of ink are silent ways to communicate with histology. Remember that whatever side of the tissue is face flat down in the cassette is what will show up on the slide.

For this example, a tissue section is inked orange on the one side and blue on the other (Fig. 1.10a, b). The pathologist wants the blue side to be seen on the microscopic slide.

Step 1: Place the blue side flat down in the cassette shown in Fig. 1.11.

Step 2: The tissue is processed and ready for embedding.

Step 3: The histo tech places the cassette on the embedding station as seen in Fig. 1.12.

Step 4: The cassette is opened, and orientation is reviewed. Notice the orange ink is still facing up in Fig. 1.13.

Step 5: The histo tech selects a mold that will fit the tissue. The mold is identified by the blue arrow in Fig. 1.14

Step 6: Transfer the tissue to the mold exactly as the tissue sits in the cassette. (Fig. 1.15a, b)

Step 7: The mold is filled with paraffin wax as shown in Fig. 1.16.

Step 8: The cassette is set on top of the mold (Fig. 1.17). The lid of the cassette is discarded.

Step 9: A small amount of paraffin wax is added to the top to fill in the cassette slots shown in Fig. 1.18.

Step 10: The mold is set on a cold plate (Fig. 1.19) to harden.

Step 11: Once the wax is hardened, the mold can be lifted away as shown in Fig. 1.20. At this point, the cassette with the tissue in it is called a block.

Step 12: The cassette is now called a block and is ready to be cut on a microtome. Notice now that the blue side (Fig. 1.21) is now visible in the block.

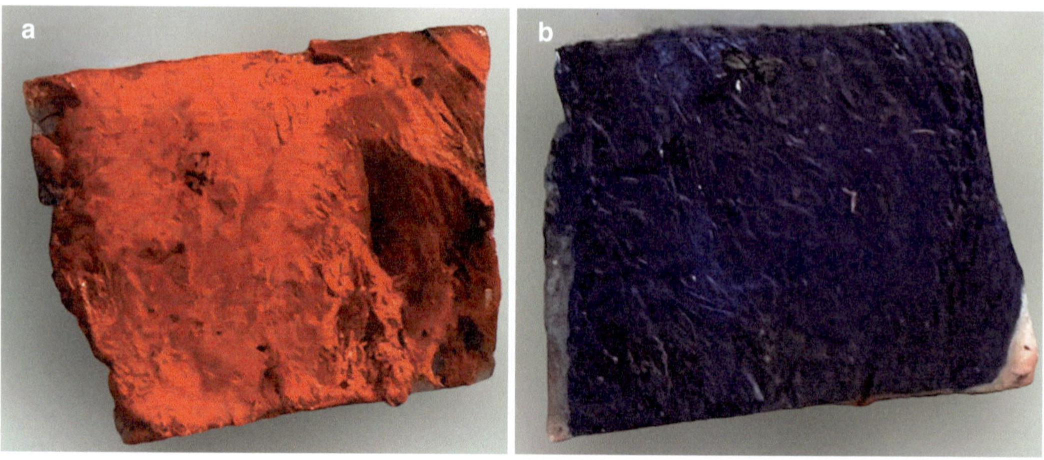

Fig. 1.10 (**a**) Orange ink side example tissue; (**b**) blue ink side example tissue

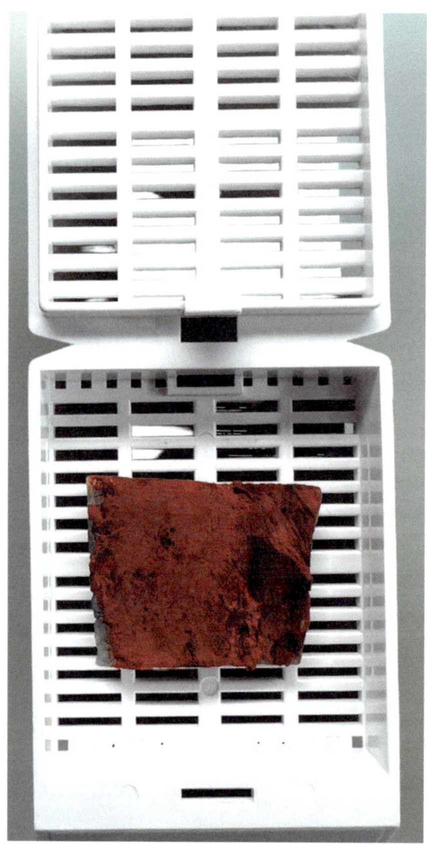

Fig. 1.11 Blue ink side example tissue placed down in the cassette

Fig. 1.12 Cassette post processing at the embedding station

Fig. 1.13 Cassette opened after processing

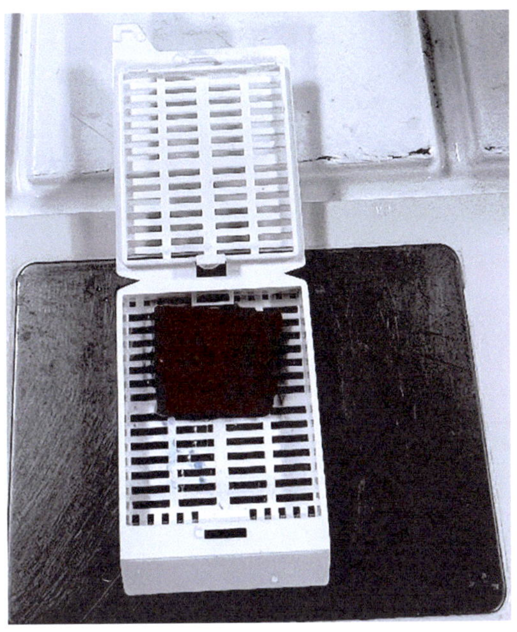

Fig. 1.14 Selection of mold tray

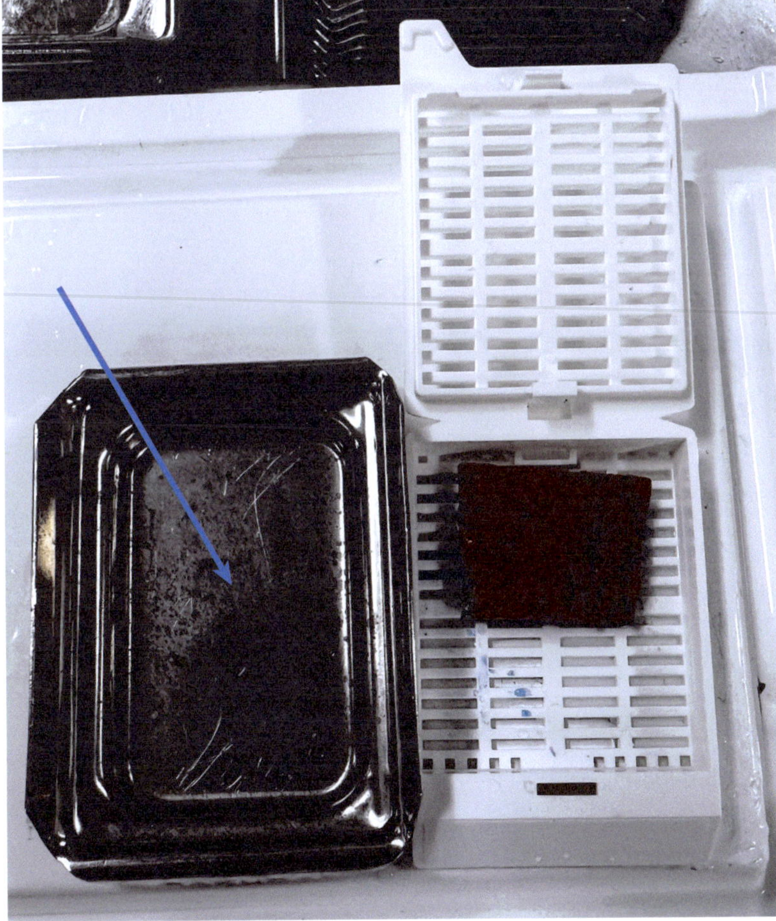

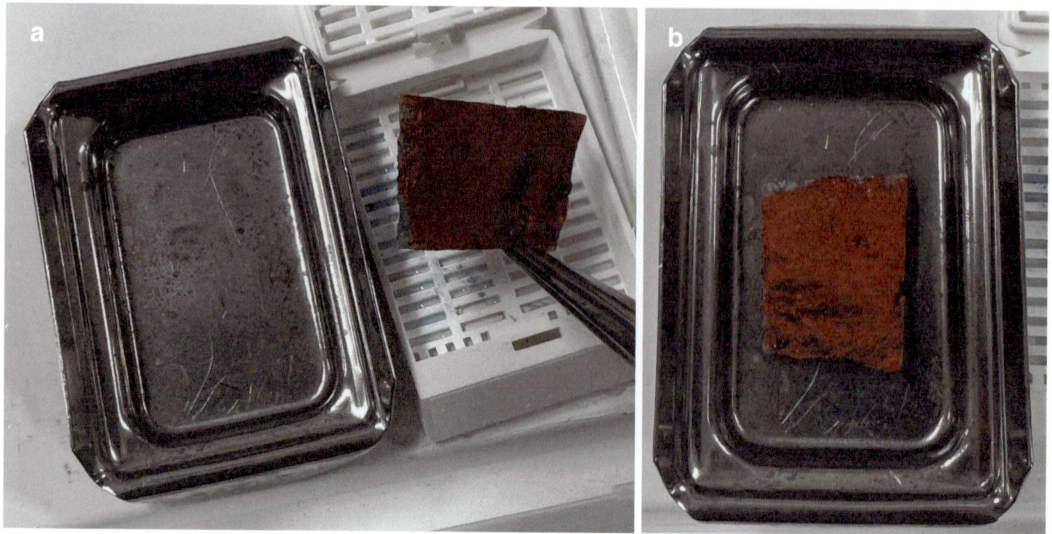

Fig. 1.15 (**a**) Pick up of example tissue; (**b**) example tissue placed in mold tray

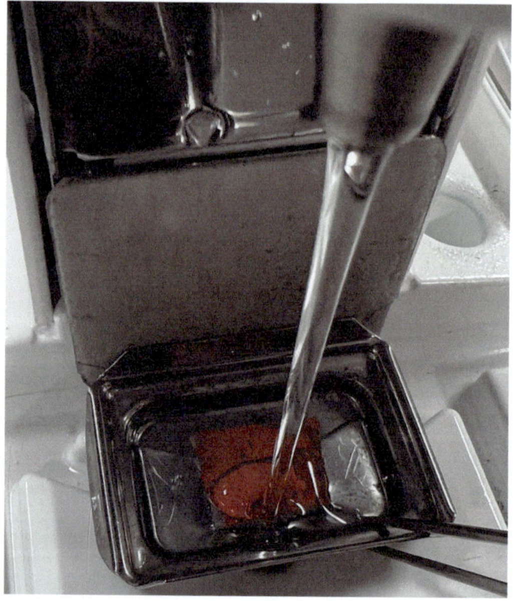

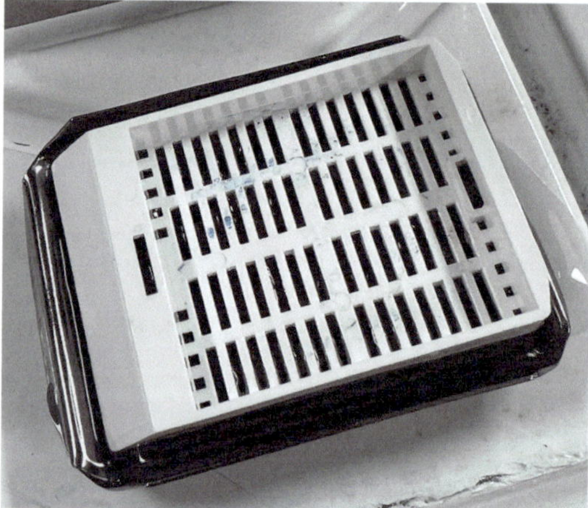

Fig. 1.17 Cassette placed onto mold tray containing example tissue

Fig. 1.16 Mold tray containing example tissue filled with paraffin wax

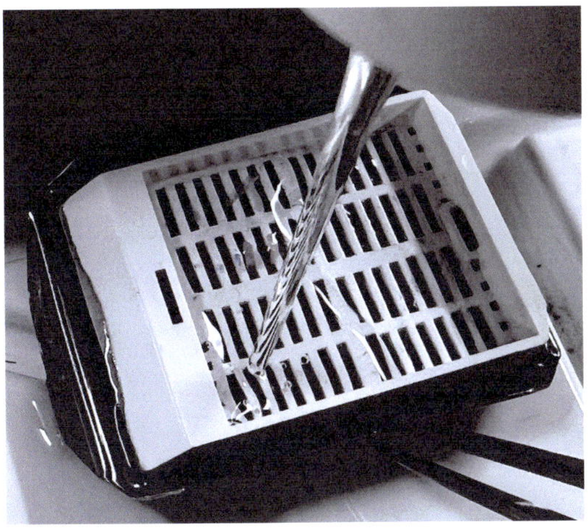

Fig. 1.18 Additional paraffin wax added to mold

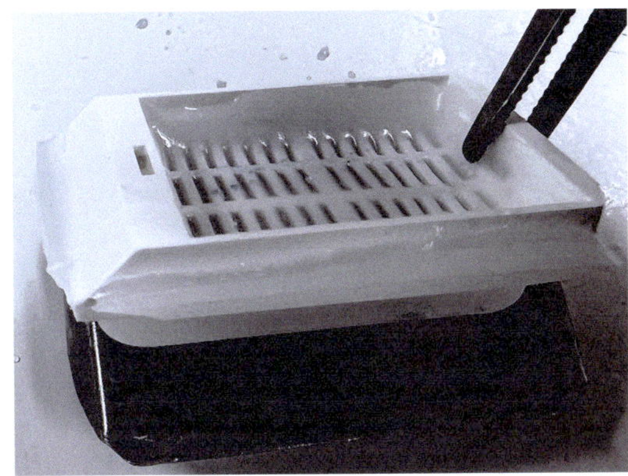

Fig. 1.20 Removal of block containing example tissue from mold tray

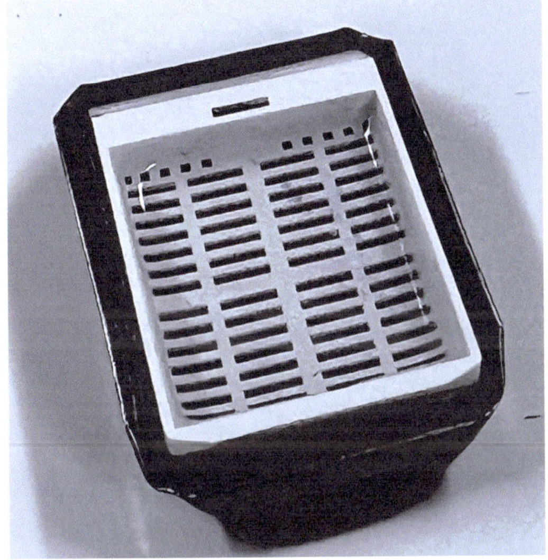

Fig. 1.19 Mold tray with example tissue cooling

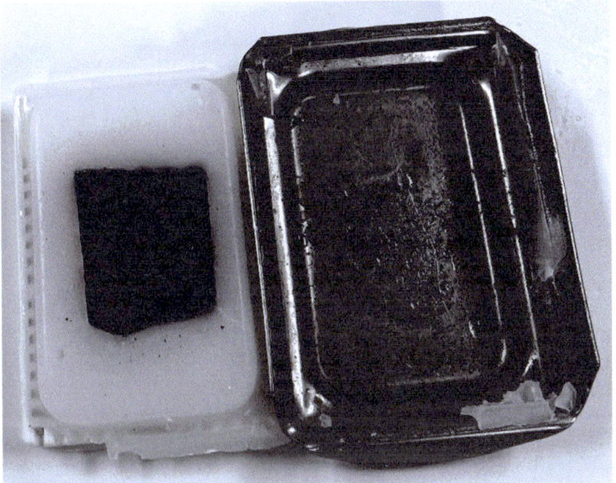

Fig. 1.21 Blue ink side example tissue exposed

1.7 Basic Use of a Cryostat

The cryostat is used to cut frozen sections during an intraoperative consultation. This is a quick way to produce microscopic slides. It is also a quick way to cut yourself. It cannot be emphasized enough that the cryostat is a dangerous piece of equipment when the grossing person is acting careless. Practice with the cryostat whenever possible to become comfortable with this piece of equipment.

Step 1: First, adjust the thick (red arrow) and thin (yellow arrow) microns to 40 micron and 6 microns; respectively (Fig. 1.22). This is the standard thicknesses but can be adjusted per situation. There are multiple brands of cryostats but they all function similarly. The chuck will be faced using the thick setting, and the thin setting is used to take the section that will be stained.

Step 2: Every cryostat has a handle lock (Fig. 1.23, blue arrow). Always make sure the handle is locked when not in use. If the handle is not locked, the cryostat arm can move, potentially trapping a finger between the chuck and the blade.

ALWAYS MAKE SURE THE HANDLE IS IN THE LOCK POSITION WHEN NOT IN USE

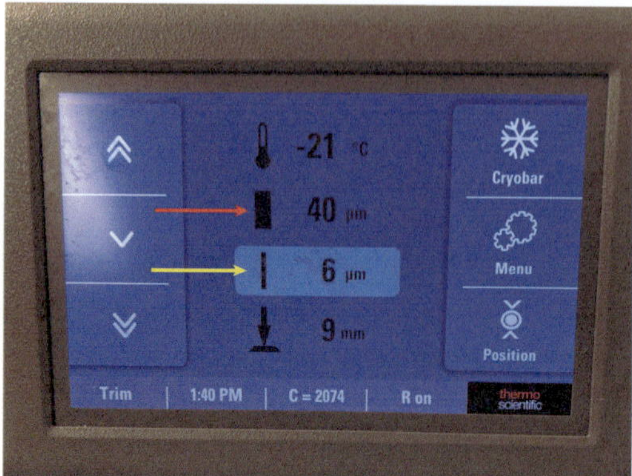

Fig. 1.22 Cryostat control screen

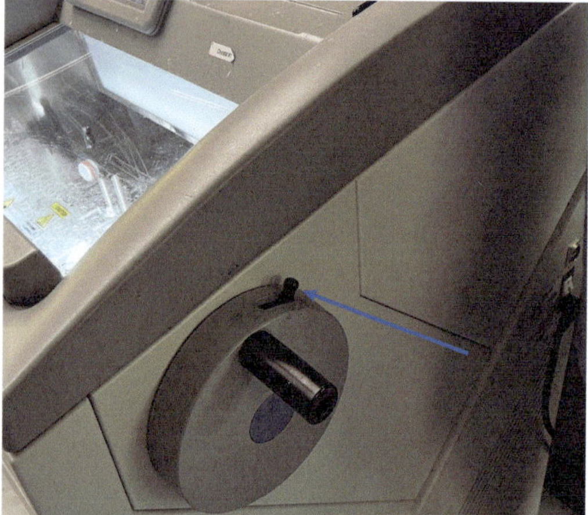

Fig. 1.23 Cryostat handle with lock

Step 3: Place a clean dry chuck (blue arrow) into the holder of the cryostat next to a heat extractor (red arrow) as seen in Fig. 1.24.

Step 4: Slowly squeeze the freeze media onto the chuck (Fig. 1.25), filling the chuck from the center to the outer metal ridge in a thin layer approximately 5–6 mm thick.

Step 5: Place the heat extractor on top of the freeze media to create a flat surface as shown in Fig. 1.26. Do not press the heat extractor down into the freeze media allowing the media to extrude off the edges of the chuck.

Step 6: Allow the freeze media to fully freeze.

Step 7: Remove the heat extractor. The freeze media should now be frozen, creating a flat, even surface shown in Fig. 1.27.

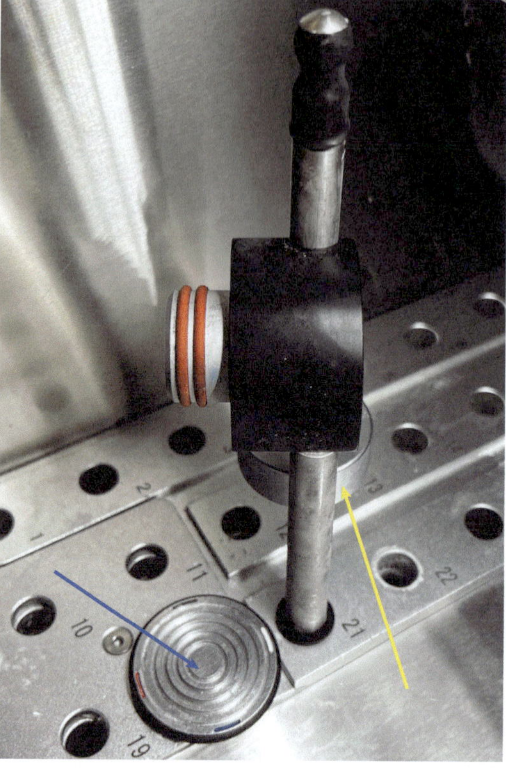

Fig. 1.24 Cryostat chuck and heat extractor

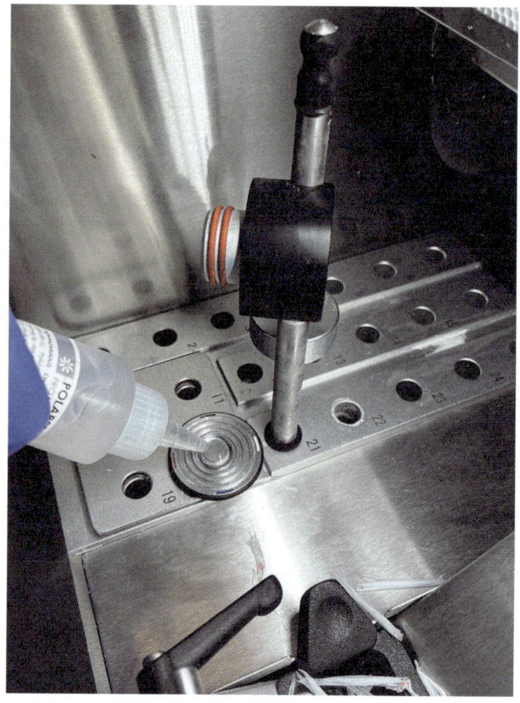

Fig. 1.25 Placing freeze media onto chuck

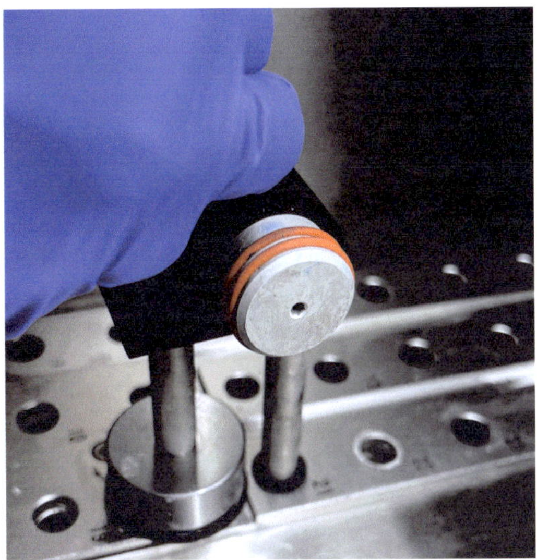

Fig. 1.26 Placing heat extractor onto chuck with freeze media

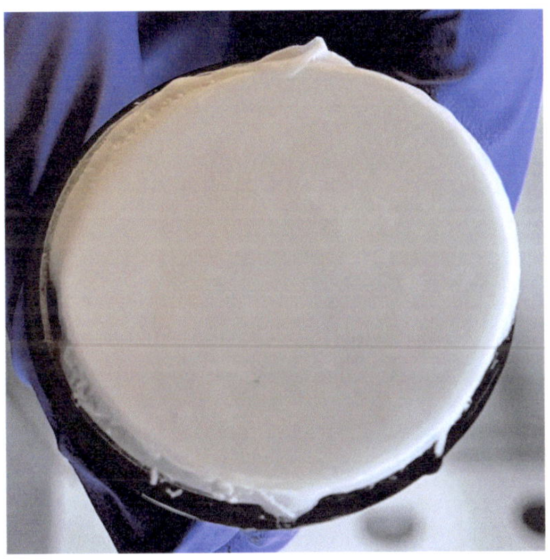

Fig. 1.27 Frozen chuck

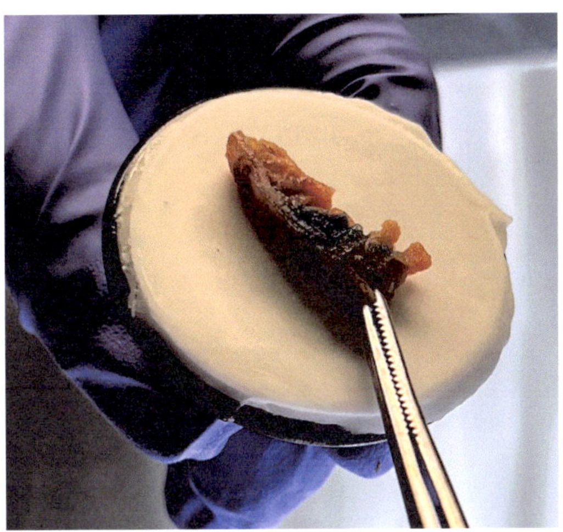

Fig. 1.28 Tissue placed on chuck

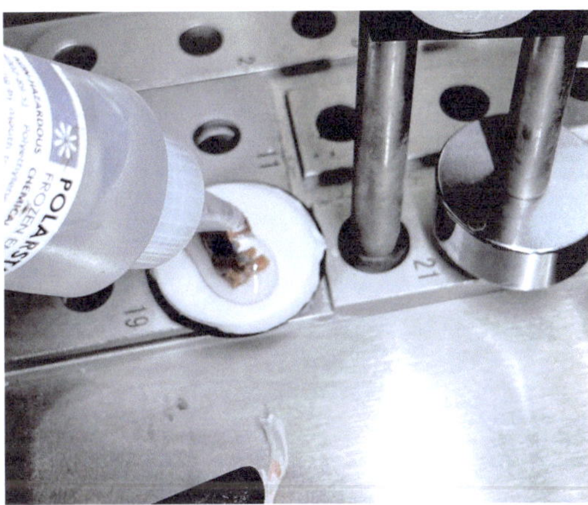

Fig. 1.29 Additional freeze media overlying the tissue

Step 8: Place the tissue on the chuck. Do not over fill the surface of the chuck. Leave an approximately 4–5 mm edge around the chuck as shown in Fig. 1.28.

Step 9: Place the chuck back in the cryostat and apply freeze media to fully cover the tissue, extending to the outer edge of the chuck. (Fig. 1.29)

Step 10: Place heat extractor back on top of the freeze media (Fig. 1.30). Again, do not press down too hard.

Step 10: Allow for the freeze media to completely freeze and then remove the heat extractor. The chuck should be flat on top and is now ready to cut as seen in Fig. 1.31.

Step 11: Place the chuck in the holder of the cryostat arm. Turn the screw handle (Fig. 1.32 blue arrow) to secure the chuck in place.

Step 12: Unlock the handle and adjust the chuck close to the blade. Advance the chuck toward the blade (blue arrow) while turning the han-

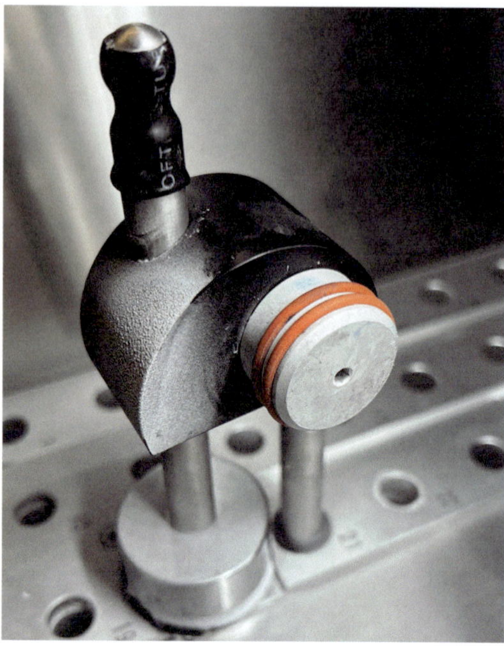

Fig. 1.30 Heat extractor placed on chuck with tissue and freeze media

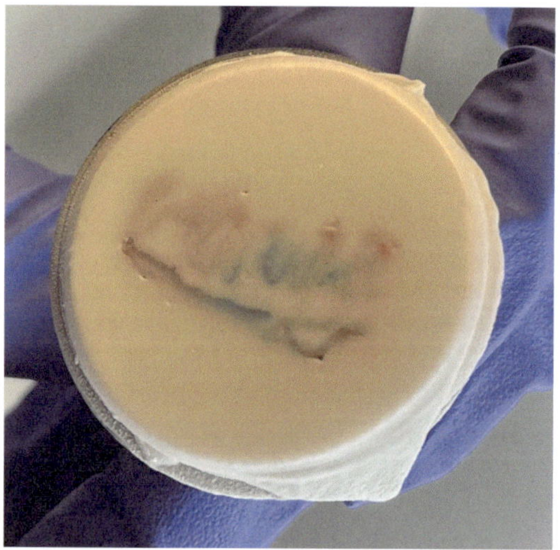

Fig. 1.31 Complete chuck

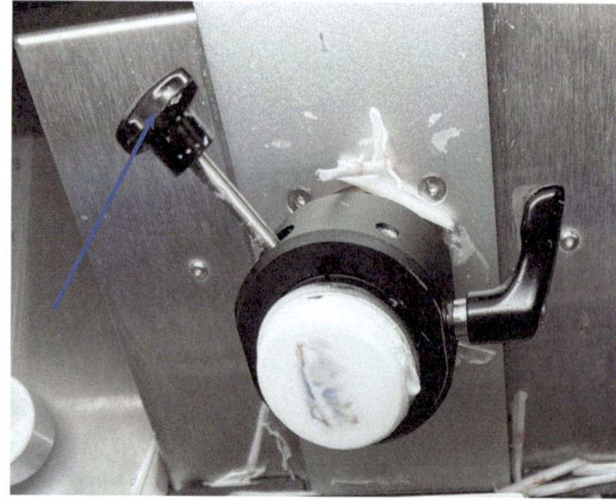

Fig. 1.32 Chuck placement in cryostat

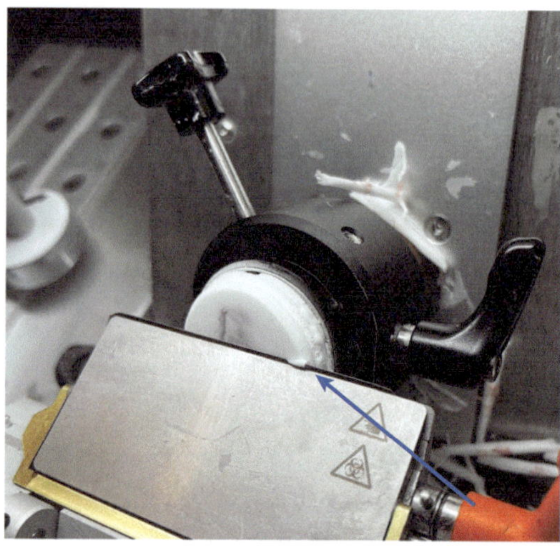

Fig. 1.33 Aligning the chuck with the cryostat blade

dle until the chuck just barely hits the blade (Fig. 1.33).

Step 13: Begin facing the chuck at 40 microns until the entire tissue is exposed. Figure 1.34 shows only a partly exposed surface of the tissue.

Step 14: Once the tissue is fully faced, as shown in Fig. 1.35, switch the microns to the thin 6 microns setting. It is best to shave off a couple of sections prior to placing a section on the slide.

Step 15: When taking a section, slowly move the handle with the right hand and pull the section out flat using a brush with the left hand shown in Fig. 1.36.

Step 16: Hold the section with the brush and pick up a slide with the right hand. (Fig. 1.37)

Step 17: Position the slide flat to the tissue picking up the section onto the slide as shown in Fig. 1.38. When the tissue is on the slide, quickly place the slide into the staining media.

Step 19: Stain and cover slip the slide. (Fig. 1.39)

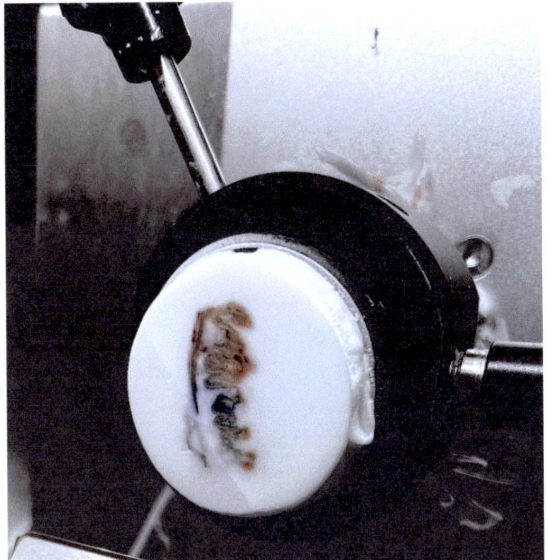

Fig. 1.34 Partially faced chuck

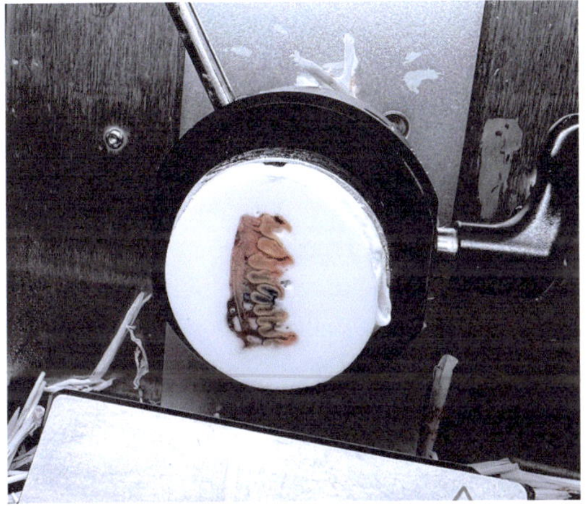

Fig. 1.35 Fully faced chuck

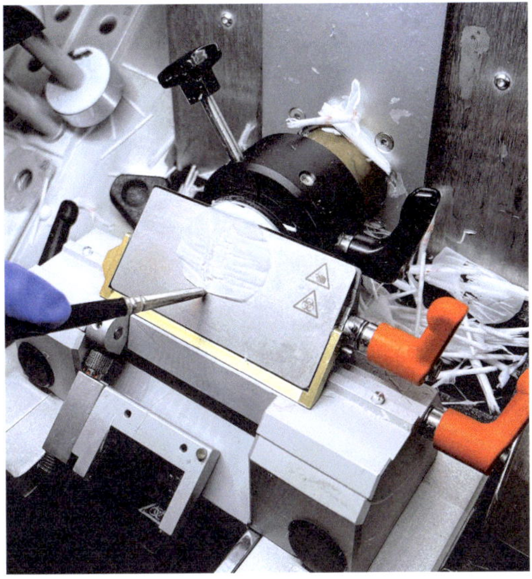

Fig. 1.36 Pulled section of tissue

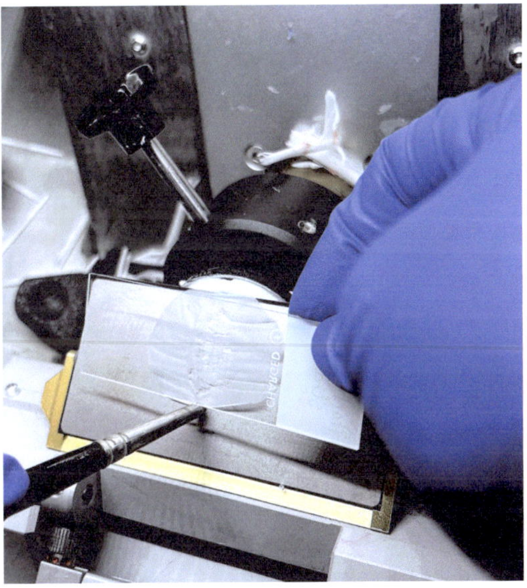

Fig. 1.37 Lining up the slide with the section of tissue

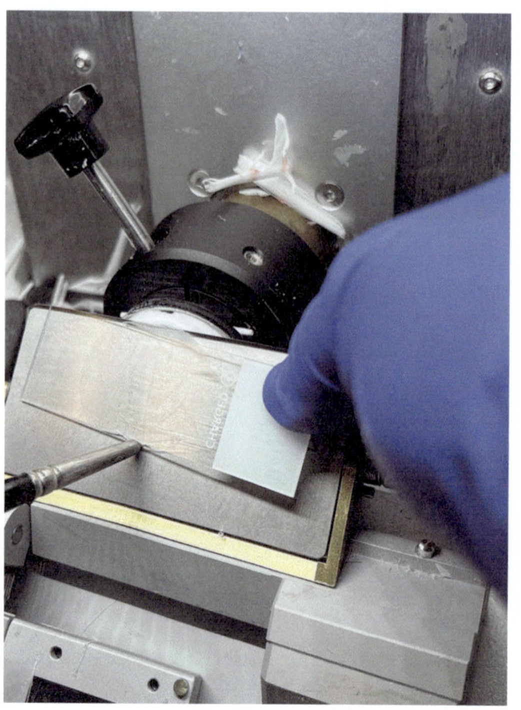

Fig. 1.38 Placing the tissue on the slide

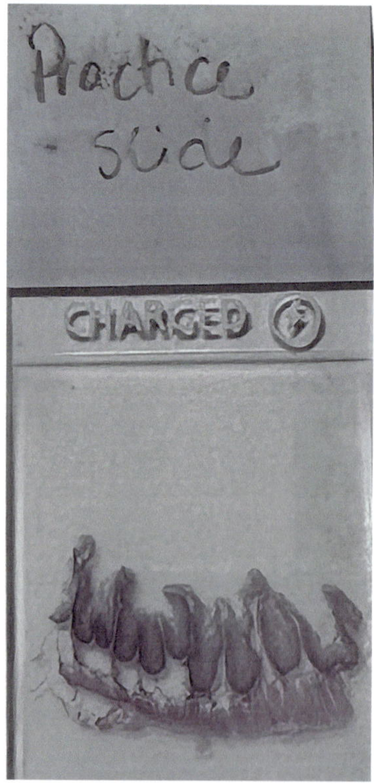

Fig. 1.39 Stained slide

1.8   Grossing and the CAP Cancer Protocols

The College of American Pathologists (CAP) created a set of cancer protocols that are considered the gold standard for grossing and signing out cancer cases. These protocols provide consistency and structure for the pathologists that, in turn, improves patient care [2]. The cancer protocols help ensure that pathology reports contain all the essential information to assist patient care [2]. Some hospitals have implemented these protocols directly into their electronic health record (EHR) system but these protocols are also available online. It is highly recommended to review these protocols before grossing any cancer case.

1.9   Trauma and Legal Cases

The surgical pathology lab is part of the chain of custody and documentation of trauma cases and potential court cases. Documentation of the specimen is crucial to the process of these types of cases. Photography and a detailed gross description along with proper section submission are keys. In these cases, always contact the physician signing out the case to view the specimen.

Cases involving gunshot, knife, traumatic wounds that could potentially become a lawsuit or court case:

1. Inform the physician who is signing out the case to view the specimen
2. Take gross photos prior to grossing and additional gross photo when specimen is open, if necessary
3. Note any trauma to the specimen with measurements
4. Submit sections providing areas of trauma

Acknowledgment The author gratefully acknowledges William P. Daley, MD, and Shivani Satia, MD, for their contribution to this chapter.

Quiz Questions

Questions

1. Which fixative is used for immunohisto-chemistry studies?
   A. Formalin
   B. Glutaraldehyde
   C. Michel's transport media
   D. RPMI
2. Which is the best method for long-term preservation of the tissue?
   A. Formalin
   B. Snap freeze
   C. Glutaraldehyde
   D. RPMI
3. Which statement is false regarding fixation of tissues?
   A. Adipose tissue and blood are the most difficult types of tissue to achieve good fixation
   B. Formalin preserves tissue by stabilizing the proteins
   C. Formalin penetrates tissue at approximately 3 mm per hour
   D. Formalin fixed tissue can be submitted for electron microscopy
4. Which statement is true for decalcifying the tissue?
   A. Before decalcifying the tissue, it should be placed in formalin
   B. Before decalcifying the tissue, it should not be placed in formalin
   C. Before decalcifying the tissue, it should be placed in glutaraldehyde
   D. Formic acid is a strong acid decalcifier
5. Which transport medium used for electron microscopy?
   A. Formalin
   B. Glutaraldehyde
   C. Michel's transport media
   D. RPMI
6. While statement is true regarding placement of the tissue in the cassette?
   A. Tissue should be filling the cassette
   B. Sections submitted in cassettes need to be thick
   C. The side of the tissue that is placed flat down on the cassette is what shows on the slide
7. The side of the tissue that is placed up on the cassette is what shows on the slide Which medium is used for cytogenetics and flow cytometry?
   A. Glutaraldehyde
   B. Formalin
   C. Michel's transport media
   D. RPMI
8. Which is the the best decalcifying agent for ancillary studies such as immunohistochemistry (IHC), fluorescence in situ hybridization (FISH), and polymerase chain reaction (PCR)?
   A. Hydrochloric acid
   B. Formic acid
   C. Nitric acid
   D. EDTA
9. Which decalcifying agent that acts the fastest?
   A. Hydrochloric acid
   B. Formic acid
   C. EDTA
   D. Glutaraldehyde
10. While statement is false regarding cases that could potentially become a lawsuit or court case?
    A. Inform the physician who is signing out the case to view the specimen
    B. No gross photos need to be submitted
    C. Any trauma to the specimen is noted with measurements
    D. Submitting sections providing areas of trauma

Answer Key

1. C

   Explanation: Zeus or Michel's transport media is the fixative used for immunohisto-chemistry (IF) studies for in vitro diagnostic use. The tissue must be received fresh or in saline before being placed in Zeus or Michel's fixative.

2. **B**

   Explanation: Snap freezing tissue is one of the best ways for long-term preservation. Snap frozen tissue can then be preserved in a −80 freezer until needed.

3. **C**

   Explanation: Formalin penetrates tissue at approximately 1mm per hour and starts fixation from the outside of the specimen, working its way in.

4. **A**

   Explanation: Before decalcifying any tissue, it must first be well fixed in formalin. Proper fixation preserves the cellular structure of the tissue before being introduced to harsh decalcification

5. **B**

   Explanation: Glutaraldehyde is used for electron microscopy. Tissue should be fresh or in saline before being placed in glutaraldehyde.

6. **C**

   Explanation: The side of the tissue that is placed flat down on the cassette is what shows on the slide. Sections submitted in cassettes need to be thin, no thicker than 4mm

7. **D**

   Explanation: RMPI is used for cytogenetic studies and flow cytometry. It is a nutritive medium that support cell viability.

8. **D**

   Explanation: EDTA is a chelating agent that works the slowest but is very gentle on the tissue and works the best for ancillary studies such as immunohistochemistry, fluorescence in situ hybridization, and polymerase chain reaction.

9. **A**

   Explanation: Hydrochloric acid and nitric acid have most rapid action solutions but if the tissue is left in these solutions for an extended period of time, it can cause loss of nuclear staining and over soften the tissue.

10. **B**

   Explanation: Taking gross photos prior to grossing and additional gross photo when the specimen is opened in cases that could potentially become a lawsuit or court case

References

1. Rolls G. An introduction to decalcification. 2023. [Online]. Available: http://www.leicabiosystems.com/us/knowledge-pathway/an-introduction-to-decalcification/
2. https://www.cap.org/protocols-and-guidelines/cancer-reporting-tools/cancer-protocol-templates. 2023. [Online]. Available: https://www.cap.org/protocols-and-guidelines/cancer-reporting-tools/cancer-protocol-templates

Grossing of Bone and Soft Tissue Specimens

Contents

Bone and soft tissue surgery can produce an array of different specimens. From small hernia sacs to major resections of multiple different bones, this subspecialty is incredibly unique. Utilizing a band-saw with a diamond blade is remarkably helpful when grossing bone but remember that bone needs to be well decalcified before submitting sections. Knowledge of the CPT codes for bone and soft tissue is necessary when grossing. Bone and soft tissue cover a large majority of the CPT codes and when tissue is decalcified, an additional charge is implemented. See Table 2.1 for CPT codes.

A. Illingworth, *Manual of Pathologic Grossing*, https://doi.org/10.1007/978-3-031-72694-1_2

Table 2.1 CPT codes

Fingers/toes, amputation traumatic	88302
Hernia sac	88302
Abscess	88304
Bone fragments, not pathologic fracture	88304
Bursa/synovial cyst	88304
Carpal tunnel tissue	88304
Cartilage shavings	88304
Dupuytren's contracture tissue	88304
Femoral head-other than fracture	88304
Ganglion cyst	88304
Intervertebral disc	88304
Joint, loose body	88304
Meniscus	88304
Pilonidal cyst/sinus	88304
Soft tissue debridement	88304
Soft tissue, lipoma	88304
Tendon/tendon sheath	88304
Bone exostosis	88305
Extremity, amputation, traumatic	88305
Femoral head, fracture	88305
Fingers/toes, amputation, non-traumatic	88305
Joint, resection	88305
Muscle biopsy	88305
Peritoneal biopsy	88305
Soft tissue, not tumor/mass/lipoma	88305
Synovium	88305
Bone and soft tissue tumor, extensive resection	88305
Bone, biopsy/curettings	88307
Bone, fragments, pathologic fracture	88307
Extremity, amputation, non-traumatic	88307
Bone resection	88309
Extremity, disarticulation	88309
Soft tissue tumor, extensive resection	88309
Decalcifying agent	88311

[1]

2.1 Bone Biopsy: Level V CPT 88307

A bone biopsy is obtaining a sample of the abnormality or lesion for diagnosis.

Step 1: Describe and measure the specimen (Fig. 2.1)

Step 2: Submit the specimen entirely as seen in Fig. 2.2.

Step 3: Decalcify bone before submitting.

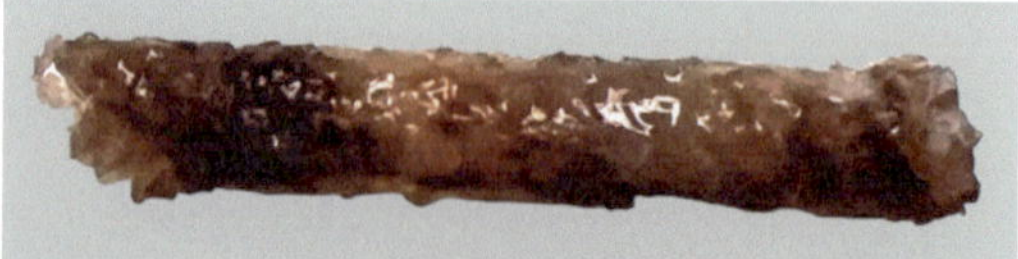

Fig. 2.1 Bone biopsy

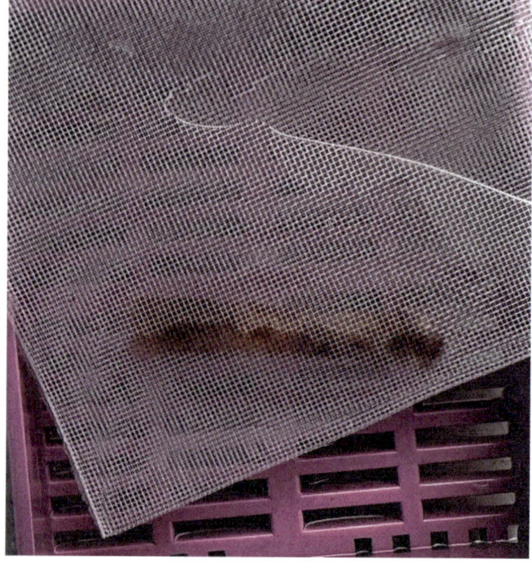

Fig. 2.2 Bone biopsy section submission

Example Dictation

Specimen A is received in formalin labeled with the patient's name, medical record number, and "bone biopsy" and consists of 1 fragment of tan-pink bone (1.2 x 0.9 x 0.5 cm) which is submitted in toto in a biopsy bag in A1, post decalcification.

2.2 Hernia Sac: Level II CPT 88302

A hernia sac is created when the abdominal wall tissue extends through a weak spot in the tissue, often between muscles and in the inguinal region. When force is applied, abdominal tissue presses on the abdominal cavity and then extrudes through the weak area producing a sac. When surgically excised, the hernia sac can arrive in the

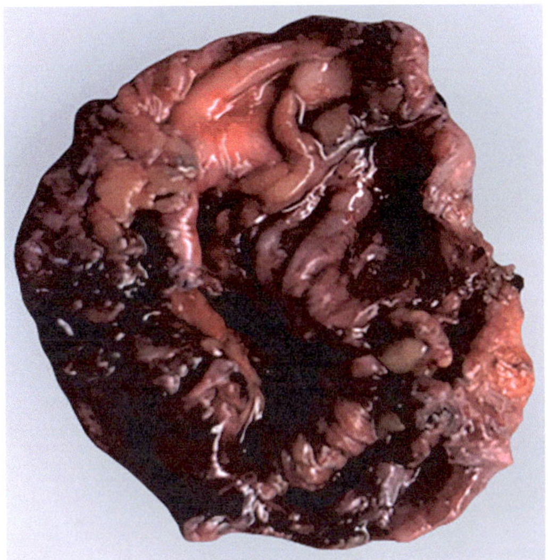

Fig. 2.3 Hernia sac

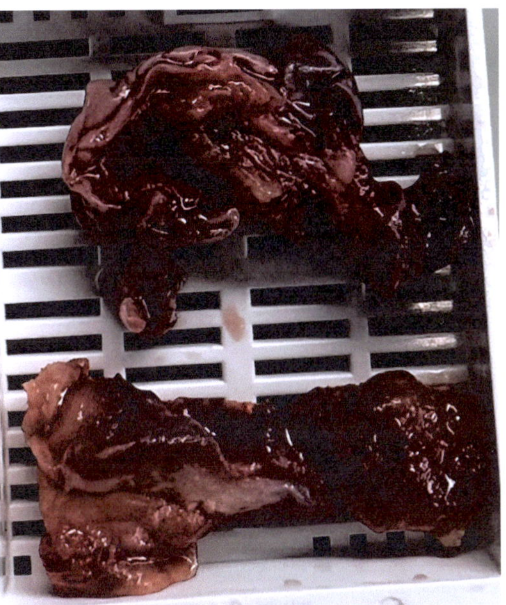

Fig. 2.4 Hernia sac sections submission

gross room intact or in fragments and can also contain other abdominal tissues such as fat.

Step 1: Describe and measure the specimen (Fig. 2.3)
Step 2: Dictate if any other structures are present. For example fat, bowel, etc.
Step 3: Submit representative sections of the hernia sac and any other structures present as seen in Fig. 2.4.

Example Dictation
Specimen A is received in formalin labeled with the patient's name, medical record number, "hernia, left" and consists of a single fragment of tan-purple fibrous tissue (4.7 x 4.1 x 0.9 cm) with a scant amount of adhered tan-yellow adipose tissue. Representative sections are submitted in A1.

2.3   Bursa: Level III CPT 88304

A bursa is a small sac filled with lubricating fluid between joints to decrease joint friction when moving. These sacs can become irritated, causing swelling. Surgically removing the bursa is an option after conservative management options like supportive measures and medications are exhausted.

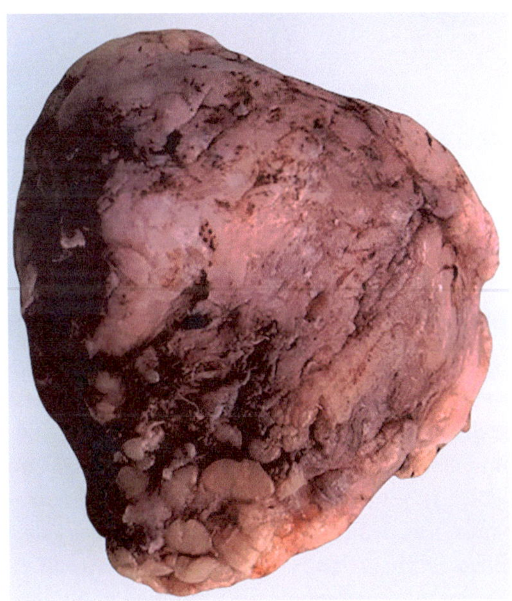

Fig. 2.5 Bursa sac

Step 1: Describe and measure the specimen. (Fig. 2.5)
Step 2: Serially section the specimen as seen in Fig. 2.6.
Step 3: Describe the internal cyst space and the presence or absence of fluid.

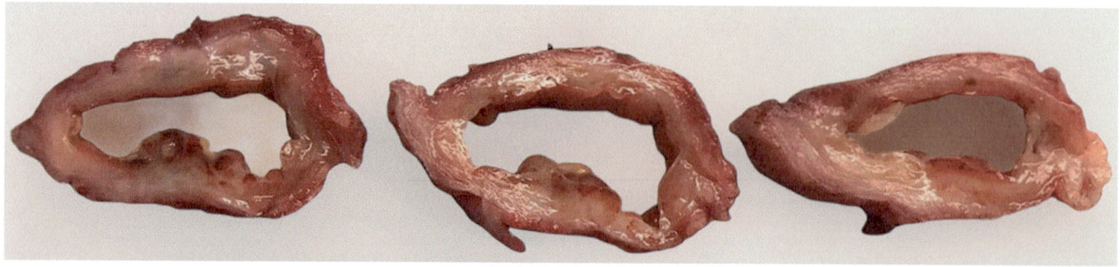

Fig. 2.6 Bursa sac, serially sectioned

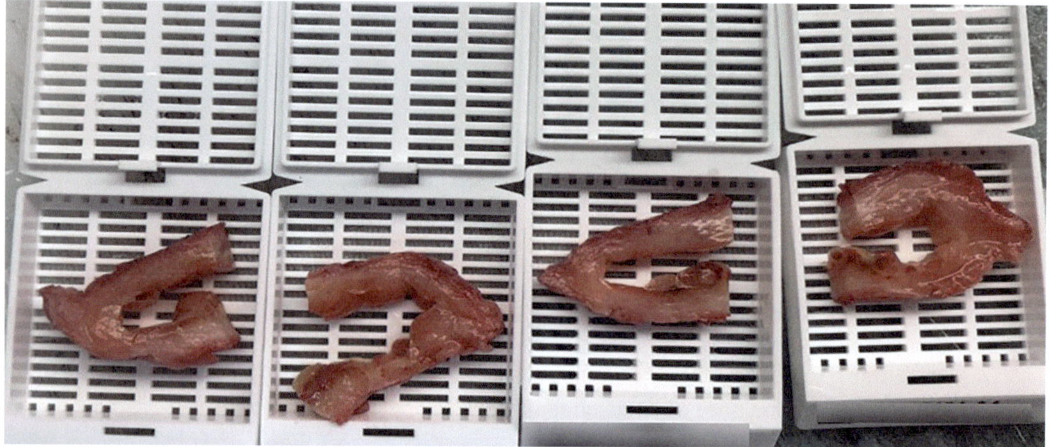

Fig. 2.7 Bursa sac sections submission

Step 4: Submit representative sections of the bursa as seen in Fig. 2.7.

Example Dictation

Specimen A is received in formalin labeled with the patient's name, medical record number, and "bursa sac" and consists of an intact, tan-yellow, unoriented soft tissue sac (7.2 x 6.2 x 2.4 cm) which is serially sectioned to reveal an internal smooth walled cystic space (2.4 x 2.2 x 2.1 cm) filled with a scant amount of clear fluid. Representative sections are submitted in A1–A4.

2.4   Lipoma: Level III CPT 88304

A lipoma is a benign fatty tumor that can grow in the subcutaneous tissue or deep in the skeletal muscle. These tumors don't require any treatment but are often removed due to the size or placement, causing issues for the patient or purely for cosmetic purposes.

Tumors greater than 5 cm in the greatest dimension have an increased risk of malignancy (liposarcoma). Therefore, the specimen needs to be sampled well to rule out malignancy.

Step 1: Describe, measure, and weigh the specimen. (Fig. 2.8)

Step 2: Ink the outer surface as seen in Fig. 2.9.

Step 3: Serially section the specimen. (Fig. 2.10)

Step 4: Describe the cut surfaces.

Step 5: Submit representative sections that include mass to the surrounding inked margin and central areas of mass. Approximately 1 section per 1 cm of the overall size of the mass is acceptable as seen in Fig. 2.11. Look for areas with necrosis, and hemorrhage and submit additional sections from different-looking/heterogeneous areas.

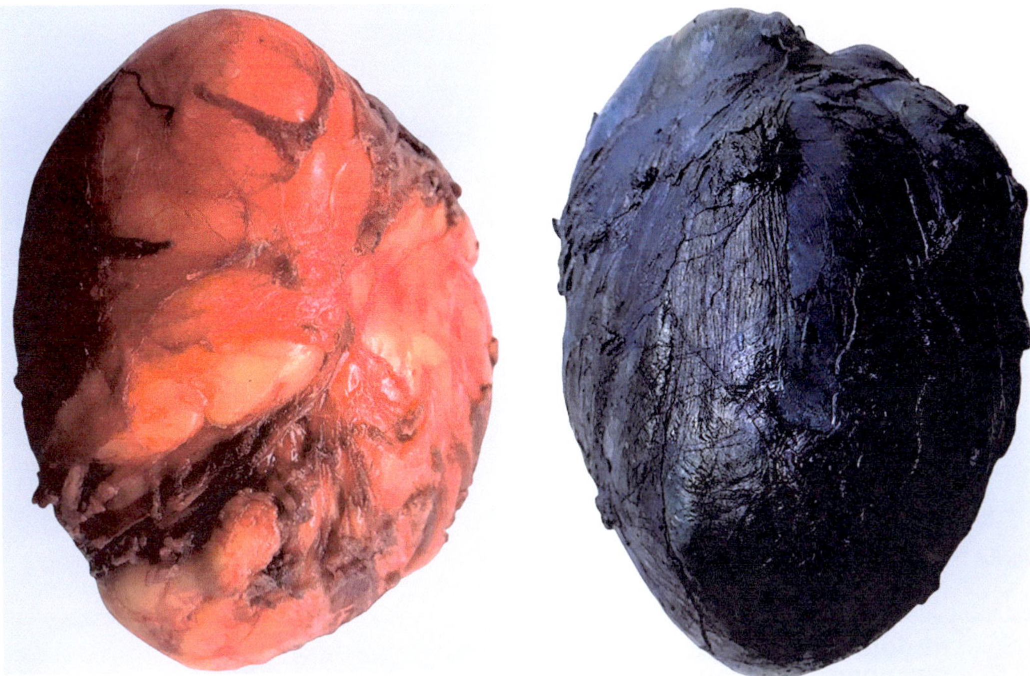

Fig. 2.8 Lipoma

Fig. 2.9 Lipoma inked

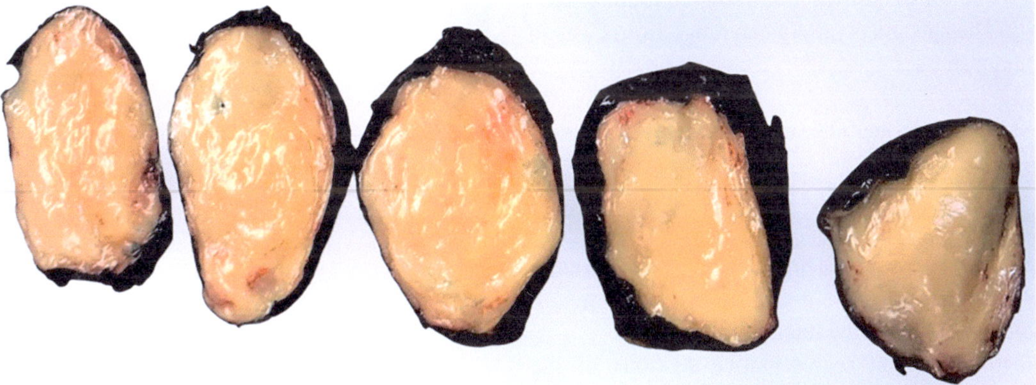

Fig. 2.10 Lipoma serially sectioned

Example Dictation

Specimen A is received in formalin labeled with the patient's name, medical record number, "R shoulder fatty mass" and consists of an unoriented mass of tan-yellow adipose tissue (10.1 x 9.5 x 9.1 cm, 145 grams) with a scant amount of adhered pink-red skeletal muscle. The specimen is entirely inked blue and is serially sectioned to reveal tan-yellow, lobulated cut surfaces with scant hemorrhage. Representative sections are submitted in A1–A10.

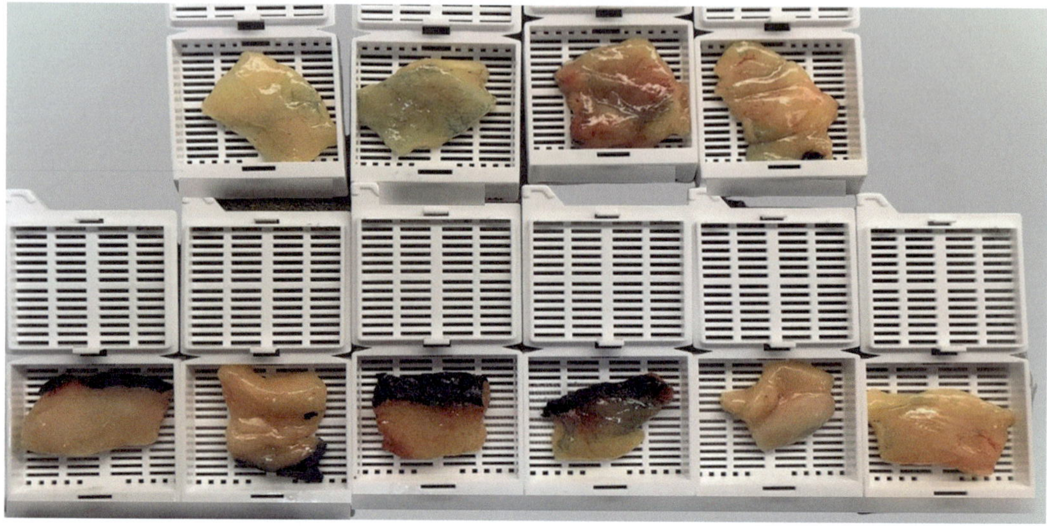

Fig. 2.11 Lipoma sections submission

2.5　Abdominal Mass: Level IV CPT 88305

The term "abdominal mass" is vague and can be any abnormal growth within the abdominal cavity. The specimen variety can range from cysts to tumor masses.

Step 1: Describe, measure, and weigh the specimen (Fig. 2.12)

Step 2: Ink the capsule or surrounding surface of the mass.

Step 3: Bivalve or serially section the mass (Fig. 2.13).

Step 4: Describe the internal cut surface.

Step 5: Submit representative sections of the mass. This will include sections of the capsule or outer surface and sections from the central area of the mass (Fig. 2.14). Attempt to submit sections from the areas which do not look necrotic grossly.

Example Dictation

Specimen A is received in formalin labeled with the patient's name, medical record number, and "abdominal mass" and consists of an intact, unori-

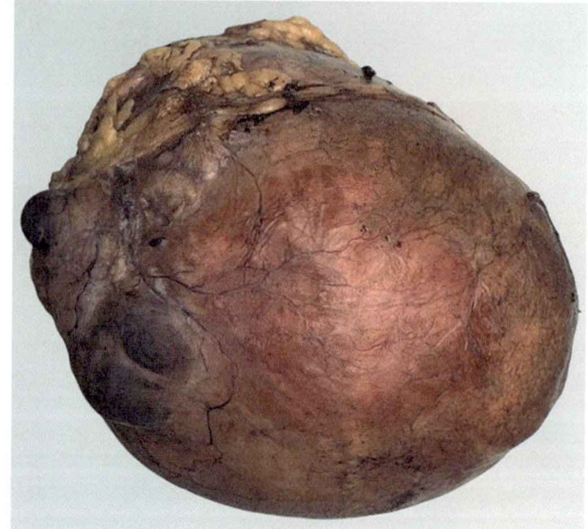

Fig. 2.12 Abdominal mass

ented mass (20.2 x 15.6 x 14.9 cm, 2104 grams) with a smooth outer surface and scant adhered adipose tissue on one side. The specimen is inked blue and bisected to reveal a marked amount of necrosis (approximately 75% of the mass), cystic areas ranging from 3.9 cm to 9.9 cm in greatest diameter, and small areas of viable tissue at the periphery of the mass capsule. Representative sections are submitted in A1–A14.

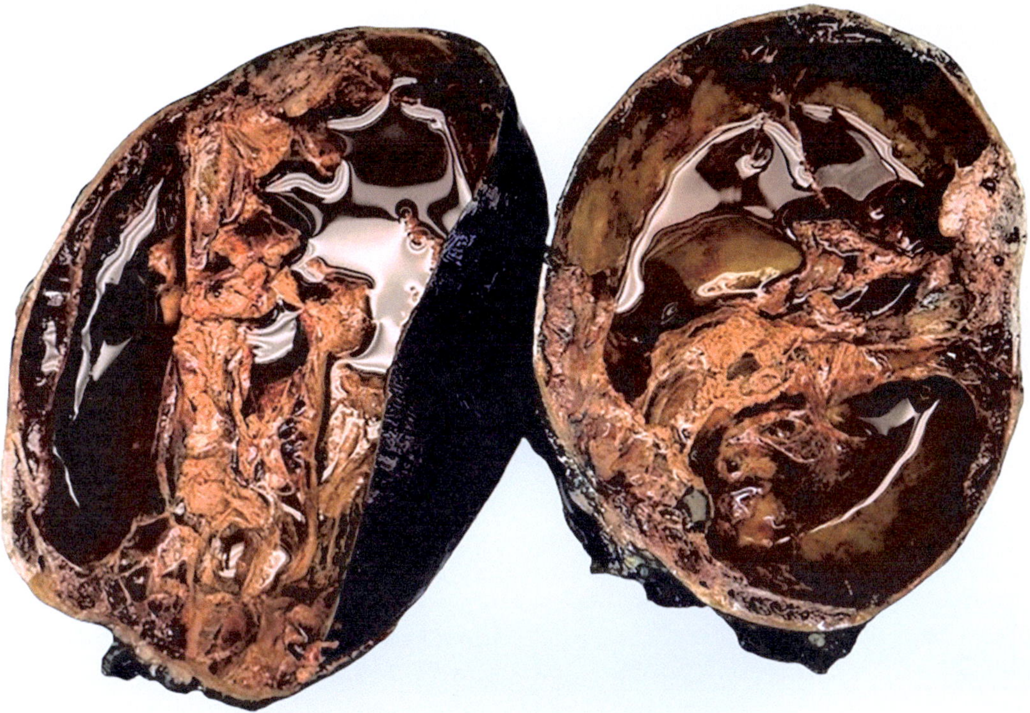

Fig. 2.13 Abdominal mass bivalved

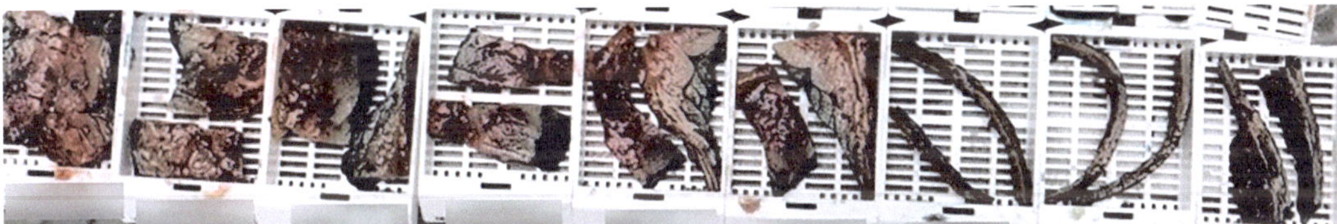

Fig. 2.14 Abdominal mass sections submission

2.6 Femoral Head Not for Fracture: Level III CPT 88304

The removal of the femoral head can be due to many causes such as arthritis, avascular necrosis, trauma, bone tumors, and metastases. This surgery requires the surgeon to remove the femoral head and a short length of the femoral neck. Occasionally, the resection can include part of the proximal femur as well. Once removed, the surgeon will replace the native, damaged femoral head with a prosthetic which should allow for normal hip function once healed.

Step 1: Describe and measure the coronal diameter of the femoral head. The blue line in Fig. 2.15 shows the coronal diameter line. Describe the extent of erosion over the articular surface.

Step 2: Measure the length of the attached femoral neck.

Step 3: Describe the resection margin. A smooth margin means the surgeon cut and removed the femoral head. A ragged, hemorrhagic margin could be due to trauma. In Fig. 2.16, the margin is cleanly transected.

Step 4: Ink the resection margin as seen in Fig. 2.17. Inking the margin isn't necessary unless a lesion is present. However, ink the margin if unsure of the pre-operative diagnosis.

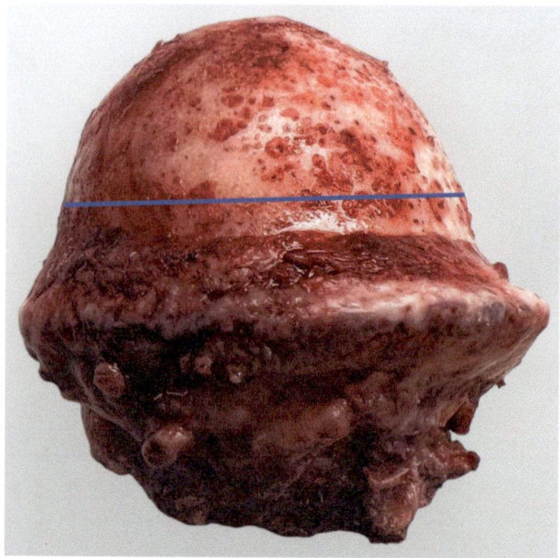

Fig. 2.15 Femoral head

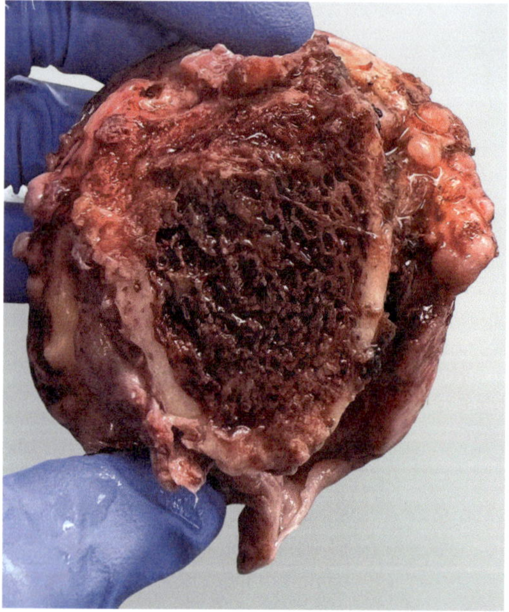

Fig. 2.16 Femoral head resection margin

Step 5: Serially section the specimen from anterior to posterior, perpendicular to the resection margin. (Fig. 2.18)

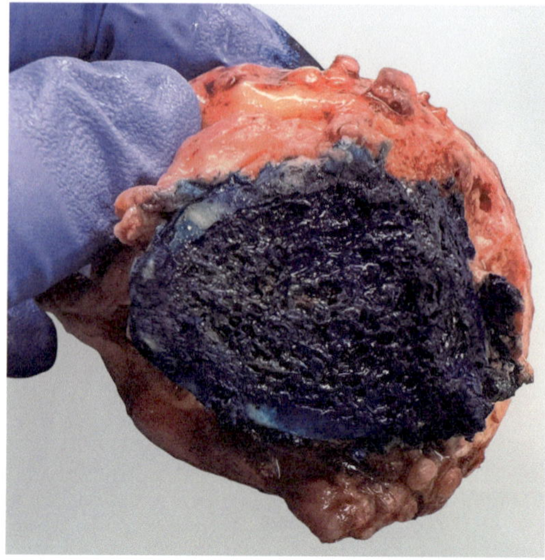

Fig. 2.17 Femoral head resection margin inked

Step 6: Describe the cut surfaces of the specimen. In Fig. 2.19, the articular surface of the bone is almost completely gone with a pale underlying area.

Step 7: Quadrisect and submit a full section. (Fig. 2.20)

Step 8: Decal the sections before submitting.

Example Dictation

Specimen A is received in formalin labeled with the patient's name, medical record number, and "right femoral head" and consists of a tan femoral head (4.5 cm in coronal diameter) with a cleanly transected femoral neck (1.1 cm in length). The specimen is sectioned to reveal tan cut surfaces with near complete erosion of the articular surface with an underlying slightly fibrous area (2.0 x 1.9 x 1.2 cm). One fullface section is quadrisected and submitted in A1–A4, post decalcification.

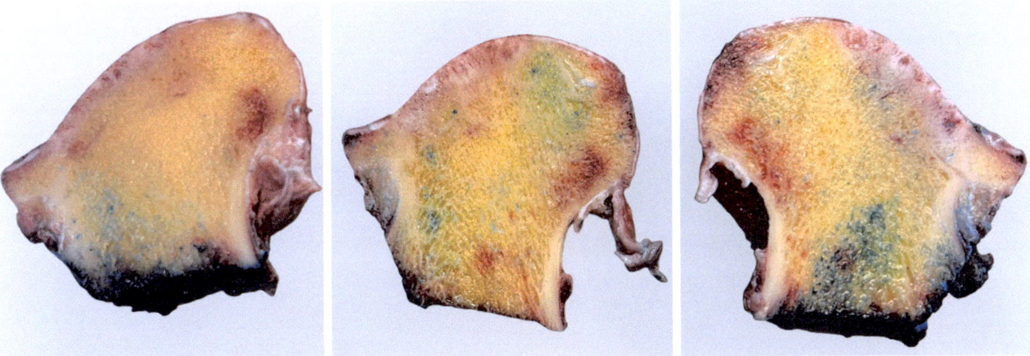

Fig. 2.18   Femoral head serially sectioned

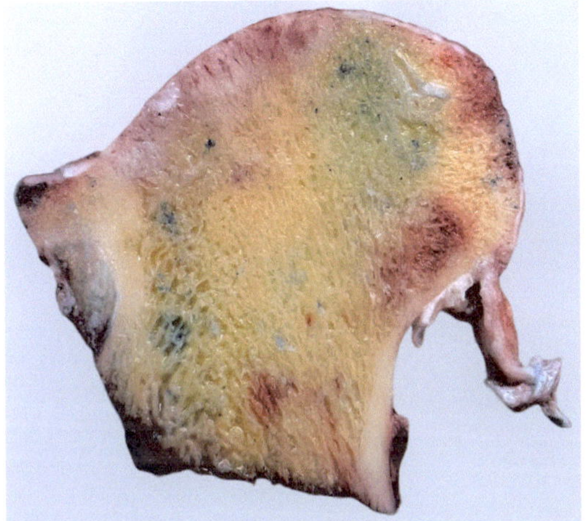

Fig. 2.19   Femoral head full section

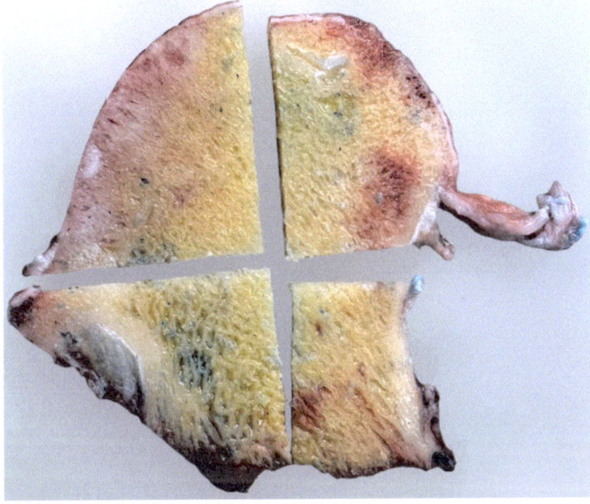

Fig. 2.20   Femoral head full section quadrisected

2.7   Osteochondroma: Level IV CPT 88305

Osteochondromas are benign growth of bone and cartilage. These lesions typically occur in large joint areas such as the knee, hip, or pelvis and are typically seen in children and young adults. Osteochondromas are removed due to pain or movement issues in the area.

Step 1: Describe and measure the specimen. (Fig. 2.21)

Step 2: Ink the resection margin of the specimen.

Step 3: Section the specimen perpendicular to the resection margin. (Fig. 2.22)

Step 4: Describe the cut surface.

Step 5: Measure the thickness of the chondral cap.

Step 6: Submit representative sections of the specimen that include the chondral cap, bone, and resection margin as seen in Fig. 2.23.

Step 7: Decalcify the specimen.

Example Dictation

Specimen A is received in formalin labeled with the patient's name, medical record number, and "right femur" and consists of an unoriented, irregular bone fragment (6.2 x 4.3 x 2.8 cm). The resection margin is inked blue, and the specimen is sectioned to reveal slight necrosis of the bone with an overlying chondral cap ranging from 0.3 to 0.5 cm thick. Representative sections are submitted in A1–A3, post decalcification.

Fig. 2.21   Osteochondroma

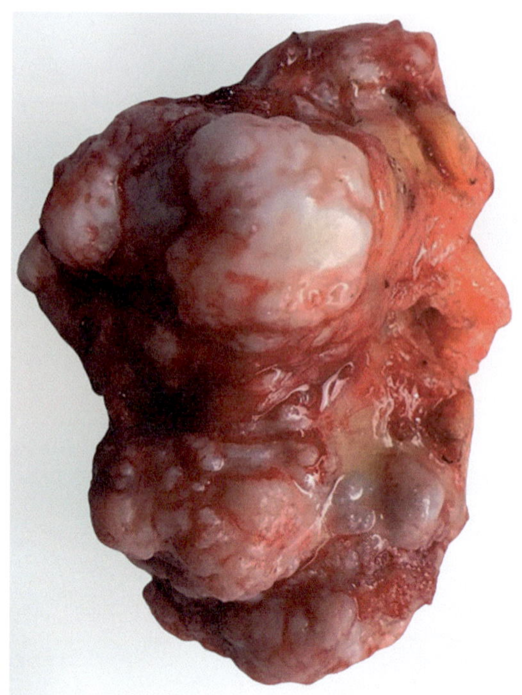

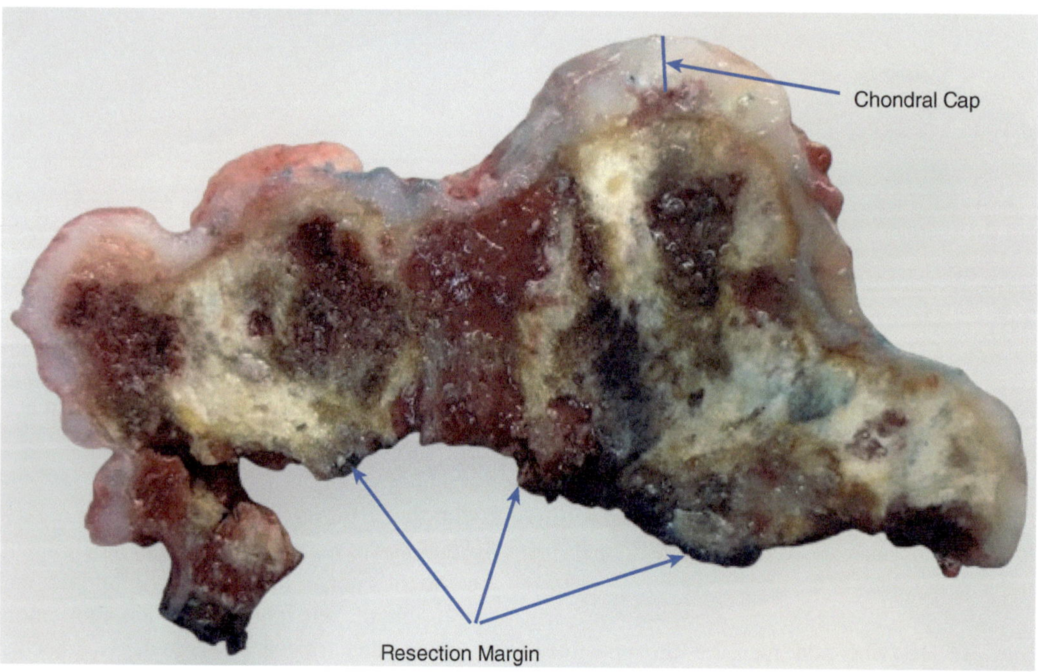

Fig. 2.22   Osteochondroma slice

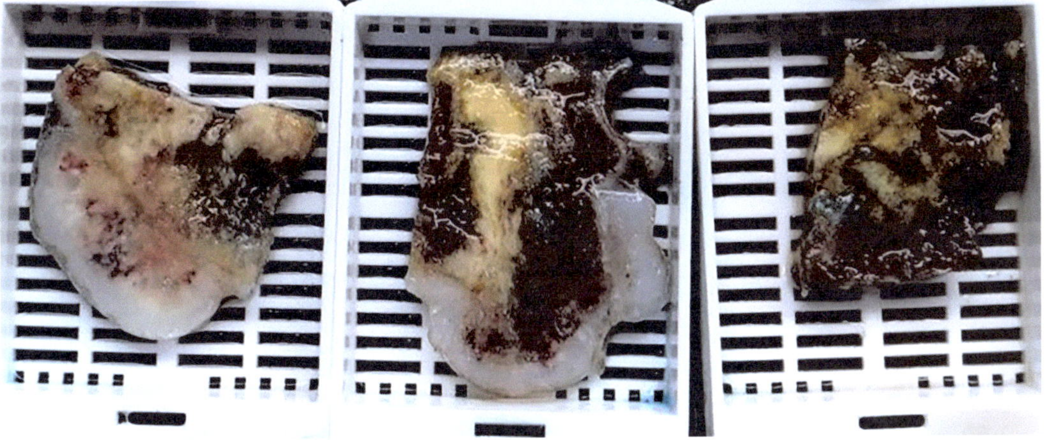

Fig. 2.23 Osteochondroma sections submission

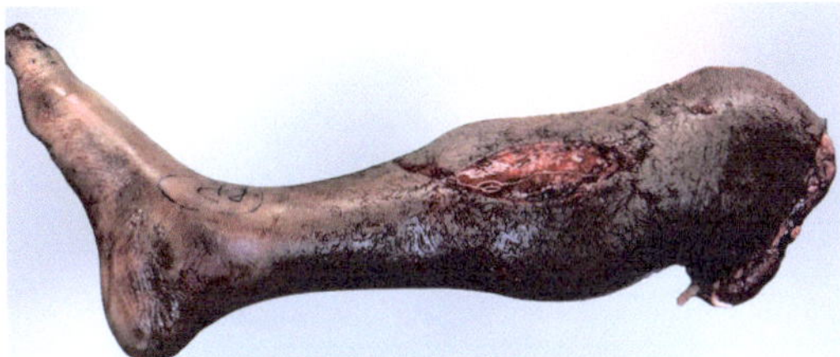

Fig. 2.24 Benign leg amputation

2.8 Leg Amputation: Level V CPT 88307

Amputations of the leg can vary from a disarticulation of the hip down to an amputation of the forefoot. They can be surgically amputated for multiple reasons, including trauma, necrotizing fasciitis, osteomyelitis, and vascular insufficiency.

Step 1: Describe and measure the leg. Include the skin color, the leg orientation, and the type of amputation (Fig. 2.24).

Step 2: Describe the resection margin (cleanly transected or ragged). Figure 2.25 shows a cleanly transected margin with no evidence of trauma. The vasculature of the leg is intricate but for surgical pathology purposes can be minimized to the femoral vascular bundle, anterior tibial vascular bundle, posterior tibial vascular bundle, and the dorsalis pedis vascular bundle. These are the main vessels that span the length of the leg. Depending on the type of amputa-

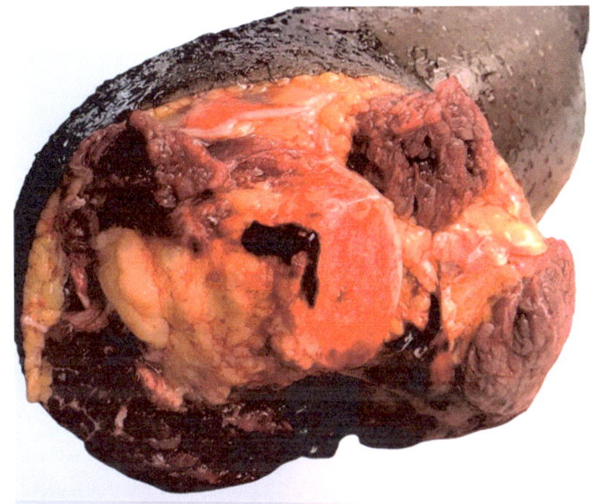

Fig. 2.25 Benign leg amputation resection margin

tion, the vascular bundle present at the resection margin is different. See Fig. 2.26, for an example, of vascular margins present with each type of amputation.

Step 3: Identify and shave the vascular margin. The vessel margin is different depending on where the leg is amputated. In Fig. 2.27, the popliteal vessel is present at the margin because the leg was amputated just above-the-knee joint.

Step 4: Shave a representative section of skin and muscle from the resection margin along with the vessel margin as shown in Fig. 2.28.

Step 5: Describe and measure any lesions on the skin surface. Then measure how close the lesion comes to the resection margin.

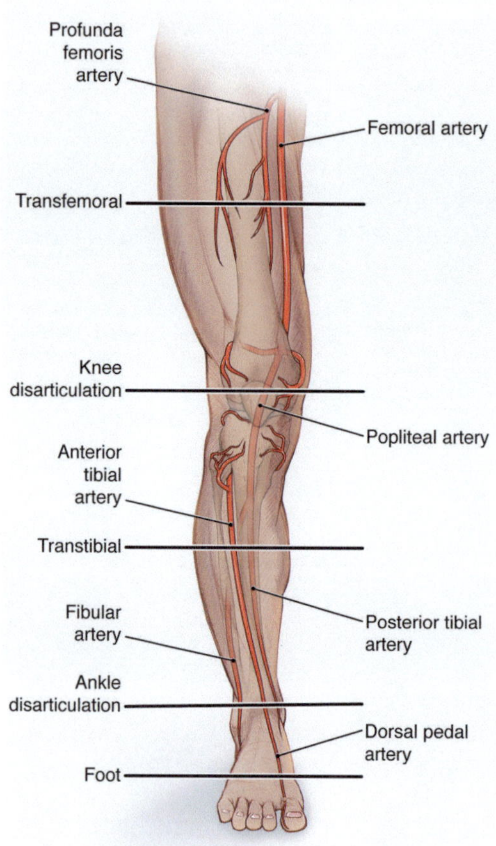

Fig. 2.26 Leg vessel illustration

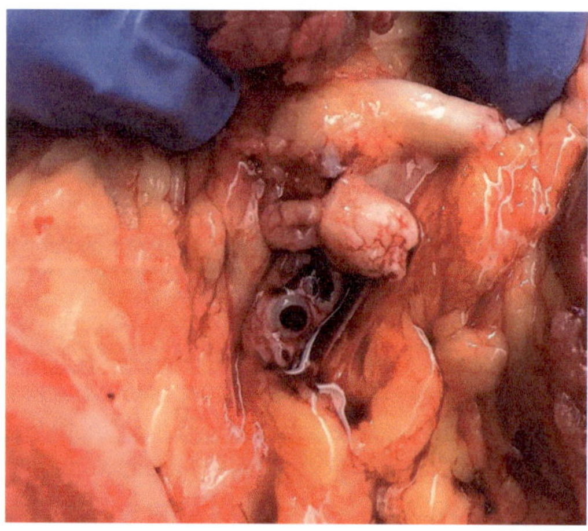

Fig. 2.27 Benign leg amputation vessel margin

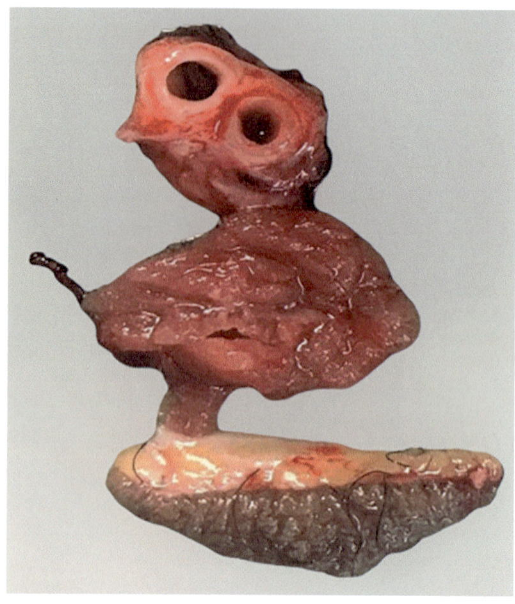

Fig. 2.28 Benign leg amputation margin section submission

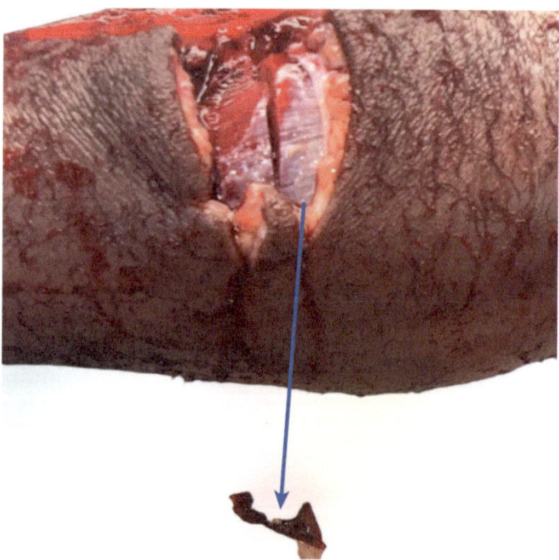

Fig. 2.29 Benign leg amputation lesion section

Step 6: Take representative sections of the lesion. Figure 2.29 shows a representative section of the lesion. The section is taken from the edge of the lesion and includes the area in relation to surrounding skin.

Step 7: Serially section and describe the anterior vascular bundle with the presence or absence of occlusion or calcification. Figure 2.30 shows the anterior vascular bundle (blue arrow) with no evidence of occlusion.

Step 8: Take multiple representative sections of the anterior vascular bundle. (Fig. 2.31)

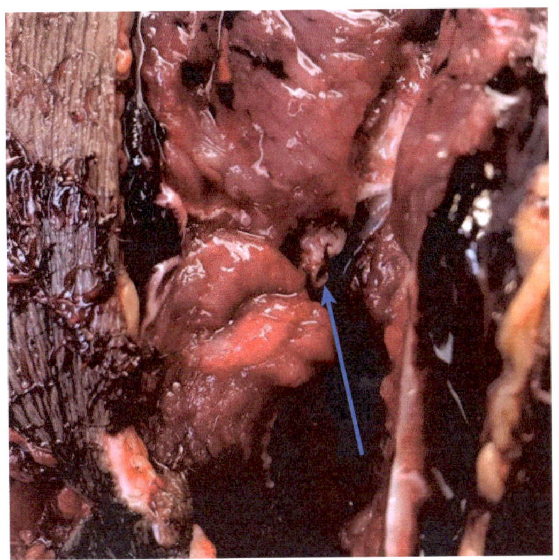

Fig. 2.30 Benign leg amputation anterior vascular bundle

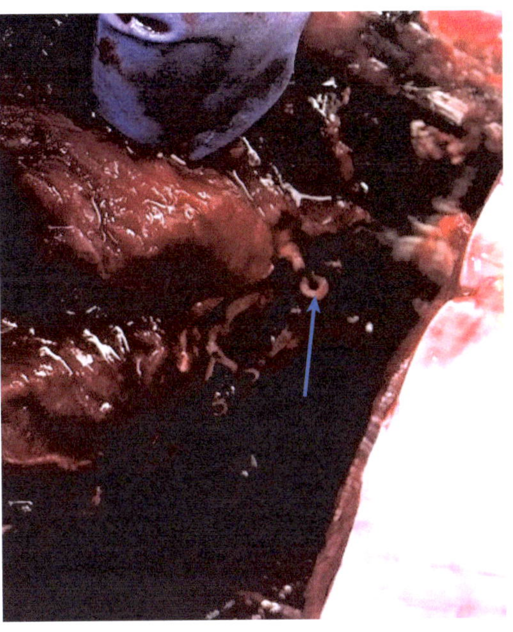

Fig. 2.32 Benign leg amputation posterior vascular bundle

Step 9: Describe the posterior vascular bundle with the presence or absence of occlusion or calcification. Figure 2.32 shows the posterior vascular bundle (blue arrow) with no evidence of occlusion.

Step 10: Take multiple representative sections of the posterior vascular bundle. (Fig. 2.33)

Step 11: Describe and take sections of the dorsalis pedis vascular bundle with the presence or absence of occlusion or calcification. Figure 2.34 shows the dorsalis pedis (blue arrow) with no evidence of occlusion.

Step 12: Submit the sections of the vessels. All vessels look similar under the microscope. The vessels can each be inked a separate color and submitted in the same cassette with ink code designation, as seen in Fig. 2.35.

Step 13: Take the bone margin. The margin can either be shaved and submitted en face or a representative portion of bone marrow can be submitted (Fig. 2.36). It is best to communicate with the pathologist as to which type of bone margin should be taken.

Step 14: Submit all sections and decalcify the bone (Fig. 2.37). If osteomyelitis is suspected, submit bone from the great toe or area of ulceration.

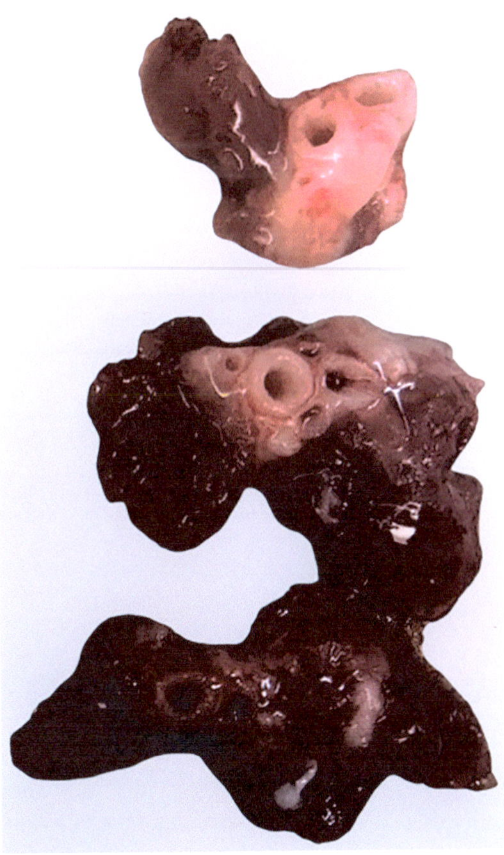

Fig. 2.31 Benign leg amputation anterior vascular bundle section submission

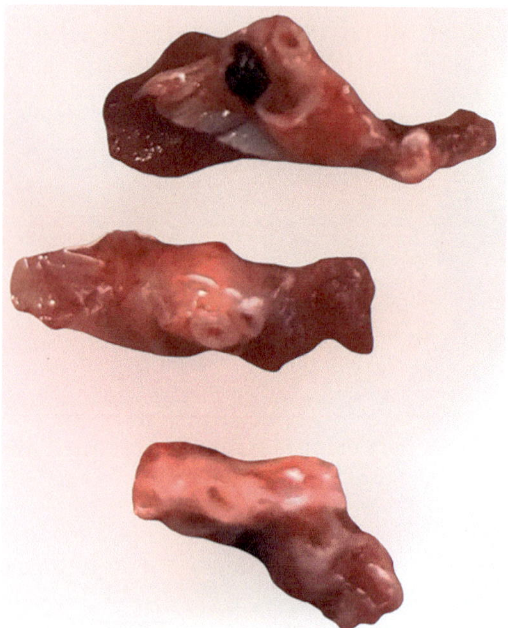

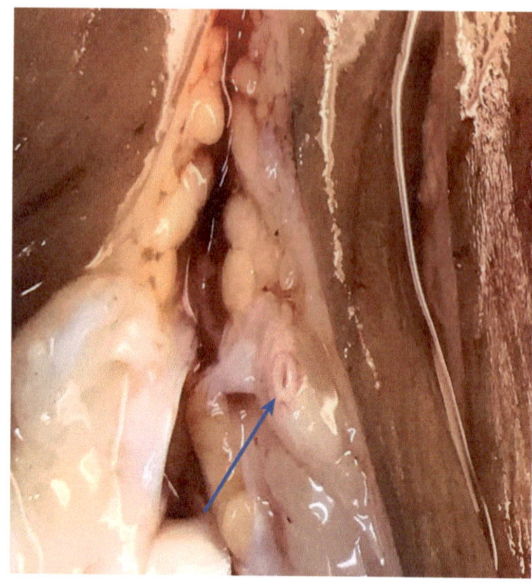

Fig. 2.34 Benign leg amputation dorsalis pedis

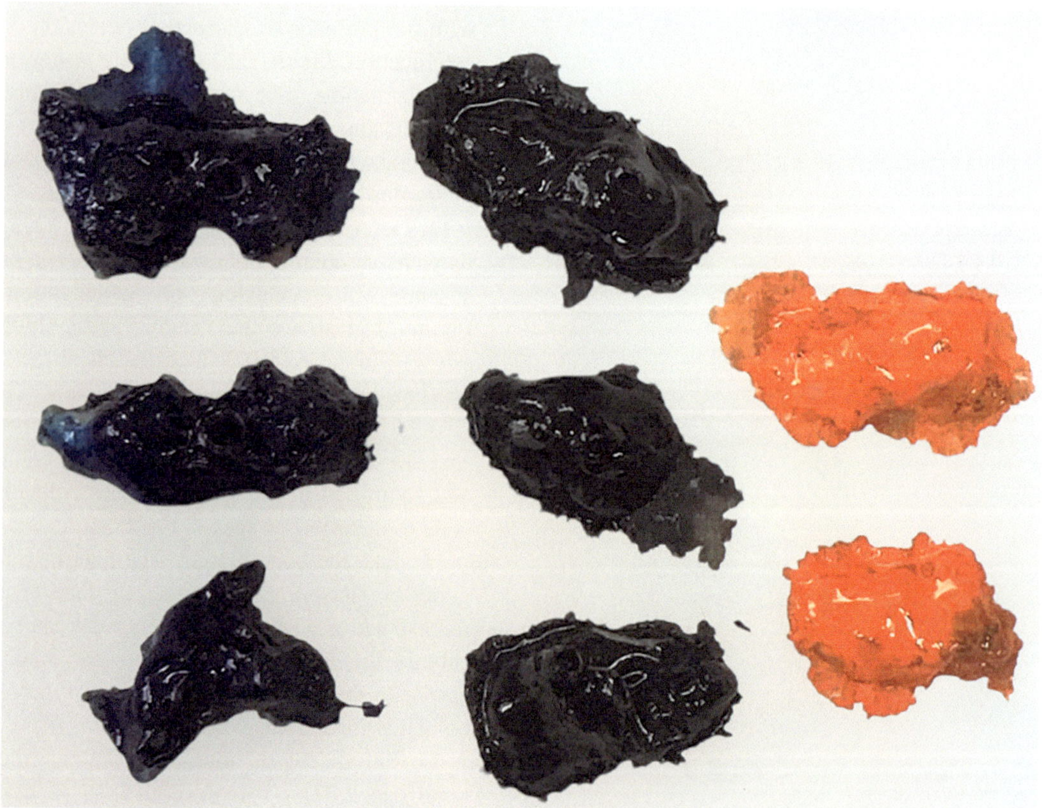

Fig. 2.33 Benign leg amputation posterior vascular bundle section submission

Fig. 2.35 Benign leg amputation vascular section submission with ink

Fig. 2.36 Benign leg amputation osseous margin

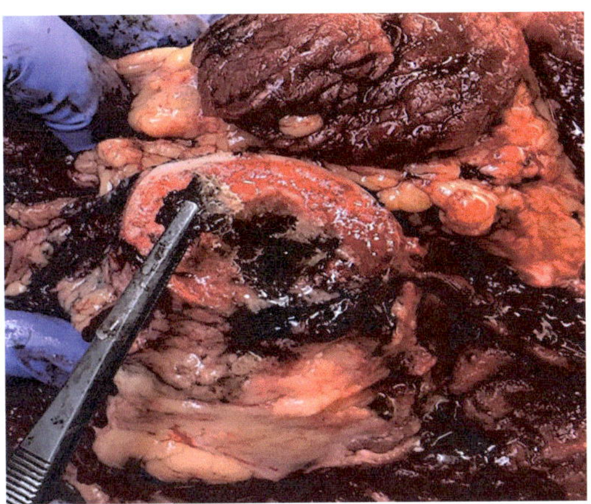

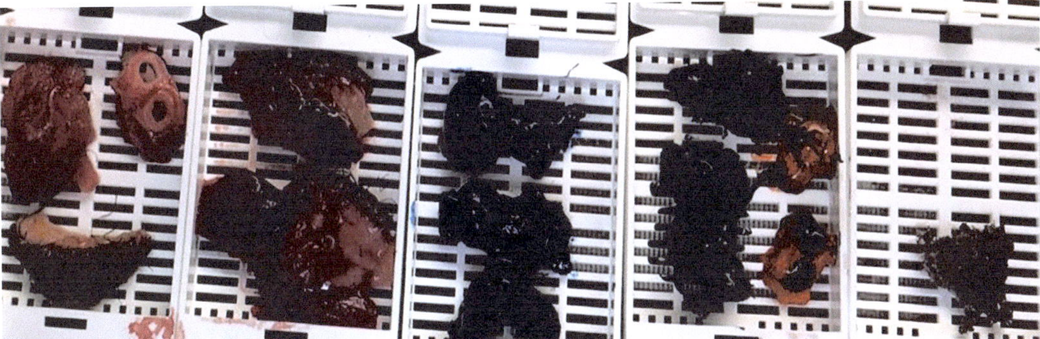

Fig. 2.37 Benign leg amputation section submission

Example Dictation

Specimen A is received fresh labeled with the patient's name, medical record number, "leg, right" and consists of a right, tan-brown above-the-knee amputation (7.5 cm from clean resection margin to knee by 45.4 cm from knee to heel by 22.1 cm from heel to great toe) with brown-gray skin and 5 nail bearing toes. There are fasciotomy sites on the medial (13.5 x 4.8 cm) and lateral (9.5 x 3.4 cm) aspects of the lower leg, coming within 11.2 cm from the soft tissue resection margin. No additional lesions are identified on the skin surface of the amputation. The anterior, posterior, dorsalis pedis, and popliteal vasculature is serially sectioned to reveal no gross occlusion.

Section code

    A 1: Skin, muscle, popliteal resection margin, en face

A 2: Representative sections of medial and lateral fasciotomy site

A 3: Anterior vascular bundle, representative (inked blue)

A 4: Posterior vascular bundle (inked black), dorsalis pedis (inked orange), representative

A 5: Bone marrow from osseous resection margin, post decalcification

2.9   Leg Stump: Level V 88307

A stump amputation revisions is when the surgeon performs a second surgery to correct any problems with the amputation site. This could include infection at the surgical margin or simply cleaning up the surgical site to better accommodate a prosthesis.

Step 1: Describe and measure the specimen. (Fig. 2.38)

Step 2: Describe the skin color and the leg orientation (left or right). The fibula is present posterior-lateral to the tibia.

Step 3: Describe any irregularities or lesions on the skin. In Fig. 2.39, the skin of the amputation is excised much lower on one side than the other. This type of excision allows for a flap of skin to be left on the proximal leg to be used as a flap to cover the open surgical wound.

Step 4: Describe the resection margin. In Fig. 2.40, the bone, skin, and soft tissue are all cleanly transected by the surgeon.

Step 5: Identify and shave the vascular margins. This is a below-the-knee stump amputation revision so the anterior (Fig. 2.41a blue arrow) and posterior (Fig. 2.41b blue arrow) vascular bundles are present at the resection margin.

Step 6: Shave a representative section of skin and muscle from the margin. The skin, muscle, and vascular margins are submitted en face. In Fig. 2.42, the anterior vascular bundle margin is inked blue to differentiate between the two vessels under the microscope on the same slide.

Step 7: Describe the previous stump amputation site where the first amputation surgery occurred. In Fig. 2.43, the skin and soft tissue is hemorrhagic and granular, and there is exposed bone present.

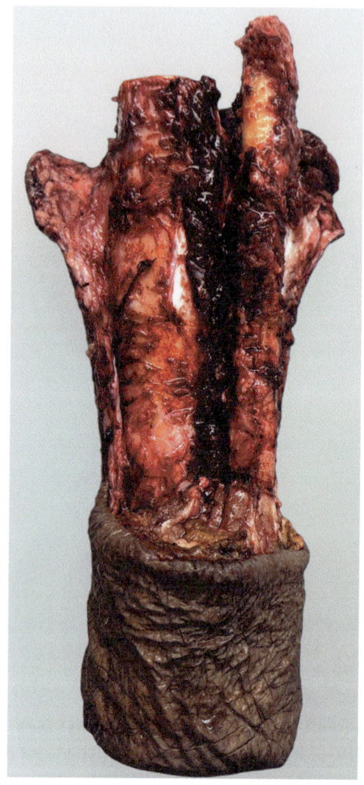

Fig. 2.39 Stump amputation revision posterior view

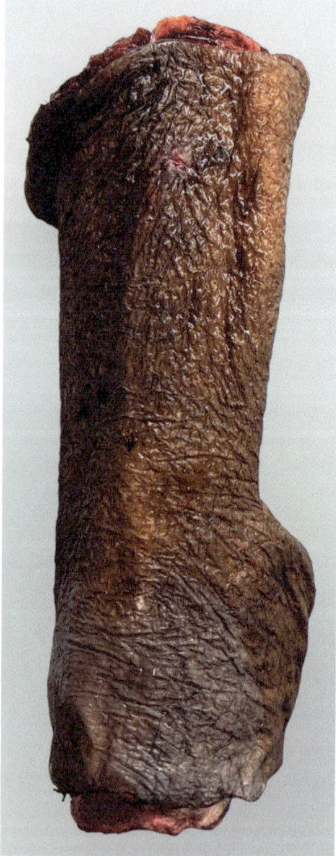

Fig. 2.38 Stump amputation revision anterior view

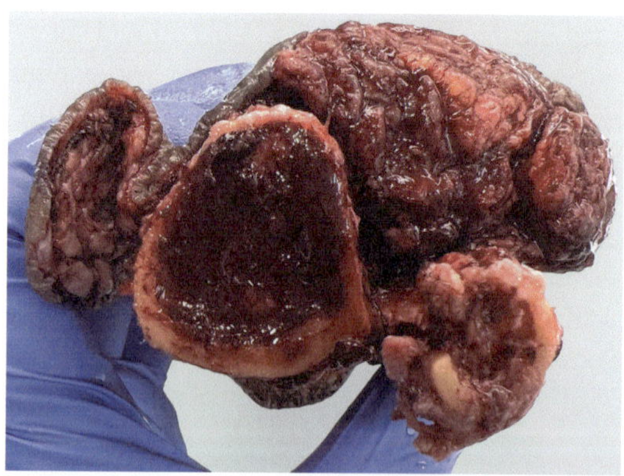

Fig. 2.40 Stump amputation revision resection margin

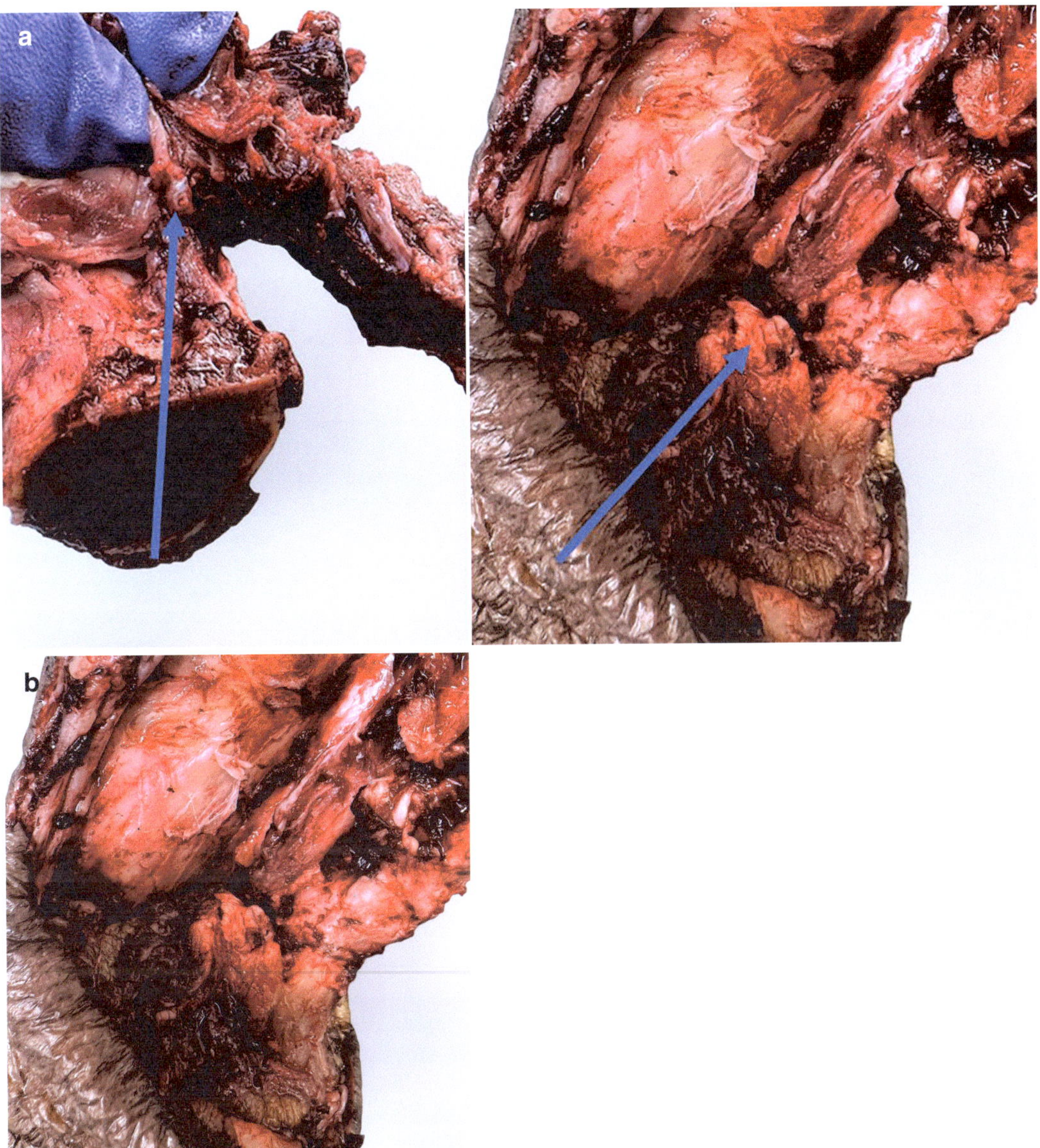

Fig. 2.41 (**a**) Stump amputation revision anterior vascular bundle margin; (**b**) stump amputation revision posterior vascular bundle margin

Step 8: Take a representative section of the bone, skin and soft tissue of the previous stump amputation site.

Step 9: Shave the true osseous margins. In Fig. 2.44, the true osseous margins are the tibia and fibula. The tibia is bisected to fit in the cassettes and both are submitted en face.

Step 10: Submit all necessary sections. Remember to decalcify the bone. (Fig. 2.45)

Example Dictation

Specimen A is received fresh labeled with the patient's name, medical record number, and "right stump" and consists of a right, tan-brown below-the-knee stump amputation revision (23.5 x 7.2 x 6.3) with a clean resection margin. The previous stump amputation site is hemorrhagic and granular with exposed bone. The anterior vascular bundle and posterior vascular bundle are sectioned to reveal slight occlusion which extends to the resection margin.

The sections are decalcified before submission. Section code

A 1: Skin, muscle, anterior vascular bundle (inked blue), and posterior vascular bundle margins, en face

A 2: Skin and soft tissue from previous amputation site, representative

A 3: Bone from previous amputation site, representative

A 4-A 5: True tibia osseous margin, bisected, en face

A 6: True fibula osseous margin, en face

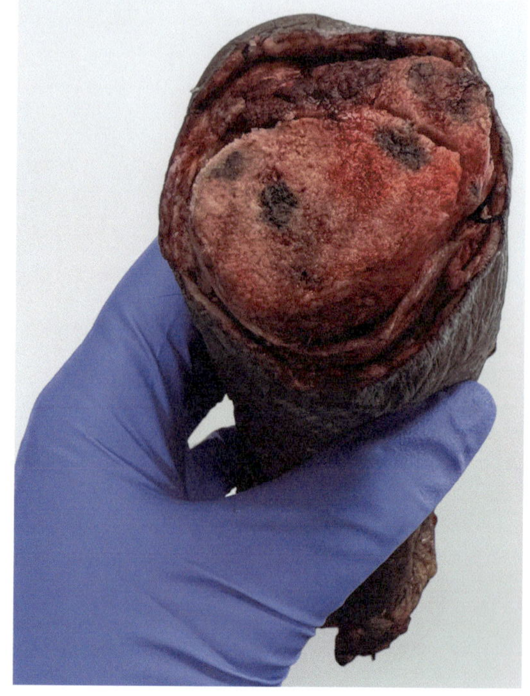

Fig. 2.43 Stump amputation revision previous amputation site

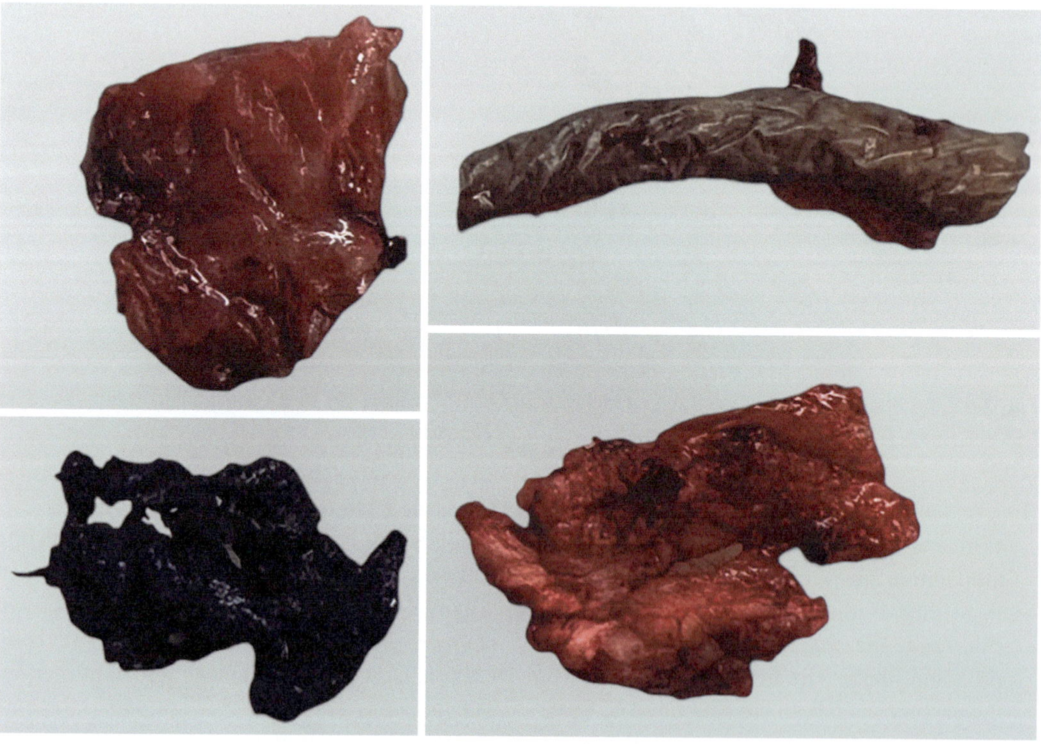

Fig. 2.42 Stump amputation revision resection margin section submission

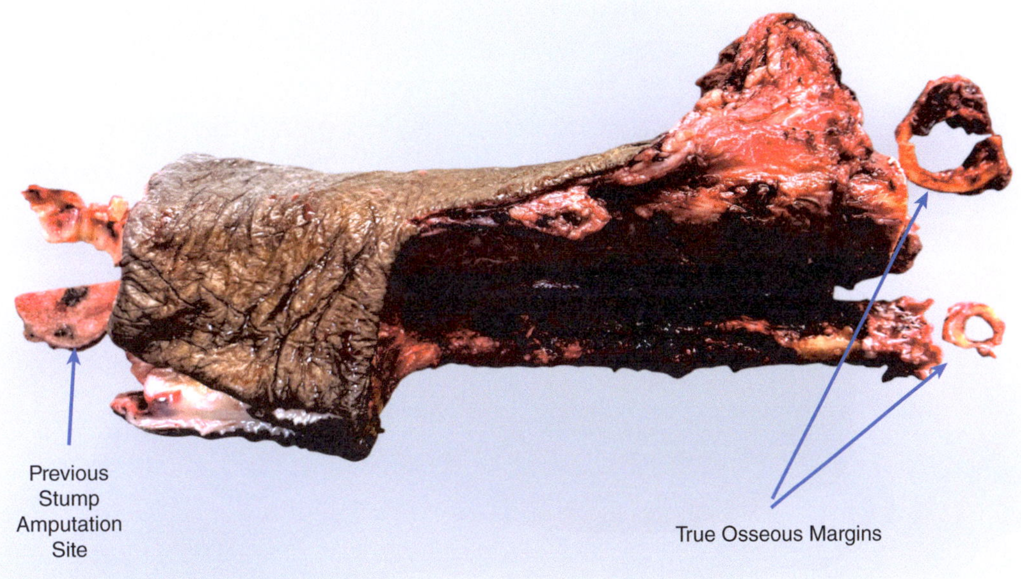

Fig. 2.44 Stump amputation revision true osseous margins

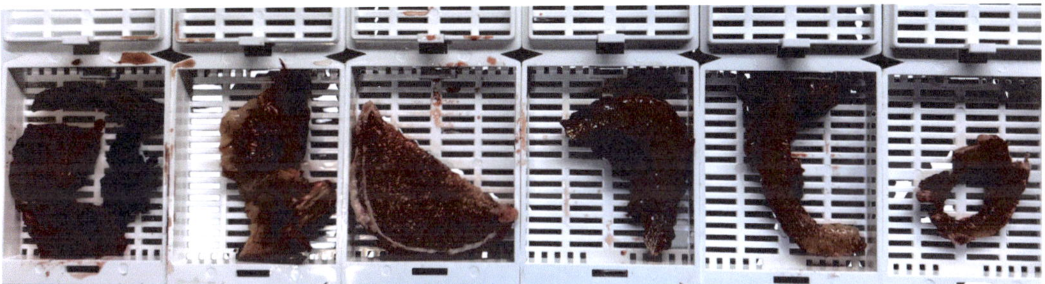

Fig. 2.45 Stump amputation revision section submission

2.10   Soft Tissue Sarcoma: Level VI CPT 88309

Sarcoma tumors of the soft tissue are tumors that arise in the adipose tissue, skeletal muscle, skin, vessels, or nerve.

Always check imaging before grossing to correlate the gross appearance (Table 2.2) and radiographic size of the tumor.

Cancer Protocol Breakdown Relative to Grossing Soft Tissue Tumors

Preresection treatment: Addressing the patient chart for chemotherapy or radiation prior to surgery is necessary to understand the lesion. Treatment before surgery should begin to necroes the lesion therefore at least some portion of the lesion should appear necrotic. Presurgical therapy can decrease the size of the tumor as well.

Procedure: Three different procedures are typically performed on bone tumors.

- An intralesional resection consists of sampling the tumor area, typically to gain a diagnosis of the tumor and leaving some tumor in the patient.
- A marginal resection removes the tumor with only the capsule or a small amount of tissue.
- A radical resection removes the entire bone and includes the surrounding soft tissues if the tumor has extended through the bone.

Table 2.2 Tumor gross appearance of soft tissue tumors

Lipoma	Yellow, lobulated tissue which looks like normal adipose tissue containing a very thin, often grossly unidentifiable capsule
Sarcoma	Solid, well-circumscribed tan-white to tan-pink mass
Liposarcoma	Yellow, lobulated mass often resembling normal adipose tissue but are paler yellow in color and slightly less lobulated than the surrounding normal adipose tissue
Angiosarcoma	Hemorrhagic area that is typically ill-defined

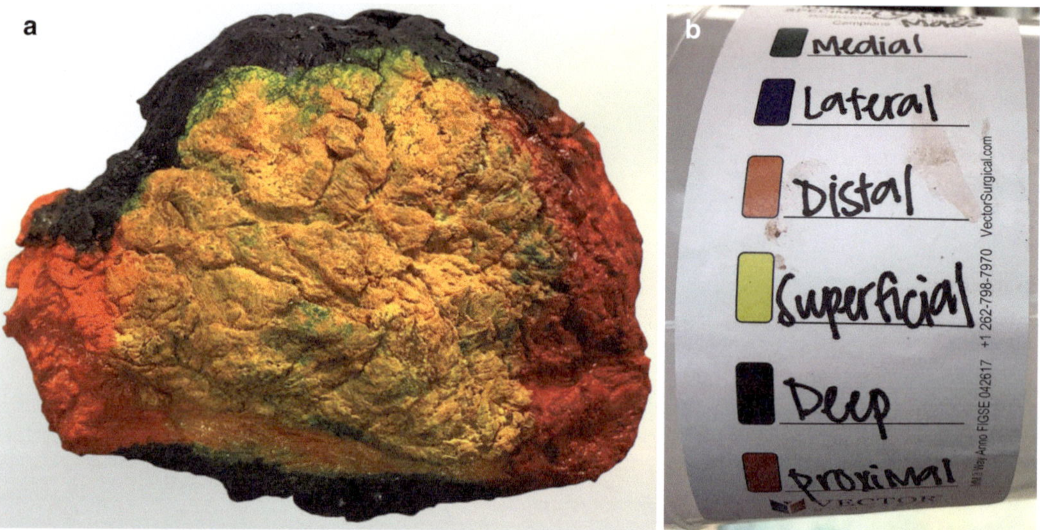

Fig. 2.46 (**a**) Soft tissue sarcoma; (**b**) ink code

Tumor focality: Identify if there is one or multiple lesions present. If multiple separate lesions are present, then count the number of separate lesions.

Tumor site: Dictate where the lesion is present in the patients and measure the distance of one lesion to another if multiple lesions are identified.

Tumor size: Measure the tumor in three dimensions in centimeters.

Necrosis: Assess the tumor and give a rough estimate of necrosis present. This is only necessary when a patient has received prior treatment before surgery.

Margin Status: All margins need to be assessed grossly and microscopically. Measure the tumor to all the margins [2].

Step 1: Describe, measure, and weigh the specimen.
Step 2: In Fig. 2.46a, the surgeon has inked the specimen in the operating room so the specimen was received in the laboratory inked with a corresponding ink code attached to the specimen container as Fig. 2.46b shows.
Step 3: Serially section the specimen. Typically sectioning perpendicular to the long axis is best. In Fig. 2.47, the specimen is serially sectioned from proximal to distal.
Step 4: Measure the mass in three dimensions and describe the mass cut surfaces.
Step 5: Measure the mass to the margins present in the slices, medial, lateral, superficial, and deep margins.
Step 6: Perpendicularly section the proximal and distal margins as shown in Fig. 2.48.
Step 7: Measure the mass to the proximal and distal margins.
Step 8: Submit a section of the mass in relation to all the margins and additional representative sections of the mass. In Fig. 2.49, 2 representative sections of the mass in relation to all the margins and representative sections of the mass. 1 section per 1 centimeter of the overall size of the mass is appropriate.

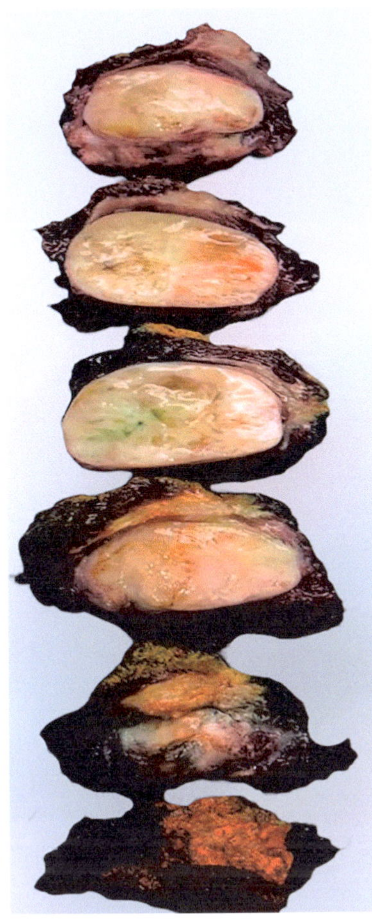

Fig. 2.47 Soft tissue sarcoma serially sectioned

Example Dictation

Specimen A is received fresh labeled with the patient's name, medical record number, "left thigh mass" and consists of a portion of red-brown skeletal muscle (10.2 x 8.3 x 6.5 cm, 248 g), oriented and previously inked per the surgeon. The specimen is serially sectioned to reveal a tan-white, firm, well-circumscribed mass (7.2 x 6.2 x 4.3 cm) which is centrally cystic. The mass comes within 0.3 cm of the deep margin, 1.1 cm from the superficial margin, 0.4 cm from the lateral margin, 0.7 cm from the medial margin, 1.5 cm from the distal margin, and 1.1 cm from the proximal margin, surrounded by red-brown skeletal muscle.

Ink code
>   Green-medial
>   Blue-lateral
>   Orange-distal
>   Yellow-superficial
>   Black-deep
>   Red-proximal

Section code
>   A 1-A 2: Mass in relation to closest proximal margin, perpendicular
>   A 3-A 4: Mass in relation to closest distal margin, perpendicular
>   A 5-A 6: Mass in relation to closest superficial margin
>   A 7-A 8: Mass in relation to closest deep margin
>   A 9-A 10: Mass in relation to closest lateral margin
>   A 11-A 12: Mass in relation to closest medial margin
>   A 13-A 14: Mass, representative (no margin present)

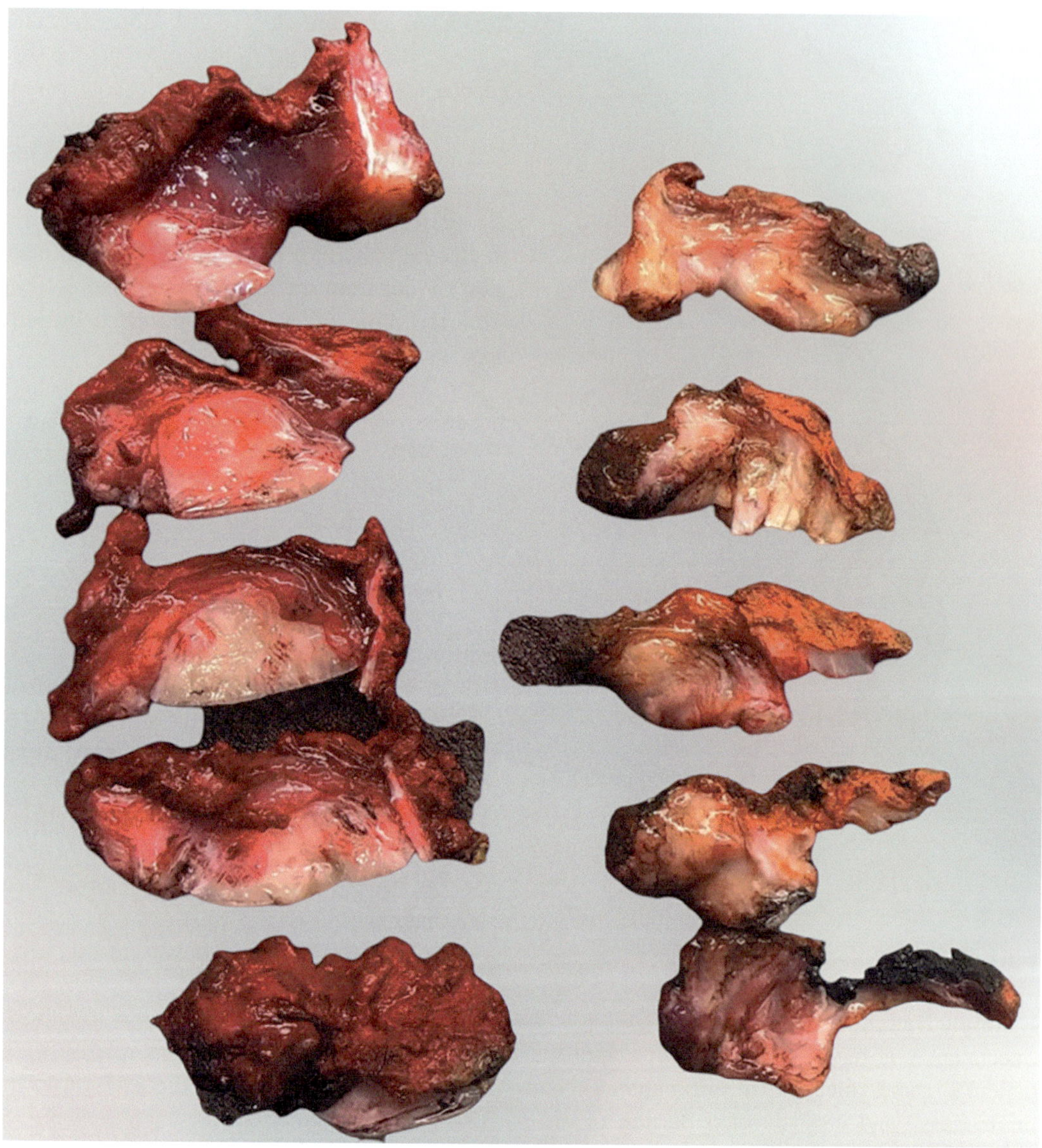

Fig. 2.48 Soft tissue sarcoma perpendicular margins

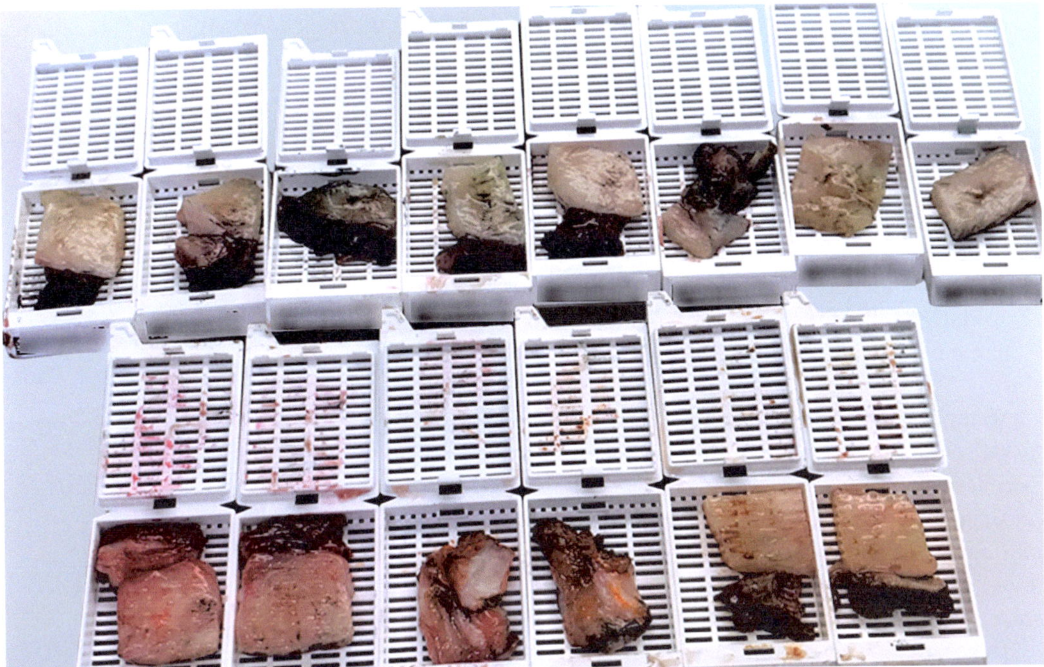

Fig. 2.49 Soft tissue sarcoma section submission

2.11   Bone Tumors: Level VI CPT 88309

Osteosarcoma is a malignant tumor that develops in bones. As the tumor grows, it can weaken the bone, leading to fractures and spreading outside of the bone. To properly assess the situation, the grossing person should first analyze the patient's imaging to determine the tumor's location, any surrounding structures it may affect, and its estimated size. Refer to Table 2.3 for guidance on the physical characteristics of bone tumors.

Cancer Protocol Breakdown Relative to Grossing Bone Tumors

Radiographic findings: Imaging is one of the more important pieces of information the grossing person can attain before grossing. The imaging allows for a better understanding of the specimen before it is grossed.

Preresection Treatment: Addressing the patient chart for chemotherapy or radiation prior to surgery is necessary to understand the lesion.

Table 2.3 Tumor gross appearance of bone tumors

Aneurysmal bone cyst (ABC)	Multiloculated cyst typically filled with clotted blood Secondary ABC-like changes can be seen in a variety of benign and malignant bone tumors
Osteochondroma	Lobulated boney projection from the bone with a semi-translucent chondral cap overly the surface
Enchondroma	White cartilaginous areas present within the bone
Giant cell tumor	Well-circumscribed pink-tan lesion within the medullary bone
Osteosarcoma	Yellow-red, hemorrhagic, and invasive lesion that may extend outside the cortical bone and into the surrounding soft tissue
Chondrosarcoma	Tan, lobulated, fleshy cartilaginous mass which can be invasive
Ewing's sarcoma	Well-circumscribed, tan mass with cystic areas and possible necrosis

Treatment before surgery should begin to necroses the lesion therefore at least some portion of the lesion should appear necrotic.

Procedure: Four different procedures are typically performed on bone tumors.

- An intralesional resection consists of sampling the tumor area, typically to gain a diagnosis of the tumor and leaving some tumor in the patient.
- A marginal resection removes the tumor with only the capsule or a small amount of tissue.
- A segmental or wide resection is a resection of a segment of bone with a lesion.
- A radical resection removes the entire bone and includes the surrounding soft tissues if the tumor has extended through the bone.

Multiple sites: Identify if the tumor is a single lesion or multiple separate lesions that are discontinuous.

Tumor site: Different sites are broken down into appendicular skeleton which includes the trunk, skull and facial bones, the pelvis, and the spine.

Tumor Size: The overall size of the tumor should be designated in centimeters.

Tumor location and extent: Describing the location, extent, and anatomic structures involved is necessary. These bone structures can include the epiphysis, metaphysis, diaphysis, cortex, and medullary cavity. Utilization of the patient's imaging is very helpful in assessing tumor involvement grossly.

Necrosis: Assess the tumor and give a rough estimate of necrosis present. This is only necessary when a patient has received prior treatment before surgery.

Margin status: All margins need to be assessed grossly and microscopically. Measure the tumor to all the margins [2].

Step 1: Describe and measure the specimen. Include the leg laterality, toes present, and type of amputation. (Fig. 2.50)

Step 2: Describe and measure any lesions on the skin surface, if applicable.

Step 3: Identify and take a shave the vessel margin and submit en face. In Fig. 2.51, the specimen is above the knee and the popliteal vessels (blue arrow) are present at the margin.

Step 4: Take a representative shave margin of the skin and muscle from the margin and submit en face. (Fig. 2.52)

Step 5: Ink the resection margin. In Fig. 2.53, the margin is inked:

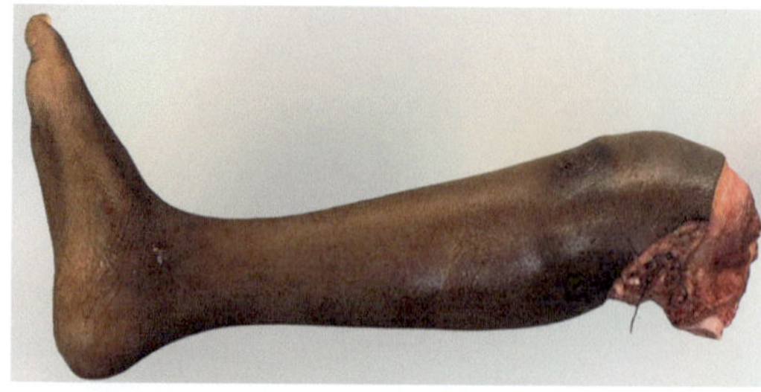

Fig. 2.50 Bone tumor leg amputation

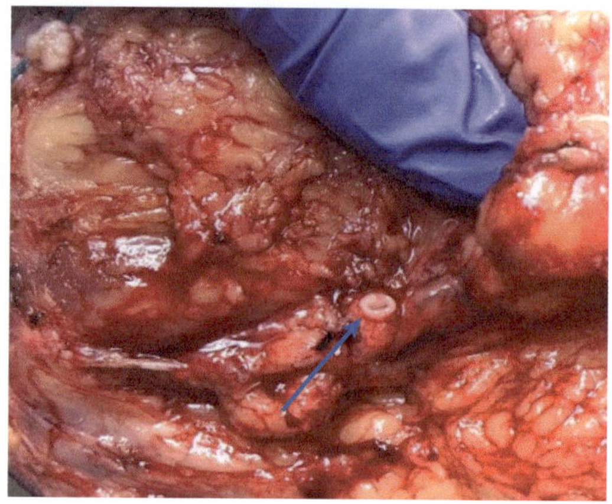

Fig. 2.51 Bone tumor vascular margin

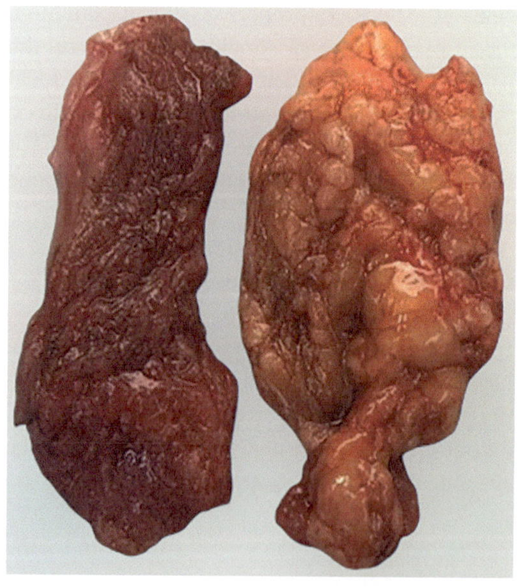

Fig. 2.52 Bone tumor skin and soft tissue margin

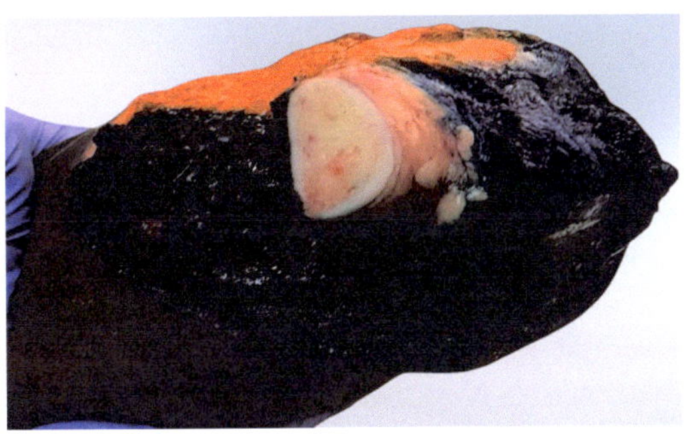

Fig. 2.53 Bone tumor resection margin

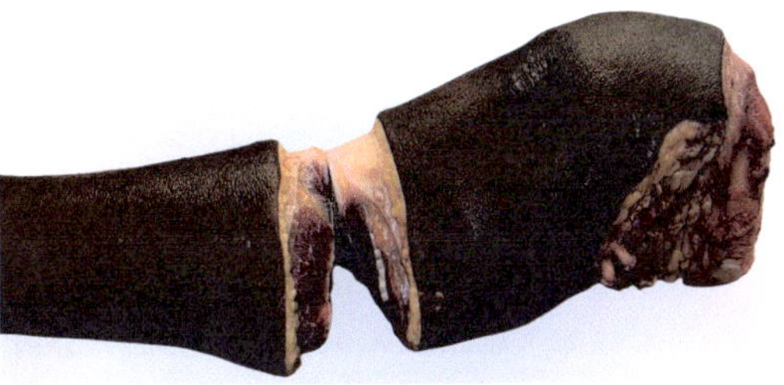

Fig. 2.54 Bone tumor leg amputation transected

Blue-anterior soft tissue
Orange-medial soft tissue
Green-lateral soft tissue
Black-posterior soft tissue

Step 6: Shave the bone margin and submit en face. In Fig. 2.53, the true osseous margin is the femur because the leg was amputated above the knee.

Step 7: In this example, the imaging states a 9 cm lesion present in the proximal tibia. Therefore, the grossing person can amputate the distal leg to allow for better manipulation of the tumor area while grossing as seen in Fig. 2.54.

Step 8: Bivalve the area with the lesion. In Fig. 2.55, the specimen is bivalved into medial and lateral halves.

Step 9: Describe the lesion (blue arrows) and measure the lesion in 3 dimensions. In Fig. 2.55, only 2 dimensions of the lesion are visible. Additional slices will be made to assess the third dimension.

Step 10: Measure the mass in relation to the true femur margin and the closest soft tissue margin.

Step 11: Take a fullfaced section of the lesion with surrounding bone and soft tissue from one of the halves. (Fig. 2.56)

Step 12: Longitudinally section the remaining medial and lateral halves. This allows for a gross view of how far the lesion extends medially and laterally.

Step 13: Measure the third dimension of the lesion. Once sectioned, the extent of tumor medial to lateral is the third dimension of the lesion as seen in Fig. 2.57 designated by the blue arrow.

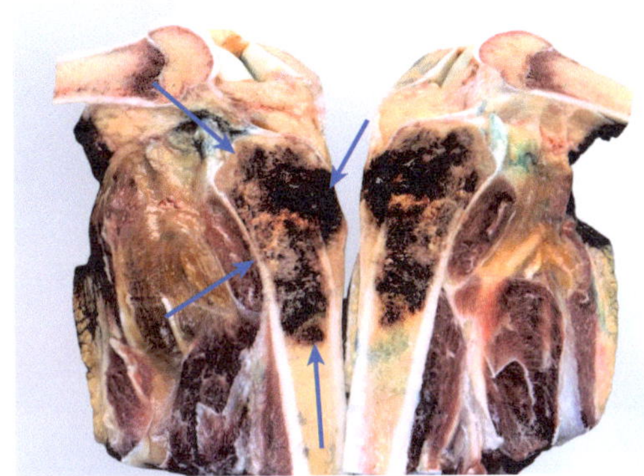

Fig. 2.55 Bone tumor bivalved

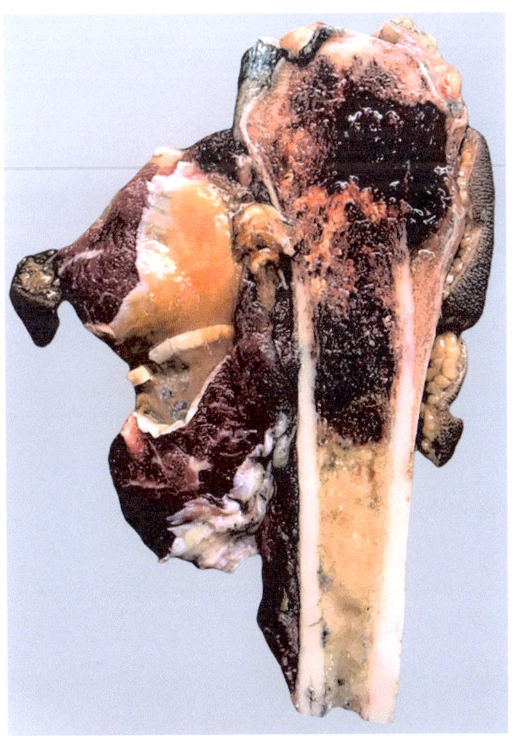

Fig. 2.56 Bone tumor full section

Step 14: Assess for extension outside the bone. When the specimen is sliced in all directions, extension outside the bone and into the soft tissue can be identified, if present. (Fig. 2.58)

Step 15: The section of the margin can be submitted using a standard section code. (Fig. 2.59)

Step 16: The full-thickness section can be mapped as seen in Fig. 2.60. To map a specimen, take a full-screen photo and label the cassette number on the photo where the section is taken.

Step 17: Map the medial and lateral slices as seen in the Fig. 2.61a and b example.

Example Dictation

Specimen A is received fresh labeled with the patient's name, medical record number, "right proximal tibia sarcoma" and consists of a right above-the-knee amputation (8.5 cm from clean resection margin to the knee by 42.5 cm from knee to heel by 21.2 cm from heel to great toe) with brown-gray skin and 5 nail bearing toes. The proximal aspect of the tibia on the anterior-medial aspect contains a well-healed scar (2.4 x 0.9 cm) surrounded by hypopigmentation (4.5 cm in diameter) which comes within 6.9 cm from the skin resection margin. There are 2 lymph node

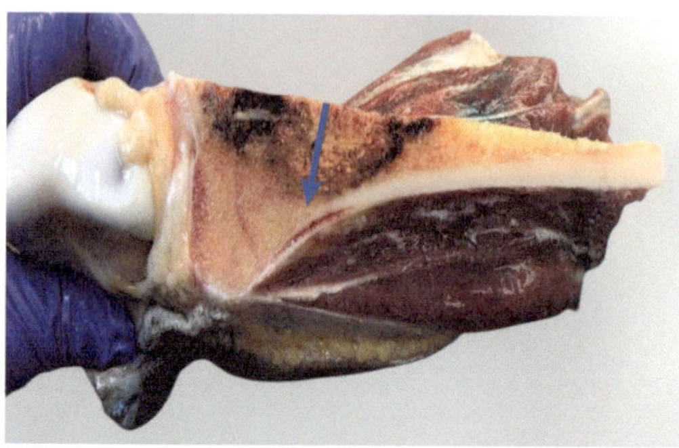

Fig. 2.57 Bone tumor longitudinal section

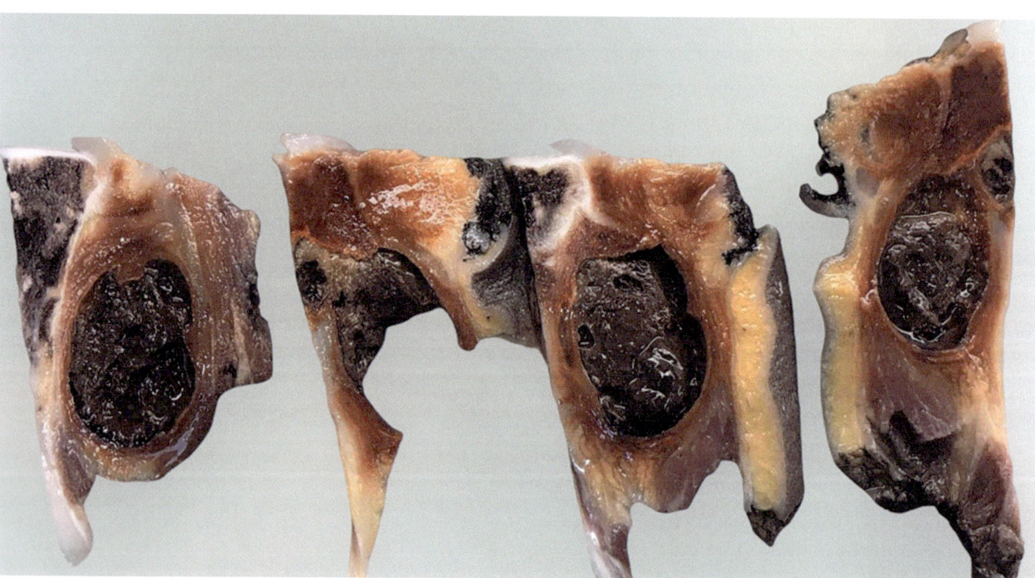

Fig. 2.58 Bone tumor extent outside of bone

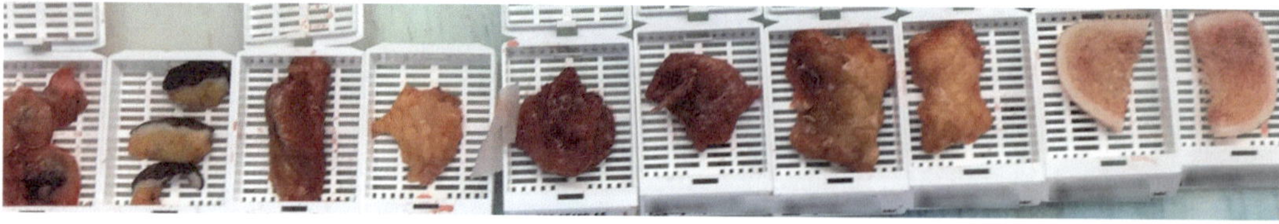

Fig. 2.59 Bone tumor section submission

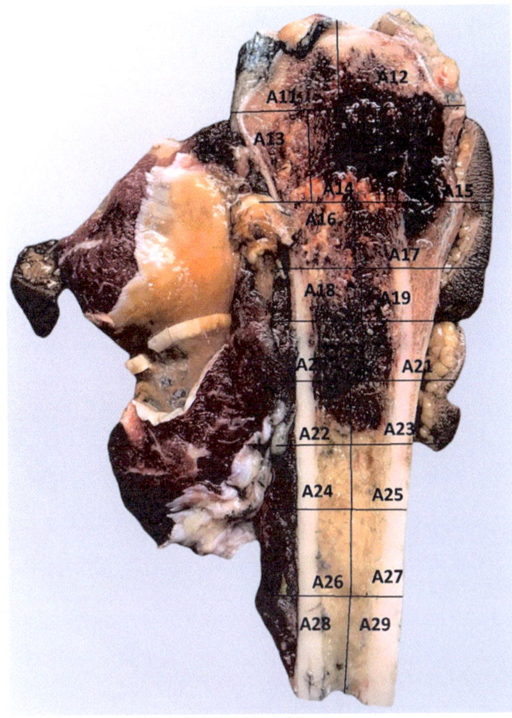

Fig. 2.60 Bone tumor full section map

candidates (0.7 cm in diameter and 0.9 cm in diameter) present abutting the popliteal vasculature margin. The tibia is bivalved to reveal an irregular, granular, red-yellow, hemorrhagic lesion (9.1 x 4.2 x 3.8 cm) present in the proximal tibia, coming within 6.3 cm from the osseous margin and 0.3 cm from the proximal tibia articular surface and extending into both the medial and lateral tibial condyle. On the anterior aspect of the tibia, there is identifiable periosteal involvement. The posterior aspect is serially sectioned to reveal a large cystic lesion (5.4 x 5.2 x 4.0 cm) which is 0.3 cm from the posterior aspect of the bone lesion with communication between and comes within 2.6 cm from the posterior soft tissue margin.

The sections are decalcified before submitting to histology.

Ink code

      Blue-anterior soft tissue
      Orange-medial soft tissue
      Green-lateral soft tissue
      Black-posterior soft tissue

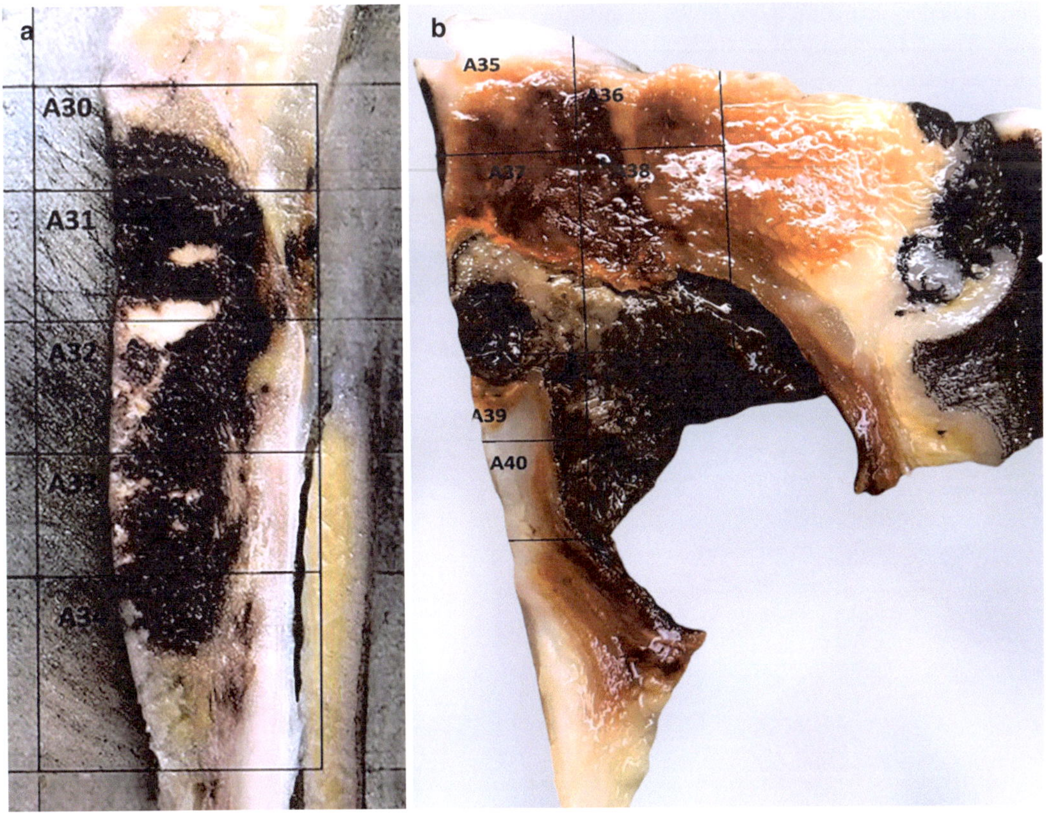

Fig. 2.61 (**a**) Bone tumor map; (**b**) bone tumor soft tissue map

Section code

A 1: Popliteal vasculature margin, en face and 2 popliteal lymph node candidates, whole

A 2: Representative skin margins, en face

A 3-A 4: Soft tissue margin which correlates en face

A 5-A 6: Femoral osseous margin, bisected, en face

A 7–A 10: Additional soft tissue margin, en face

A 11–A 29: Fullface anterior-posterior section with photograph mapping

A 30–A 34: Mass in relation to lateral aspect with photograph mapping

A 35–A 40: Representative sections of tibia in relation to posterior-medial hemorrhagic cystic lesion with photograph mapping

2.12 Separate Tumor Margins: Level IV CPT 88305

Occasionally surgeons will send separate oriented margins that correlate with the main specimen. These fragments of tissue are considered the true margins.

Step 1: Describe and measure the specimen.

Step 2: Dictate how the specimen is oriented. In Fig. 2.62, the black ink designates the true margin.

Step 3: Ink the specimen. In Fig. 2.63, the true margin is inked black and the remaining false margin is inked orange.

Step 4: Serially section the specimen perpendicular to the true margin. In Fig. 2.64, both the orange false margin and the black true margin can be seen.

Step 5: Submit the specimen entirely.

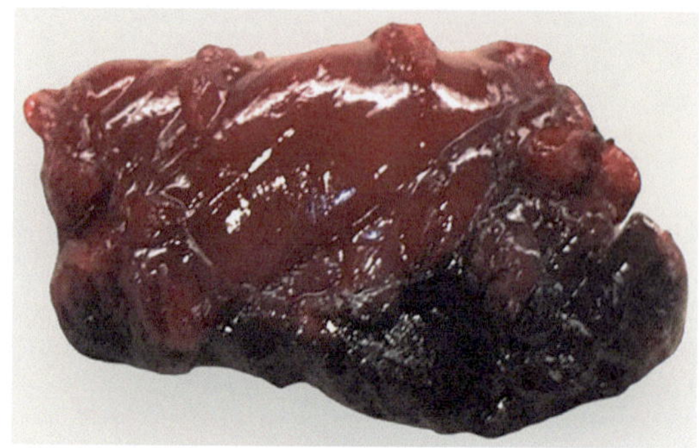

Fig. 2.62 Separate margin

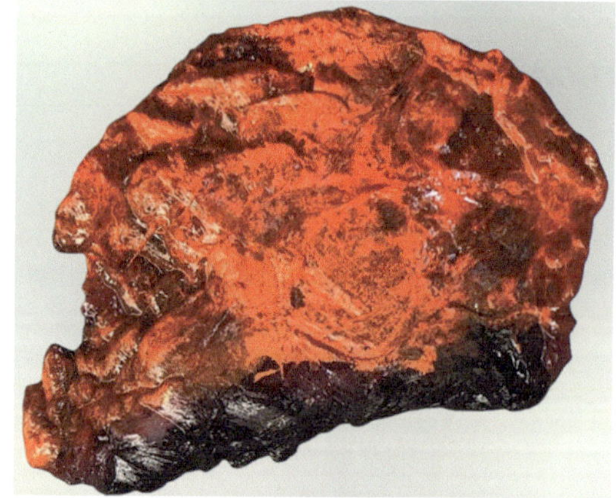

Fig. 2.63 Separate margin inked

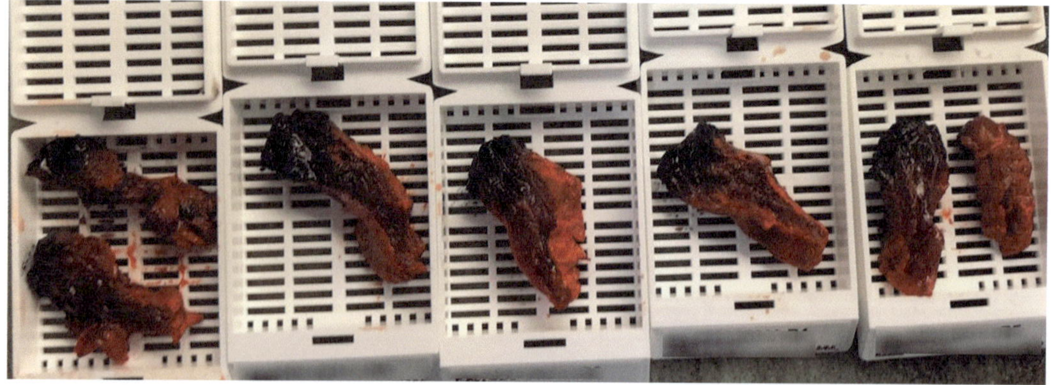

Fig. 2.64 Separate margin section submission

Example Dictation

Specimen A is received fresh labeled with the patient's name, medical record number, "medial margin" and consists of a single fragment of pink-red skeletal muscle (4.1 x 2.2 x 1.0 cm) with ink on the one side designating the true margin. The specimen is serially sectioned to reveal red-brown cut surfaces. The specimen is submitted entirely in A 1–A 5.

Ink code

> Black-true margin
> Orange-false margin

Acknowledgments The author gratefully acknowledges Youssef Al Hmada, MD, and Navdeep Kaur, MD, for their contribution to this chapter.

Quiz Questions

1. The pathologic process shown in the picture can be seen in all conditions except:
   Figure 2.65a Quiz question 1a
   Figure 2.65b Quiz Question 1b
   A. Papillary synovial hyperplasia
   B. Synovial lipomatosis
   C. Degenerative joint disease
   D. Synovial sarcoma

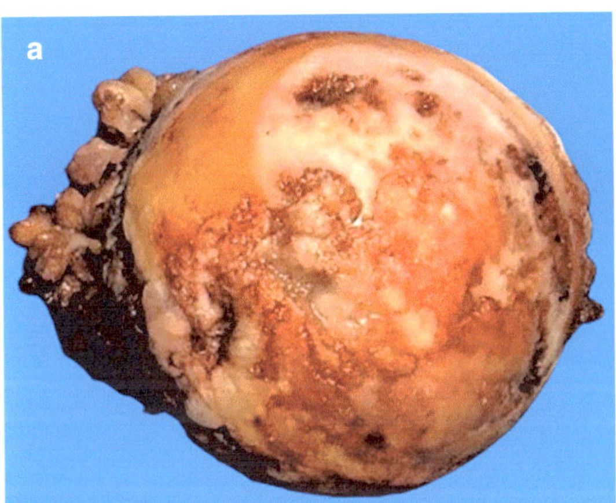
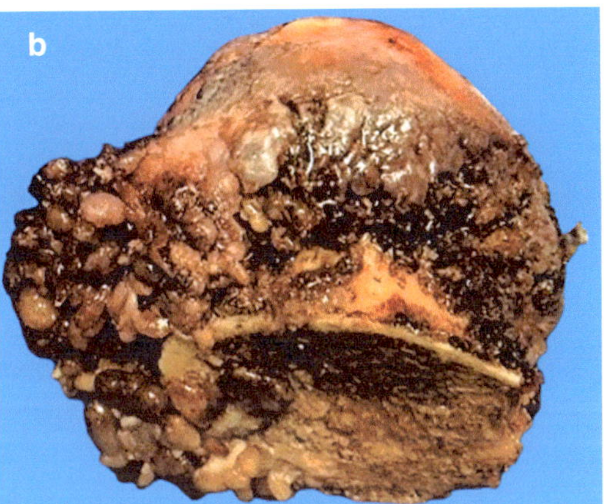

Fig. 2.65 (**a**) Quiz question 1a; (**b**) Quiz question 1b

2. The picture shows resected 13.1 cm, well circumscribed soft tissue mass/sarcoma in the arm. What would be pT category in this case?
   Figure 2.66 Quiz question 2

   A. pT1
   B. pT2
   C. pT3
   D. pT4

Fig. 2.66 Quiz question 2

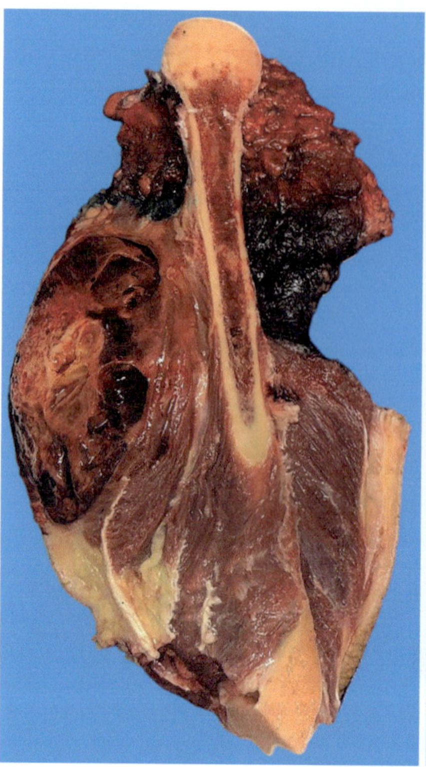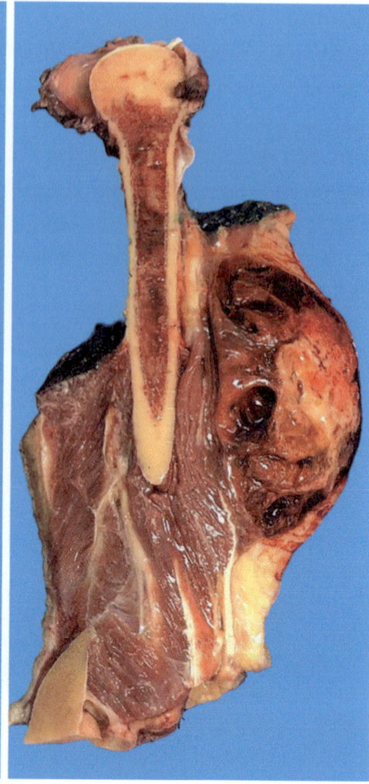

3. The surgeon calls you regarding handing over a fresh thigh sarcoma specimen after hours. What should be your next step?
   A. Receive the specimen and leave it in gross room for the assigned resident to gross next day
   B. Receive the specimen and place it in formalin
   C. Receive the specimen and bisect/open it before fixing it in formalin
   D. Receive the specimen and place it in decalcification agent

4. Which is the best agent in which bone specimen can be placed for getting adequate results of molecular testing?
   A. Hydrochloric acid
   B. EDTA
   C. Formical
   D. Formalin

5. All of the following regarding the given measurement in the following picture are true except?

Figure 2.67 Quiz Question 5

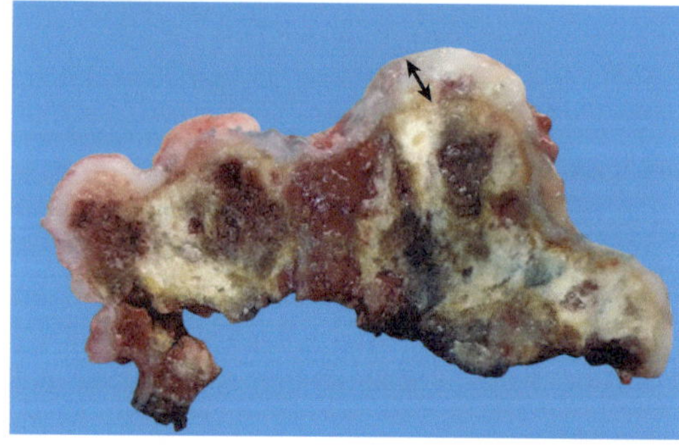

Fig. 2.67 Quiz question 5

   A. Increased cartilage cap thickness is an indication of malignant degeneration
   B. Normal cartilage cap thickness is less than 2 cm in adults
   C. This measurement has no clinical significance
   D. This picture depicts cartilaginous neoplasm

6. Which is the most likely pathology in the given bivalved specimen from the shoulder joint?

> Figure 2.68 Quiz question 6

A. Conventional osteosarcoma
B. Chondrosarcoma
C. Giant cell tumor of bone
D. Chondroblastoma

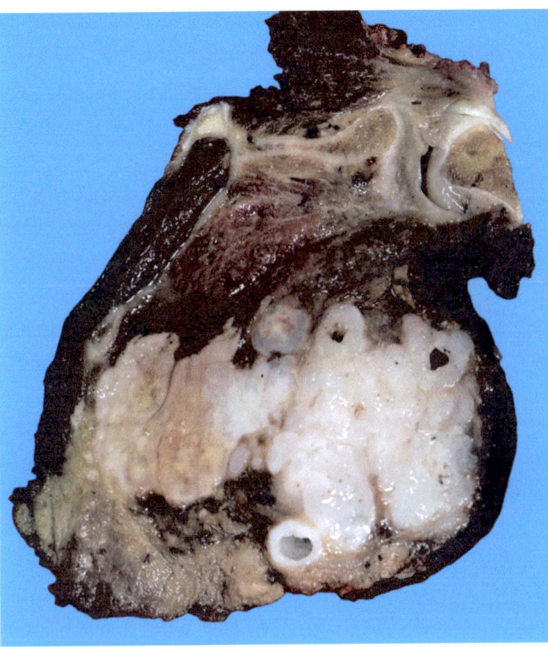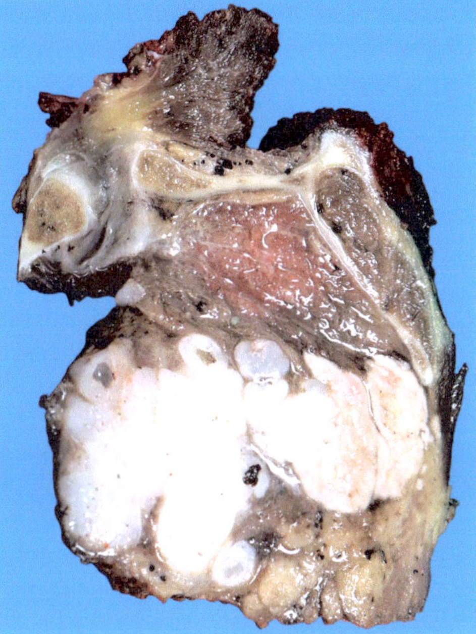

Fig. 2.68 Quiz question 6

7. Which vascular section is submitted in above-the-knee amputation, but not in below-the-knee amputations?
   A. Popliteal artery
   B. Anterior vascular bundle
   C. Posterior vascular bundle
   D. Femoral artery

8. You receive a soft tissue mass in the gross room. The clinical history favors this mass to be a lipoma. All of the following options favor this to be a malignant lesion except?
   A. Size >5 cm
   B. Tan-yellow lobulated cut surfaces
   C. Hemorrhagic areas
   D. Necrotic areas

9. Multiloculated cyst filled with clotted blood is the most likely gross description of which pathologic process?

   A. Angiosarcoma
   B. Aneurysmal bone cyst
   C. Osteosarcoma
   D. Giant cell tumor of bone

10. A marginal resection in bone and soft tissue is best described as
   A. Sampling the tumor area to gain a diagnosis of the tumor and leaving some tumor in the patient.
   B. Resection of the entire bone, including the surrounding soft tissues if the tumor involves it
   C. Resection of a segment of bone with a lesion
   D. Resecting the tumor with only the capsule or a small amount of tissue

Answer Key

1. D. Synovial sarcoma is a misnomer. Despite the name, the cells of origin are not synovial. It is a malignant soft tissue tumor of unknown cell differentiation. This is why "D" is the correct answer. Meanwhile, the other options don't fit the diagnosis. The picture shows a patchy eroded surface with loss of articular cartilage, classically seen in degenerative joint disease (DJD), along with villous projections (synovial overgrowth) predominantly at one end. Synovial overgrowth can be seen in DJD when synovium overgrows the meniscus due to chronic irritation. Synovial lipomatosis can also be seen in DJD or inflammatory conditions where synovium has a bright villonodular appearance as sub-synovial connective tissue is replaced by adipose tissue.

2. C. Trunk and extremities soft tissue tumors are staged pT3 if more than 10 cm and less than or equal to 15 cm in greatest dimension. This is why "C" is the correct answer. Meanwhile, the other options don't fit the diagnosis. The tumor is staged pT1 when 5 cm or less in greatest dimension, pT2 when more than 5 cm and less than or equal to 10 cm in greatest dimension, pT4: tumor more than 15 cm in greatest dimension.

3. C. A Sarcoma specimen needs to be bisected or serially sectioned before placing it in formalin for better fixation. Fixation is the crucial step in pathology for better evaluation of the gross specimen and for microscopic and immunohistochemical analysis. This is why "C" is the correct answer. Keeping the tissue fresh for 24 hours will cause tissue autolysis and affect tissue quality. Placing the tissue into formalin without bisecting/serially sectioning will not cause proper tissue preservation. Placing the tissue directly into the decal without fixation protects the cellular elements from harsh effects caused by the acids used in decalcifying agents.

4. B, EDTA is an acid-free chelating agent which binds calcium in the bone, making the bone soft enough to be sectioned for H&E

analysis. This method of decalcifying bone is prolonged but gentle and maintains the nuclear antigenicity required for molecular testing. This is why "C" is the correct answer. Hydrochloric acid is the conventional method used for decalcification, but it damages DNA, RNA, and proteins and compromises molecular testing. Formical is a mixture of formic acid and formalin and is gentler than hydrochloric acid, but it also somewhat destroys nucleic acids.

5. C. Measurement of cartilage cap thickness is of clinical relevance. That is why "C" is the correct answer. The picture shows osteochondroma, a benign cartilaginous with a cap thickness of less than 2 cm. Cartilage cap thickness > 2 cm in adults might reflect cancerous transformation.

6. B. The picture shows a large lobulated, fleshy cartilaginous mass, which favors it to be a malignant cartilaginous tumor. That is why "B" is the correct answer. To further elaborate, this is a case of dedifferentiated chondrosarcoma, and two different-looking areas can be appreciated grossly. The white cartilaginous area is a well-differentiated component, whereas the tan-yellow area is a dedifferentiated component. Chondroblastoma is a benign cartilaginous neoplasm usually well-demarcated and less than 5 cm. Osteosarcoma and giant cell tumor of the bone are malignant bone tumor that appears red-yellow with hemorrhagic areas mainly affecting the long bones.

7. A. The popliteal artery is an extension of the femoral arteries, starting in the middle of the thigh and running behind your knees before dividing into anterior and posterior tibial arteries. That is why "A" is the correct answer. Anterior and posterior vascular bundles are submitted in both above and below-knee amputations. The femoral artery is not present in both of these resection specimens.

8. B. Tan-yellow lobulated cut surfaces can be seen in lipoma and its malignant counterpart, liposarcoma. That is why "B" is the correct answer. Lipomas with homogenous cut surfaces are usually less than 5 cm in the great-

est dimension. However, liposarcomas can have heterogeneous surfaces with areas of hemorrhage and necrosis. Therefore, adequate specimen sampling is of utmost importance in these cases.

9. B. An aneurysmal bone cyst is a large hemorrhagic multicystic mass separated by fibrous septae. That is why B is the correct answer. Angiosarcoma is a dark red, hemorrhagic, ill-defined lesion that is not multicystic. Many benign or malignant tumors-like osteosarcoma and giant cell tumor of bone can undergo secondary aneurysmal bone cyst-like changes. However, it is less likely compared to a primary aneurysmal bone cyst.

10. D. A marginal resection removes the tumor with only the capsule or a small amount of tissue. That is why "D" is the correct answer. An intralesional resection consists of sampling the tumor area, typically to gain a diagnosis of the tumor and leaving some tumor in the patient. A radical resection removes the entire bone and includes the surrounding soft tissues if the tumor has extended through the bone. Segmental or wide resection is a resection of a segment of bone with a lesion.

References

1. UMHS Department of Pathology: specimen to charge code rapid finder list. 2011.
2. College of American Pathologists. June 2021. [Online]. Available: https://www.cap.org/protocols-and-guidelines/cancer-reporting-tools/cancer-protocol-templates. Accessed 7 July 2023.

Grossing of Breast Specimens

Contents

Breast specimens are straightforward when grossing if the proper methodology is applied to all specimens. Apart from different modalities of biopsies, the surgery could be directed for a single or multiple lesion and status post-chemotherapy cases. Mostly, the lesions are small and not grossly visible on mastectomy/excision specimens; hence, biopsy site clips (see Fig. 3.1) help identify the lesion. Using an X-ray machine is the superlative way to find the incredibly small biopsy site clips in breast specimens, but not every gross room has access to these machines.

All excisional breast specimens, including lumpectomies and mastectomies, require thorough investigation. A schematic approach should include acquiring clinical information, radiological findings, and surgical Op notes. Radiology gives information regarding the size, location, borders, and impression. The radiological findings are especially helpful in cases of status post-chemotherapy to compare the size of the mass pre- and post-chemotherapy. It helps in terms of microscopic examination and accurate staging of the patient.

All breast excisional specimens must be inked properly as lumpectomy margin status is critical. The specimens must be thinly sliced as numerous lesions are small and may not be visualized on thicker sections. The cut surface must be dried so that they are not greasy and shiny, for better visualization of the lesions. Attention should be paid for the presence of cysts, masses, location of lesions, architecture distortion, biopsy clips, and calcifications.

Fixing the specimen for 6–72 hours before processing is important because breast specimens require ample formalin fixation. Adequate fixa-

Fig. 3.1 Breast clips

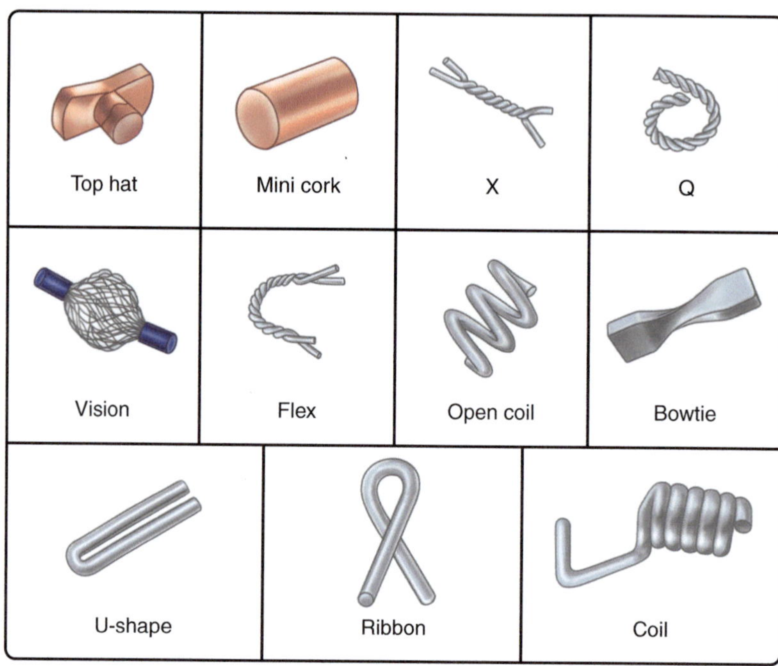

Table 3.1 CPT codes [1]

Breast biopsy	88305
Breast reduction	88305
Breast margin	
Breast excision	88307
Breast mastectomy, partial/simple/prophylactic	88307
Breast mastectomy with regional lymph nodes	88309
Sentinel node	88307

tion helps in the preservation of histology and antigenicity retrieval. Documentation of the adequate (6–72 hours) formalin fixation time of the tissue is required to perform ER, PR, and Her2 studies. Some common errors in submitting the tissue for processing are too much fat tissue, improper fixation (including over fixation and under fixation), thick sections, large sections in one cassette, and a stitch or clip within the tissue. See Table 3.1 for CPT codes.

3.1 Breast Biopsy—Level IV CPT 88305

A breast biopsy is when a needle is placed into the breast lesion, and samples of the lesion are removed. Different modalities of obtaining biop-

sies exist, including ultrasound, stereotactic, and MRI guided. For larger lesions, radiologists prefer to perform ultrasound-guided biopsies because the target is easier to locate and helps provide a thicker sample that can be used for optimal preservation of biomolecules for molecular assays since ischemia time is less. Stereotactic biopsies are often used when the target has calcifications or an architecture distortion. The pathologist must make sure that calcifications are visible on the microscopic examination. Additional levels from the block must be obtained if calcifications are absent, or X-raying the blocks should be considered. MRI-guided biopsies are used when lesions are small, and the radiologist is trying to assess the extent of the disease.

After removing the samples, a small breast biopsy clip is placed in the biopsy site, by the radiologist, so it can be easily identified on later imaging, if necessary.

Step 1: Describe and measure the biopsy cores. Often the cores are counted up to 5+ and can then be dictated as an aggregate. In Fig. 3.2, 3 tan cores are present.

Step 2: Place the biopsy cores in a biopsy bag and submit them entirely (Fig. 3.3). If necessary,

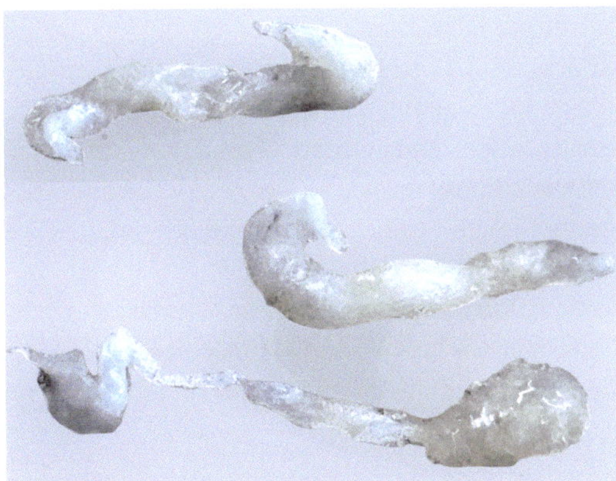

Fig. 3.2 Breast biopsy cores

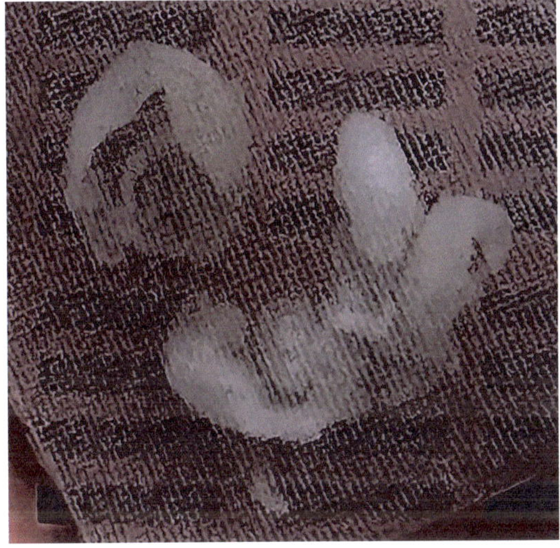

Fig. 3.3 Breast biopsy cores in biopsy bag

divide the cores into multiple cassettes. Do not overfill the cassettes. Fatty breast tissue is tricky for histology to section, and overfilling the cassette makes that even more challenging.

Step 3: Dictate the time the specimen is fixed in formalin before submitting for processing.

Unstained tissue slides are usually cut in between levels by histology; however, sometimes, the tissue is small, and if the radiologist suspects cancer, ductal carcinoma in situ (DCIS), or architecture distortion, the prosector can order a few additional unstained slides, which could be used for biomarker or further immunohistochemical studies.

Example Dictation

Specimen A is received in formalin labeled with the patient's name, medical record number, "right breast biopsy" and consists of 3 tan cores (1.2 × 1.6 × 0.2 cm) in aggregate which is submitted entirely in a biopsy bag in A1.

Remember to include: According to ASCO/CAP Guidelines related to HER2 testing in breast cancer recommendations, cytologic, biopsy, and resection specimens must be placed in formalin promptly (within 1 hour) and fixed in 10% neutral buffered formalin for 6 to 72 hours.

3.2 Breast Reduction

Breast reduction is the removal of breast tissue and areas of skin to minimize the size of the breast. These procedures are often done for breast asymmetry, congenital conditions, or back pain. The specimen weight is the most critical part of grossing the breast reduction. It can be used to assure both the right and left breast had appropriate amounts of tissue removed. If the specimen has already been weighed in the operating room, there is no need to weigh the specimen again, and that weight can be used in the pathology report. The weights are used for insurance purposes for reimbursements.

Radiology and clinical notes must be reviewed before examining the specimen, especially in patients older than 40. If a previous biopsy was performed or a radiologist has identified lesions in the respective breast, they must be correlated with the gross examination. The specimen should be measured and thinly sliced (1 cm) to look for abnormal areas, including masses, cysts, and irregularities. If none of these anomalous areas are found, 2–3 sections from white fibrous breast tissue submitted in the same cassette are enough for histopathological examination. Rarely, in situ and invasive carcinoma are found in these specimens. If a malignant lesion is found on the initial sections, the cut surfaces of the specimen must be examined again, and additional sections must be submitted.

Step 1: Dictate, measure, and weigh the specimen. Figure 3.4 is an aggregate tan-yellow tissue.

Step 2: Dictate the skin color and dimension of the skin if present.

Step 3: Serially section all tissue fragments and grossly assess for any lesions or cysts.

Step 4: Submit a section of skin and two sections of breast tissue. Breast tissue is the white fibrous tissue spanning through the yellow adipose tissue (Fig. 3.5).

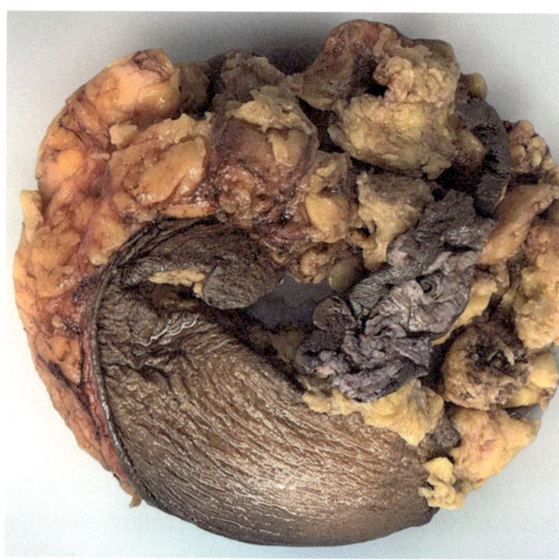

Fig. 3.4 Breast reduction tissue

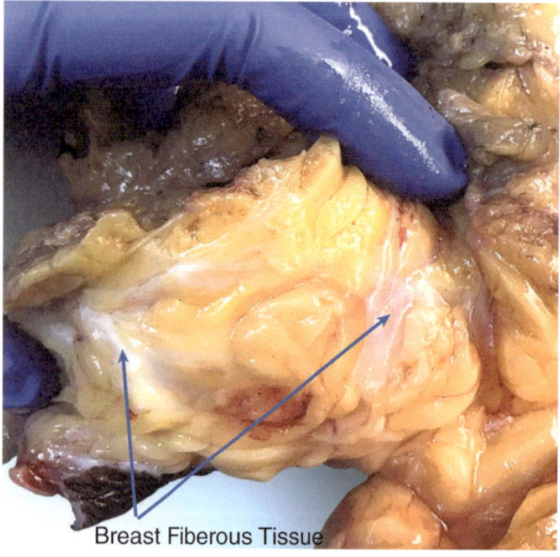

Fig. 3.5 Tan-white areas of breast tissue

Example Dictation

Specimen A is received in formalin labeled with the patient's name, medical record number, "right breast tissue" and consists of an aggregate of tan-yellow adipose tissue (21.4 × 20.2 × 6.4 cm, 1124 grams) with overlying tan-brown skin. The aggregate is serially sectioned to reveal tan-yellow, lobulated cut surfaces. No masses, cysts, heterogenous areas, or irregularities are identified. Representative sections are submitted in A1.

3.3 Breast Excision—Level V CPT 88307

A lumpectomy is the removal of a breast mass and additional surrounding breast tissue with the intent to remove the entire lesion. The surrounding normal breast tissue is the margin around the mass. Lumpectomy specimens are typically received oriented and inked accordingly. The specimen should be inked after thoroughly examining the radiology and OP note. There is usually a wire present in the specimen. Before cutting the specimen, the wire should be removed, and the specimen should be serially sectioned. After sectioning, find the clip area if visible grossly. If not visible, the specimen should be X-rayed, and the slice containing the clip must be submitted with the closest margin. Each lumpectomy should be treated according to clinical need. Sometimes, the lumpectomy can be submitted in less than ten cassettes; if so, the entire lumpectomy can be submitted to evaluate all margins and any area of invasion. If the lumpectomy as a whole cannot be submitted in 10 or fewer cassettes, the specimen must be discussed with the attending pathologist. This is because radiation treatment is dependent on DICS extent. Greater than 70% of the specimen must be submitted. If the lumpectomy is status post-chemotherapy, the entire tumor bed and adjacent slices must be submitted. For benign lesions, such as complex sclerosing lesions, fibroadenoma, or intraductal papilloma, 2–3 sections from clip areas are sufficient for microscopic examination. After submitting the targeted lesion, attention should be paid to abnormal areas visible on cut surfaces. If another lesion is grossly identified, the distance between these two lesions and the distance from margin must be documented. See Table 3.2 for gross descriptions of breast lesions.

Step 1: X-ray the specimen to identify the presence of a biopsy clip. The localizing needle can be removed before or after the X-ray. In Fig. 3.5, a Q-clip, Hourglass clip, and the localizing needle can be identified (Fig. 3.6).

Step 2: Describe, measure, and weigh the specimen.

Step 3: Describe and measure the attached skin, if present.

Step 4: Dictate how the specimen is oriented. In Fig. 3.7, the lumpectomy specimen contains breast tissue, tan-pink skin, and 2 black stitches for orientation.

Table 3.2 Tumor gross appearance

Fibroadenoma or benign phyllodes	Tan-white, firm, fibrous, well-circumscribed, and whorled cut surfaces
Borderline or malignant phyllodes	Tan-white, firm, fibrous masses with slit-like spaces, pushing borders, and possible areas of necrosis and hemorrhage
Ductal carcinoma in situ	Can form a mass or not. Travels along with ducts and forms small nodules. Mass-type lesions are typically solid, firm, ill-defined areas
Invasive ductal carcinoma	Tan-white or tan-yellow, ill-defined and stellate lesions
Invasive lobular carcinoma	Markedly ill-defined tan-yellow lesion. Typically challenging to define grossly

Step 5: Orient the specimen and ink appropriately. Figure 3.8 shows six ink colors orienting the lumpectomy.

Step 6: Serially section the specimen (Fig. 3.9). Typically sectioning along the long axis works best.

Step 7: Describe and measure the lesion. It is best to find the biopsy clip at this point because it cannot be submitted for histology.

Step 8: Measure the distance of the lesion to all of the margins.

Step 9: If necessary, X-ray the slices to identify which slice the clip is in. In Fig. 3.10, two different clips are seen and are present in the same lesion.

Step 10: Communicate with the pathologist about section submission. If the lesion is small, it can typically be submitted entirely in relation to all surrounding margins. In cases where the margin is too far away to fit in a cassette, a representative section of that margin can be submitted without the lesion. (Fig. 3.11).

Example Dictation

Specimen A is received in formalin labeled with patient's name, medical record number, "excision of left breast mass" and consists of a single fragment of tan-yellow adipose tissue (6.1 × 4.5 × 2.9 cm, 36 g) oriented with a long stitch designating lateral, a short stitch designating superior and a double stitch designating deep, with an overlying ellipse of tan-pink skin (4.4 × 1.3 cm). The specimen is serially sectioned to reveal a firm, centrally hemorrhagic mass (1.5 × 1.4 × 0.9 cm)

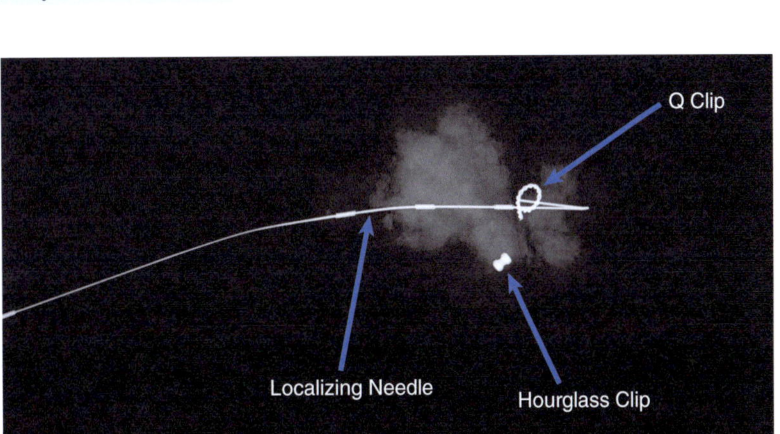

Fig. 3.6 X-ray with 2 biopsy clips and localizing needle

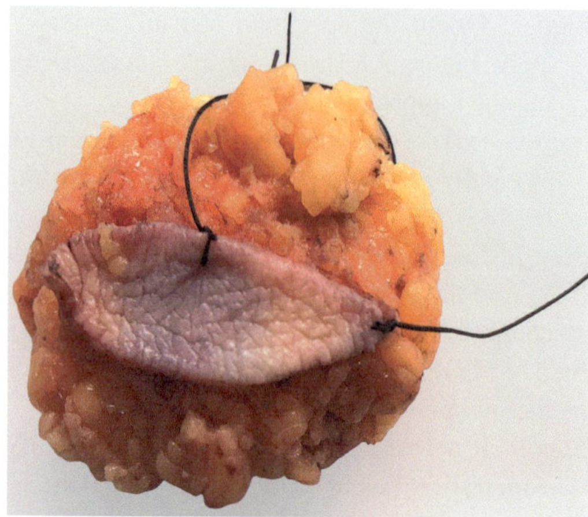

Fig. 3.7 Oriented lumpectomy

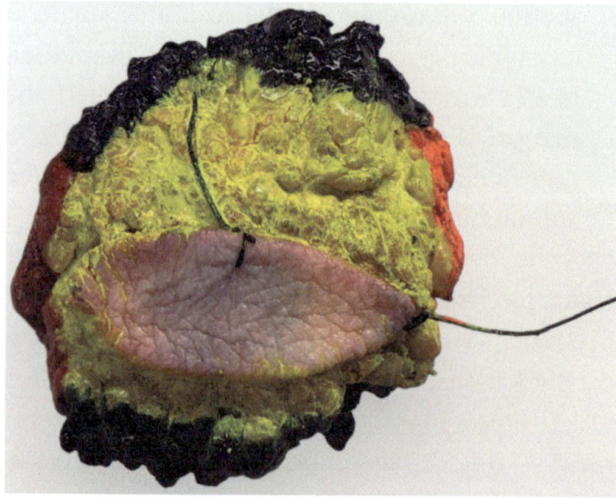

Fig. 3.8 Inked lumpectomy specimen

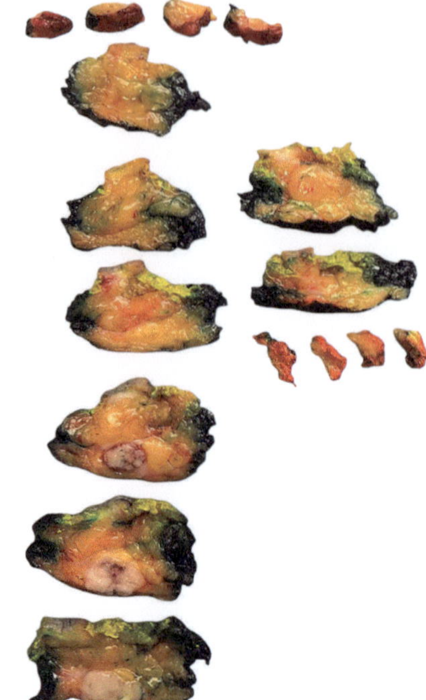

Fig. 3.9 Lumpectomy serially sectioned

with 2 biopsy clips, which comes within 2.2 cm of
the medial margin, 1.6 cm from the lateral margin,
1.6 cm from the superficial margin, 0.1 cm from
the deep margin, 0.9 cm from the superior margin,
and 1.4 cm from the inferior margin, surrounded
by tan-yellow, lobulated cut surfaces.

Ink code:
    Blue: superior
    Green: inferior
    Yellow: superficial
    Black: deep
    Red: medial
    Orange: lateral

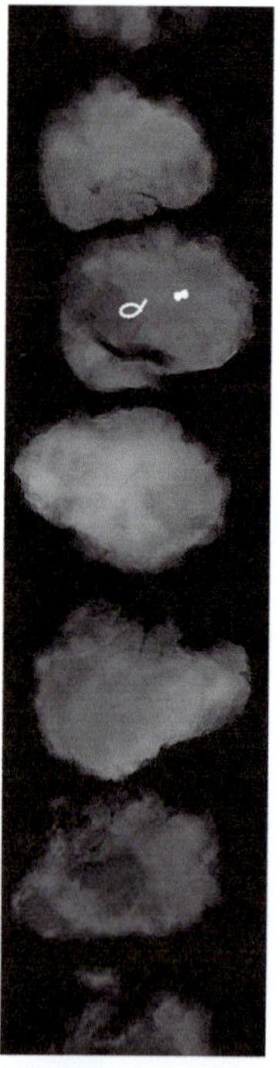

Fig. 3.10 X-ray of serially sectioned lumpectomy

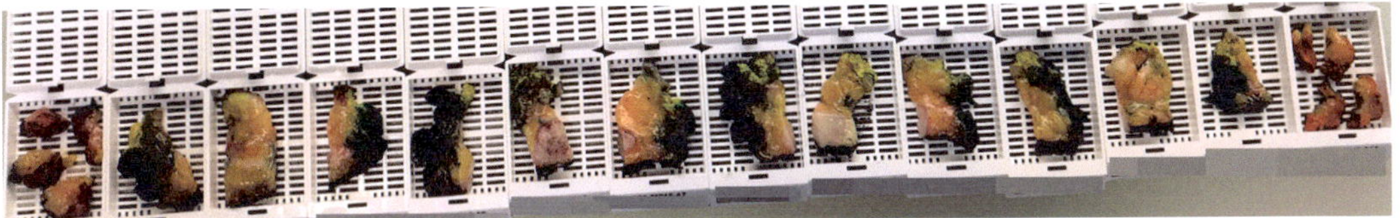

Fig. 3.11 Lumpectomy sections

Section code:
> A 1: Medial margin, perpendicular
> A 2-A 13: Mass entirely from medial to lateral (1 slice per 3 cassettes, trisected, clips sites in A4-A5)
> A 14: Lateral margin, perpendicular

Remember to include: According to ASCO/CAP Guidelines related to HER2 testing in breast cancer recommendations, cytologic, biopsy, and resection specimens must be placed in formalin promptly (within 1 hour) and fixed in 10% neutral buffered formalin for 6 to 72 hours.

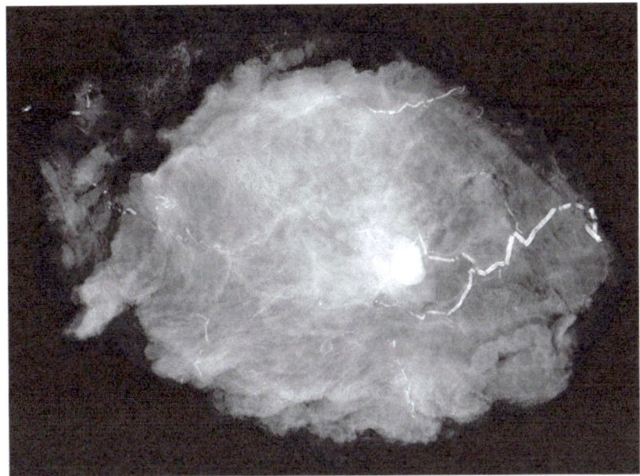

Fig. 3.12 X-ray of mastectomy

3.4 Prophylactic Mastectomy— Level V CPT 88307

Prophylactic breast specimens are the removal of a non-cancerous breast. These specimens are typically done as a compliment to the opposing cancerous breast. BRCA+ patients will often have bilateral prophylactic mastectomies to reduce cancer risk. There are a couple of different methods for grossing mastectomy specimens. For this example, the technique used keeps the specimen orientation intact, but it can sometimes be more challenging to visualize the lesion and margins in a breast with a mass. The main aim of prosector is to correlate with radiology and thinly slice the breast tissue to look for abnormal areas, including irregularities, heterogenous areas, masses, and cystic areas. These areas should be sampled. If abnormal areas are not seen, then four sections in two cassettes per breast are sufficient for the documentation purposes.

Step 1: If there is access to an X-ray machine, X-ray the breast to ensure there are no clips. In Fig. 3.12, a linear area of calcification can be noted but no biopsy clip is identified.

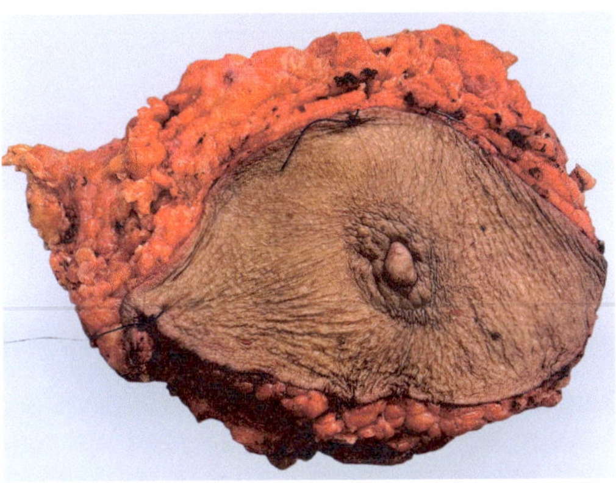

Fig. 3.13 Oriented mastectomy

Step 2: Describe, measure, and weigh the breast.

Step 3: Describe and measure the skin, nipple, areola, and any skin lesions or scars present.

Step 4: Orient the specimen and dictate how the specimen is oriented. In Fig. 3.13, the entire breast is excised with overlying tan skin, nipple, and 2 black orientation stitches.

Step 5: Ink the specimen and spray fixative.
> Superior-blue (Fig. 3.14a upper inner and upper outer quadrant).
> Inferior- green (Fig. 3.14a lower inner and lower outer quadrant).

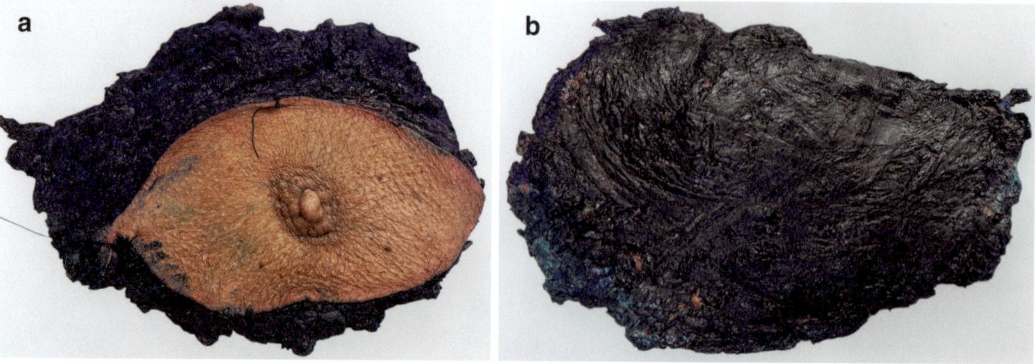

Fig. 3.14 (**a**) Inked mastectomy anterior view; (**b**) inked mastectomy posterior view

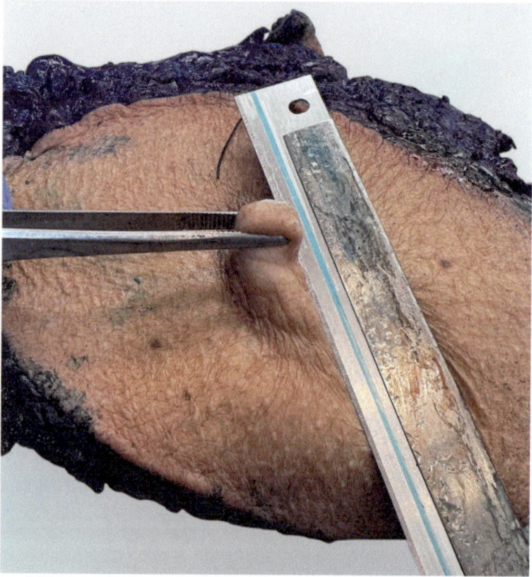

Fig. 3.15 Nipple sectioning

Posterior-black (Fig. 3.14b deep).

Step 6: Amputate the nipple from the breast as seen in Fig. 3.15.

Step 7: Trisect or serially section the nipple as seen in Fig. 3.16.

Step 8: Place the skin surface of the breast down on the cutting board and serially section the breast medial to lateral, leaving the skin surface intact (Fig. 3.17). This allows the breast slices to remain together, bound by the skin.

Step 9: Identify any areas of concern. Measure the overall size and how close they come to the closest margin. If no lesions are identified, describe the general cut surface of the breast as seen in Fig. 3.18.

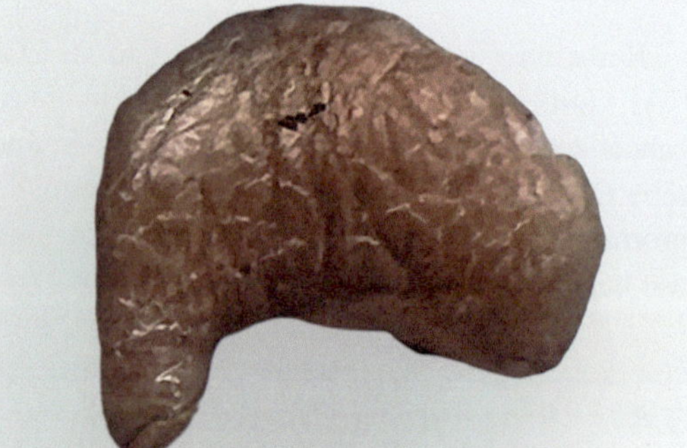

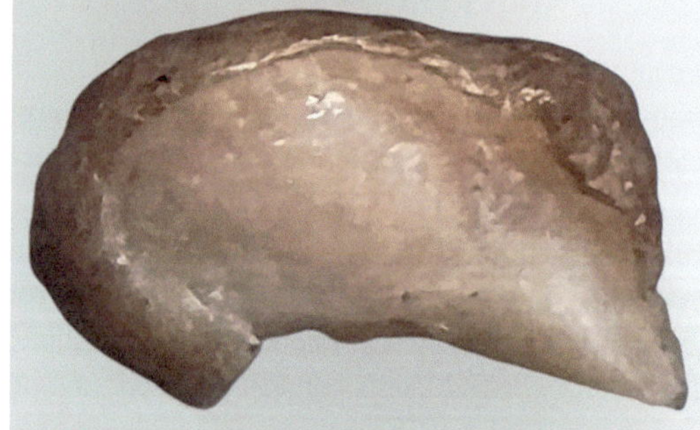

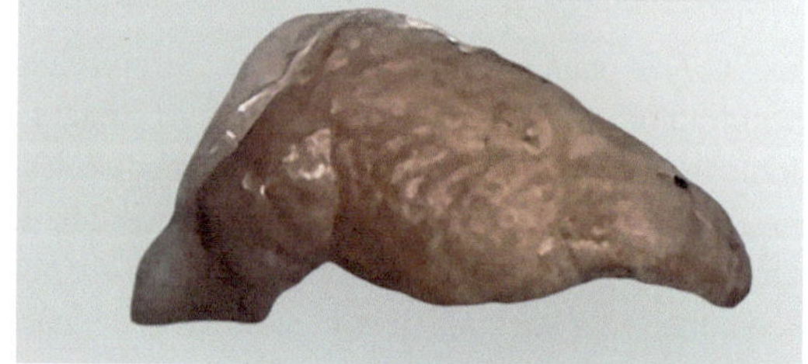

Fig. 3.16 Nipple trisected

Step 10: Submit representative sections per quadrant of the prophylactic breast (Fig. 3.19). Take sections of the tan-white, fibrous areas

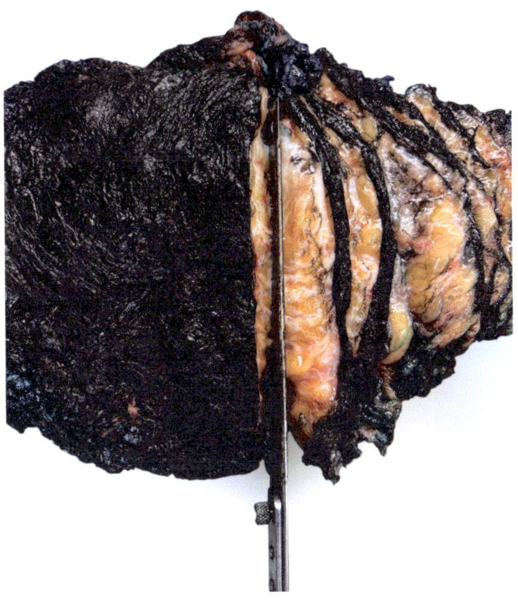

Fig. 3.17 Serial sectioning of the specimen

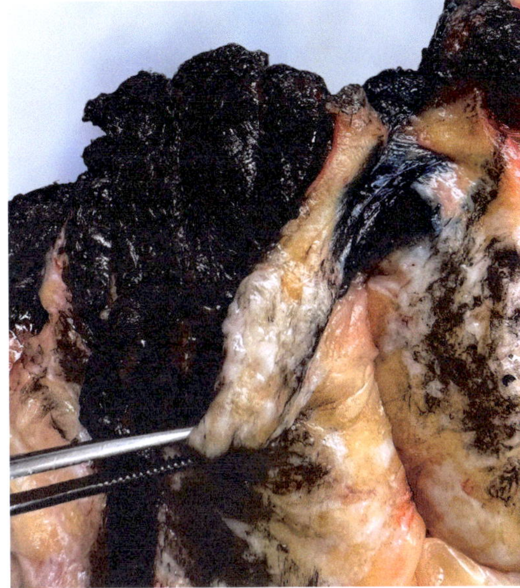

Fig. 3.18 White breast tissue

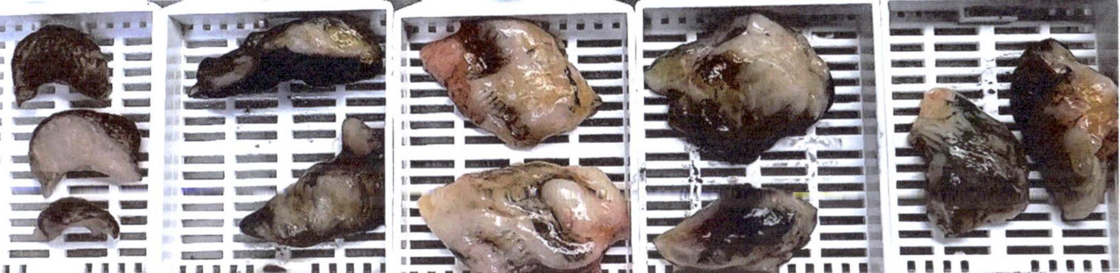

Fig. 3.19 Prophylactic mastectomy sections

representing breast tissue (ducts, etc.). The yellow areas are adipose tissue.

Example Dictation

Specimen A is received in formalin labeled with patient's name, medical record number, "left breast" and consists of a simple mastectomy (19.9 × 19.5 × 3.7 cm, 778 g) with an overlying tan-brown ellipse of skin (19.1 × 5.5 cm) with an everted nipple (1.3 cm in diameter). The specimen is oriented with a single stitch designating superior and a double stitch designating lateral. The specimen is serially sectioned to reveal tan-yellow, lobulated cut surfaces.

Ink code
  Blue: superior
  Green: inferior
  Black: deep

Section code
  A 1: Nipple, serially sectioned
  A 2: Upper inner quadrant, representative
  A 3: Lower inner quadrant, representative
  A 4: Upper outer quadrant, representative
  A 5: Lower outer quadrant, representative

Remember to include: According to ASCO/CAP Guidelines related to HER2 testing in breast cancer recommendations, cytologic, biopsy, and resection specimens must be placed in formalin promptly (within 1 hour) and fixed in 10% neutral buffered formalin for 6 to 72 hours.

3.5 Breast Mastectomy with Regional Lymph Nodes—Level VI CPT 88309

A mastectomy with the removal of axillary lymph nodes is performed to remove the breast with cancer and the associated lymph nodes. In this example, the method used to gross the breast allows for better visualization, but specimen orientation can be lost without careful attention. This is also the best method if an X-ray machine is available.

A comprehensive approach, including reviewing the radiology first, helps before cutting the specimen. The specimen must be first radiographed to find the area with the clip(s). Once clips are identified, the next step should be inking, weighing, and measuring. After thinly slicing the specimen, look for clips, and document their location and distance from other clips and margins. In status post-chemotherapy cases, the tumor is sometimes not visible, a photograph with annotation of the tumor bed (Fig. 3.20) can help during the microscopic examination.

A mastectomy specimen can be challenging if multiple lesions are present within the same breast. Most of the time, the margins are negative because the entire breast tissue is removed. However, anatomically breast tissue can extend into the skeletal muscle on the posterior surface. Those areas could have foci of DCIS at the margin. Therefore, close attention should be paid to the posterior margin while examining the cut surfaces. Trailing ducts or nodules close to the posterior margin should be submitted for microscopic examination.

Cancer Protocol Breakdown Relative to Grossing Breast

Procedure: There are multiple different ways to excise a breast. See Table 3.3 for examples.

Quadrants: Upper-inner, lower-inner, upper-outer, lower-outer (Fig. 3.21).

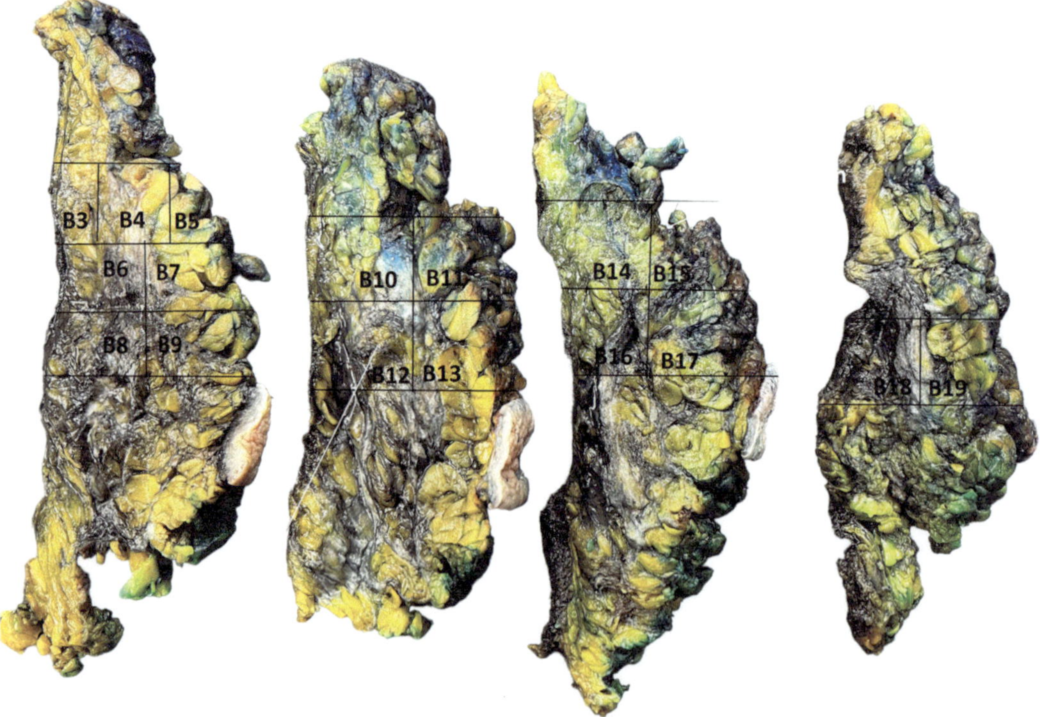

Fig. 3.20 Example of annotation of sections submitted

Clock: The central upper aspect of the breast is 12 o'clock and moves clockwise around the breast (Fig. 3.21).

Tumor Size: The overall size of the mass is measured to the millimeter, so be specific.

Table 3.3 Breast procedures [2]

Prophylactic	Removal of all breast tissue before cancer is identified
Nipple sparing	Removal of all breast tissue with no overlying nipple, areola, or skin
Skin sparing	Removal of all breast tissue with nipple and areola but minimal or no overlying skin
Simple	Removal of all breast tissue with nipple, areola, and a variable amount of overlying skin
Modified radical	Removal of all breast tissue with the nipple, areola, skin, and axillary lymph nodes
Radical	Removal of all breast tissue with the nipple, areola, skin, lymph nodes, and some underlying chest wall muscle

Important tumor size measurement considerations:

pT1: Tumor ≤20 mm in greatest dimension,

pT2: Tumor >20 mm but ≤50 mm in greatest dimension,

pT3: Tumor >50 mm in greatest dimension,

pT4: Tumor of any size with direct extension to the chest wall and/or to the skin (ulceration or skin nodules) [2].

Tumor focality: Some specimens have multifocal lesions. If multiple lesions are identified close together, then it is considered multifocal. If possible, assess the number of foci and the distance between the various lesions [2].

Skin satellite foci: Always evaluate the skin surface for lesions or scars. If lesions or scars are identified, submit sections [2].

Margins: Measure the distance of the lesion from all margins.

Lymph nodes: Submit all lymph nodes identified. See Table 3.4 for examples.

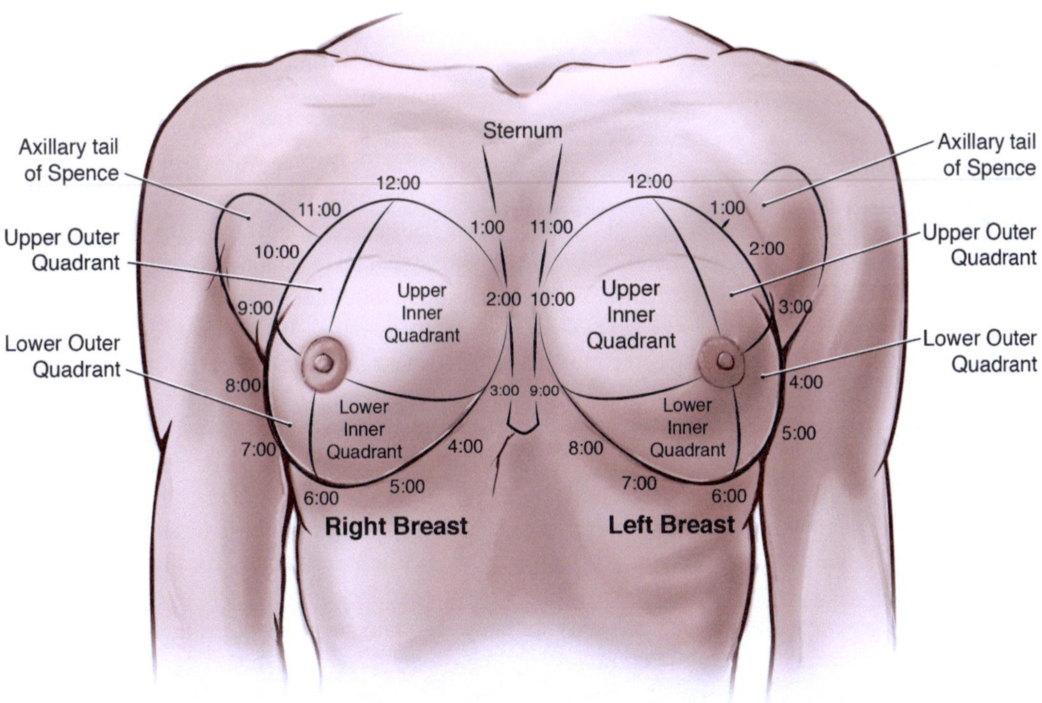

Fig. 3.21 Illustration of breast orientation

Table 3.4 Types of lymph nodes [2]

Axillary lymph nodes	Removed by en bloc resection of axillary tissue. Levels I: Low-axilla Level II: Mid-axilla Level III: Apical axilla or infraclavicular nodes
Intramammary nodes	Present within breast tissue: Most commonly found in the upper outer quadrant
Sentinel lymph nodes	Identified by the surgeon by uptake of radiotracer or dye or both

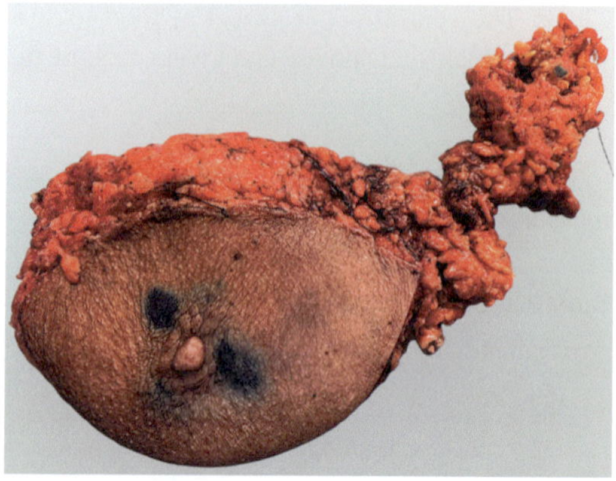

Fig. 3.23 Oriented modified radical mastectomy

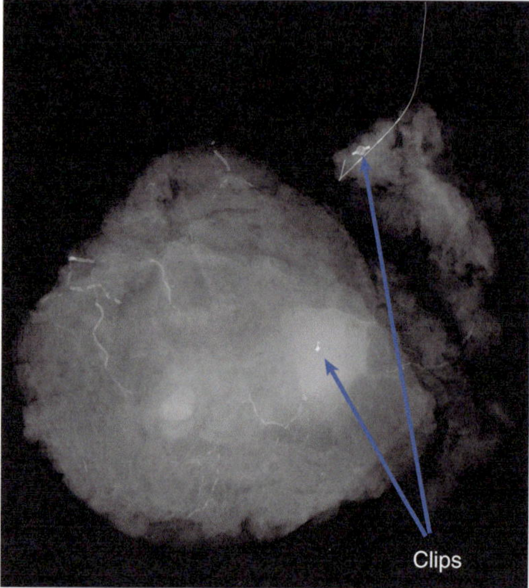

Fig. 3.22 X-ray of mastectomy with axillary tail

Step 1: If an X-ray machine is available, X-ray the breast to identify the biopsy clips. This allows for a general idea of where the clip is located. In Fig. 3.22, there is a coil clip in the breast and a vision clip in the axillary tail with a localizing needle.

Step 2: Describe, measure, and weigh the breast.

Step 3: Describe and measure the skin and nipple and any skin lesions or scars present.

Step 4: Orient the specimen and dictate how the specimen is oriented. Figure 3.23 contains a single black surgical stitch designating the axillary tail which is positioned superior-lateral in the body.

Step 5: Palpate the specimen to identify any palpable masses and whether they correlate with imaging.

Step 6: Ink the specimen.
   Superior: blue (Fig. 3.24a upper inner and upper outer quadrant).
   Inferior: green (Fig. 3.24a lower inner and lower outer quadrant).
   Posterior: black (Fig. 3.24b deep).

Step 7: Amputate the nipple from the breast as seen in Fig. 3.25.

Step 8: Trisect or serially section the nipple as seen in Fig. 3.26 or horizontally section the nipple. If unsure, communicate with the pathologist.

Step 9: Amputate the axillary tail and set it to the side (Fig. 3.27). Measure it separately as well.

Step 10: Place the skin surface of the breast down on the cutting board and serially section the breast medial to lateral, making complete cuts through the skin surface (Fig. 3.28).

Step 11: Lay out each slice on a flat surface from medial to lateral as seen in Fig. 3.29, taking care not to lose the orientation.

Step 12: Identify the mass. (Fig. 3.30). Figure 3.31 shows the X-ray of the same slices with the clip.

Step 13: Describe and measure the mass.

Step 14: Measure the mass to anterior-superior, anterior-inferior, deep, medial, lateral margins, and the nipple.

Step 15: Dictate which quadrant the mass is present.

Step 16: Describe the location of the clip according to the orientation.

Step 17: Take sections of the mass in relation to the closest margin. In Fig. 3.32, a full section of the mass is quadrisected and submitted.

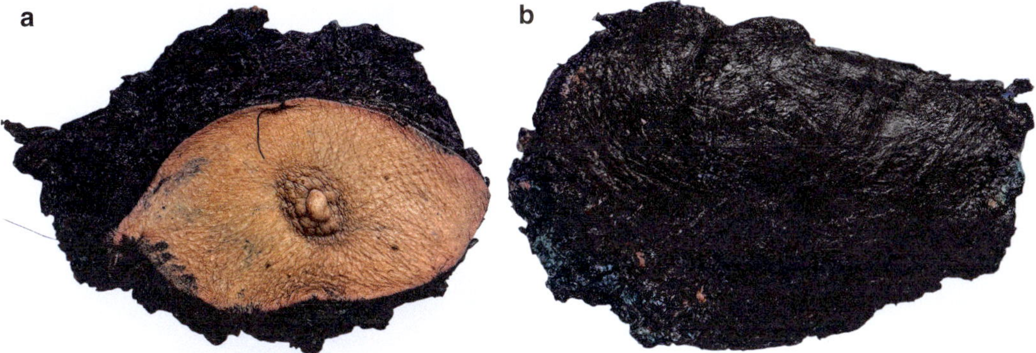

Fig. 3.24 (**a**) Inked mastectomy anterior view; (**b**) inked mastectomy posterior view

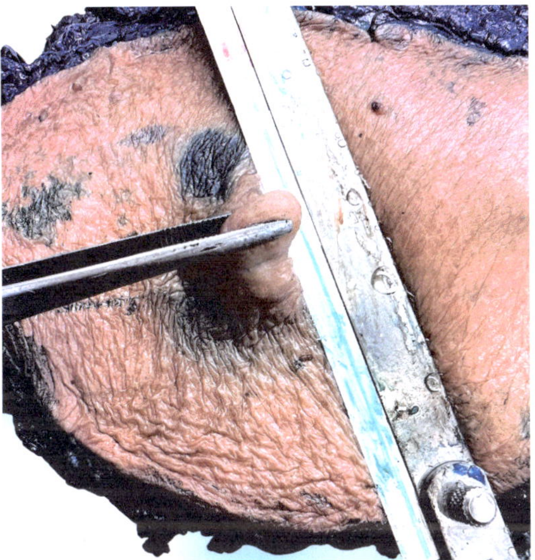

Fig. 3.25 Nipple sectioning

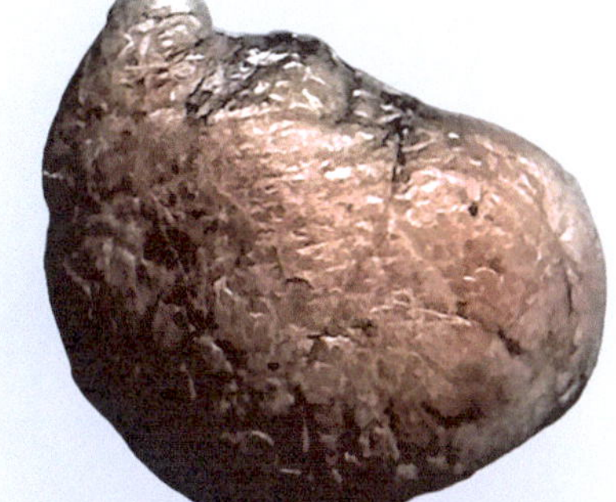

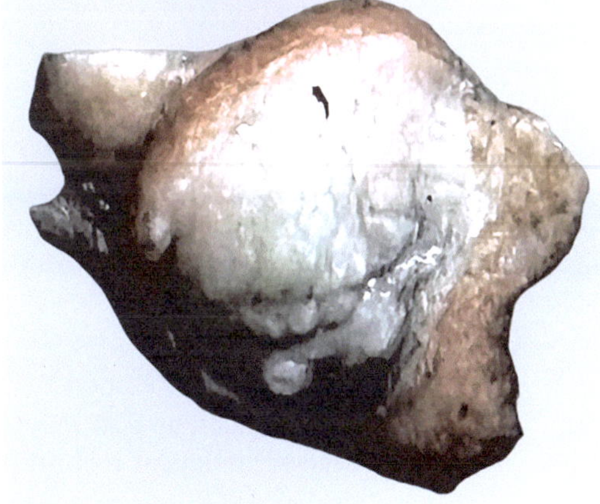

Fig. 3.26 Horizontal sections of nipple

This shows the mass in relation to the skin surface and the deep margin, which is the closest margin.

Step 18: Take additional representative sections of the quadrants of the breast that are uninvolved.

Step 19: Palpate for lymph nodes in the axillary tail (Fig. 3.33). Record the range of size of all nodes and the size of grossly positive nodes. Submit all lymph nodes identified and areas suggestive of extra-nodal extension. Tumor deposits in the axillary tail/ fat adjacent to the breast may be completely replaced lymph nodes and are considered lymph node metastasis. Submit representative sections of the larger lymph nodes, if necessary.

Always dictate how the lymph nodes are submitted.

3 lymph node candidates, whole

1 lymph node candidate, bisected

If larger/matted lymph nodes are present, serially section and submit representative section. If small enough, submit it entirely.

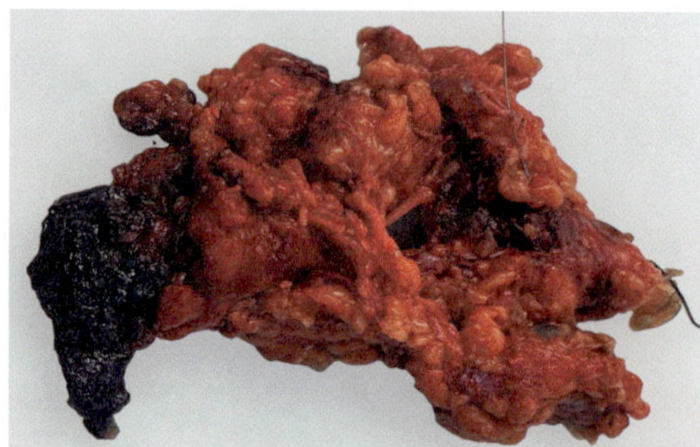

Fig. 3.27 Axillary tail amputated

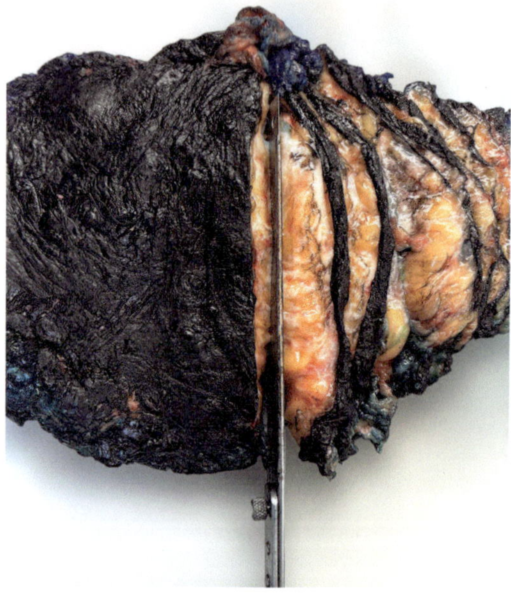

Fig. 3.28 Serial sectioning of specimen

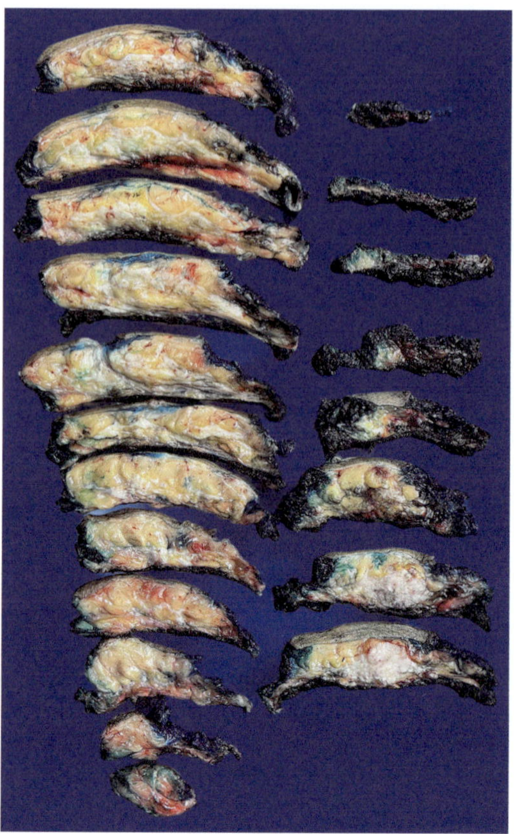

Fig. 3.29 Serial sectioning of specimen with each slice laid out

1 matted lymph node, serially sectioned.

Step 20: The mass should be submitted entirely if the patient has received treatment before. If the patient hasn't had previous treatment, representative mass can be submitted—approximately 1 section per 1 cm of the overall mass size (Fig. 3.34).

Example Dictation

Specimen A is received in formalin labeled with patient's name, medical record number, "left breast" and consists of a modified radical mastectomy (22.6 × 19.8 × 4.7 cm, 1128 g) with an overlying ellipse of tan-brown skin (19.8 × 10.2 cm) with an everted nipple (1.1 cm in diameter) and attached axillary tail (15.2 × 4.2 × 2.2 cm). The specimen is oriented with a single stitch designating superior and a double stitch designating lateral. The specimen is serially sectioned to reveal a firm well-circumscribed lesion (3.9 × 3.5 × 2.8 cm) with a biopsy clip, present in the lower outer quadrant at approximately 5 o'clock, coming within 0.9 cm from the deep margin, 2.1 cm form the anterior-superior margin, 3.5 cm from the anterior-inferior margin, and 3.1 cm from the nipple. The remaining cut surfaces are tan-yellow and lobulated with no additional lesions identified. The axillary tail is palpable for 21 lymph node candidates ranging from 0.4 to 3.2 cm, with a biopsy clip present in the largest lymph node.

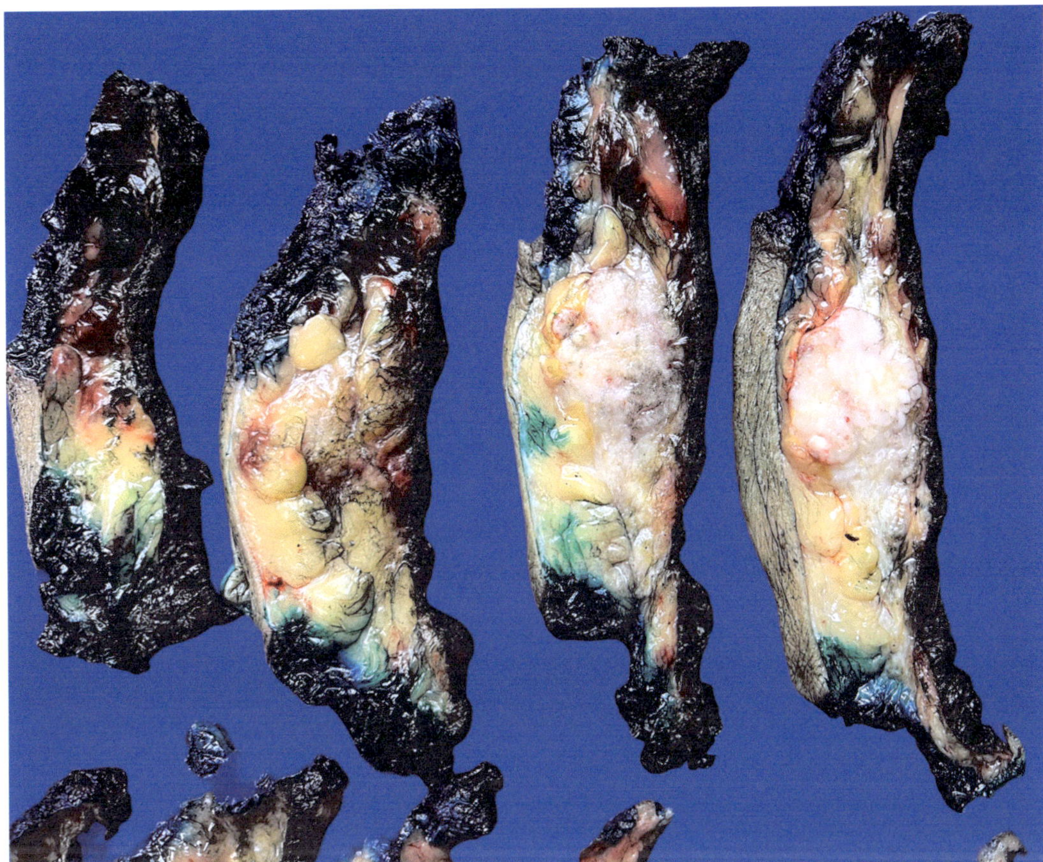

Fig. 3.30 Slices with mass

Ink code

    Blue: anterior-superior
    Green: anterior-inferior
    Black: deep

A 1: Nipple, serially sectioned

A 2-A 5: Full face section of mass in relation to the skin surface and deep margin, quadrisected with biopsy site

A 6-A 9: Full face section of mass in relation to the skin surface and deep margin, quadrisected

A 10: Upper inner quadrant, representative

A 11: Upper outer quadrant, representative

A 12: Lower inner quadrant, representative

A 13- A 14: 5 lymph node candidates per cassette, whole

A 15- A 24: 1 lymph node candidate per cassette, bisected

A 25-A 27: 1 lymph node candidate, trisected with biopsy site

Remember to include: According to ASCO/CAP Guidelines related to HER2 testing in breast cancer recommendations, cytologic, biopsy, and resection specimens must be placed in formalin promptly (within 1 hour) and fixed in 10% neutral buffered formalin for 6 to 72 hours.

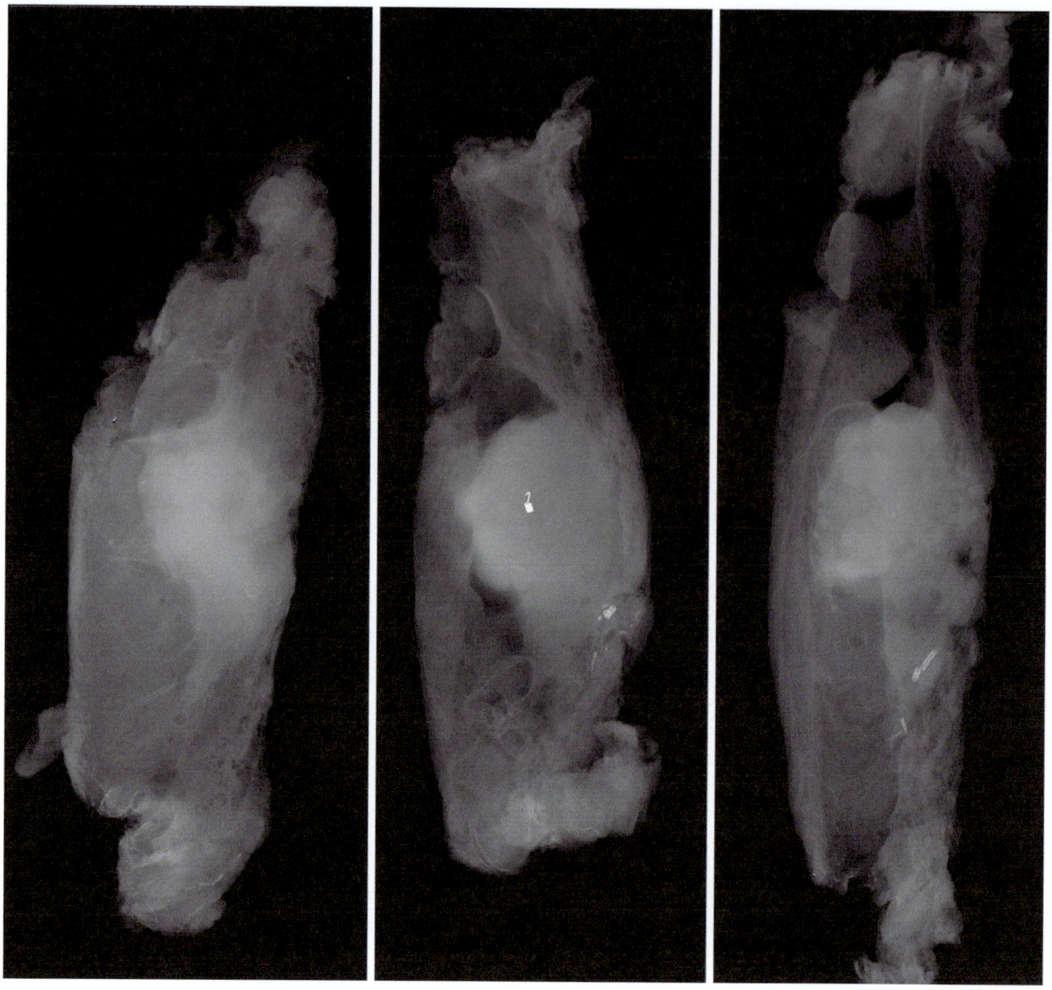

Fig. 3.31 X-ray of slices with coil clip

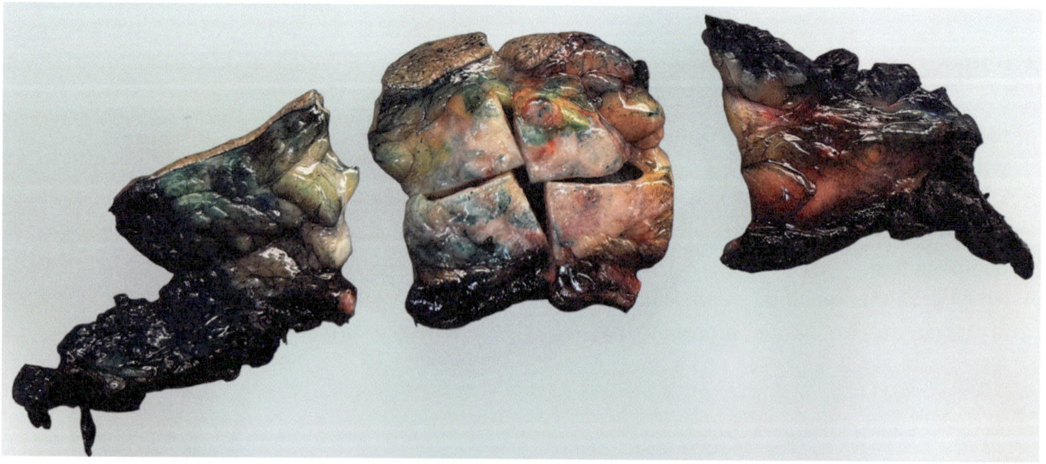

Fig. 3.32 Quadrisected section

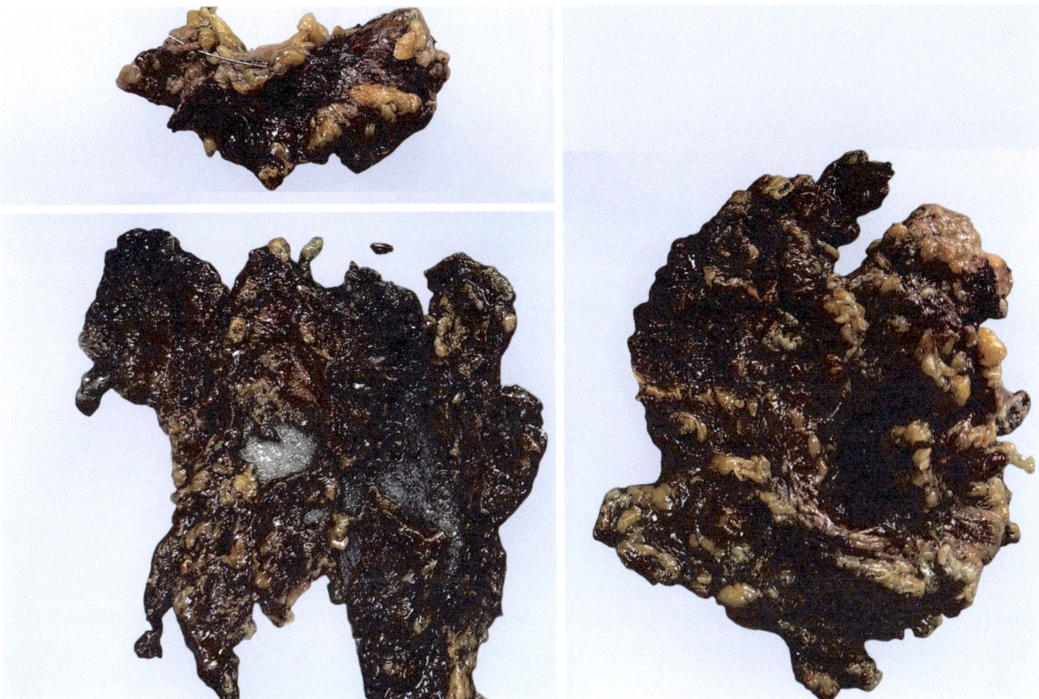

Fig. 3.33 Axillary tail assessed for lymph nodes

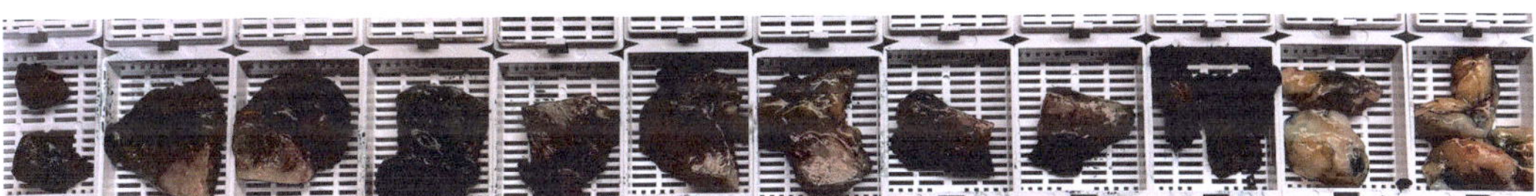

Fig. 3.34 Mastectomy sections

3.6 Breast Margin—Level V CPT 88307

Additional breast margins can be received separately depending on the surgeon. Occasionally, a surgeon may perform a second surgery to remove an additional margin if the original specimen has positive margins.

Step 1: Describe, measure, and weigh the specimen.

Step 2: Orient the specimen. In Fig. 3.35, the stitch designates the new true margin. Notice in Fig. 3.35b that the false margin is slightly cauterized. Cautery marks the previous resection site, which is now the false margin.

Step 3: Ink the true margin (Fig. 3.36a blue ink) and the false margin (Fig. 3.36b orange ink). Choose two different colors, one for each margin.

Step 4: Serially section the specimen keeping the slices in order (Fig. 3.37).

Step 5: Describe the cut surfaces of the specimen. If any lesions are identified, describe, measure the size and how close it comes to the true margin.

Step 6: Margins should be submitted entirely and in sequential order (Fig. 3.38). If the tissue is

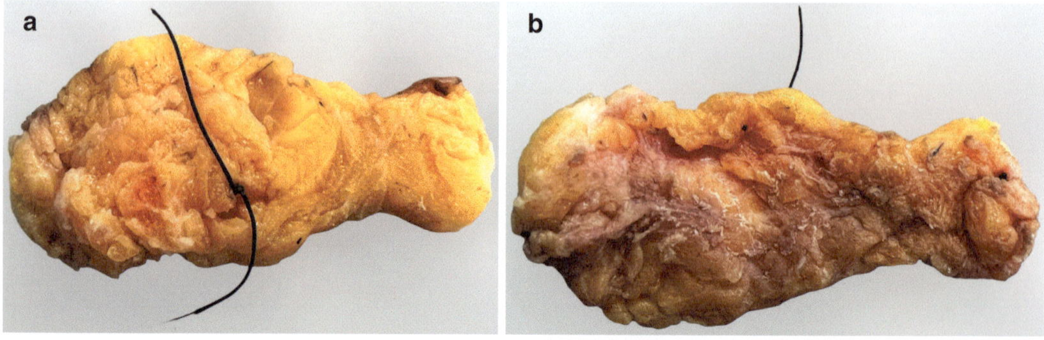

Fig. 3.35 (**a**) Stitch on true margin. (**b**) False margin

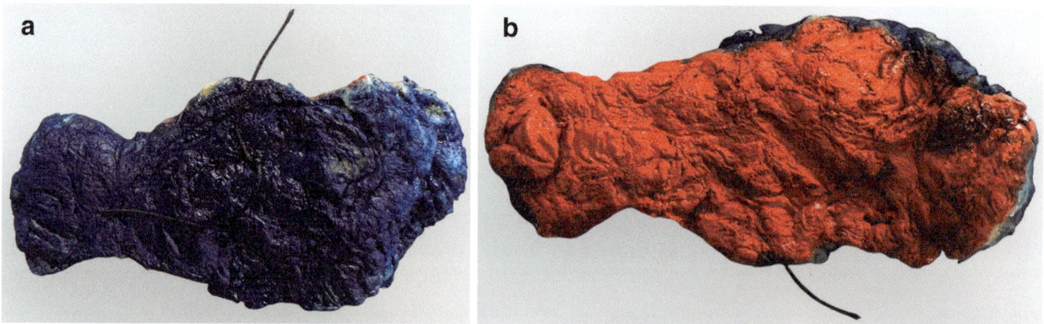

Fig. 3.36 (**a**) True margin inked. (**b**) False margin inked

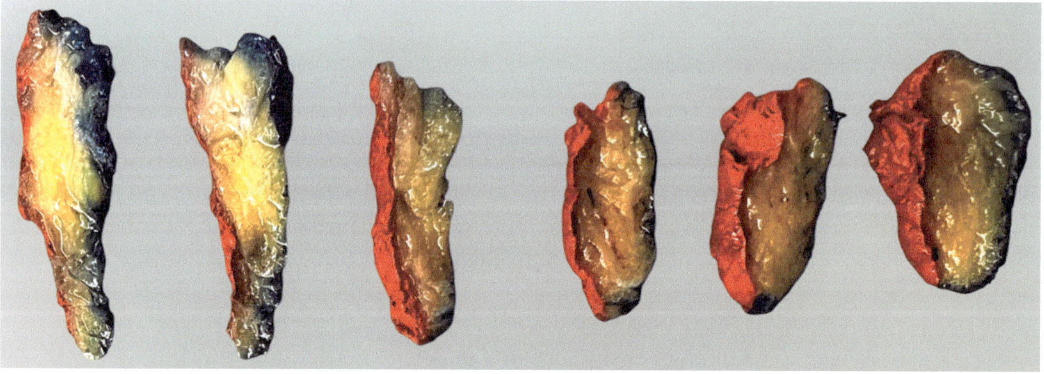

Fig. 3.37 Serial section of specimen

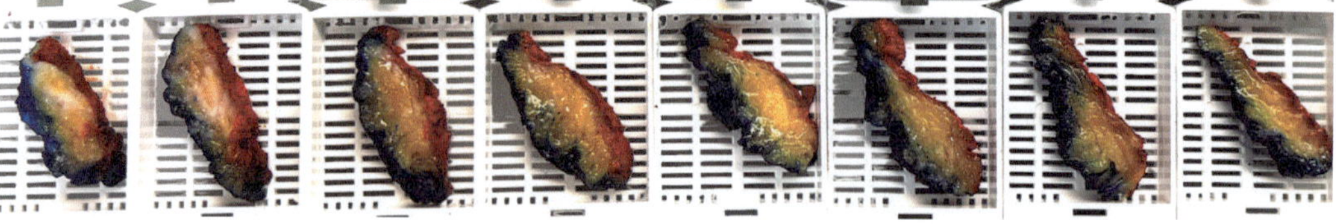

Fig. 3.38 Sections submitted

large, communicate with the pathologist for further instruction.

Example Dictation

Specimen A is received in formalin labeled with patients' name, medical record number, "new superior margin" and consists of a single fragment of tan-yellow adipose tissue (5.9 × 2.1 × 1.3 cm, 14 g) with a stitch designating the true superior margin. The specimen is serially sectioned to reveal tan-yellow, lobulated cut surfaces. The specimen is sequentially submitted, entirely in A1-A8.

Ink code
> Blue: True superior margin
> Orange: False margin

3.7 Sentinel Nodes—Level V CPT 88307

The sentinel node is the lymph node most likely to acquire cancer cells first. Often, surgeons inject a radioactive dye into the area of the cancerous lesion and follow the dye to the first node(s) that registers on the radiation detector. Those lymph node(s) are removed and assessed microscopically for cancer cells. An axillary dissection is necessary if cancer is identified within the sentinel node.

Step 1: Describe and measure the lymph node (Fig. 3.39).

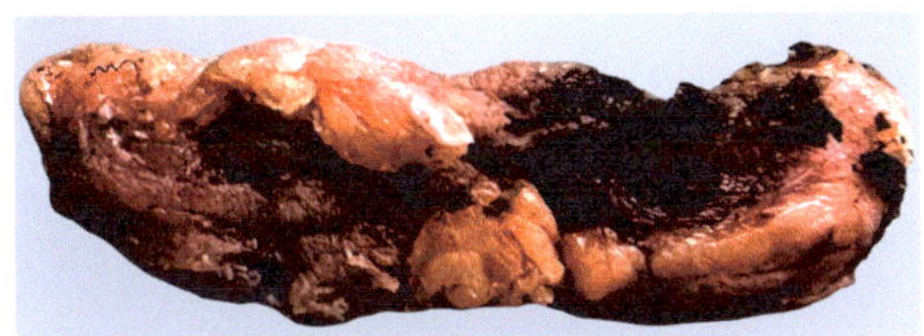

Fig. 3.39 Lymph node

Step 2: Serially section the lymph node in approximately 2 mm thick sections (Fig. 3.40).
Step 3: Submit the lymph node entirely (Fig. 3.41).

Multiple fragments/lymph node candidates should be measured separately but if there are more than 3, they can be measured in aggregate. All candidates are serially sectioned individually and submitted entirely.

Example Dictation

Specimen A is received in formalin labeled with patient's name, medical record number, "left breast sentinel node #1" and consists of a single lymph node candidate (1.6 × 0.6 × 0.5 cm) which is serially sectioned and submitted entirely in A1-A2.

Acknowledgments The author gratefully ackno wledges Muhammad Masood Hassan, MD, and Javaria A. Khan, MD, for their contribution to this chapter.

Fig. 3.40 Serial section of lymph node

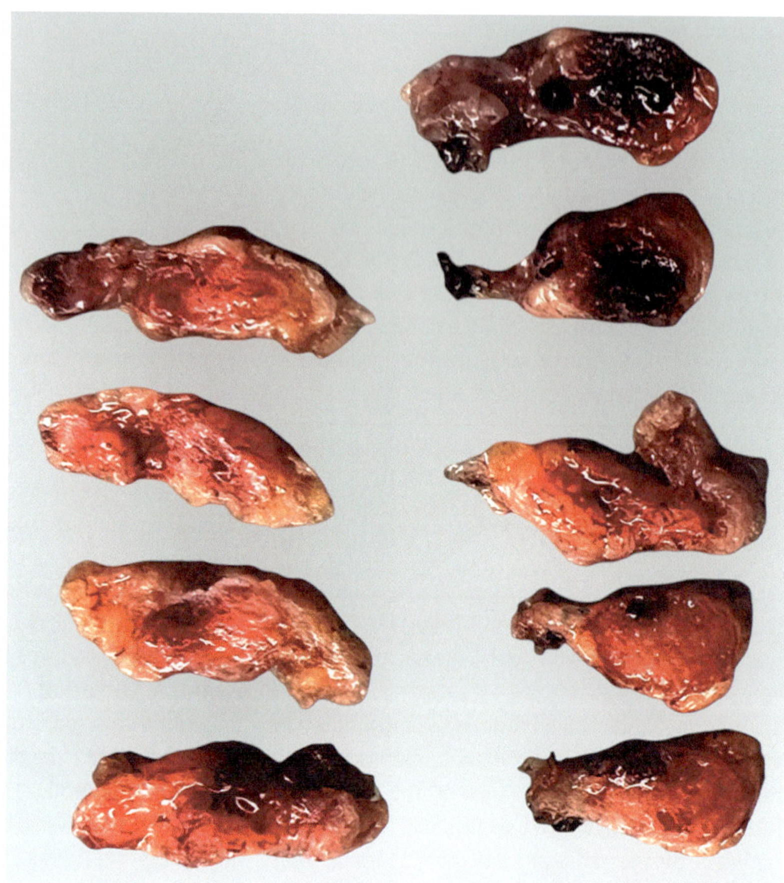

Fig. 3.41 Sections submitted

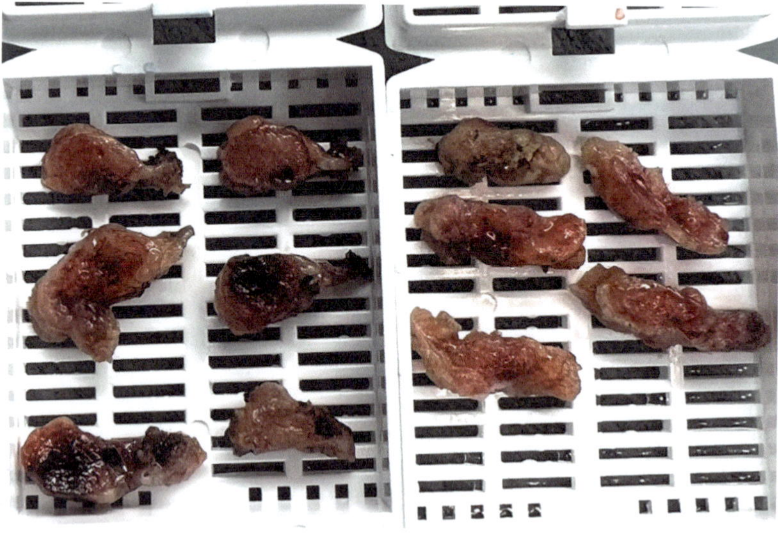

Quiz Questions

1. What mastectomy containing breast, skin, nipple, and axillary tail is called?
   (a) Radical mastectomy
   (b) Simple mastectomy
   (c) Skin sparing mastectomy
   (d) Modified radical mastectomy
2. What is the proper formalin fixation time for breast tissue?
   (a) 6–24 hrs
   (b) 24–72 hrs
   (c) 6–72 hrs
   (d) 24–48 hrs
3. How many margins are part of a lumpectomy?
   (a) 6
   (b) 8
   (c) 4
   (d) 3
4. On the X-ray, you see this biopsy clip. What is the name of this clip?
   Fig. 3.42 X-ray of Clip
   (a) Top hat clip
   (b) Ribbon slip
   (c) Bowtie clip
   (d) Vision clip

5. Upon completing a lumpectomy, you receive a tan-white, firm, fibrous, and whorled 5 cm mass. What is your gross diagnosis?
   (a) Invasive ductal carcinoma
   (b) Adenoma
   (c) Benign cyst
   (d) Invasive lobular carcinoma
6. What kind of mastectomy is pictured here:
   Fig. 3.43 Anterior view of breast
   (a) Nipple-sparing mastectomy
   (b) Skin sparing mastectomy
   (c) Simple mastectomy
   (d) Modified radical mastectomy

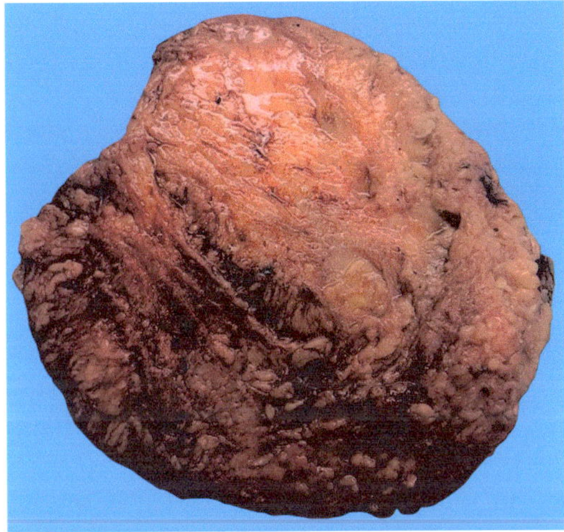

Fig. 3.43 Quiz question 6, anterior view of breast

Fig. 3.42 Quiz question 4

7. You receive a sentinel lymph node from a right radical mastectomy That is 1.2 × 1.0 × 1.0 cm. How do you gross the lymph node?
   (a) Bivalve the lymph node and submit one-half of the specimen
   (b) Serially section the lymph node in 2 mm slices and submit every other slice
   (c) Trisect the lymph node and submit entirely
   (d) Serially section the lymph node in 2 mm slices and submit entirely

8. Imaging describes a 3 cm mass at 2 o'clock in the left breast. What quadrant is this?
   (a) Upper outer
   (b) Lower outer
   (c) Upper inner
   (d) Lower inner

9. Imaging describes a 2.5 cm mass at 2 o'clock in the right breast. What quadrant is this?
   (a) Upper inner
   (b) Lower inner
   (c) Upper outer
   (d) Lower outer

10. You receive a modified radical mastectomy and notice blue dye coloring the central aspect of the specimen. What is the medical reason for using this dye?
   (a) Identifying the sentinel lymph node
   (b) Identifying the mass
   (c) Differentiating the difference between cancer and benign masses
   (d) Designating the nipple

Answer Key

1. *(d) Modified radical mastectomy*

   Explanation: A modified radical mastectomy removes the breast tissue, some skin, the nipple, and the axillary tail, so "(d)" is the correct answer. A radical mastectomy also includes all those structures but contains pectoralis muscle as well. A nipple-sparing mastectomy consists of the nipple and areola but not the additional surrounding skin, whereas a simple mastectomy includes the nipple, areola, and some overlying skin.

2. *(c) 6–72 hr.*

   Explanation: According to ASCO/CAP Guidelines related to HER2 testing in breast cancer recommendations, cytologic, biopsy, and resection specimens must be placed in formalin promptly (within 1 hour) and fixed in 10% neutral buffered formalin for 6–72 hours. This makes option "(c)" the correct answer.

3. *(a) 6*

   Explanation: A lumpectomy is an excision of a portion of the breast, so the entire periphery of the specimen is a margin. Utilizing standard medical orientation, the tissue is typically oriented: anterior, posterior, superior, inferior, medial, and lateral. Each individual margin is inked separately, so there are six margins with six different ink colors, rendering option A as the correct answer.

4. *(d) Vision clip*

   Explanation: A vision clip is a small circle of mesh with two short metal ends extending from opposite sides. This makes option "(d)" the correct choice. A top hat clip looks like a very small; "T." A ribbon clip is a segment of wire looped around and crossed over at the end like a ribbon you would wear on your lapel. A bowtie clip looks like a flat clip that has been twisted in the middle.

5. *(b) Adenoma*

   Explanation: An adenoma is a tan-white, firm, fibrous mass with tan-white, whorled cut surfaces, which makes option "(b)" the best choice. Invasive ductal carcinoma appears as a tan-white or tan-yellow, ill-defined, stellate lesion. Invasive lobular carcinoma is a markedly ill-defined tan-yellow lesion that is often difficult to identify from the periphery grossly. A Benign cyst would contain fluid or soft material within the cyst wall and would not be a solid cut surface.

6. *(a) Nipple sparing*

   Explanation: The photo shows a mastectomy with no overlying skin, nipple, or areola. This is called a nipple-sparing mastectomy making option "(a)" correct. A prophylactic mastectomy is the removal of all breast tissue before cancer is identified. A skin-sparing mastectomy is the removal of all breast tissue with nipple and areola but minimal or no overlying skin. A simple mastectomy is the removal of all breast tissue with the nipple, areola, and a variable amount of overlying skin. A modified radical mastectomy is the removal of all breast tissue with the nipple, areola, skin, and axillary lymph nodes. A radical mastectomy is the removal of all breast tissue with the nipple, areola, skin, lymph nodes, and some underlying chest wall muscles.

7. *(d) Serially section the lymph node in 2 mm slices and submit entirely*

    Explanation: All sentinel lymph nodes for all types of specimens are serially sectioned into 2 mm slices. This allows for the most surface area of the lymph node to be microscopically examined, so "(d)" is the right choice.

8. *(a) Upper outer quadrant*

    Explanation: Identify the clock orientation by facing the patient and moving around the periphery of the correct breast (right vs. left) in a clockwise fashion. 2 o'clock of the left breast is the upper outer quadrant of the left breast which makes "(a)" the correct answer.

9. *(a) Upper inner quadrant*

    Explanation: Identify the clock orientation by facing the patient and moving around the periphery of the correct breast (right vs. left) in a clockwise fashion. 2 o'clock of the right breast is the upper inner quadrant of the right breast which makes "(a)" the correct answer.

10. *(a) Identifying the sentinel lymph node.*

    Explanation: The sentinel node is the lymph node most likely to acquire cancer cells first. Surgeons can inject a radioactive dye into the area of the cancerous lesion and follow the dye to the first node that registers on the radiation detector or grossly turns the color of the dye. Those lymph node(s) are removed and assessed microscopically for cancer cells. An axillary dissection is necessary if cancer is identified within the sentinel node.

References

1. "FirstPath," 2009–2023. [Online]. https://www.first-pathlab.com/cpt-codes/. Accessed on 2 Jun 2023.
2. "Protocol for the Examination of Resection Specimens from," College of American Pathologists, 2023.

Grossing of Cardiac and Thoracic Specimens

4

Contents

Welcome to the guide on grossing techniques for cardiothoracic specimens. In this section, we will explore the examination and dissection of heart, lung, and mediastinal specimens obtained from surgical specimens and autopsies.

Accurate assessment and thorough sampling of cardiothoracic specimens are crucial for diagnosis and patient care. This chapter covers the fundamental principles, techniques, and considerations involved in the gross examination of these specimens.

This chapter addresses challenges, specimen handling, documentation including CPT codes (Table 4.1), and macroscopic evaluation of neoplastic and non-neoplastic conditions within the thoracic cavity.

© The Author(s), under exclusive license to Springer Nature Switzerland AG 2024
A. Illingworth, *Manual of Pathologic Grossing*, https://doi.org/10.1007/978-3-031-72694-1_4

Table 4.1 CPT codes

Plaque	88304
Aneurysm	88304
Heart biopsy	88307
Heart leaflets	88305
Heart explant	88309
Lung biopsy	88305
Lung lymph node (1 node)	88305
Lung lymph node packet (2+ nodes)	88307
Lung wedge	88307
Long lobectomy	88309
Mediastinal mass	88307
Thymus tumor	88307

[1]

4.1   Heart Biopsy: Level V CPT 88307

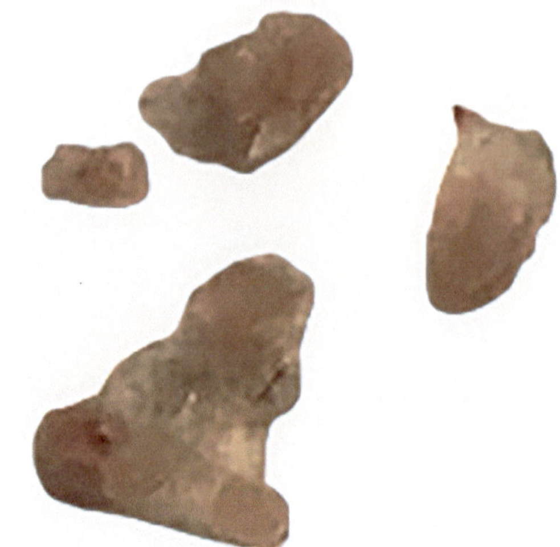

Fig. 4.1 Heart biopsy

A biopsy of the heart involves taking a few small samples of cardiac muscle, typically taken from the septal aspect of the right ventricle. This is most often performed in heart transplant patients for the evaluation of potential rejection, but may also be performed for the assessment of myocarditis, sarcoidosis, and amyloidosis. Three fragments of cardiac muscle are considered an acceptable biopsy but four fragments are considered optimal so it is important to count the number of fragments present in the specimen container. A separate fragment of cardiac muscle may be received in special media for immunofluorescence studies.

Step 1: Count the number of fragments, describe and measure the aggregate. In Fig. 4.1, there are 4 separate fragments, which is optimal.

Step 2: Submit all tissue in a biopsy bag. (Fig. 4.2)

Example Dictation

Specimen A is received in formalin labeled with patient's name, medical record number, "heart biopsy" and consists of 4 fragments of tan-brown tissue (0.5 × 0.4 × 0.2 cm). The specimen is submitted entirely in a biopsy bag in A1.

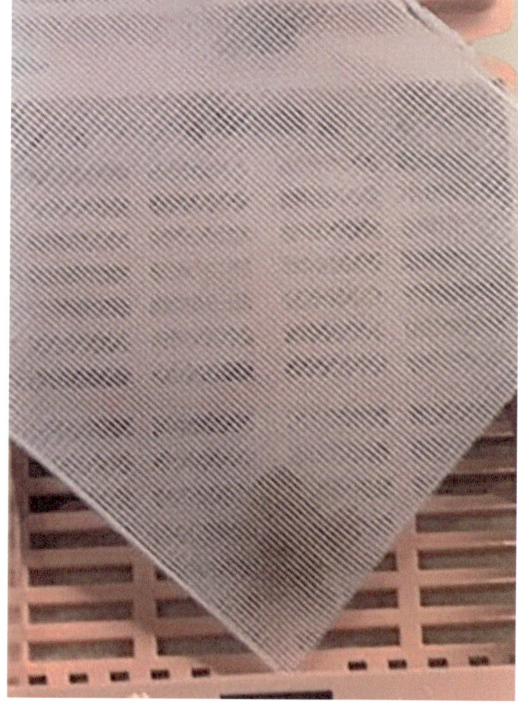

Fig. 4.2 Heart biopsy section submission

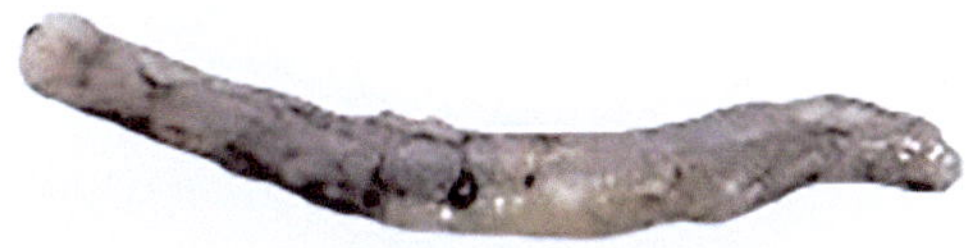

Fig. 4.3 Temporal artery biopsy

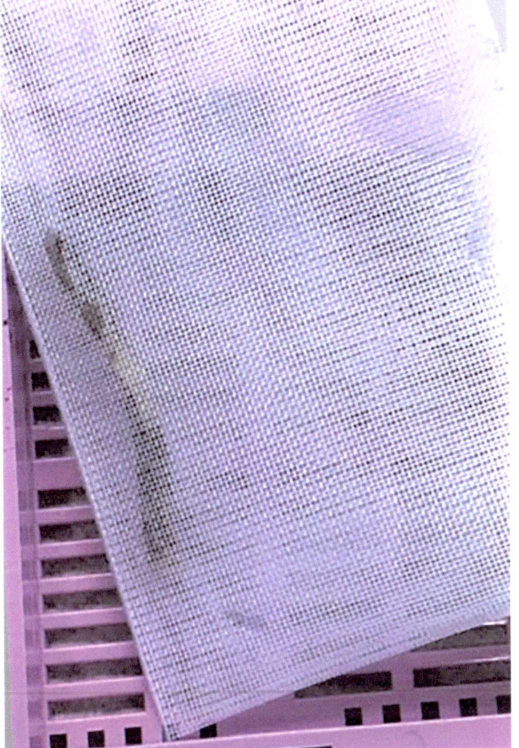

Fig. 4.4 Temporal artery biopsy section submission

4.2   Temporal Artery Biopsy: Level IV CPT 88305

A temporal artery biopsy is the removal of a short segment of temporal artery for potential diagnosis of giant cell arteritis (GCA). GCA is inflammation of the artery that can cause severe headaches and skewed vision.

Step 1: Describe and measure the temporal artery segment. (Fig. 4.3)

Step 2: Temporal artery biopsies can be submitted in two ways. The first option is to submit the specimen whole as seen in Fig. 4.4. When submitted whole, the histotechnologist will serially section the biopsy and embed the sections such that cross sections of the artery are demonstrated on the slide. The second option is to serially section the specimen in the gross room.

Allowing the histotechnology to section and embed at the same time will produce slides with the artery lumen embedded correctly. The orientation of the specimen can occasionally be lost while processing if sectioned in the gross room.

Example Dictation

Specimen A is received in formalin labeled with patient's name, medical record number, "temporal artery" and consists of a segment of tan artery (2.8 × 0.3 × 0.3 cm). The specimen is submitted in toto in A1.

4.3   Plaque: Level III CPT 88304

Plaque refers to the accumulation of cholesterol within the walls of blood vessels. It is a key feature in the development of atherosclerosis, a progressive condition characterized by narrowing of the arterial lumen as the plaque enlarges. During gross examination, plaques are identified as tan-yellow, raised or irregular areas along the inner surface of arteries. The central core of a plaque may calcify, necessitating the need for decalcification.

Step 1: Describe and measure the specimen. The specimen can be one or many fragments as seen in Fig. 4.5.

Step 2: Submit representative sections in one cassette.

Example Dictation

Specimen A is received in formalin labeled with patient's name, medical record number, "plaque" and consists of an aggregate of yellow-tan, focally hemorrhagic plaque material (2.8 × 1.4 × 1.2 cm). Representative sections are submitted in A1.

Document the presence of calcification, and the specimen is decalcified.

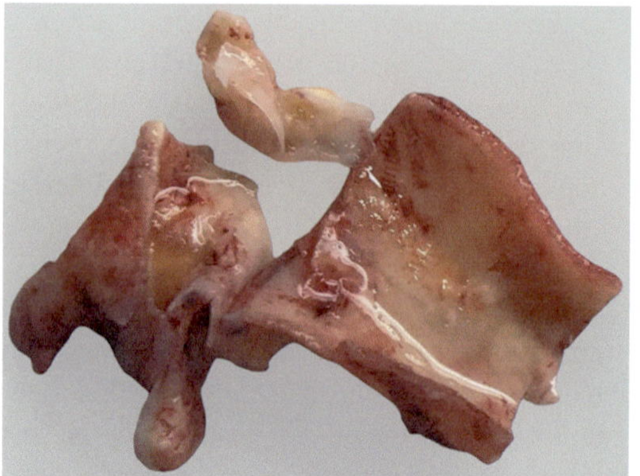

Fig. 4.5 Plaque

Fig. 4.6 Heart valve leaflet

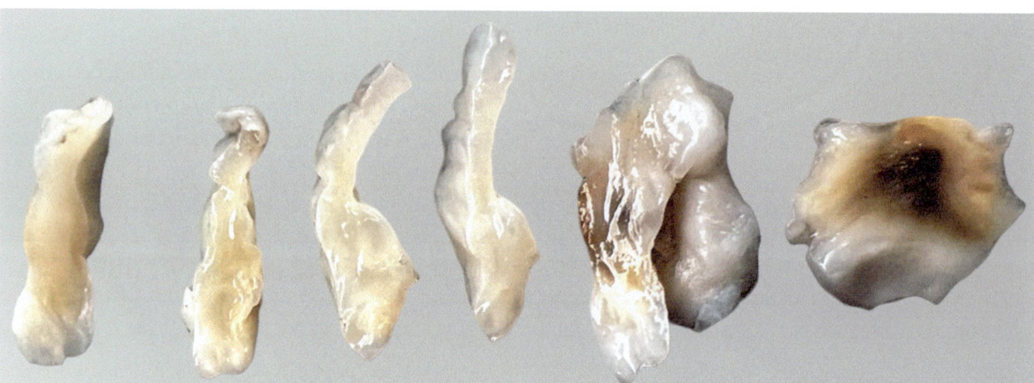

Fig. 4.7 Heart leaflet serially sectioned

4.4   Heart Valve: Level IV CPT 88305

Heart valve leaflets can be surgically removed for stenosis or regurgitation and replaced with a prosthetic valve. This procedure aims to restore proper valve function and alleviate associated symptoms, improving the patient's quality of life.

Step 1: Describe and measure the specimen noting any evidence of thickening or calcification of the leaflet. (Fig. 4.6)
Step 2: Serially section the specimen such as in Fig. 4.7.
Step 3: Submit representative sections. (Fig. 4.8)

Specimen A is received in formalin labeled with patient's name, medical record number, "aortic valve leaflet" and consists of a single fragment of thick tan-yellow tissue (1.9 × 1.1 × 0.5 cm)

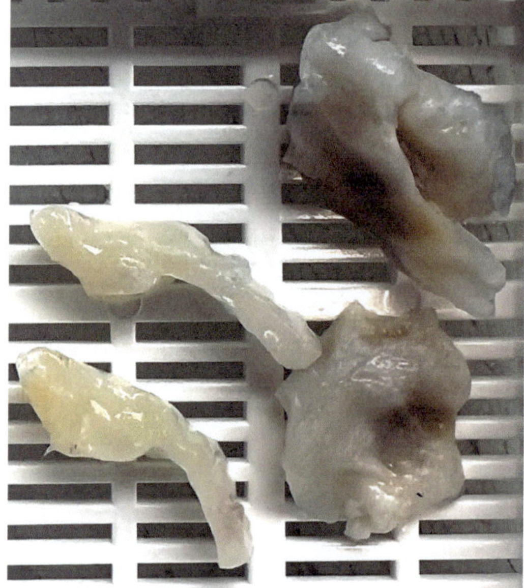

Fig. 4.8 Heart leaflet section submission

with scant calcification. Representative sections are submitted in A1.

Document the presence of calcification, and that the specimen is decalcified.

4.5 Aortic Dissection: Level III CPT 88304

Aortic dissection is a condition characterized by a tear in the layers of the aortic wall. It typically occurs due to damage to the innermost layer, known as the intima, leading to the formation of a false channel within the aortic wall. During gross examination, the tear is identified as a longitudinal or transverse disruption in the aorta. Histopathological examination confirms the diagnosis and assesses the degree of intimal disruption, degeneration, and inflammation. Accurate grossing and pathological examination play a crucial role in guiding clinical management and interventions.

Step 1: Describe and measure the specimen. In Fig. 4.9, the aortic tissue was removed in fragments.

Step 2: Describe any identifiable separation of the aortic layers or evidence of blood. In Fig. 4.10, the layers of the aorta have grossly separated.

Step 3: Submit representative sections of the areas where the aortic layers have separated (Fig. 4.11).

Example Dictation

Specimen A is received in formalin labeled with patient's name, medical record number, "aorta" and consists of 2 fragments of ragged tan-yellow aortic tissue (4.6 × 3.0 × 1.9 cm) with separation of the aortic layers. Representative sections are submitted in A1.

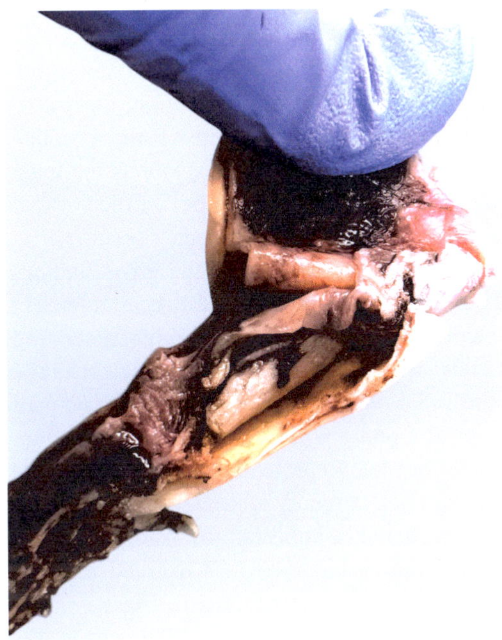

Fig. 4.10 Aortic dissection separation of aortic layers

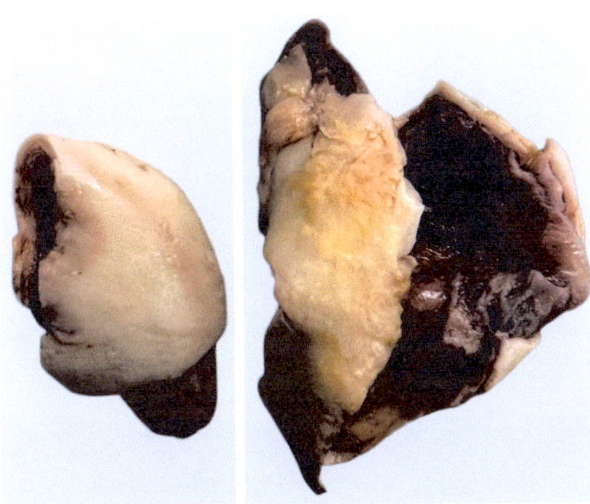

Fig. 4.9 Aortic dissection

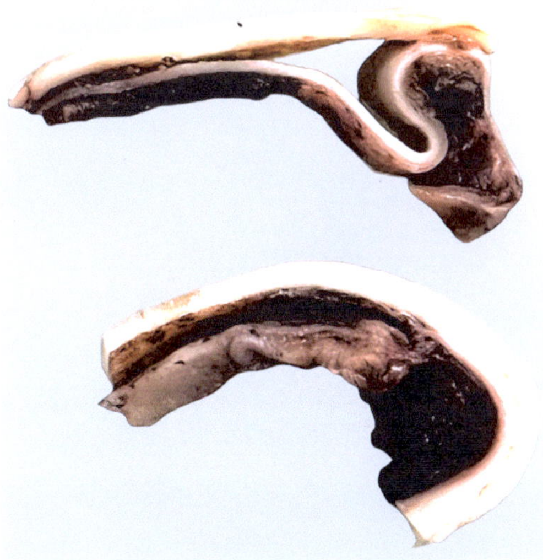

Fig. 4.11 Aortic dissection section submission

4.6 Heart Explant: Level VI CPT 88309

Heart failure, cardiomyopathy, and arrhythmia are broad categories of cardiac conditions that can ultimately necessitate a heart transplant as a life-saving treatment option. Grossing a heart transplant requires a comprehensive understanding of the anatomic structures of the heart. During gross examination, the explanted heart is carefully inspected for macroscopic abnormalities, such as hypertrophy, dilatation, fibrosis, or inflammation. The condition of the coronary arteries and their branches, as well as the integrity and functionality of the cardiac valves should be thoroughly evaluated.

Precise documentation of the gross findings, including measurements of the heart's weight, chamber dimensions, valve circumferences, wall thicknesses, and any other pathologic changes observed, is vital for generating an accurate pathological report and facilitating further investigations if needed. Representative samples from the myocardium, coronary arteries, and any areas of interest should be collected for histopathological examination, which provides detailed information about the underlying structural and cellular changes.

Step 1: Describe and measure the heart (Fig. 4.12a shows the anterior aspect of the heart and Fig. 4.12b shows the posterior aspect).

Step 2: Weigh the heart.

Step 3: Orient the heart. The heart is best oriented using the atria, aorta, and pulmonary truck. The right and left atria sit most posterior with the aorta in the middle and the pulmonary truck at the most anterior aspect. In heart explant specimens, portions of the atria may be surgically absent. See Fig. 4.13 for orientation.

The main arteries of the heart all stem from the aorta and span in different directions. Assess Fig. 4.14 for vessel illustration.

Step 4: Identify and take sections of the left anterior descending artery (LAD). The LAD is present on the anterior-left aspect of the heart as seen by the probe in Fig. 4.15a. This vessel can be resected from the heart or serially section in situ as seen in Fig. 4.15b. Note any stenosis of the LAD and submit representative sections demonstrating the maximum area of stenosis.

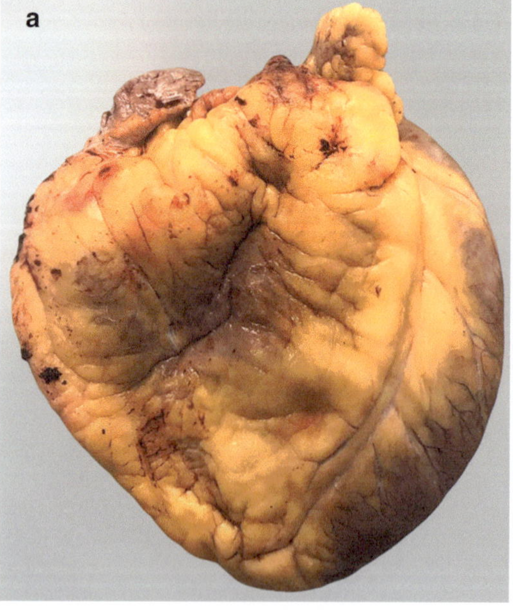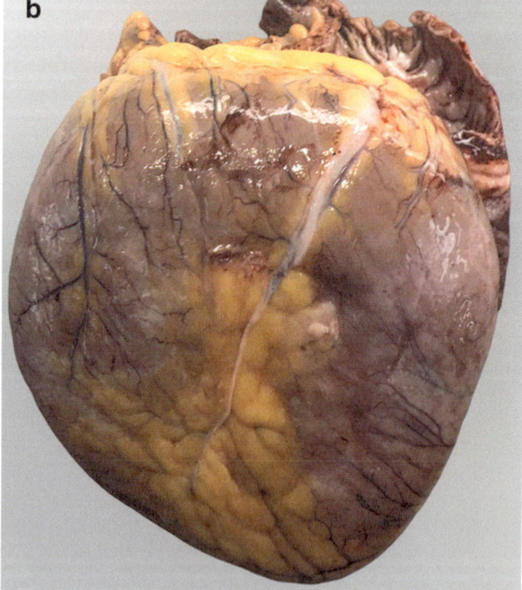

Fig. 4.12 (**a**) Heart anterior view; (**b**) heart posterior view

Fig. 4.13 Heart orientation

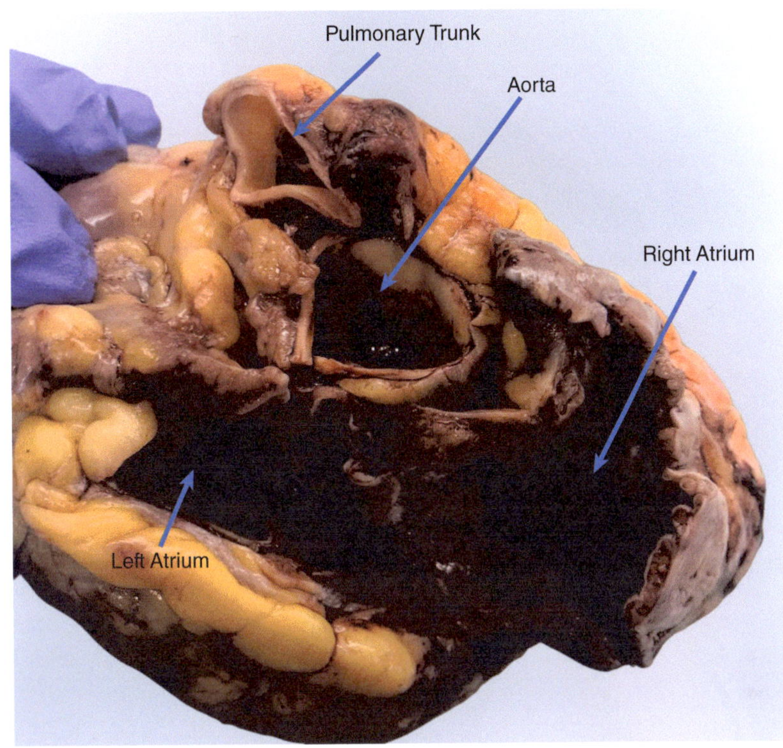

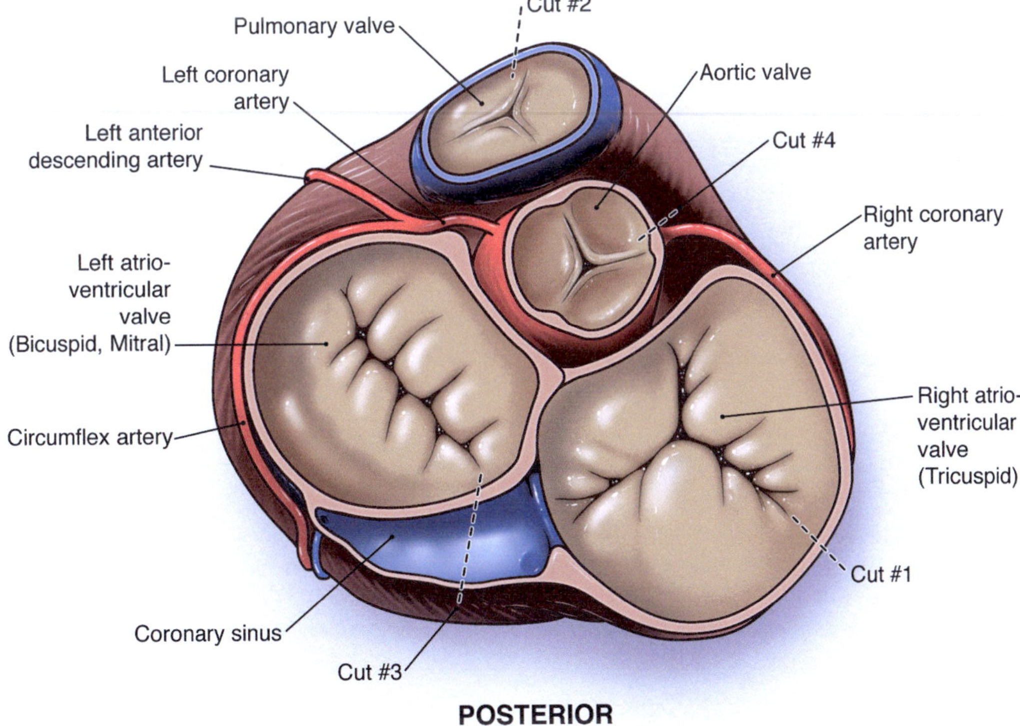

Fig. 4.14 Heart vessels, superior view

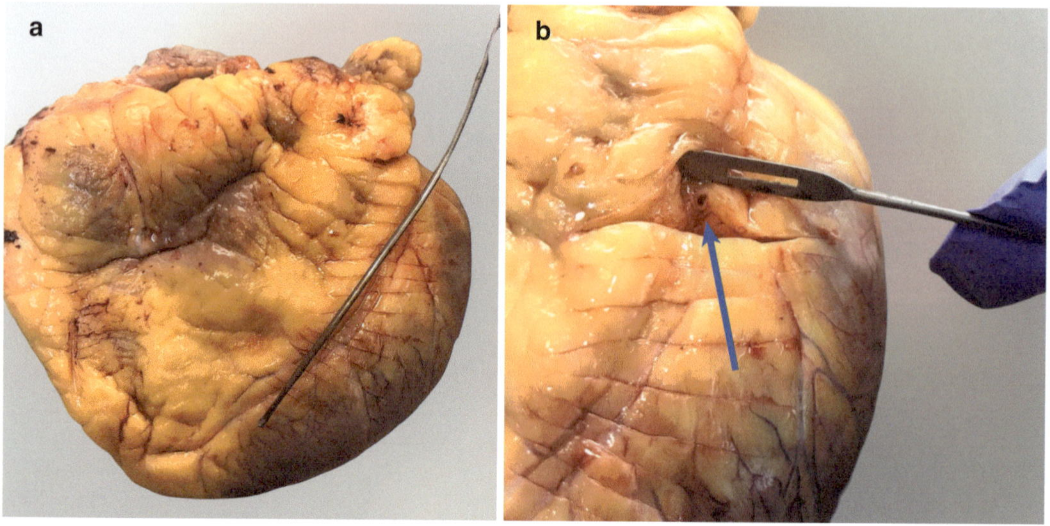

Fig. 4.15 (**a**) Heart LAD; (**b**) heart LAD serially sectioned

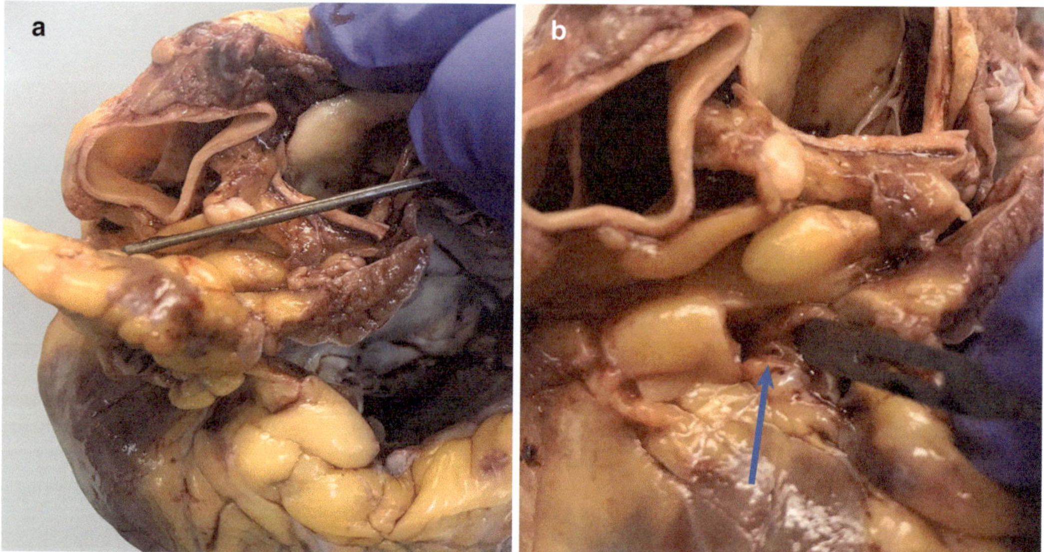

Fig. 4.16 (**a**) Heart left coronary; (**b**) heart left coronary serially sectioned

Step 5: Identify and take sections of the left coronary artery. The left coronary artery extends from the left ostium (as seen by the probe in Fig. 4.16a) of the aorta and bifurcates into the LAD (tracking anteriorly) and the left circumflex (tracking posteriorly) arteries. Section the left coronary artery and assess for stenosis (Fig. 4.16b blue arrow).

Step 6: Identify and take sections of the left circumflex artery. The left circumflex artery wraps around the posterior aspect of the heart (as seen by the probe in Fig. 4.17a) from the left side. Section the circumflex artery and assess for stenosis (Fig. 4.17b blue arrow).

Step 7: Identify and take sections of the right coronary artery. The right coronary artery extends from the right ostium of the aorta as seen by the arrow in Fig. 4.18a. Section the right coronary artery and assess for stenosis as seen in Fig. 4.18b.

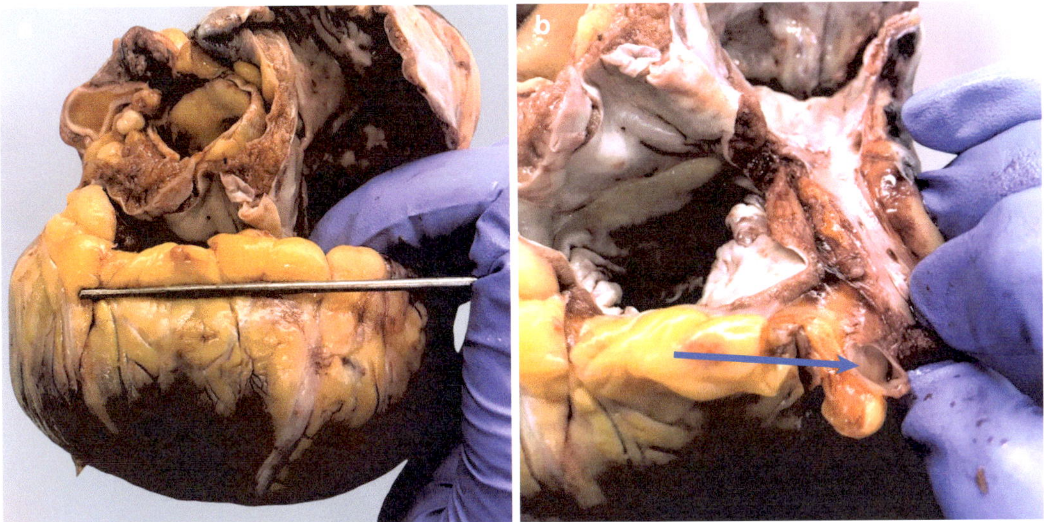

Fig. 4.17 (**a**) Heart, left circumflex; (**b**) heart, left circumflex serially sectioned

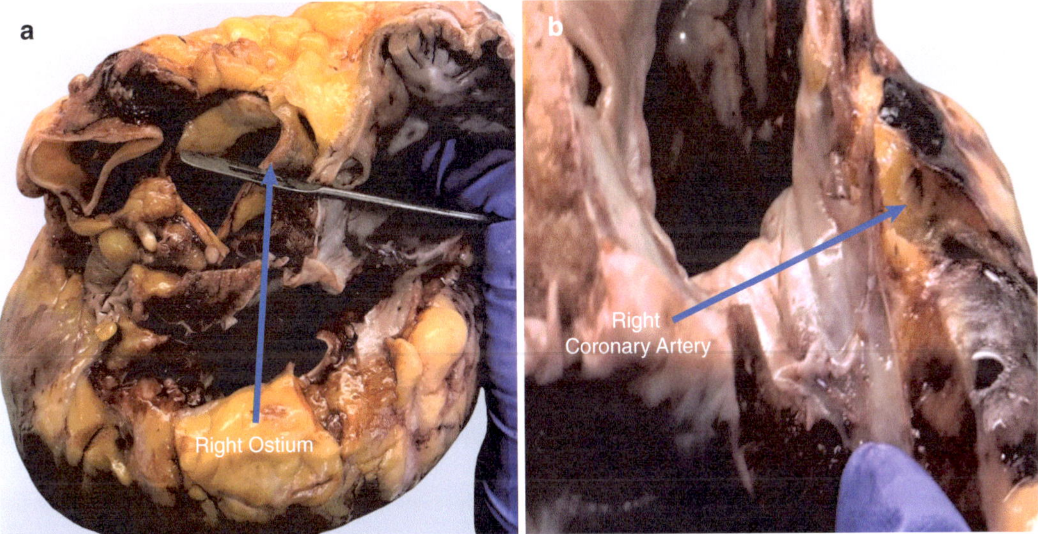

Fig. 4.18 (**a**) Heart right ostia; (**b**) heart right coronary artery

Step 8: Serially section the ventricles (inferior aspect) of the heart from the apex to the papillary muscles as seen in Fig. 4.19. Lay out each slice and assess for lesions and infarcts. Measure the diameters of the right and left ventricles.

Step 9: Measure the thickness of all the heart wall aspects and the ventricular septum (Fig. 4.20).

Step 10: Measure the diameter of the right and left ventricle.

Step 11: Submit one representative section of each of the cardiac walls.

Step 12: Open the aorta by lines of flow. This means following the flow of blood that would pass through the heart and opening the heart valves in the direction that blood flows through the heart. Pay very close attention while cutting. Once entirely open, it can become overwhelming to keep correct orientation. Refer back to Fig. 4.14 for an illustration of the cuts made to open the heart.

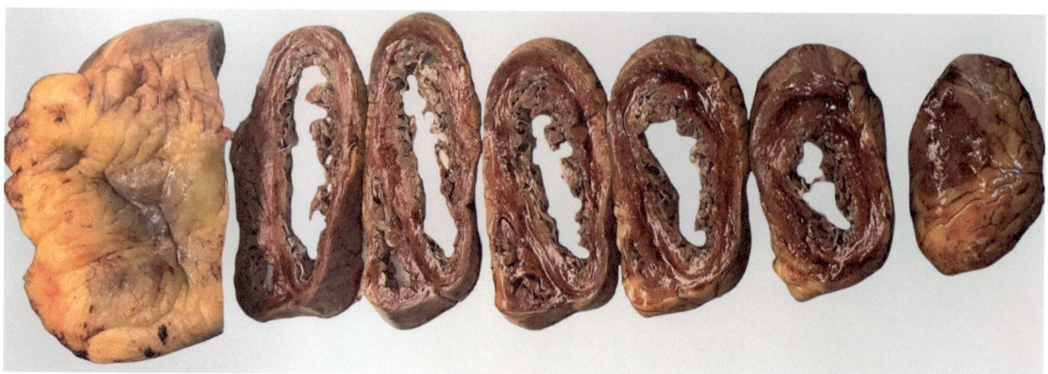

Fig. 4.19 Heart ventricles serially sectioned

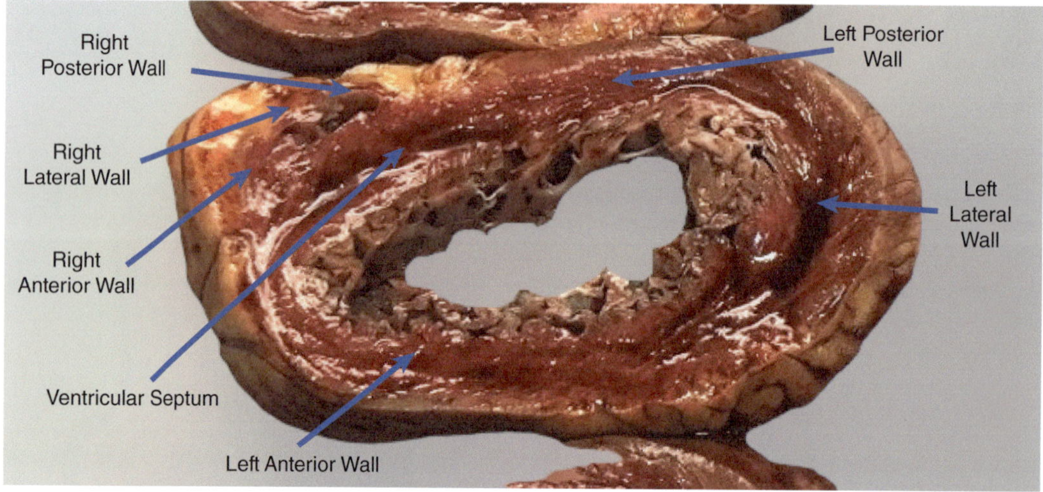

Fig. 4.20 Heart measurements

Step 13: Lines of flow step 1- on the posterior aspect of the heart cut from the remaining right ventricle up through the right atrium, exposing the tricuspid valve (Fig. 4.21). Measure the circumference of the tricuspid valve and note any calcifications or areas of valve thickening.

Step 14: Lines of flow step 2- from the anterior surface of the heart cut from the right ventricle up and out the pulmonary truck, exposing the pulmonary valve (Fig. 4.22). Measure the circumference and note any calcifications or thickening.

Step 15: Lines of flow step 3- from the posterior aspect of the heart open from the remainder of the left ventricle up through the left atrium, exposing the mitral valve (Fig. 4.23). Measure the circumference of the mitral valve and note any calcifications or valve thickening.

Step 16: Lines of flow step 4- from the anterior aspect of the heart open from the remaining left atrium up and out the aorta, exposing the aortic valve (Fig. 4.24). Measure the circumference of the aortic valve and note any calcifications or valve thickening.

Step 17: Sections of the valves are not typically submitted unless pathology is identified grossly. Consult attending pathologist.

Example Dictation

Specimen A is received in formalin labeled with patient's name, medical record number, "heart explant" and consists of an intact heart (14.9 × 13.6 × 7.5 cm, 489 g). The left coronary artery, left anterior descending artery, circumflex artery, and right coronary artery are serially sectioned to reveal no gross stenosis. The ventricles

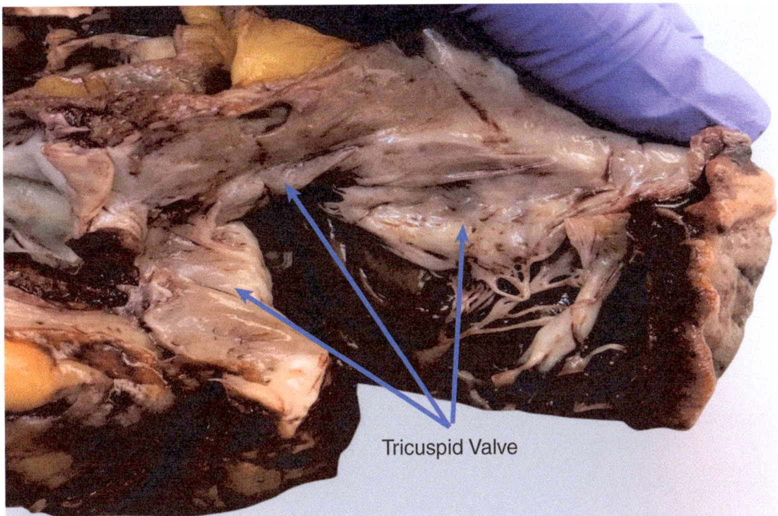

Fig. 4.21 Heart, tricuspid valve

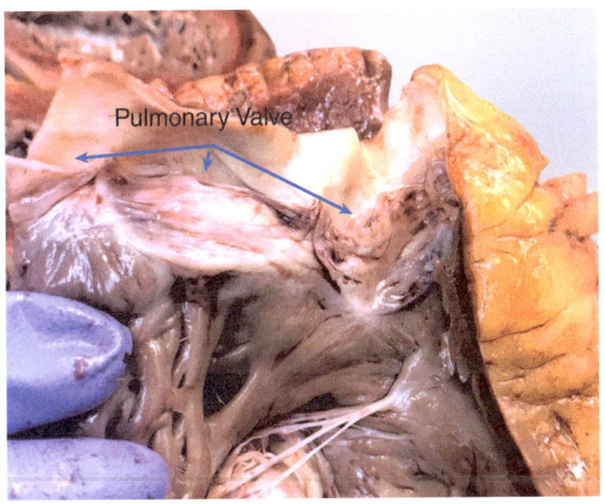

Fig. 4.22 Heart, pulmonary valve

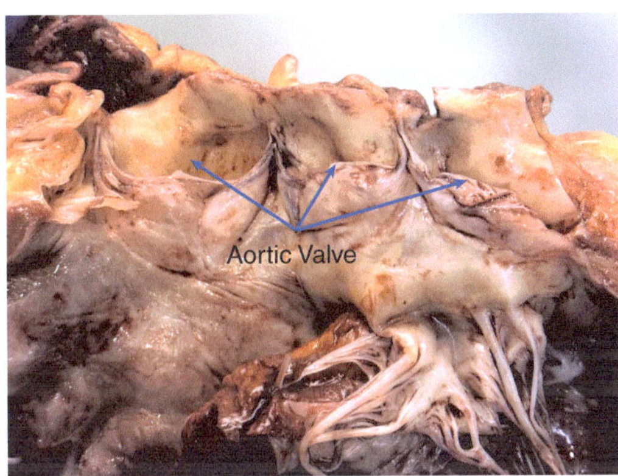

Fig. 4.24 Heart aortic valve

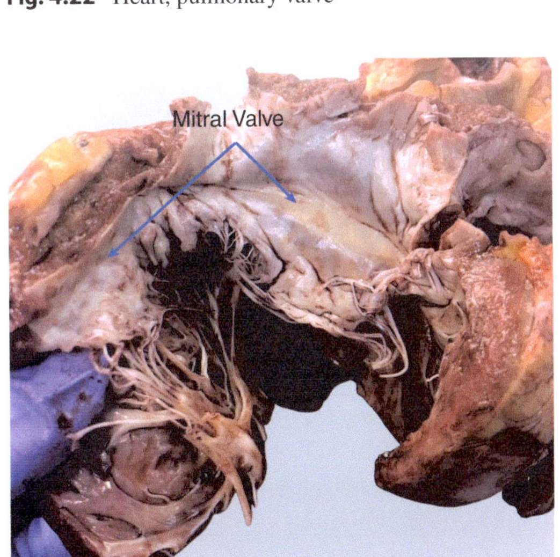

Fig. 4.23 Heart, mitral valve

are serially sectioned from the apex, superiorly to reveal a dilated left ventricle approximately 8.8 cm in diameter and a scantly dilated right ventricle of 2.7 cm with no evidence of scarring on cut surface. The ventricle walls are tan-brown with no evidence of infarct with a ventricular septum of 1.1 cm thick. The right anterior, lateral, and poster ventricular walls are 1.3 cm, 0.9 cm, 0.5 cm, respectively. The left anterior, lateral, and posterior ventricular walls are 1.0 cm, 1.9 cm, and 0.9 cm, respectively. The remainder of the heart is opened by lines of flow to reveal a tricuspid valve circumference of 8.7 cm, a pulmonary valve circumference of 8.4 cm, a mitral valve circumference of 7.5 cm, and aortic valve of 7.4 cm, with no distinct calcifications of these valves.

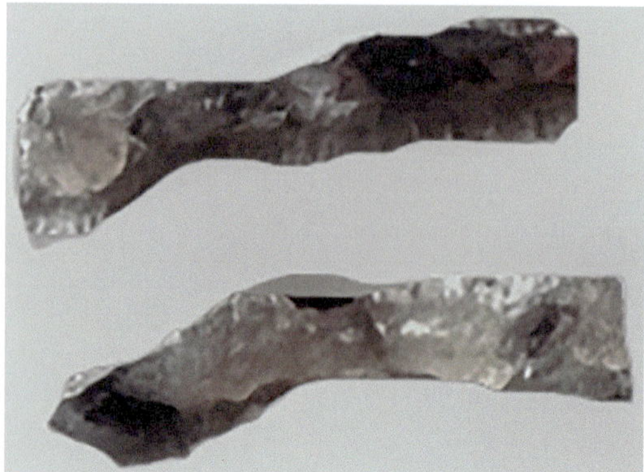

Fig. 4.25 Lung biopsy

Section code
A 1: Left anterior descending artery, representative
A 2: Left coronary artery, representative
A 3: Left circumflex artery, representative
A 4: Right coronary artery, representative
A 5: Anterior aspect of left ventricle
A 6: Lateral aspect of left ventricle
A 7: Posterior aspect of left ventricle
A 8: Lateral aspect of right ventricle
A 9: Ventricular septum, representative

4.7 Lung Biopsy: Level IV CPT 88305

When an abnormal area is detected in the lung during imaging, a biopsy is often necessary for diagnostic purposes. The procedure involves using a needle to target the specific abnormal area of the lung with the guidance of imaging techniques.

Step 1: Describe and measure the specimen. The specimen can be one or many fragments or cores as shown in Fig. 4.25.
Step 2: Submit the specimen entirely in one or more cassettes as seen in Fig. 4.26.

Example Dictation
Specimen A is received in formalin labeled with patient's name, medical record number, "left lower lung biopsy" and consists of 2 tan, hemorrhagic cores (0.8 and 0.9 cm in length and 0.1 cm in diameter). The specimen is submitted entirely in A1.

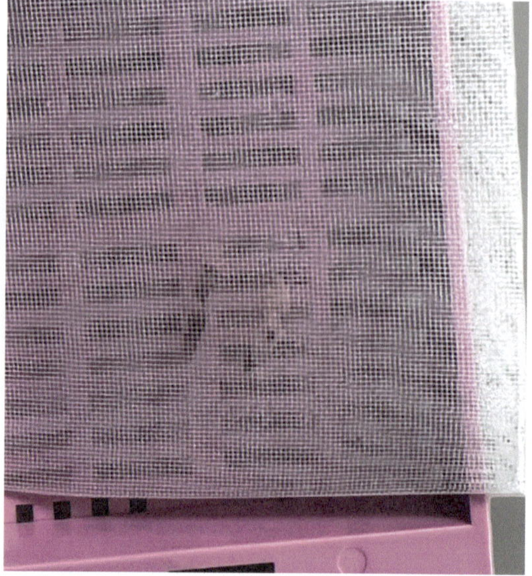

Fig. 4.26 Lung biopsy section submission

4.8 Lung Lymph Nodes: Level V CPT 88307

Lymph nodes of the lung hilar or mediastinum can be removed during surgery to assess for metastases. The specimens obtained can either be 1 intact lymph node, 1 fragmented lymph node or a packet of multiple lymph nodes. Ten lymph nodes are required.

Step 1: Describe and count the number of fragments. In Fig. 4.27, the specimen is labeled as "10R lymph node" which means this is 1 lymph node which has fragmented into multiple pieces when resected and should only be counted as 1 lymph node, not multiple lymph nodes.
Step 2: Measure the lymph node or aggregate of lymph nodes.
Step 3: Submit entirely. (Fig. 4.28).

Specimen A is received in formalin labeled with patient's name, medical record number, "10R lymph node" and consists of 2 fragments of yellow-brown tissue (1.8 × 0.9 × 0.4 cm) which is submitted entirely in A1.

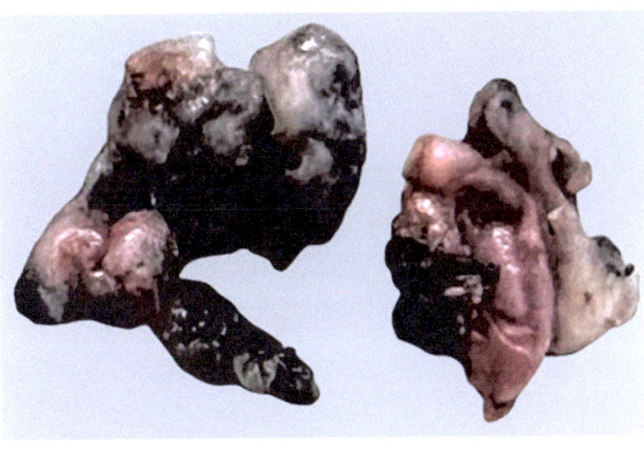

Fig. 4.27 Lung lymph node

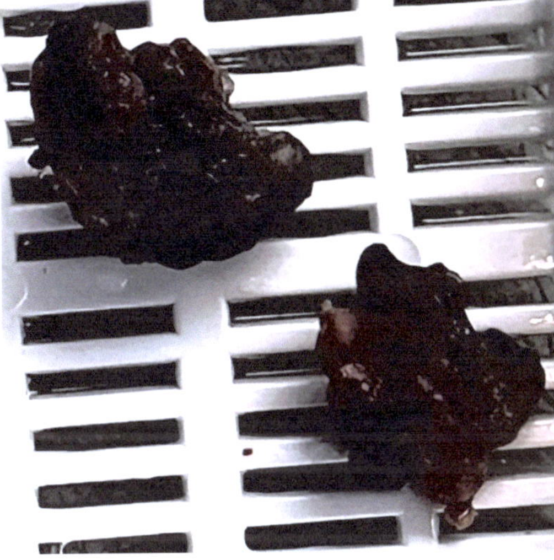

Fig. 4.28 Lung lymph nodes section submission

4.9   Lung Wedge: Level V CPT 88307

A lung wedge resection is a surgical procedure commonly performed to remove a localized abnormality or lesion from the lung (see Table 4.2 for tumor gross appearance). This portion can be of any size depending on the area of abnormality. However, a wedge resection is done for abnormalities or lesions identified in the peripheral lung.

Synoptic Breakdown Relative to Grossing for Both Lung Wedge and Lobectomy Specimens Procedures:

Wedge resection: Removing a wedge-shaped area of lung that includes the abnormal area.

Table 4.2 Tumor gross appearance of lung lesions

Tuberculosis	Firm, tan, diffusely scattered, irregularly sized nodules
Mesothelioma	Diffuse, dense, thick mass encasing the lung, extending into the interlobar fissures
Hamartoma	Pale, firm, round to multilobulated, well-circumscribed nodule
Granuloma	Tan-white, firm nodule
Adenocarcinoma	Firm, gray-white, ill-defined mass with hemorrhage, and necrosis
Squamous cell carcinoma	Tan-yellow cavitary mass with hemorrhage and central necrosis
Small cell carcinoma	Tan-white, soft, friable mass with necrotic areas
Carcinoid tumor	Tan-yellow, well circumscribed, firm, round mass

Segmentectomy: Similar to a wedge but is typically a larger portion of the lung lobe.

Completion lobectomy: Removes the remaining lung lobe after the wedge resection or segmentectomy.

Sleeve lobectomy: Removes the lung tumor and part of the airway and then reconnects the 2 remaining airways of either side of the resection.

Bilobectomy: Removal of two adjacent lung lobes (right lung only).

Pneumonectomy: Removal of the entire lung [2].

Laterality: Include the laterality in the dictation [2].

Tumor focality: Dictate how many separate nodules are included in the specimen [2].

Tumor site: This includes the upper, middle, and lower lobes, the main bronchus, bronchus intermedius, and lobar bronchus [2].

Tumor size: Measure the lesion in three dimensions [2].

Visceral pleura invasion: Dictate if the lesion abuts or invades through the pleura of the lung.

Direct invasion of adjacent structures: Dictate if the lesion extends outside the lung and invades into any adjacent structures [2].

Margins: Dictate how close the lesion comes to the lung hilum and the parenchymal resection margin (if present). Surgical removal of the entire lung lobe is performed for lesions present close to the lung hilum but are also performed for diffuse disease such as COPD or infection [2].

pT Staging

pT0: No evidence of primary tumor

pTis (SCIS): Squamous cell carcinoma in situ (SCIS)

pT1: Tumor less than or equal to 3 cm in greatest dimension, surrounded by lung or visceral pleura, without bronchoscopic evidence of invasion more proximal than the lobar bronchus (i.e., not in the main bronchus)

pT2: Tumor greater than 3 cm but less than or equal to 5 cm or having any of the following features: Involves the main bronchus regardless of distance to the carina, but without involvement of the carina; OR invades visceral pleura; OR associated with atelectasis or obstructive pneumonitis that extends to the hilar region, involving part or all of the lung T2 tumors with these features are classified as T2a if less than or equal to 4 cm or if the size cannot be determined and T2b if greater than 4 cm but less than or equal to 5 cm

pT3: Tumor greater than 5 cm but less than or equal to 7 cm in greatest dimension; or directly invading any of the following: parietal pleura, chest wall, phrenic nerve, parietal pericardium; or separate tumor nodule(s) in the same lobe as the primary

pT4: Tumor greater than 7 cm in greatest dimension; or tumor of any size invading one or more of the following: diaphragm, mediastinum, heart, great vessels, trachea, recurrent laryngeal nerve, esophagus, vertebral body or carina; or separate tumor nodule(s) in an ipsilateral lobe different from that of the primary [2]

Step 1: Describe and measure the specimen. A lung wedge is typically a portion of unoriented lung with a staple line along one side where the surgeon cuts to remove the specimen from the remaining lung (Fig. 4.29).

Step 2: Describe and measure any defects or puckering on the pleural surface. In Fig. 4.30, a small puckering is present on the pleural surface (blue arrow).

Step 3: Measure the distance of the puckered area to the staple line.

Step 4: Remove the staple line. Cut as close to the staples as possible as shown in Fig. 4.31.

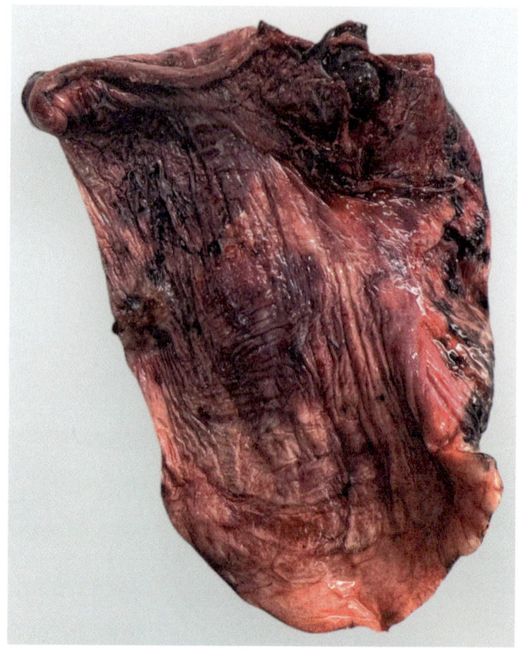

Fig. 4.29 Lung wedge

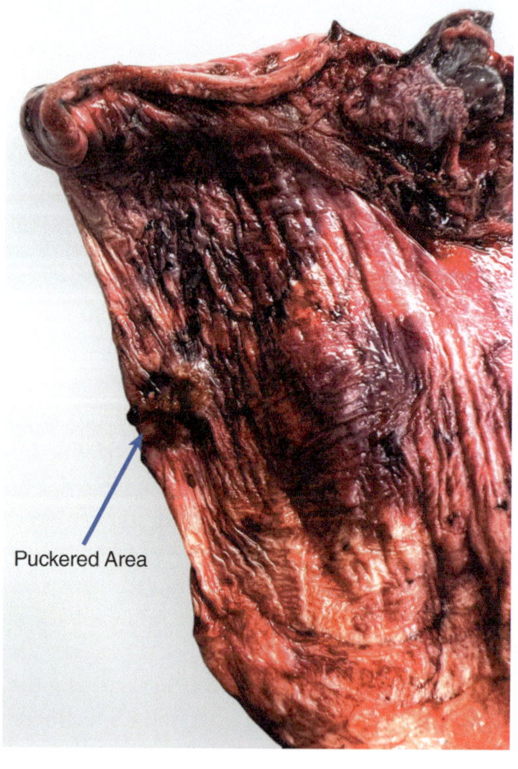

Fig. 4.30 Lung wedge pleural puckering

The underlying parenchyma is now the resection margin.

Step 5: Ink the resection margin and the puckered area on the pleural surface. In Fig. 4.32, the resection margin is inked blue and the puckered area is inked green.

Step 6: For this specimen, the resection margin is far from the lesion so the resection margin can be shaved and submitted en face as shown in Fig. 4.33 blue arrow. Remember, if the lesion is close to the resection margin (approximately 2 cm or less), taking perpendicular sections of the lesion in relation to the resection margin is best.

Step 7: Serially section the specimen perpendicular to the resection margin and lay out each slice flat for best visualization as seen in Fig. 4.34.

Step 8: Identify, describe, and measure the lesion. In Fig. 4.35, the lesion correlates with the puckered area of the pleural surface (blue arrow).

Step 9: Submit sections of the lesion in relation to the resection margin and pleural surface (Fig. 4.36). In this example, the lesion is small and present in one slice only. Only one section of the lesion in relation to the pleural surface can be submitted. If the lesion is larger, submit one section per every one centimeter of the overall mass size in relation to the resection margin and the pleural surface, if applicable. For solid tumors, one section per every one centimeter of the overall mass size in relation to the resection margin and the pleural surface

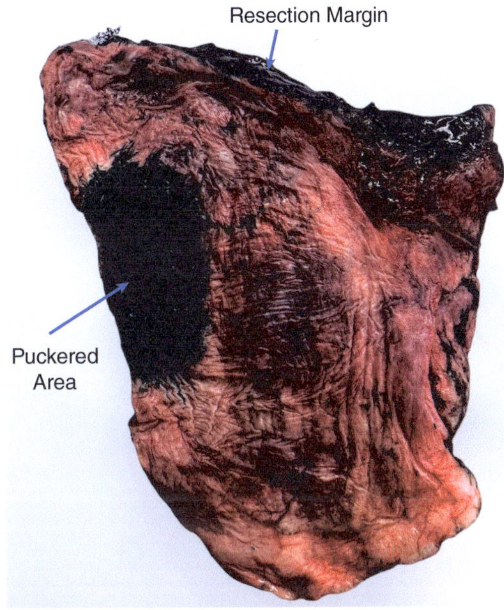

Fig. 4.32 Lung wedge ink

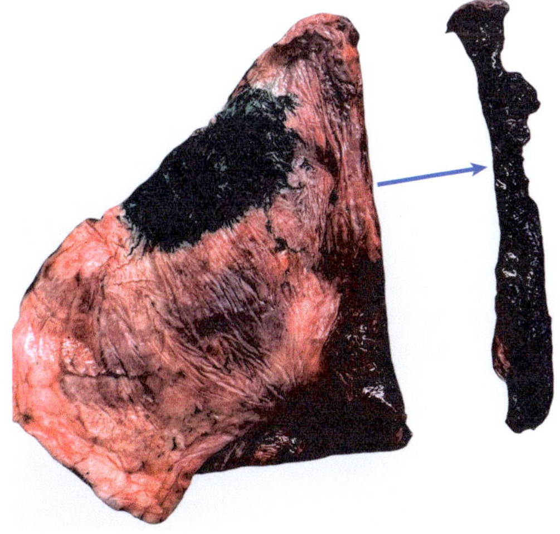

Fig. 4.33 Lung wedge shave parenchymal margin

Fig. 4.31 Lung wedge parenchymal staple line

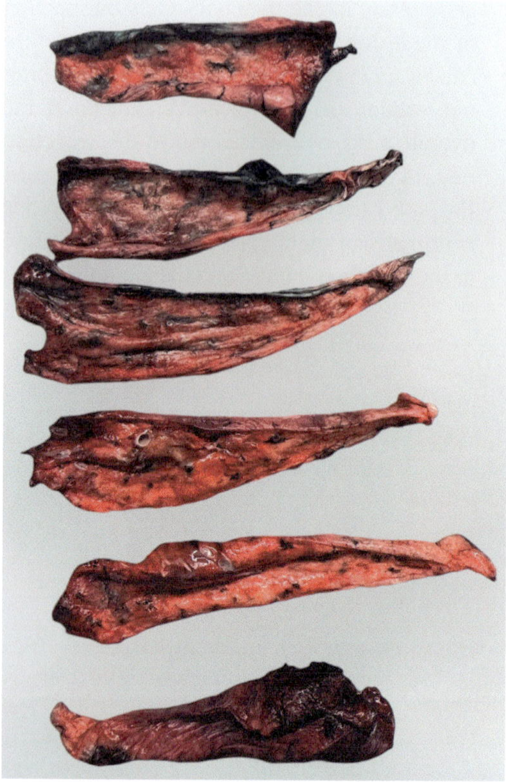

Fig. 4.34 Lung wedge serially sectioned

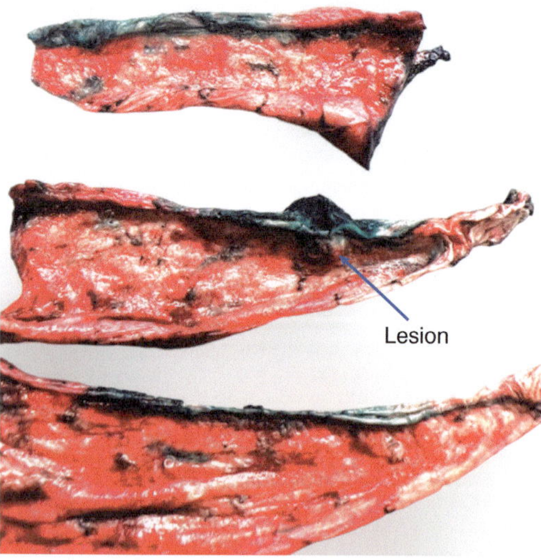

Fig. 4.35 Lung wedge lesion

should be submitted, if applicable. If the lesion is status-post treatment, the lesion should be submitted entirely. Communicate with the pathologist.

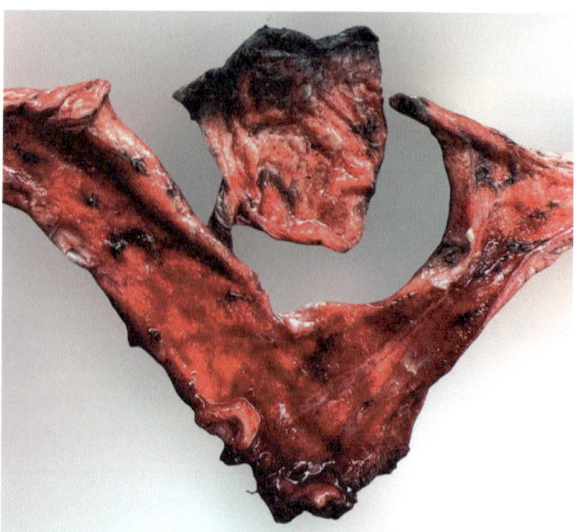

Fig. 4.36 Lung wedge lesion section

Step 10: Submit the resection margin either en face or perpendicular in relation to the lesion, the lesion in relation to the pleural surface, and a section of unremarkable lung. (Fig. 4.37)

Example Dictation

Specimen A is received in formalin labeled with patient's name, medical record number, "right lower lobe lung wedge" and consists of an intact tan-purple lung wedge (9.6 × 7.1 × 2.5 cm) with a single parenchymal staple line margin (9.5 cm in length) along one edge. The pleural surface contains a single area of puckering (1.2 × 1.0 cm) which comes within 5.2 cm of the resection margin. The specimen is serially sectioned to reveal a tan-white, round, firm, well-circumscribed nodule (1.2 × 1.0 × 0.8 cm) which abuts the pleural surface, correlating with the previously mentioned puckered area. The nodule comes within 5.1 cm from the resection margin. The remaining lung parenchyma is red-brown with no additional lesions identified.

Ink code

    Blue: Resection margin

    Green: Puckered area on pleural surface

Section code

    A 1–A 3: Resection margin, trisected, en face

    A 4: Nodule entirely in relation to pleural surface

    A 5-A 6: Unremarkable lung, representative

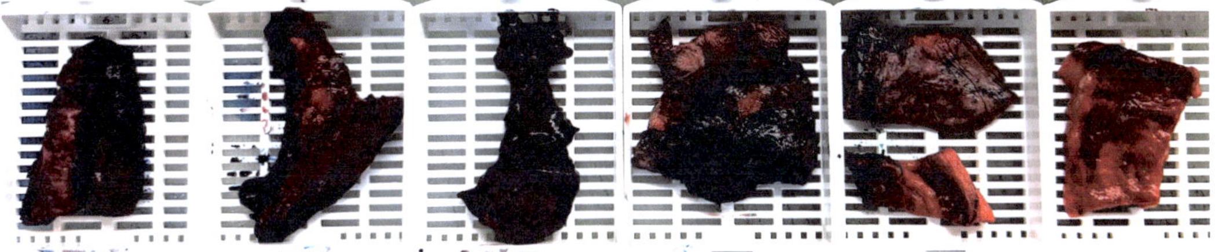

Fig. 4.37 Lung wedge section submission

4.10   Lung Lobectomy: Level VI CPT 88309

A lobectomy is the surgical removal of the entire lobe of the lung which is useful for varied benign and malignant lung diseases. Any chronic infectious process not controlled with antibiotic therapy can benefit from surgical resection. Tuberculosis is the most common reason for lobectomy. Also, developmental anomalies like congenital bronchial atresia, pulmonary sequestration, bronchogenic cyst, and congenital cystic adenomatous malformation can be an indication for a lobectomy. It is the standard surgical approach for stage I-II non–small cell lung carcinoma. Other less common neoplastic indications include mucoepidermoid tumors, adenoid cystic tumors, and sarcomas.

Step 1: Describe and measure the lung lobe.

Step 2: Identify the hilum and shave the margins which include the bronchus, vascular margins, and parenchymal margin. Figure 4.38 shows the parenchymal margin staple line. This is where the surgeon transected one lung lobe from the adjacent lobe.

Step 3: The parenchymal margin can be submitted in two different ways.

> Option 1: If the lesion is far from the parenchymal margin, the margin can be shaved and submitted en face.

> Option 2: If the lesion is close to the parenchymal margin, remove the staple line as close to the staples as possible and ink the underlying margin. Sections of the lesion in relation to the margin will be submitted after the lung is serially sectioned (After Step 9).

Step 4: Assess the pleural surface and describe and measure any areas of puckering. Figure 4.39 shows an area of puckering on the

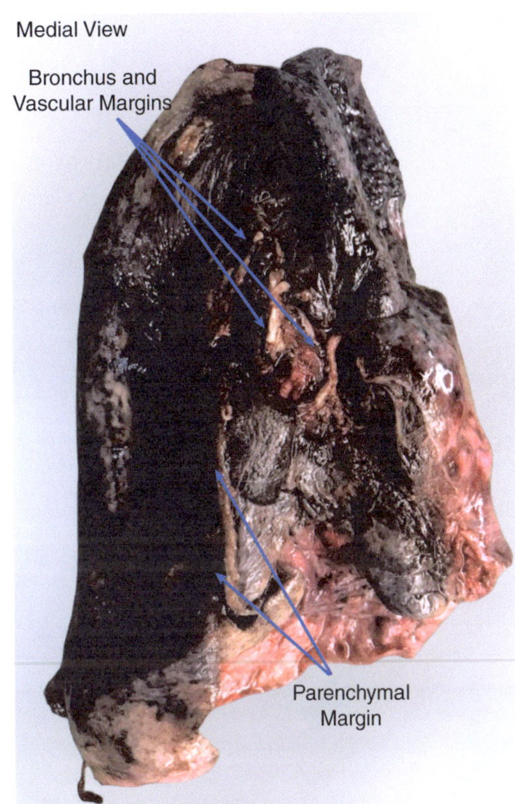

Fig. 4.38 Lobectomy

pleural surface on the lateral side of the lung circled in blue.

Step 5: Remove any hilar lymph nodes and submit. In Fig. 4.40, there is one hilar lymph node designated with a blue arrow. Hilar lymph nodes are ill-defined and can take practice to identify.

Step 6: Ink the hilum and parenchymal margin in two different colors. Figure 4.41 shows the hilum inked in blue and the parenchymal margin inked in orange. Inking two different colors will help the grossing person identify these anatomic structures once the lung is sliced.

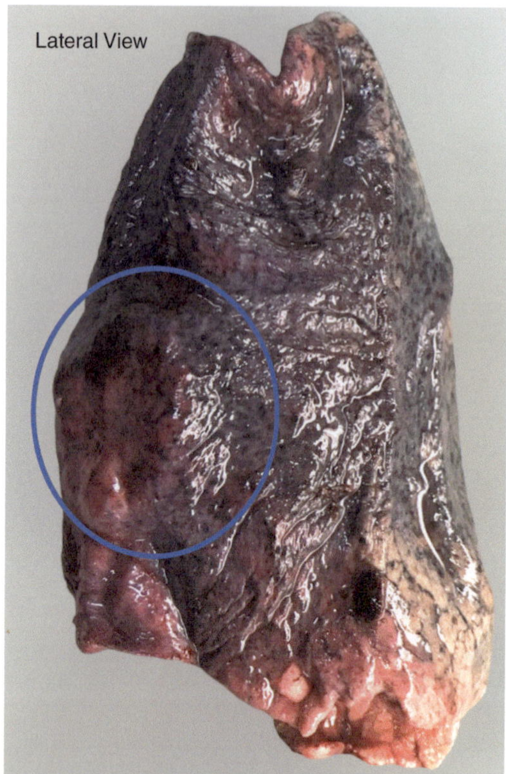

Fig. 4.39 Lobectomy pleural puckering

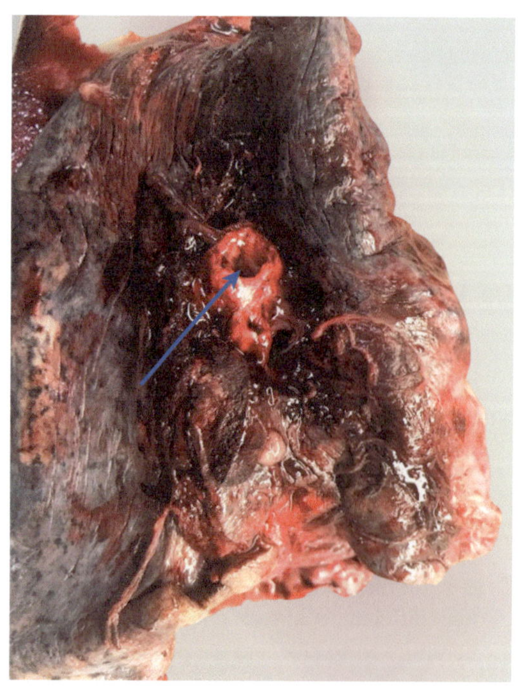

Fig. 4.40 lobectomy hilar lymph nodes

Step 7: Ink a separate color over the puckered area on the pleural surface shown in Fig. 4.42.

Step 8: Inflate the lung with formalin using a syringe and fix for a minimum of 2 hours (Fig. 4.43). Fill the syringe with formalin and

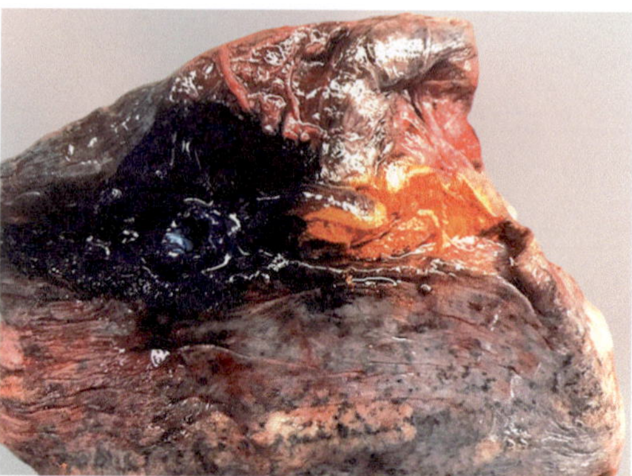

Fig. 4.41 Lobectomy hilar and parenchymal margin ink

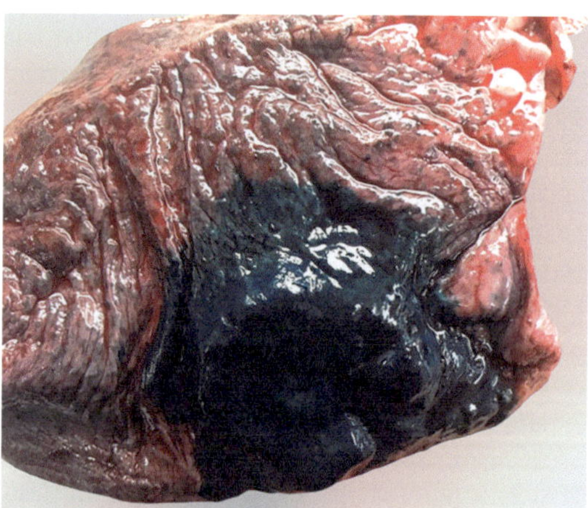

Fig. 4.42 Lobectomy pleural puckering inked

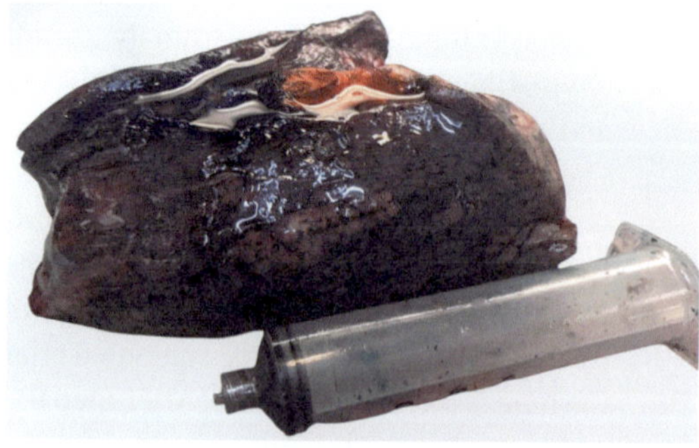

Fig. 4.43 Lobectomy fixation

place the syringe into the bronchioles. Press the plunger, filling the lung with formalin. This can be done multiple times until the lung appears inflated.

This step is optional and dependent on the preference of the pathologists.

Step 9: Serially section the lung and lay each slice flat as shown in Fig. 4.44.

Step 10: Describe and measure the lesion in three dimensions.

Step 11: Measure the lesion to the closest hilar and parenchymal margins and state if the lesion abuts or invades through the pleural surface. For this example, the lesion is close to the hilar margin and abuts the pleural surface. In Fig. 4.45, blue ink, orange ink, and green ink are present and can be measured. In case where patients received neoadjuvant therapy, the tumor or tumor bed size should be documented for the approximate percentage of necrosis. If the size of the tumor/tumor bed is less than 3 cm, it should be submitted entirely. When larger than 3 cm, a fullface section should be submitted so as to identify the greatest dimension of the tumor. A 1 cm section of uninvolved lung parenchyma adjacent to the tumor/tumor bed should also be submitted so as to accurately identify the true edges of the tumors.

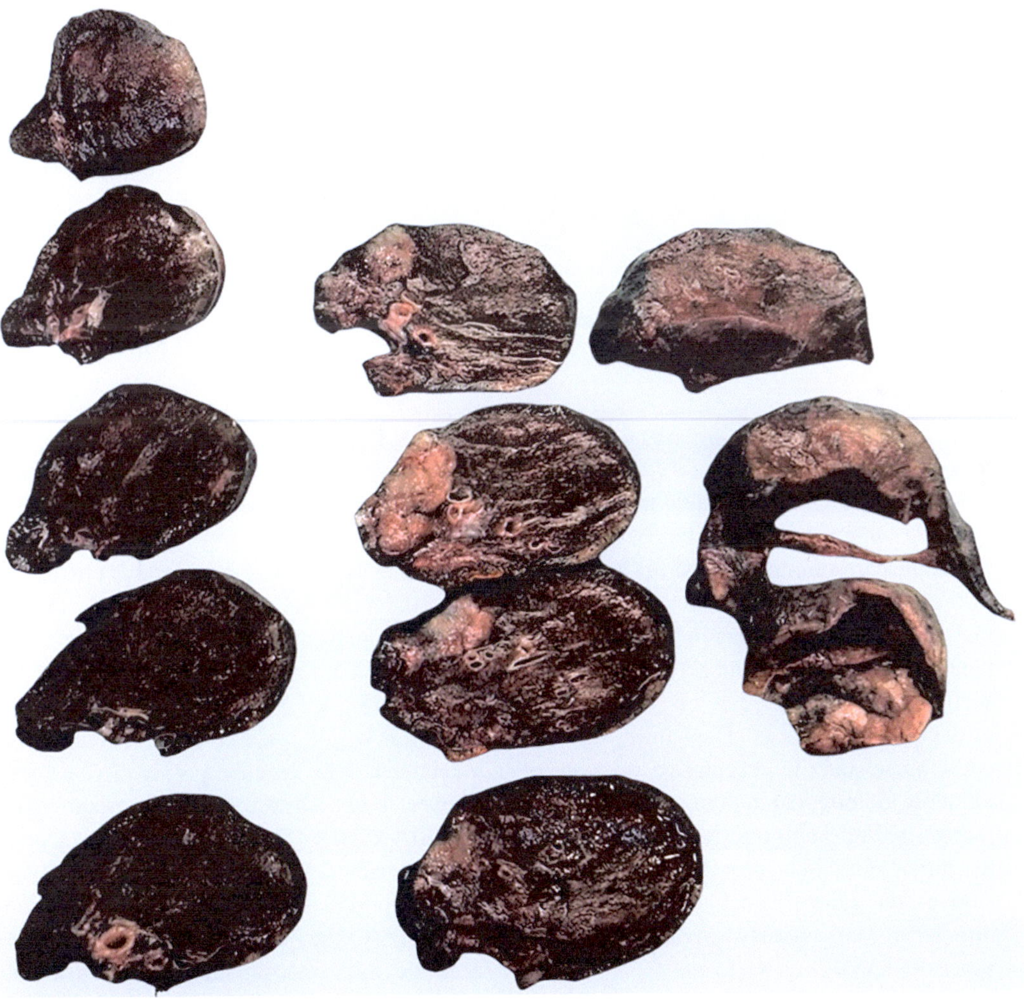

Fig. 4.44 Lobectomy serially sectioned

Fig. 4.45 Lobectomy section with lesion

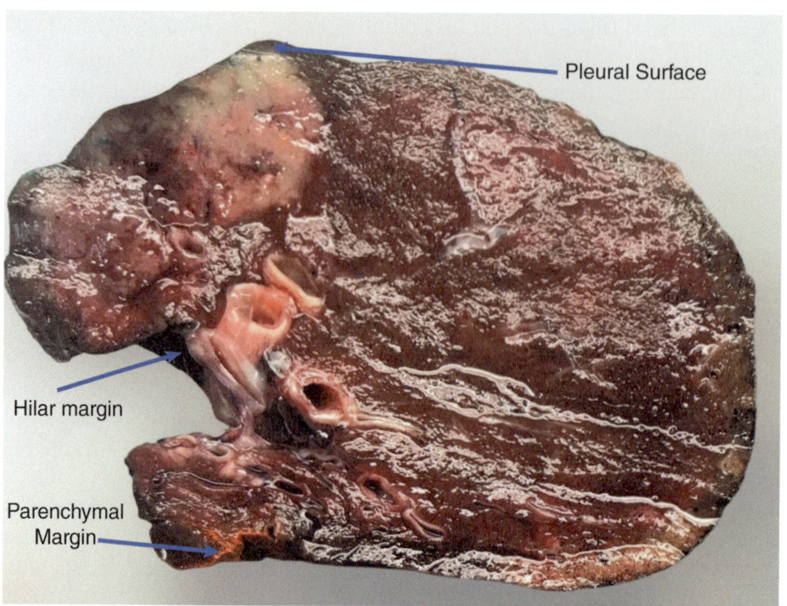

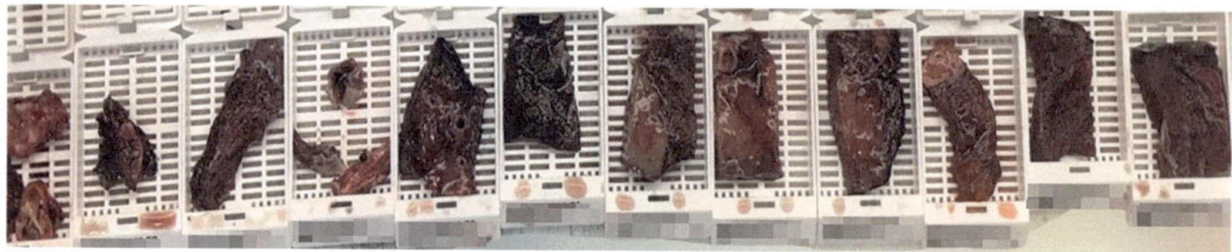

Fig. 4.46 lobectomy section submission

Step 12: Assess and palpate the remaining lung for additional nodules.

Step 13: The hilar bronchus and vascular margins are submitted. The hilar lymph node candidates are submitted. Lesions in relation to the closest margins (hilar and parenchymal) are submitted. Lesion in relation to pleural surface is submitted. Then, a fullface section of the lesion can be submitted to measure overall size. Depending on the pathologist, one representative section of uninvolved lung parenchyma close to the tumor (within 3 cm) and further away from the tumor should be submitted. The submission of the lung parenchyma close to the tumor can help identify spread through air spaces (STAS). (Fig. 4.46)

Example Dictation

Specimen A is received in formalin labeled with patient's name, medical record number, "right lower lobe" and consists of an intact tan-purple lower lung lobe (15.2 × 9.3 × 3.2 cm) with a single parenchymal staple line margin (4.5 cm in length) present extending from the hilum. Opposite the hilum, there is a single area of puckering (3.5 × 3.3 cm). The hilum is palpable for 2 hilar lymph node candidates (0.5–0.8 cm in diameter). The specimen is serially sectioned to reveal a tan-white, firm, well-circumscribed mass (0.4 × 3.6 × 1.9 cm) with focal black areas. The mass abuts the pleural surface, correlating with the previously mentioned puckered area. Additionally, the mass comes within 0.9 cm from the hilar margin and 1.9 cm from the parenchymal margin, present in the mid aspect of the lung lobe. The remaining lung parenchyma is red-brown with no additional lesions identified.

Ink code
>   Blue: hilum
>   Orange: parenchymal margin
>   Green: pleural surface over area of puckering

Section code
>   A 1: Bronchial and vascular margins, en face
>   A 2:2 Hilar lymph node candidates, whole
>   A 3: Parenchymal margin, en face
>   A 4-A 5: Mass in relation to closest hilar margin, perpendicular
>   A 6–A 8:1 Full-thickness section of mass, trisected
>   A 9: Mass in relation to closest parenchymal margin
>   A 10: Unremarkable lung, representative

4.11 Thymectomy: Level V CPT 88307

A thymectomy is most commonly performed for myasthenia gravis or the presence of a thymoma however, other malignant lesions or cysts can also occur in the thymus (See Table 4.3 for tumor gross appearance of thymus). The thymus deteriorates with age and it becomes difficult to identify the thymic tissue from the surrounding adipose tissue. Specimens are often fragmented or unoriented due to the ill-defined nature of the surgery.

Table 4.3 Tumor gross appearance of thymus

Myasthenia gravis	Enlarged thymic gland
Thymoma	Tan-gray, lobulated, encapsulated lesion
Lymphoma	Tan-gray solid mass with cystic areas
Thymic carcinoma	Poorly defined, infiltrative mass with areas of hemorrhage, necrosis, and cystic degeneration

Synoptic Breakdown Relative to Grossing Thymus

Procedure: A thymectomy is the removal of the entire thymus, and a partial thymectomy is the removal of only part of the thymus. The specimen order form or the surgeon's notes may help identify the type of procedure performed [3].

Tumor size: Measure the lesion in three dimensions [3].

Sites involved by direct tumor invasion: Describe invasion of the lesion. The lesion can invade through the thymus and surrounding soft tissue and into any adjacent structures such as pleural, superior vena cava, chest wall, aorta, myocardium, esophagus, etc. [3]

Margin status: Measure the lesion to the closest margin if unoriented. If the thymus is oriented measure the lesion to all the designated margins. In most thymectomy specimens, the posterior surface is the true margin. The margins of any attach structures such as the lung, pericardium, and pleura should also be noted and sectioned [3]

pT Staging

pT1: Tumor encapsulated or extending into the mediastinal fat; may involve the mediastinal pleura

pT1a: Tumor with no mediastinal pleura involvement

pT1b: Tumor with direct invasion of mediastinal pleura

pT2: Tumor with direct invasion of the pericardium

pT3: Tumor with direct invasion into any of the following: lung, brachiocephalic vein, superior vena cava, phrenic nerve, chest wall, or extrapericardial pulmonary artery or veins

pT4: Tumor with invasion into any of the following: aorta, arch vessels, intrapericardial pulmonary artery, myocardium, trachea, esophagus [3]

Step 1: Describe, measure, and weigh the specimen.

Step 2: Thymus usually comes unoriented or minimally oriented. It is best to contact the pathologist to view the specimen before inking.

Step 3: Ink the specimen. In Fig. 4.47, the specimen is unoriented and therefore is entirely inked blue.

Step 4: Serially section the thymus.

Step 5: Describe the lesion (if any) and measure the lesion in three dimensions. In Fig. 4.48, the blue arrows designate the lesion.

Step 6: Measure the lesion to the closest oriented or unoriented margins.

Step 7: Submit sections of the lesion in relation to the closest margins. Typically, 1 section for every 1 cm of lesion can be submitted, i.e., a 5-cm lesion should have 5 sections submitted.

Example Dictation

Specimen A is received in formalin labeled with the patient's name, medical record number, "thymus" and consists of a slightly ragged, unoriented fragment of gland and soft tissue (19.4 × 12.1 × 2.6 cm, 38 grams) which is entirely inked blue and serially sectioned to reveal a firm, tan-pink, focally hemorrhagic mass (9.4 × 6.3 × 1.4 cm) with tan-yellow necrosis at one edge. The mass comes within 0.2 cm of

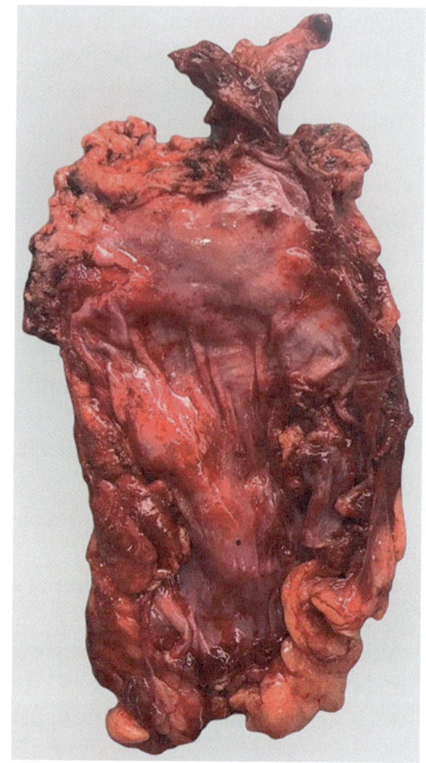

Fig. 4.47 Thymus

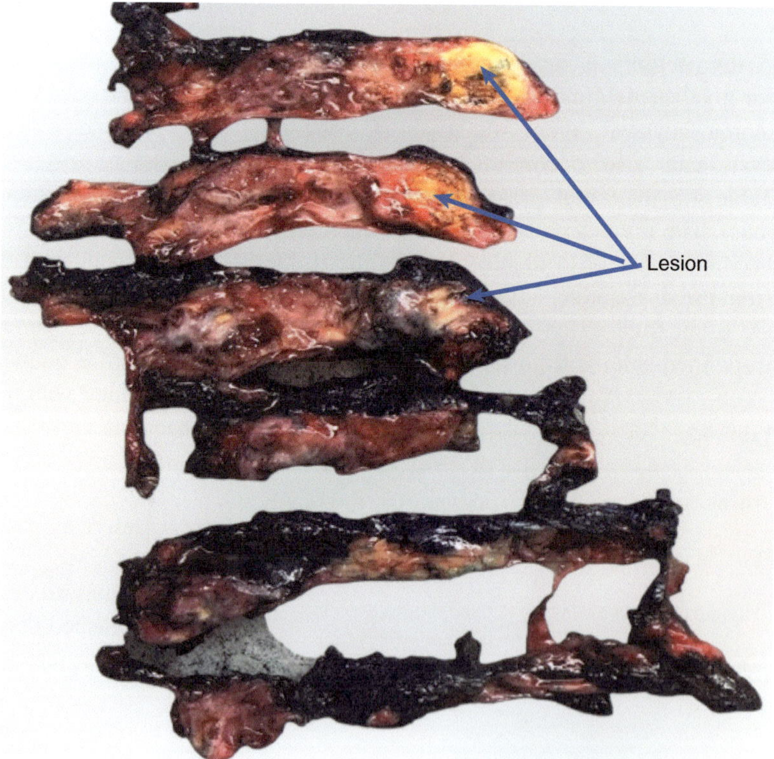

Fig. 4.48 Thymus serially sectioned

the closest unoriented margin and is surrounded by tan-yellow adipose and glandular tissue. Representative sections are submitted in A1–A20.

Acknowledgments The author gratefully acknowledges Syed Hussain Abbas, MD, William P. Daley, MD, and Selcuk Erturk, MD, for their contribution to this chapter.

Quiz Questions

1. A lung wedge resection is performed for a peripheral lung lesion. Upon gross examination, the lesion is described as a tan-white, round, firm, well-circumscribed nodule measuring $2.0 \times 1.5 \times 1.2$ cm. The lesion is located 0.5 cm away from the parenchymal resection margin. How should the lesion be sampled for histopathological examination?
   A) Submit the entire lesion in one cassette
   B) Submit perpendicular sections of the lesion in relation to the parenchymal resection margin
   C) Submit one section per centimeter of the lesion's size
   D) Submit the lesion entirely, along with en face parenchymal resection margin

2. A heart biopsy is performed for a patient with cardiomyopathy. The specimen contains four separate fragments of tan-brown tissue, each measuring $0.5 \times 0.4 \times 0.2$ cm. How should the specimen be submitted for processing?
   A) Submit all tissue in a biopsy bag in one cassette
   B) Submit representative sections in one cassette
   C) Submit the largest fragment only in one cassette
   D) Submit each fragment in biopsy bag in different cassettes

3. A plaque specimen is received, consisting of an aggregate of yellow-tan, focally hemorrhagic material measuring $2.8 \times 1.4 \times 1.2$ cm. How should representative sections of the plaque be submitted?

A) Submit all sections in one cassette
B) Submit multiple cassettes with different sections of the plaque
C) Submit one representative section in a single cassette
D) Submit sections from the hemorrhagic areas only

4. During the gross examination of a lung lobectomy specimen, a diffuse, dense, thick mass encasing the lung is identified. The mass extends into the interlobar fissures. What is the most likely diagnosis?
   A) Tuberculosis
   B) Mesothelioma
   C) Hamartoma
   D) Granuloma

5. A heart valve leaflet is surgically removed for stenosis. The fragment measures $1.9 \times 1.1 \times 0.5$ cm and shows scant calcification. What is the appropriate CPT code for this procedure?
   A) 88,304
   B) 88,305
   C) 88,307
   D) 88,309.

6. What are the 4 valves of the heart?
   A) Tricuspid, right coronary, circumflex, aortic
   B) Atrium, pulmonary, ventricle, left anterior descending
   C) Ostia, pulmonary, circumflex, tricuspid
   D) Tricuspid, mitral, pulmonary, aortic

7. How many fragments of tissue are considered optimal for a heart biopsy?
   A) 4
   B) 1
   C) 3
   D) 4

8. You receive this specimen (Fig. 4.49) on your gross bench. What is the resection margin?
   A) Pleural surface
   B) Parenchymal margin
   C) Bronchial margin
   D) Vascular margin

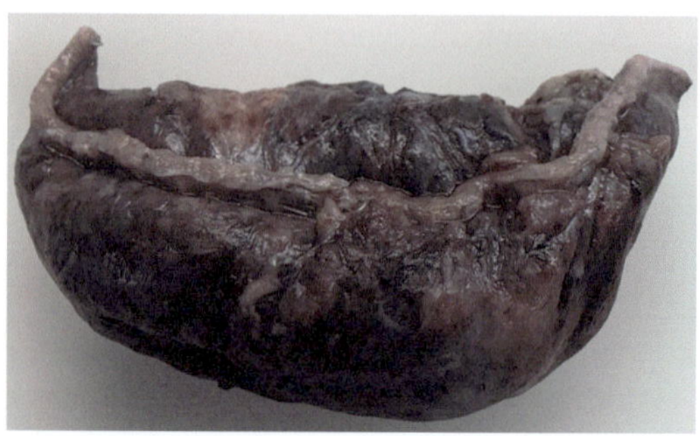

Fig. 4.49 Quiz question 8

9. How many heart biopsy fragments is considered optimal?
   A) 2
   B) 3
   C) 4
   D) 5

10. A lung is serially sectioned and a tan-white mass is identified measuring 2.2 × 1.9 × 1.4 cm present in the middle of the specimen. What is the pT stage for this mass?
   A) pT0
   B) pT1
   C) pT2
   D) pT3

Answer Key

1. B- Submit perpendicular sections of the lesion in relation to the parenchymal resection margin.

   Explanation: Submit perpendicular sections of the lesion in relation to the resection margin. When sampling a peripheral lung lesion for histopathological examination, it is important to submit perpendicular sections of the lesion in relation to the resection margin if the lesion is close to resection margin. This approach allows for more accurate evaluation of the tumor's relationship to the margins and helps assess the extent of invasion and adequacy of resection.

2. A- Submit all tissue in a biopsy bag in one cassette

   Explanation: Submit all tissue in a biopsy bag in one cassette. When dealing with heart biopsy specimens, it is generally recommended to submit the biopsies entirely in one cassette

for histopathological examination. This approach ensures adequate sampling of the tissue and allows for comprehensive evaluation of the myocardium, including assessment for inflammation, fibrosis, and other pathological changes associated with cardiomyopathy.

3. C- Submit one representative section in a single cassette

   Explanation: Submit one representative section in a single cassette. When dealing with plaque specimens, it is generally recommended to submit one representative section in a single cassette for histopathological examination. This approach ensures that a representative portion of the plaque, including areas of interest, such as areas of hemorrhage, is evaluated while minimizing the number of cassettes used.

4. B- Mesothelioma

   Explanation: The presence of a diffuse, dense, thick mass encasing the lung and extending into the interlobar fissures is indicative of mesothelioma. Whereas tuberculosis presents as diffusely scattered nodules, hamartoma firm, multilobulated, well-circumscribed nodule, and granuloma presents as a tan, firm nodule.

5. B- 88305

   Explanation: CPT code 88305 corresponds to the examination and pathological evaluation of a heart valve leaflet. In this scenario, a heart valve leaflet is surgically removed for stenosis. The provided fragment size of 1.9 × 1.1 × 0.5 cm and the presence of scant calcification indicate that a more detailed examination and evaluation of the specimen are required. CPT code 88305 specifically describes the comprehensive examination of a heart valve leaflet including gross and microscopic evaluation, interpretation, and preparation of a pathology report, which aligns with the given scenario.

6. D- Tricuspid, mitral, pulmonary, aortic

   Explanation: The correct answer is the tricuspid, mitral, pulmonary, aortic valves. The right coronary artery and left anterior descending artery are vessels of the heart and the ostia are the orifice of the aorta the lead to the right a left coronary artery. The antrum and ventricles are the heart chambers.

7. D- 4

Explanation: Four fragments of tissue are considered optimal for a heart biopsy, so A is correct. 3 fragments are acceptable. More fragments are always good but less is considered suboptimal.

8. B- Parenchymal margin

Explanation: Lung wedge resections from the periphery of the lung contain a parenchymal margin only, so B is correct. The pleura surrounds the rest of the specimen but is not a true margin. The bronchial and vascular margins are present on a lobectomy or pneumonectomy but typically not on a lung wedge resection.

9. C- 4

Explanation: Three fragments of heart are considered acceptable but 4 fragments are optimal, so C is correct. It is important to count the number of fragments received while grossing to document if the sample is unacceptable, acceptable, or optimal.

10. B- pT1

Explanation: pT1 is a tumor less than or equal to 3 cm in greatest dimension, so B is the correct answer. pT2 tumor is greater than 3 cm but less than or equal to 5 cm. pT3 tumor is greater than 5 cm but less than or equal to 7 cm in greatest dimension. pT4 tumor is greater than 7 cm in greatest dimension.

References

1. FirstPath. 2009–2023. [Online]. Available: https://www.firstpathlab.com/cpt-codes/. Accessed 2 Jun 2023.
2. Protocol for the examination of resection specimens from. College of American Pathologists; 2022.
3. Protocol for the examination of specimens from patients with. College of American Pathologists; 2021.

Grossing of Gastrointestinal Specimens

5

Contents

Gastrointestinal grossing includes a wide variety of specimens from esophagus to rectum. A logical and problem-solving approach to grossing gastrointestinal specimens is presented. The presence or absence of circumferential radial margins varies along the luminal gastrointestinal tract which makes grossing gastrointestinal specimens unique among the grossing of other organ systems. Proper orientation and sectioning of polyps, Hirschsprung's specimens, and diverticu-

Table 5.1 CPT codes [1]

GI biopsy	88305
GI polyp	88305
Appendix incidental	88302
Appendix other than incidental	88304
Omentum biopsy	88305
Esophagus resection	88309
Stomach resection not for tumor	88307
Stomach resection for tumor	88309
Colostomy	88304
GI diverticulum	88304
Colon resection not for tumor	88307
Colon resection for tumor	88309
Total colon	88309

losis among others have been covered. Step by step grossing, pictures, and an example dictation with respective CPT codes (see Table 5.1) have been included for reader's understanding.

5.1 Gastrointestinal Biopsies: Level IV CPT 88305

Gastrointestinal (GI) biopsy is a vague term for sampling any area from the esophagus to the rectum. These samples are taken during endoscopy for a multitude of reasons from constipation to malignancy. Almost all GI biopsies are handled the same way.

Step 1: Describe the tissue, count the number of fragments, and give a three-dimensional measurement. In Fig. 5.1, there is 1 fragment of tissue. If the number of fragments is greater than 5, the specimen can be dictated as an aggregate.

Step 2: State how the biopsy is submitted in cassettes and submit the tissue entirely as shown in Fig. 5.2.

Example Dictation

Specimen A is received in formalin labeled with patient's name, medical record number, "cecum biopsy" and consists of 1 tan-brown tissue fragment ($0.6 \times 0.5 \times 0.2$ cm) which is submitted in toto in a biopsy bag in A1.

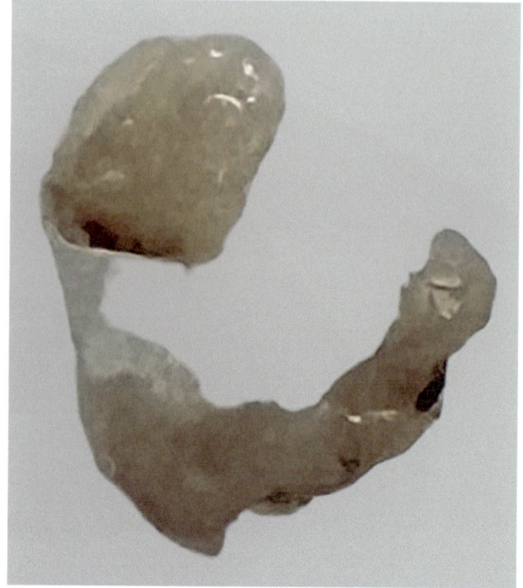

Fig. 5.1 GI biopsy

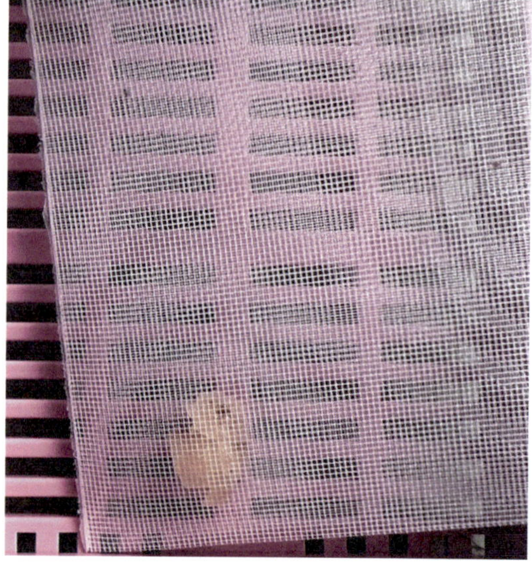

Fig. 5.2 GI biopsy cassette submission in a biopsy bag

5.2 Gastrointestinal Polyps: Level IV CPT 88305

Polyps of the GI tract are removed from the mucosa at the base of the polyp. The base of the polyp is the resection margin.

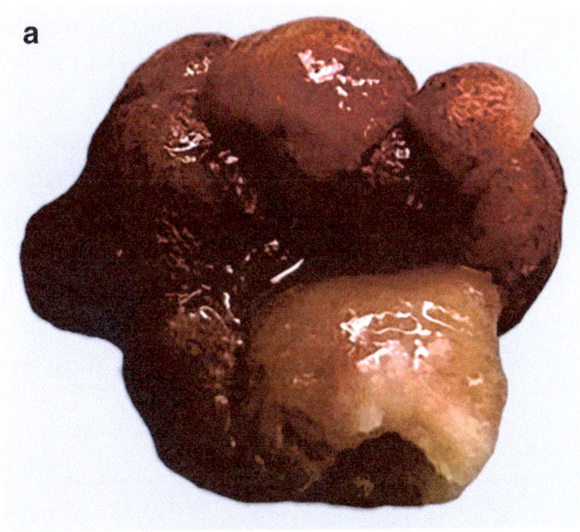

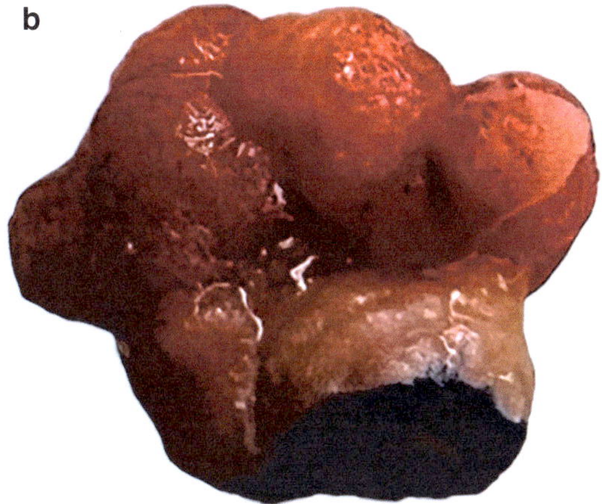

Fig. 5.3 (**a**) Polyp, (**b**) Polyp with inked margin

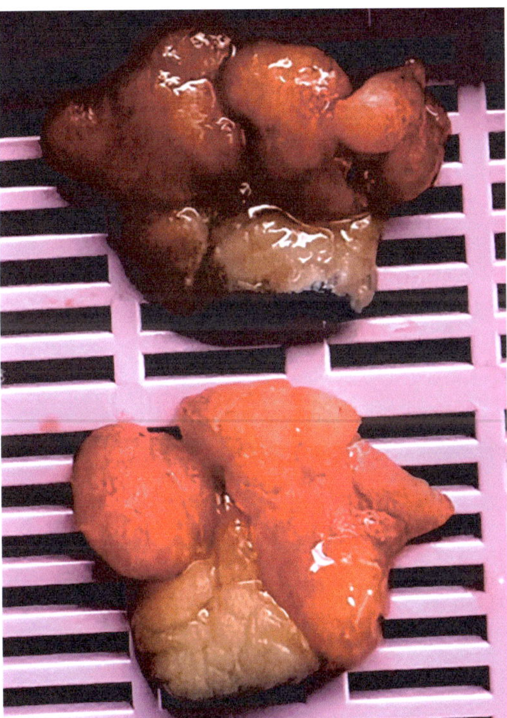

Fig. 5.4 Polyp section submission

Step 1: Describe and measure the polyp (Fig. 5.3a).

Step 2: Ink the resection margin of the polyp as seen in Fig. 5.3b.

Step 3: Section the polyp perpendicular to the margin so ink is present on both sections and submit entirely. In Fig. 5.4, the polyp is small and can be bisected to fit in one cassette. The larger the polyp the more sections are necessary.

Example Dictation

Specimen A is received in formalin labeled with patient's name, medical record number, "colon polyp" and consists of an unoriented, tan-pink, pedunculated polyp (1.1 × 0.9 × 0.5 cm). The resection margin is inked blue, and the specimen is bisected and submitted entirely in A1.

5.3 Endoscopic Submucosal Dissection (ESD): Level V CPT 88307

An endoscopic submucosal dissection (ESD) is a procedure used to remove growths from within the gastrointestinal tract. These procedures use endoscopic tools to remove the growth and the underlying submucosa. This is different from endoscopic mucosal resection (EMR) which uses a wire loop to snare the growth often leading to a resection of fragments instead of a whole resection where the margins can be evaluated [2].

Step 1: Describe, orient, and measure the specimen. In Fig. 5.5, the surgeon pinned the specimen flat and labeled "S" for superior, "I" for inferior, "R" for right and "L" for left.

Step 2: Describe and measure the lesion as seen by the blue arrow in Fig. 5.5.

Step 3: Measure how close the lesion comes to all peripheral margins.

Step 4: Ink the resection margins. In Fig. 5.6, the right side of the deep margin is inked orange, and the left side of the deep margin is inked blue.

Step 5: Serially section the specimen and measure the greatest depth of invasion if grossly identifiable. In Fig. 5.7, the specimen is sectioned from superior to inferior. Leave the end margins longer, approximately 0.5–0.8 cm in length.

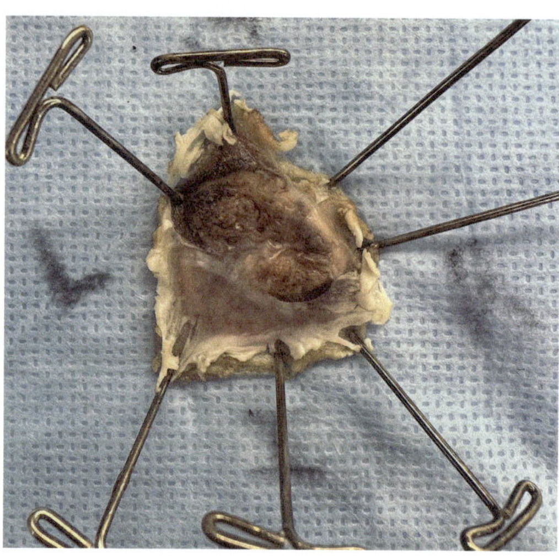

Fig. 5.5 ESD oriented

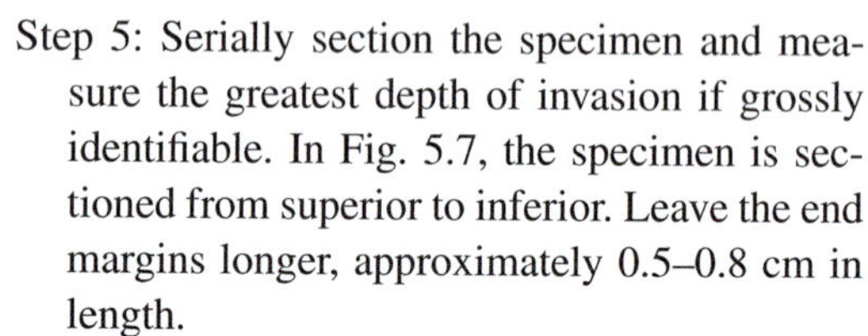

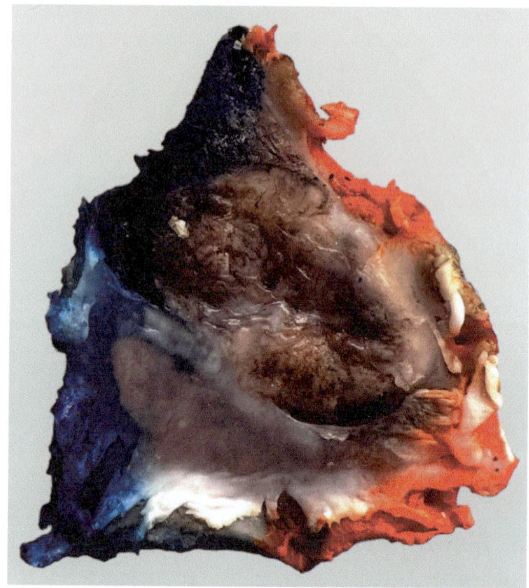

Fig. 5.6 ESD inked

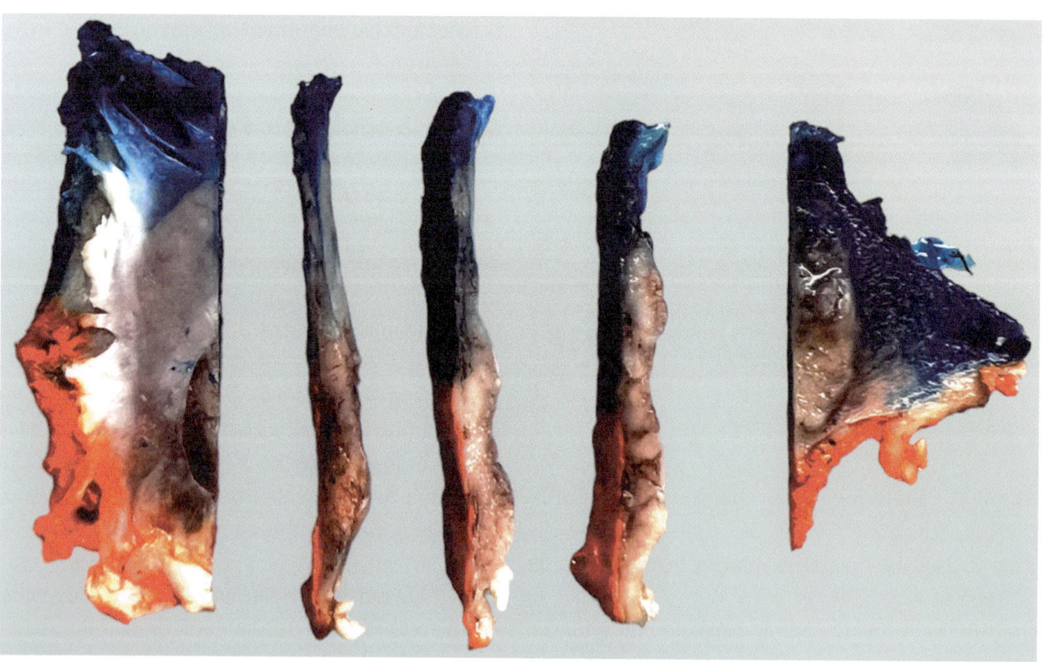

Fig. 5.7 ESD serially sectioned

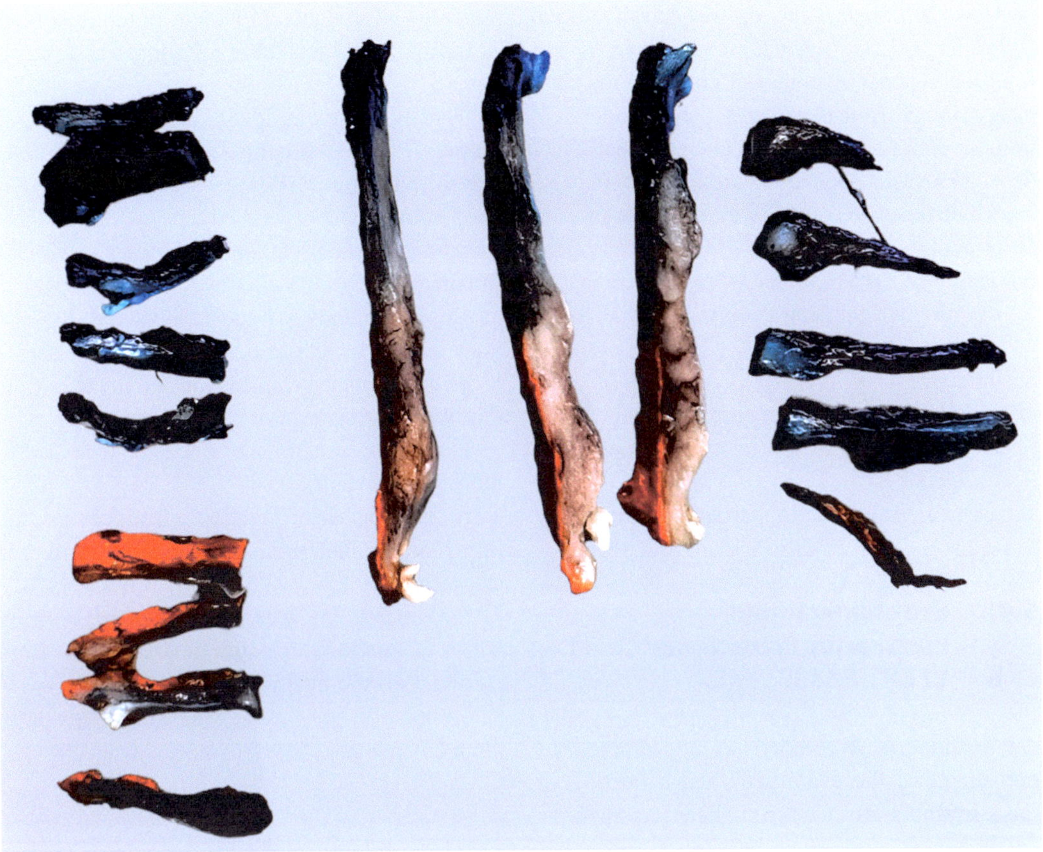

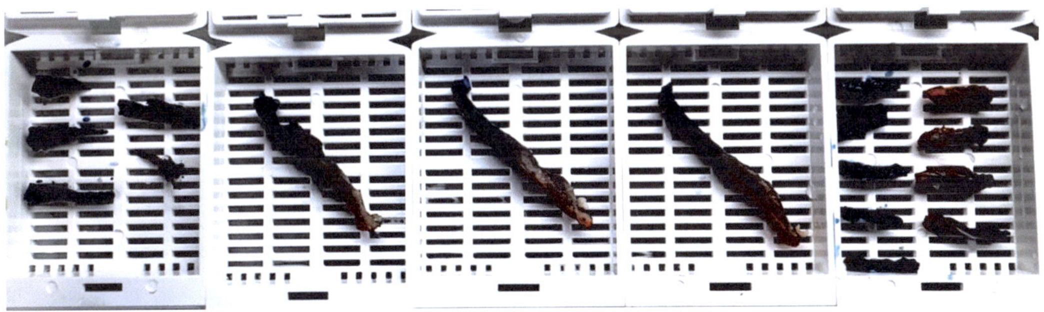

Fig. 5.8 ESD perpendicular margins

Fig. 5.9 ESD section submission

Step 6: Perpendicularly section the end margins. In Fig. 5.8, the superior and inferior margins are perpendicularly sectioned. These sections are submitted on edge.

Step 7: Submit the specimen entirely as shown in Fig. 5.9.

Example Dictation

Specimen A is received in formalin labeled with patient's name, medical record number, "ESD" and consists of a tan excision of mucosa (3.8 × 2.4 × 0.3 cm) oriented per the surgeon as left, right, superior, and inferior. The mucosal surface contains a single, raised, red-brown lesion (1.9 × 1.1 × 0.2 cm) which comes within 0.5 cm from the superior margin, 0.3 cm from the right margin, 0.6 cm from the inferior margin, and 0.2 cm from the left margin. The specimen is serially sectioned to reveal a depth of invasion of 0.2 cm coming within less than 0.1 cm of the deep margin.

Ink code

> Orange: right deep margin
> Blue: left deep margin

Section code

> A1: superior margin, perpendicular
> A2–A4: body of specimen from superior to inferior
> A5: inferior margin, perpendicular

## 5.4	Esophagectomy/ Esophagogastrectomy: Level VI CPT 88309

An esophagogastrectomy is the removal of part or all of the esophagus and a portion of the proximal stomach for diseases such as Barrett's esophagus with high grade dysplasia or malignancy (see Table 5.2 for gross descriptions).

Cancer Protocol for the Examination of Specimens from Patients with Carcinoma of the Esophagus

Location of the tumor (See Fig. 5.10 for illustration):

Upper esophagus: Cancers located in the cervical and upper thoracic esophagus (proximal).

Mid esophagus: Cancers located in the middle thoracic esophagus.

Distal esophagus: Cancers located in the lower thoracic esophagus.

Esophagogastric junction: Defined as the junction of the tubular esophagus and the stomach.

Proximal stomach/cardia: Portion of stomach which is less than or equal to 2 cm distal from esophagogastric junction [3].

Tumor size and extent: Measure the lesion in three dimensions.

Table 5.2 Gross appearance of esophagus tumors [3]

Adenocarcinoma	Stricturing, polypoid, fungating, ulcerative, or diffusely infiltrative lesions
Squamous cell carcinoma	Fungating/exophytic/polypoid lesions
	Ulcerative or infiltrative (intramural causing thick, rigid esophageal wall with luminal narrowing)
	Most esophageal squamous carcinomas are identified in the middle 1/3

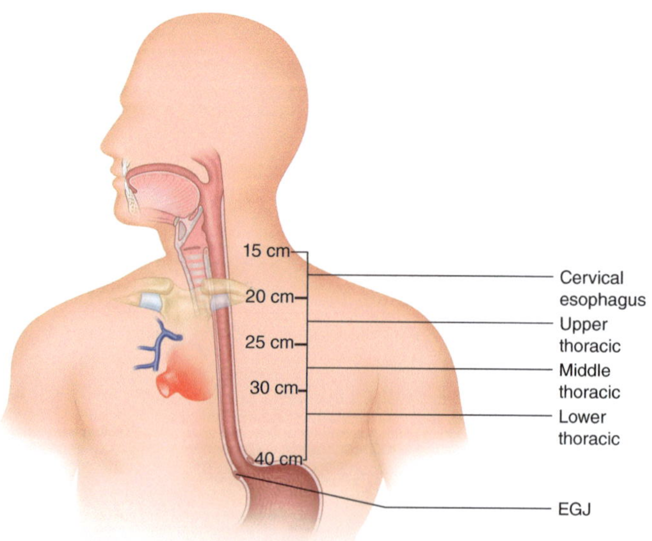

Fig. 5.10 Esophagus anatomic areas

Relationship of tumor to esophagogastric junction (EGJ): Measure the distance of the lesion center to the EGJ [3].

Tumors involving the EGJ that have a midpoint within the proximal 2 cm of the cardia/proximal stomach are to be staged as esophageal cancers. Cancers whose center is more than 2 cm distal from the EGJ, even if EGJ is involved, should be staged using the stomach cancer protocol [3].

Margin status: Margins include the proximal, distal, and radial margins. The radial margin represents the adventitial soft tissue margin closest to the deepest penetration of tumor. Sections to evaluate the proximal and distal resections margins can be obtained in 2 orientations: en face sections parallel to the margin or longitudinal sections perpendicular to the margin. Depending on the distance of the tumor to the margin, select the orientation(s) that will most clearly demonstrate the status of the margin [3].

Tumor extent: The depth of invasion of the tumor/mass is measured. Also assess for tumor extension into the pleura, pericardium, azygos vein, diaphragm, peritoneum, or other adjacent structures, such as the aorta, vertebral body, or airway if applicable [3].

pT Category

pT0: No evidence of primary tumor

   pTis: High grade dysplasia

   pT1a: Tumor invades the lamina propria or muscularis mucosae

   pT1b: Tumor invades the submucosa

   pT2: Tumor invades the muscularis propria

   pT3: Tumor invades adventitia

   pT4a: Tumor invades the pleura, pericardium, azygos vein, diaphragm, or peritoneum

   pT4b: Tumor invades other adjacent structures, such as the aorta, vertebral body, or airway [3]

Step 1: Describe, measure, and orient the specimen. In Fig. 5.11, the esophagus is narrower than the proximal stomach aspect of the specimen so the narrow portion is the esophagus and the wide portion is the stomach.

Step 2: Shave the proximal and distal margins and submit en face. Figure 5.12a shows the

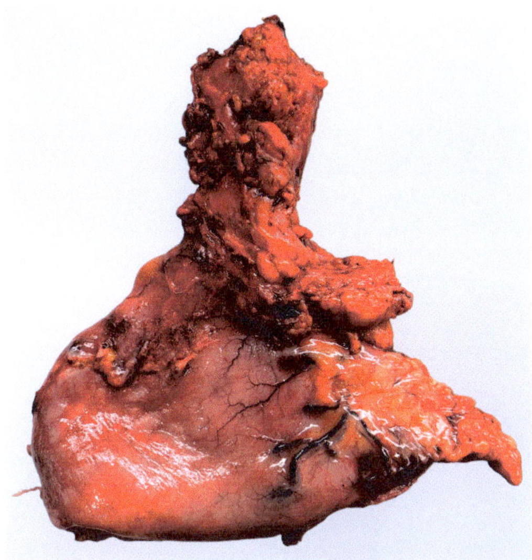

Fig. 5.11 Esophagogastrectomy specimen

proximal margin shaved, and Fig. 5.12b shows the stapled resection margin of the distal margin. Another option is to open and ink the proximal and distal margins of the specimen first and take margins after. This allows for visualization of the lesion. If the lesion is close to a margin, then perpendicular sections of the lesion in relation to the margin would be best.

Step 3: Ink the surrounding margin as shown in Fig. 5.13. The entire outer circumference of the esophagus is a margin.

Step 4: Open the specimen as shown in Fig. 5.14.

Step 5: Describe and measure the lesion. In Fig. 5.15, the lesion is designated with a blue arrow.

Step 6: Fix the specimen in formalin. It is best to fix the specimen for a few hours at minimum for optimal sections but not required if the lesion area is firm.

Step 7: Amputate the lesion as seen in Fig. 5.16. If the lesion is close to the margin, then amputate the lesion with the closest margin. In Fig. 5.16, the lesion is in relation to the proximal margin.

Step 8: Serially section the lesion perpendicular to the margin. (Fig. 5.17)

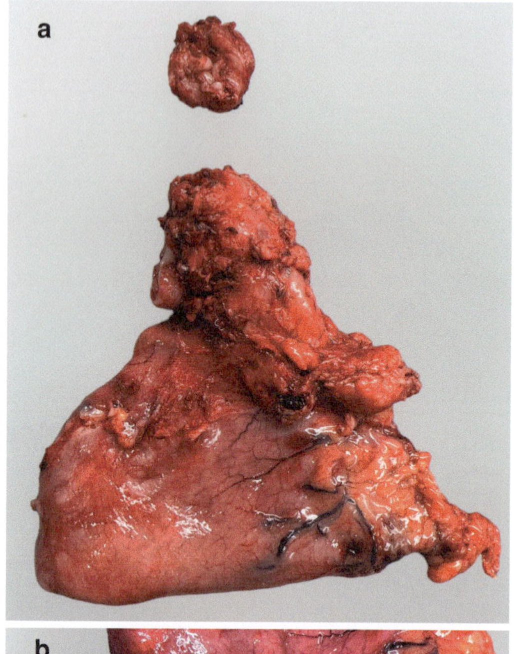

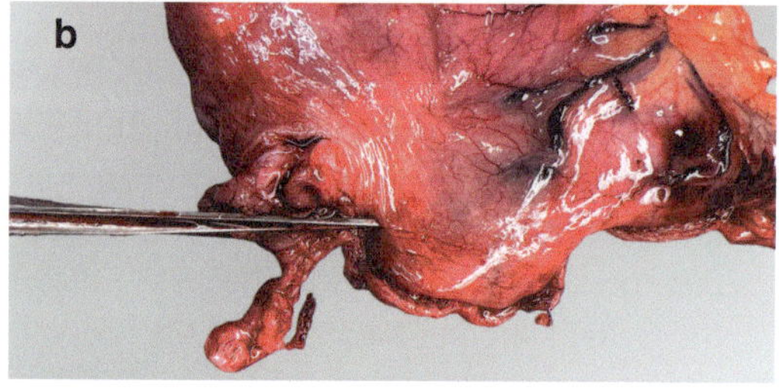

Fig. 5.12 (**a**) Proximal margin, (**b**) Distal margin

Step 9: Identify the greatest depth of invasion. In Fig. 5.18, the ulcerated lesion reveals a depth of invasion into the surrounding serosal surface without invasion through the serosa.

Step 10: Submit the lesion entirely. If the lesion is large, communicate with the pathologist for section submission.

Step 11: Submit representative unremarkable esophagus and stomach sections.

Step 12: Remove all remaining adipose tissue and palpate for lymph nodes. In Fig. 5.19, an aggregate of adipose tissue is removed from the remainder of the specimen and palpated. Fifteen lymph nodes are required.

Example Dictation

Specimen A is received in formalin labeled with patient's name, medical record number, "esophagus and stomach" and consists of a pink-red esophagogastrostomy (18.6 × 8.7 × 3.2 cm). The

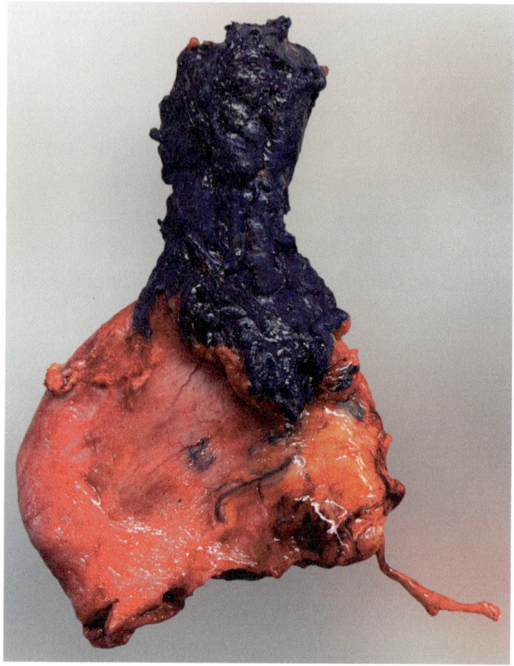

Fig. 5.13 Inked margin of specimen

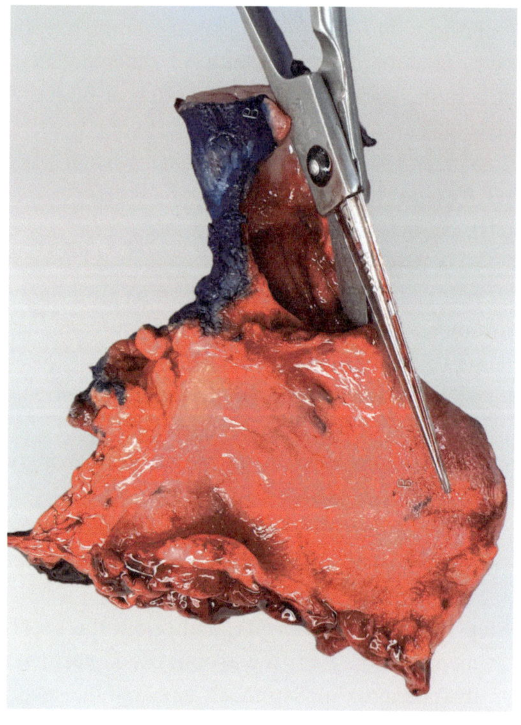

Fig. 5.14 Opening the specimen

surrounding esophageal soft tissue is inked blue, and the specimen is opened to reveal an ulcerative, pink-red, ill-defined lesion (2.7 × 1.4 cm) present at the gastroesophageal junction coming within 0.9 cm from the proximal margin and 16.3 cm from the distal margin. The lesion is serially sectioned to reveal a focal area of invasion (0.6 cm) into the serosa without invasion into the soft tissue coming within 0.5 cm of the peripheral margin. The remaining esophageal mucosa is pale-pink and smooth, and the gastric mucosa is hemorrhagic and dusky. The surrounding adipose

tissue is palpable for 15 lymph node candidates ranging from 0.1 to 0.5 cm.

Section code

A 1: Proximal margin, en face
A2–A4: Distal margin, en face
A5: Lesser curvature radial margin, en face
A6 Greater curvature radial margin, en face
A7–A13: Lesion, entirely
A14: Stomach, representative
A15–A17: Five lymph node candidates per cassette, whole

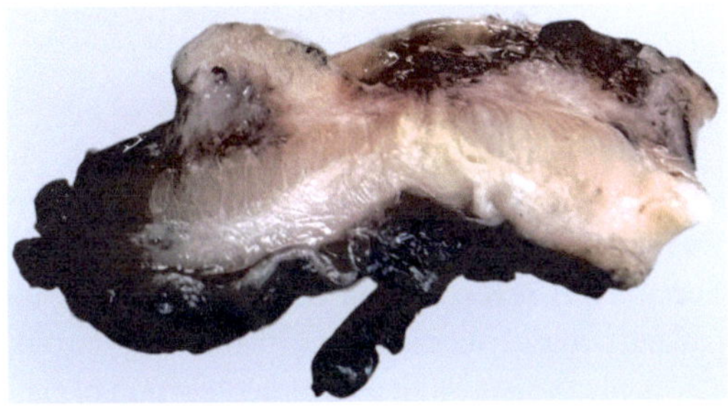

Fig. 5.18   Section with greatest extent of invasion

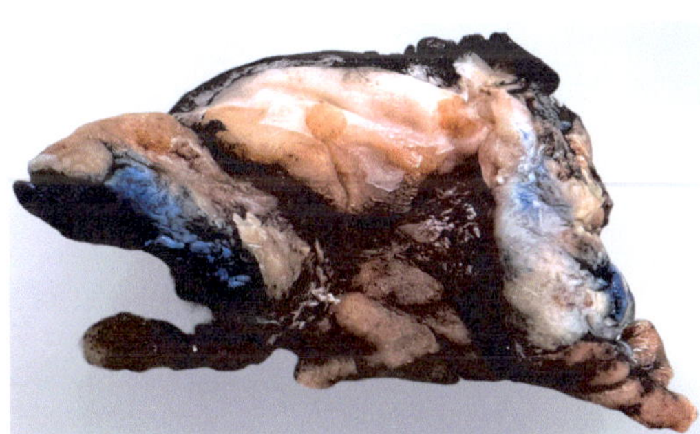

Fig. 5.15   Specimen with lesion

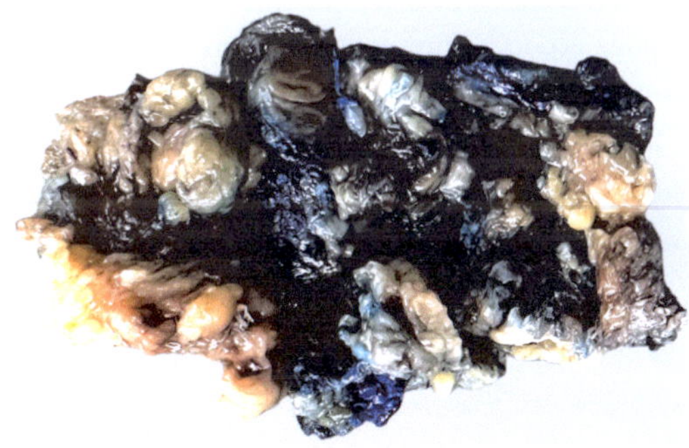

Fig. 5.16   Lesion post fixation

Fig. 5.19   Adipose tissue for lymph nodes

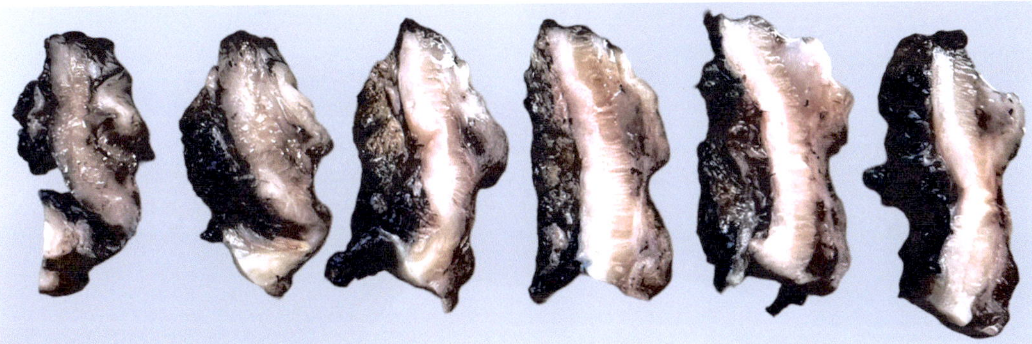

Fig. 5.17   Lesion in relation to proximal margin perpendicularly sectioned

5.5 Stomach for Obesity: Level V CPT 88307

A sleeve gastrectomy is an elective surgery typically performed for obesity. The procedure is the removal of a portion of the stomach to reduce the stomach overall size resulting in probable weight loss.

Step 1: Describe and measure the specimen (Fig. 5.20).
Step 2: Remove the staple line and open the specimen as shown in Fig. 5.21.
Step 3: Describe the mucosal surface identifying any lesions.
Step 4: Submit representative sections as shown in Fig. 5.22.

Example Dictation

Specimen A is received in formalin labeled with patient's name, medical record number, "stomach" and consists of an unoriented portion of tan-pink stomach (17.4 × 3.9 × 2.8 cm) which is opened to reveal tan-pink rugal folds which are slightly dusky toward one unoriented end. No lesions are identified within. Representative sections are submitted in A1.

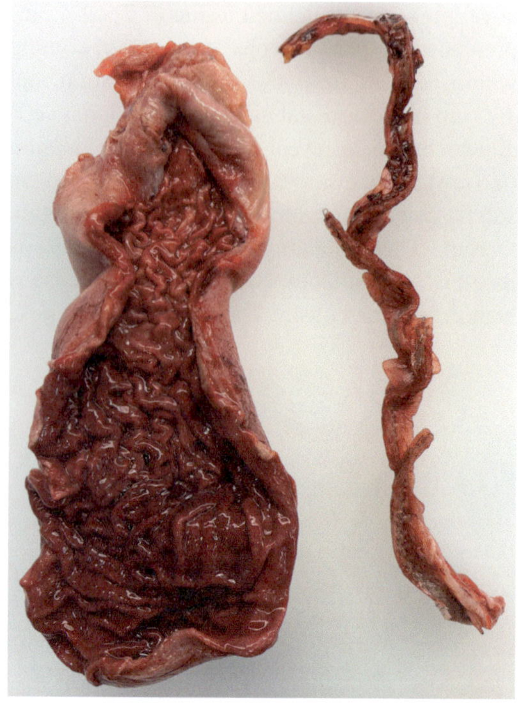

Fig. 5.21 Gastric sleeve opened

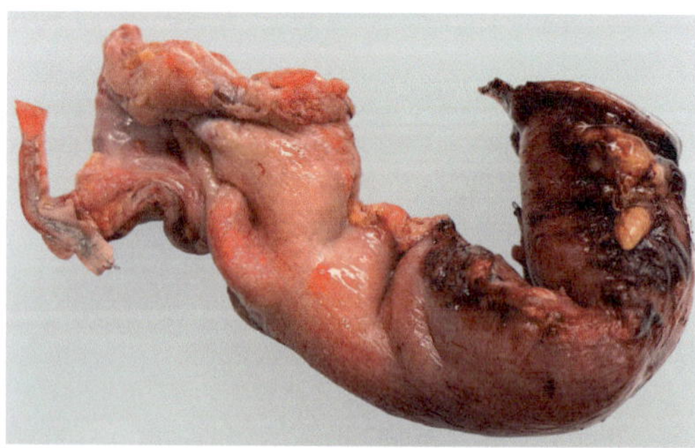

Fig. 5.20 Gastric sleeve

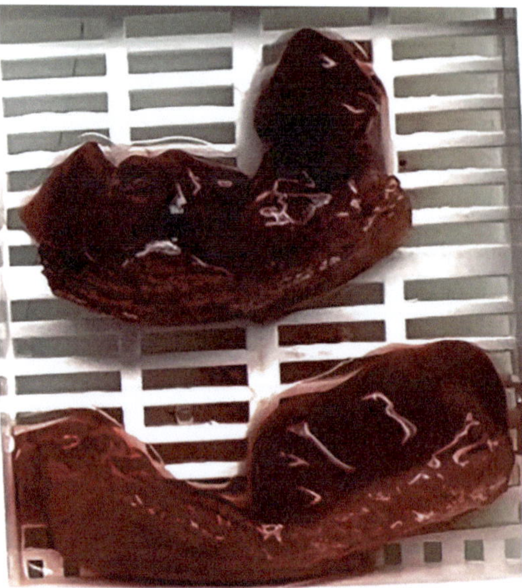

Fig. 5.22 Gastric sleeve section submission

5.6 Stomach for GIST: Level VI CPT 88309

Gastrointestinal Stromal Tumor (GIST) is a digestive system tumor that occurs in the GI tract but most often in the stomach. They typically appear as a mass protruding from within the serosa with overlying mucosa.

Cancer Protocol Relative to Grossing GIST
Procedure:

Local resection: Removal of the tumor.
Resection: Removal of the tumor with clear surrounding margins.
Metastasectomy: Removal of a tumor metastasis [4]

Tumor focality: Dictate if the tumor is unifocal or multifocal. If multifocal, dictate the number of separate nodules and the range of size [4].

Tumor site: Dictate where the tumor is located. GIST can occur anywhere along the GI tract [4].

Margin status: If the specimen is oriented, measure the tumor to the proximal, distal, and radial margin, if applicable [4].

pT Category
pT0: No evidence of primary tumor
pT1: Tumor 2 cm or less
pT2: Tumor more than 2 cm but not more than 5 cm
pT3: Tumor more than 5 cm but not more than 10 cm
pT4: Tumor more than 10 cm in greatest dimension [4]

Step 1: Describe and measure the specimen. In Fig. 5.23, there is a mass (blue arrow) protruding from the serosal surface from the small portion of the stomach (red arrow).

Step 2: Remove the staple line (Fig. 5.24a) and ink the stomach margin as seen in Fig. 5.24b.

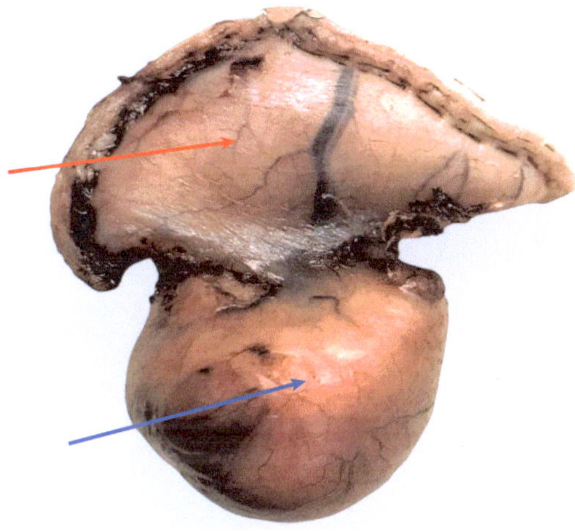

Fig. 5.23 Stomach resection for GIST

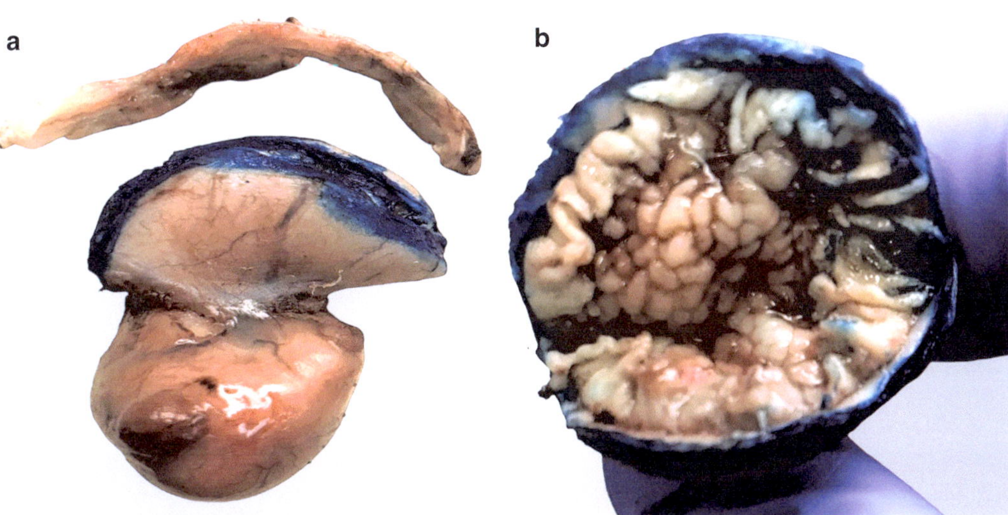

Fig. 5.24 (**a**) Staple line removed; (**b**) gastric resection margin inked

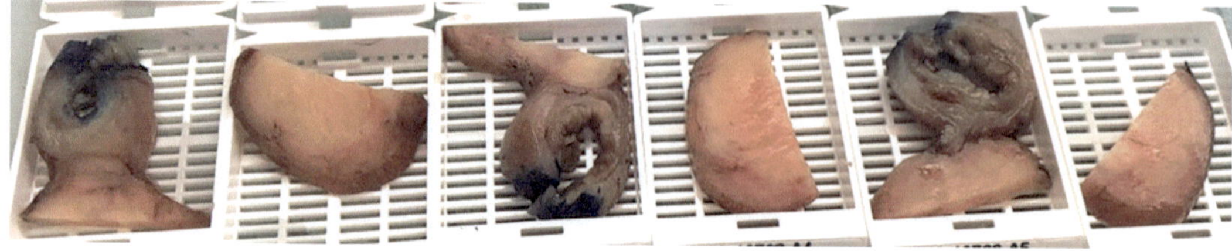

Fig. 5.26 Stomach for GIST section submission

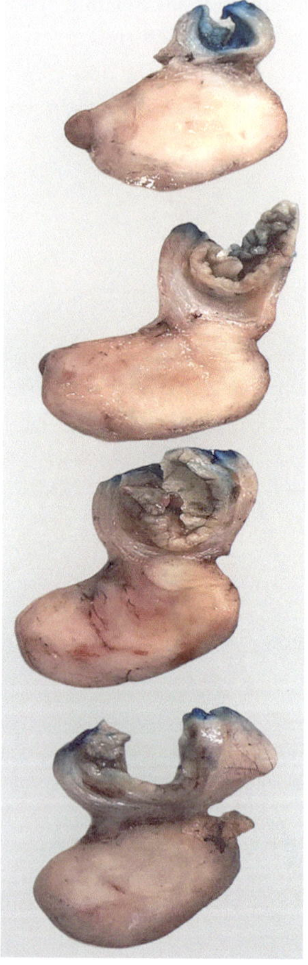

Fig. 5.25 Stomach serially sectioned

Step 3: Serially section the specimen perpendicular to the stomach resection margin as seen in Fig. 5.25.

Step 4: Describe the surface of the nodule and if mucosa and serosa are visible on either side.

Step 5: Submit representative sections of the mass in relation to the stomach margin. (Fig. 5.26)

Example Dictation

Specimen A is received in formalin labeled with patient's name, medical record number, "stomach" and consists of an unoriented portion of tan stomach (3.8 × 2.4 × 2.0 cm) with an attached tan-brown, smooth, bulging nodule (3.6 × 2.7 × 2.2 cm) present opposite to the margin. The staple line is removed from the margin, and the underlying margin is inked blue. The specimen is serially sectioned to reveal solid, tan-white cut surfaces of the nodule which arises from the serosal aspect of the specimen and comes within 1.5 cm from the resection margin. Representative sections are submitted in A1–A6.

5.7   Stomach for Tumor: Level VI CPT 88309

A partial or total gastrectomy is performed for malignancies identified in the stomach (see Table 5.3 for gross descriptions). The surgery removes some or all of the stomach and typically regional lymph nodes or adjacent structures depending on the extent of tumor in the abdomen.

Cancer Protocol for Carcinoma of the Stomach

Procedure description

Partial gastrectomy: Removal of a portion of stomach

Complete gastrectomy: Removal of the entire stomach

[5]

Tumor site: Tumor location should be described in relation to the following landmarks:

Gastric region: cardia, fundus, body, antrum, pylorus

Table 5.3   Gross appearance of stomach tumors [5]

Ulcer	Red-pink crater with raised everted edges
Carcinoma, intestinal type	Tumors can vary in size from no macroscopic mass to an exophytic polypoid or gastric wall thickening/stricturing
Carcinoma, signet right cell type/diffuse type	Very early stage lesions may not produce any visible abnormalities/lesions More advanced lesions—thickening, ulceration or just rigid, leather bottle-like stomach (linitis plastica); may cause pyloric obstruction Typically invades the submucosa at an early phase and the tumor cells often spread in the stomach wall instead of growing as a tumor protruding into the lumen Marked thickening of the gastric wall with loss of rugal folds
Neuroendocrine tumors	Small, sharply outlined polyps and nodules, covered by flattened mucosa
GIST	Well-circumscribed, fleshy lesion with tan-pink cut surfaces, which may show hemorrhage or cystic degeneration

Greater curvature, lesser curvature
Anterior wall, posterior wall [5]

Tumor size: Measure the lesion in 3 dimensions [5].

Tumor extent: Depth of invasion of the tumor/mass is measured and dictate if tumor penetrates the subserosal connective tissue or serosa or adjacent structures [5].

Margin status: Proximal, distal, omental (radial) margin of greater and lesser curvature [5].

Sections to evaluate the proximal and distal resections margins can be obtained in 2 orientations: (1) en face sections parallel to the margin or (2) longitudinal sections perpendicular to the margin [5].

pT Category

pT0: No evidence of primary tumor

pTis: Carcinoma in situ: intraepithelial tumor without invasion of the lamina propria, high grade dysplasia

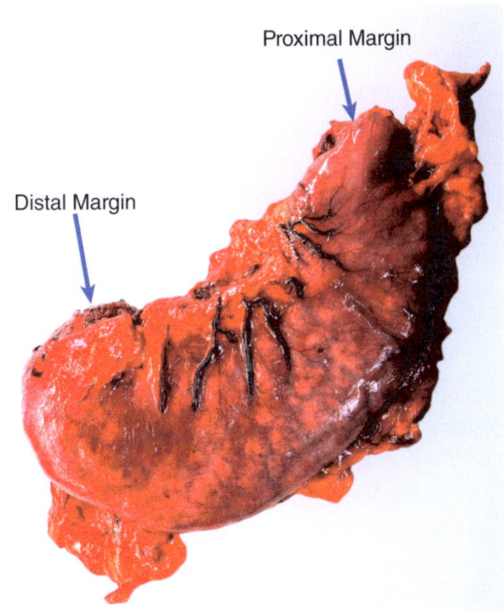

Fig. 5.27   Gastrectomy

pT1a: Tumor invades the lamina propria or muscularis mucosae

pT1b: Tumor invades the submucosa

pT2: Tumor invades the muscularis propria

pT3: Tumor penetrates the subserosal connective tissue without invasion of the visceral peritoneum or adjacent structures

pT4a: Tumor invades the serosa

pT4b: Tumor invades adjacent structures/organs [5]

Step 1: Describe and measure the specimen. (Fig. 5.27)

Step 2: Orient the specimen. The proximal margin typically is smaller in diameter and may contain a small portion of esophagus.

Step 3: Submit the proximal (Fig. 5.28a) and distal (Fig. 5.28b) margins en face. The specimen can also be opened first and if the lesion is close to a margin, then that margin can be submitted perpendicular in relation to the lesion.

Step 4: Shave the radial margin of the lesser and greater curvature and submit en face as shown in Fig. 5.29.

Step 5: Open the specimen as shown in Fig. 5.30. The standard is to open the stomach along the greater curvature due to most ulcers and lesions being present in the lesser curvature. In this example, the majority of the lesion is present in the greater curvature so the stomach was opened along the lesser curvature.

Step 6: Describe and measure the lesion. In Fig. 5.31, the cancerous lesion is designated by the blue arrow with innumerable polyps surrounding the cancerous lesion.

Step 7: Measure the lesion to the proximal and distal margins. In this example, the cancerous lesion is measured to the proximal and distal margins and the polypoid area is also measured to the proximal and distal margins.

Step 8: Fix the specimen. Pin the specimen to a wax board as shown in Fig. 5.32a. Fill a large container with formalin and submerge the specimen in the fixative with the wax board on top as shown in Fig. 5.32b. It is best to fix these specimens overnight, if possible.

Step 9: Ink the proximal (blue ink) and distal (orange ink) margins as shown in Fig. 5.33a.

Step 10: Ink the serosal surface where the lesion is located. The overall lesion is large so the

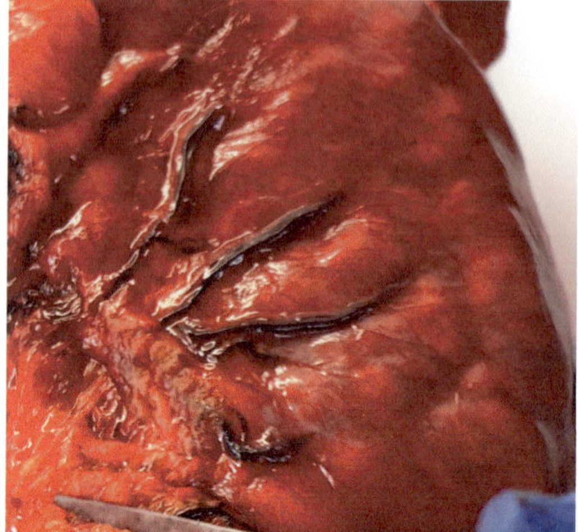

Fig. 5.30 Opening gastrectomy

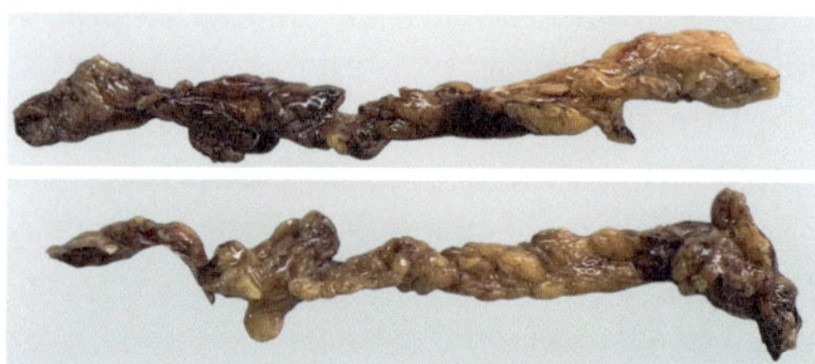

Fig. 5.29 Radial margins

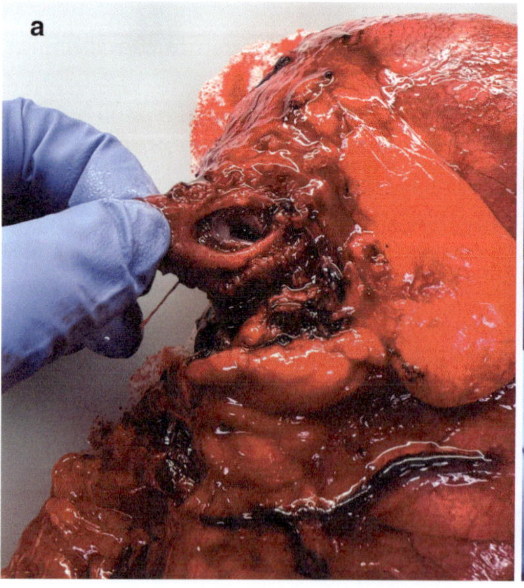

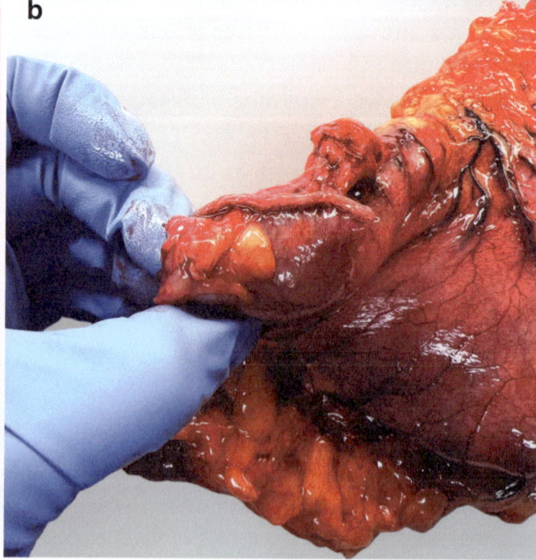

Fig. 5.28 (**a**) Proximal margin; (**b**) distal margin

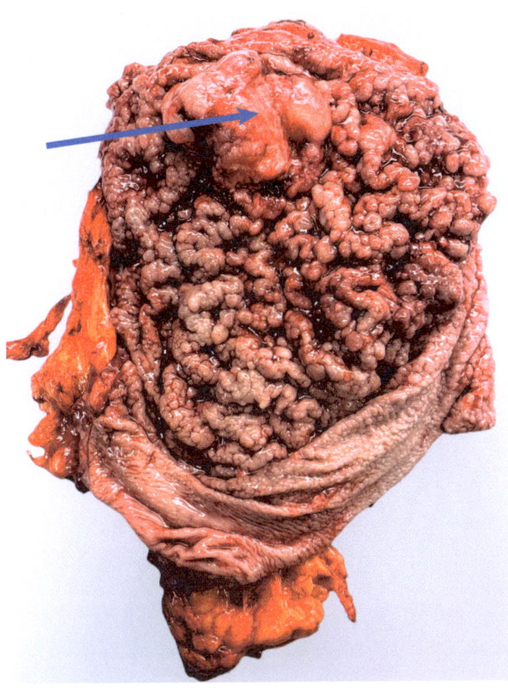

Fig. 5.31 Gastrectomy opened

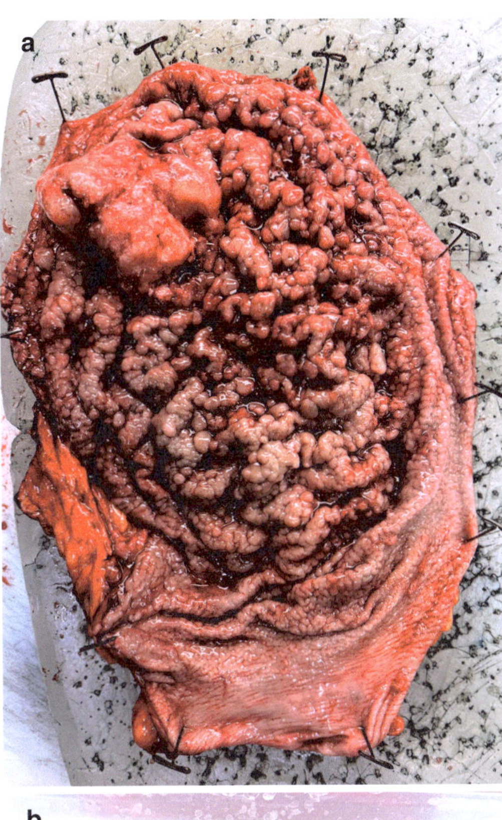

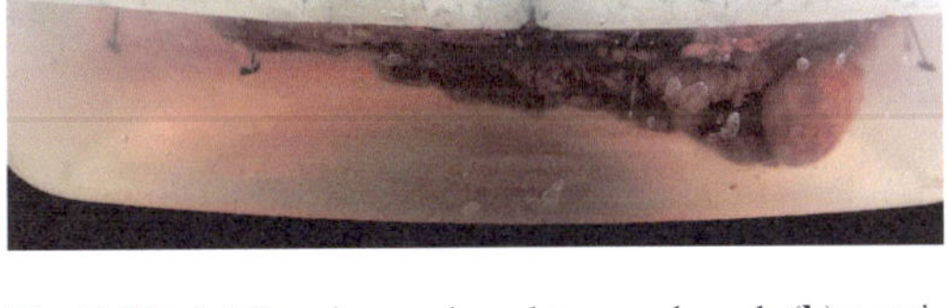

Fig. 5.32 (**a**) Specimen pinned to wax board; (**b**) specimen in formalin

majority of the serosal surface is inked as shown in Fig. 5.33b.

Step 11: Serially section the specimen from proximal to distal as shown in Fig. 5.34a.

Figure 5.34b. Lay each slice flat for an optimal view of the lesion.

Step 12: Identify and measure the greatest depth of invasion. In Fig. 5.35, the lesion invades into the serosa but does not invade outside the stomach as noted by the blue arrow.

Step 13: Representative sections of the cancerous lesion with the greatest depth of invasion are submitted.

Step 14: Assess the remainder of the polyps and identify any additional areas of invasion.

Step 15: Submit ample representative sections of the surrounding polyps. (Fig. 5.36)

Step 16: Submit representative sections of the uninvolved stomach.

Step 17: Remove the remainder of the adipose tissue as shown in Fig. 5.37 and palpate for lymph nodes.

Example Dictation

Specimen A is received in fortmalin labeled with the patient's name, medical record number, "total gastrectomy" and consists of a tan-red stomach (25.1 × 12.3 × 2.2 cm). The stomach is opened along the greater curvature to reveal a large, polypoid, ill-defined area (15.2 × 11.5 cm) containing small polyps ranging from 0.1 to 0.7 cm, present within the greater curvature fundus and body, with a large raised, friable tan-brown polypoid mass (6.9 × 5.2 × 2.5 cm) present superiorly

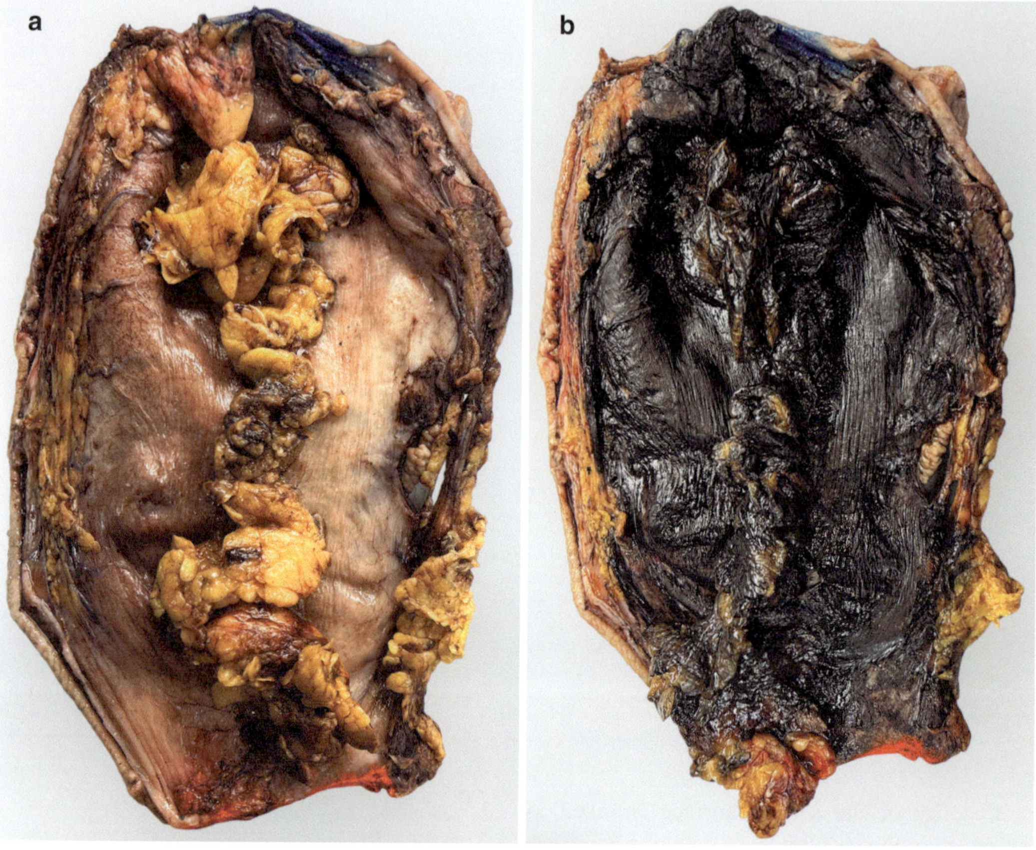

Fig. 5.33 (**a**) Proximal and distal margin inked; (**b**) serosal surface inked

within the aggregate. The polypoid area comes within 2.1 cm of the proximal margin and 8.5 cm from the distal margin. The polypoid mass comes within 4.2 cm of the proximal margin and 10.1 cm from the distal margin. The specimen is serially sectioned to reveal a greatest depth of invasion of the polypoid mass is 0.3 cm, coming within 0.1 cm of the serosal surface, with invasion through the mucosa and into the submucosa. The surrounding polyps are confined to the mucosal surface, without involvement into the submucosa or serosal surface. The surrounding adipose tissue is palpable for 5 lymph node candidates ranging from 0.1 to 0.7 cm.

Ink code

    Black: serosa
    Blue: proximal margin
    Orange: distal margin

Section code

    A 1-A 2: Frozen section remnant proximal margin, bisected, en face

    A 3: Distal margin, en face

    A4–A6: Lesser curvature omental margin, en face

    A7–A9: Greater curvature omental margin, en face

    A10–A12: Mass in relation to proximal false margin, perpendicular

    A 13–A 15: Fullface section of polypoid mass in relation to serosal surface, trisected with greatest depth of invasion

    A 16–A 18: Fullface section of polypoid mass in relation to serosal surface, trisected

    A 19–A 22: Representative sections polypoid area surrounding the mass, representative

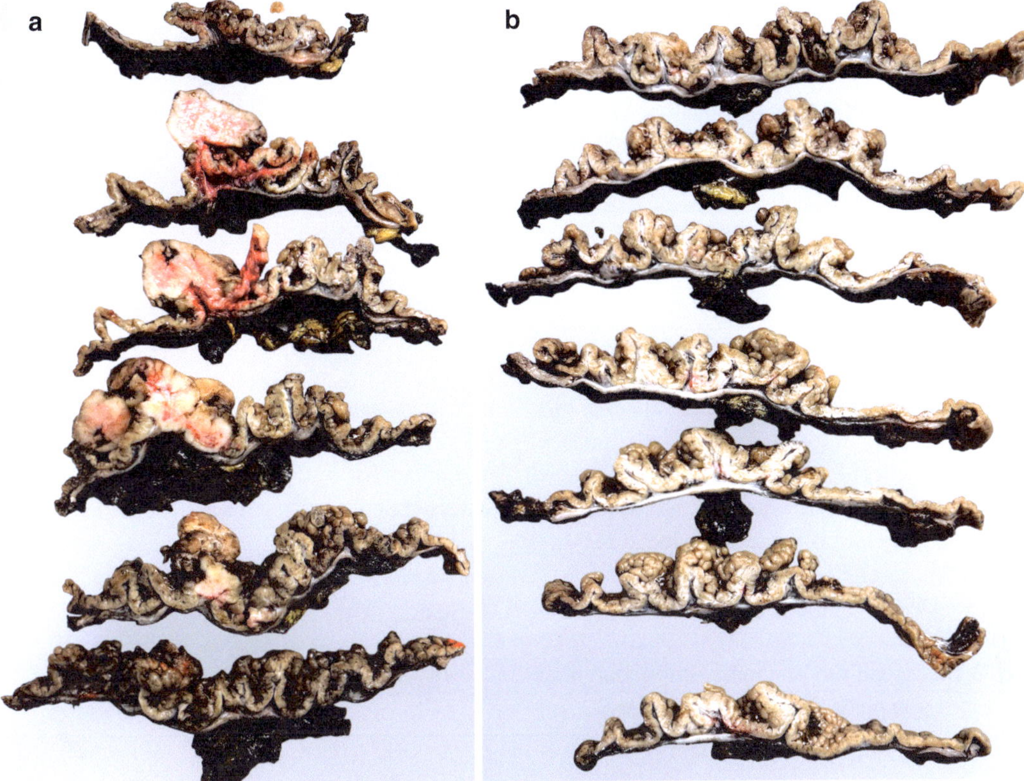

Fig. 5.34 (**a**) Cancerous lesion serially sectioned; (**b**) surrounding polyps serially sectioned

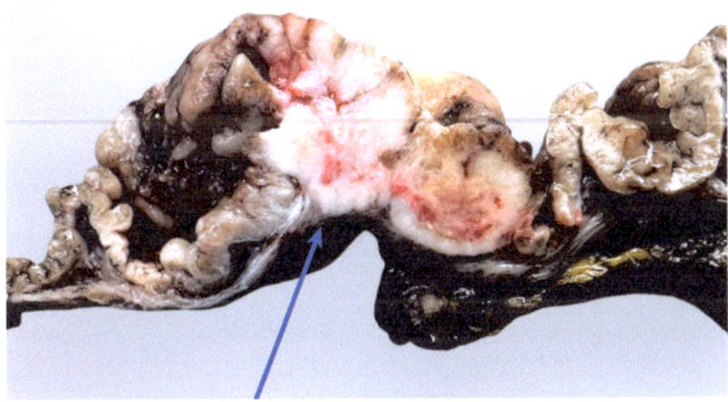

Fig. 5.35 Section of cancerous lesion with greatest depth of invasion

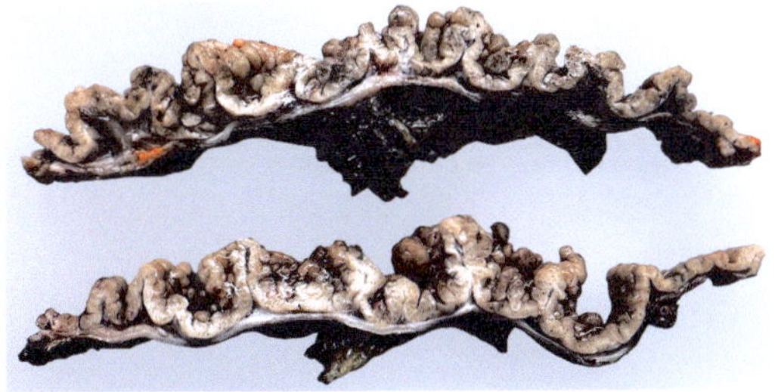

Fig. 5.36 Sections of surrounding polyps

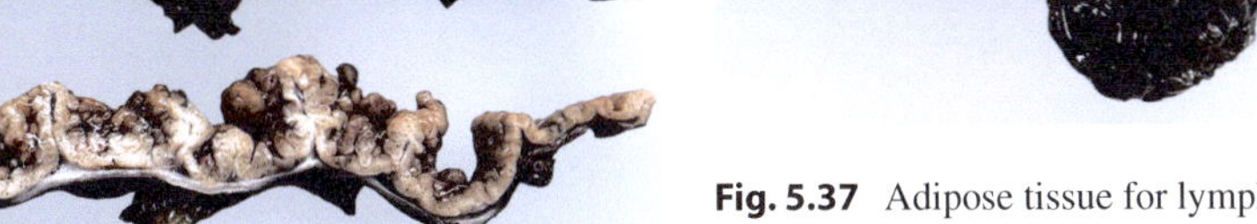

Fig. 5.37 Adipose tissue for lymph nodes

A 23–A 34: Representative sections of polypoid area inferior to mass
A 35:3 lymph node candidates, whole
A 36: 2 lymph node candidates, whole
A 37–A 56: Adipose tissue for lymph nodes

5.8 Appendix: Level III CPT 88304

The appendix is a very common specimen received in the surgical pathology lab. An appendectomy is performed to remove the appendix for issues such as appendicitis or malignancy. However, the appendix is sometimes removed incidentally while the surgeon is performing another surgery and is in the same location.

Step 1: Describe and measure the appendix (Fig. 5.38).
Step 2: Shave and submit the resection margin en face. If you place all sections in 1 cassette, ink the resection margin to designate.

Step 3: Serially section the appendix from proximal to distal.
Step 4: The tip of the appendix is bisected longitudinally as shown in Fig. 5.39 by the blue arrow.
Step 5: Submit both tip halves, the resection margin (inked) and one or two representative cross sections of appendix as shown in Fig. 5.40.

Example Dictation
Specimen A is received in formalin labeled with patient's name, medical record number, "appendix" and consists of a pink-red appendix (7.2 × 1.0 × 1.0 cm) with minimal attached mesoappendix and scant exudate and dilated vessels spanning the serosal surface. The speci-

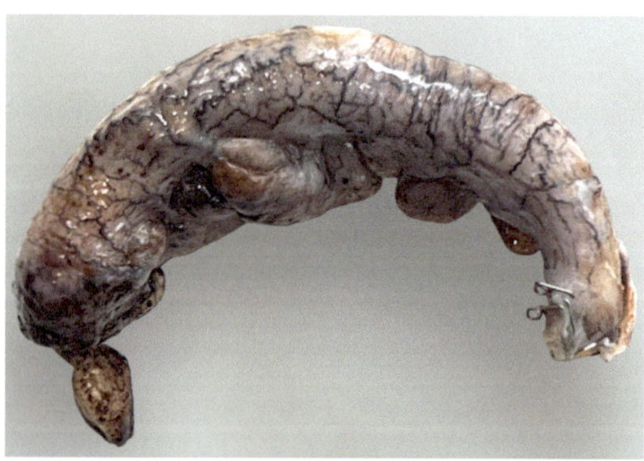

Fig. 5.38 Appendix

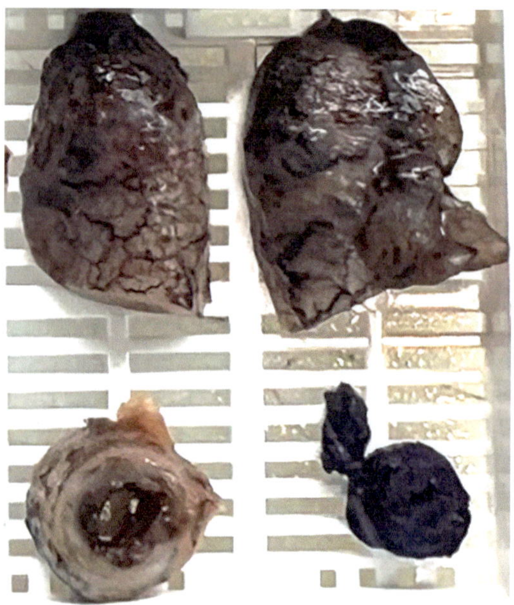

Fig. 5.40 Appendix section submission

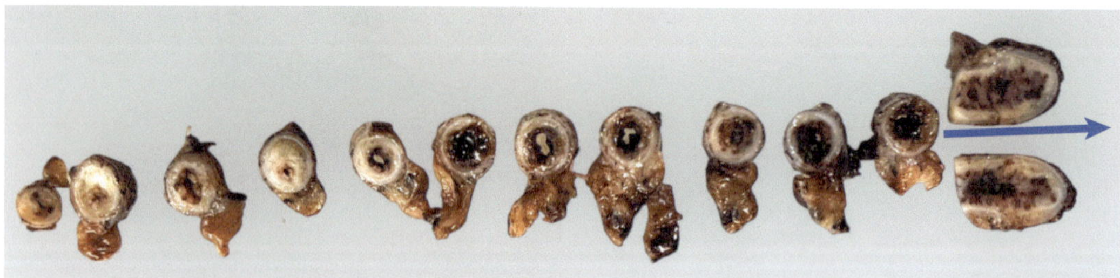

Fig. 5.39 Serially sectioned appendix and appendiceal tip bisected

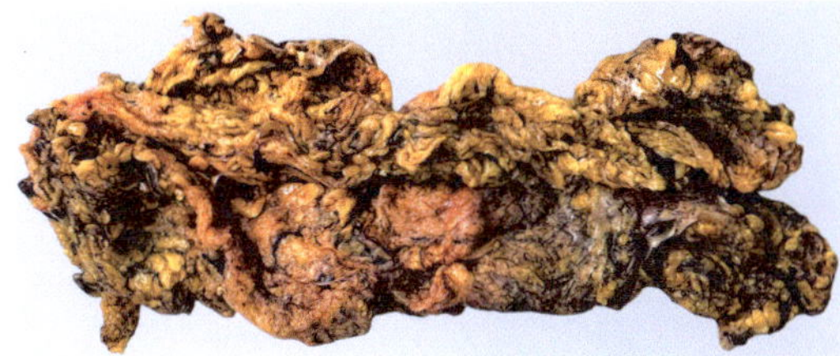

Fig. 5.41 Omentum

men is serially sectioned to reveal a slightly dilated, hemorrhagic lumen filled with red-brown material. No nodules are identified at the appendiceal tip. The tip, bisected, margin enface, and representative appendix is submitted in A1 (margin inked blue).

5.9 Omentum: Level IV CPT 88305

The omentum is occasionally removed during surgery to allow for a clearer surgical field. However, omentum is often resected as part of pathologic staging. Identifying tumor in the omentum will up-stage the patient.

Step 1: Describe, measure, and weight the specimen. (Fig. 5.41)

Step 2: Serially section the specimen as shown in Fig. 5.42.

Step 3: Assess for nodules present within the omentum. If present, measure and describe the nodules.

Step 4: Submit representative sections of the specimen as seen in Fig. 5.43. If nodules are present, submit representative sections of the nodules.

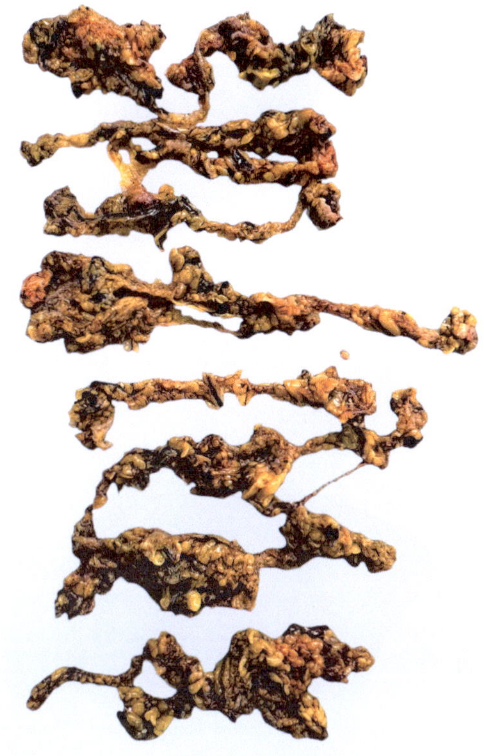

Fig. 5.42 Omentum serially sectioned

Example Dictation

Specimen A is received in formalin labeled with patient's name, medical record number, "omentum" and consists of an unoriented fragment of tan-yellow adipose tissue ($10.4 \times 5.9 \times 2.6$ cm, 42 g) which is serially sectioned to reveal tan-yellow, lacey, lobulated cut surfaces with no nodules present. Representative sections are submitted in A1–A3.

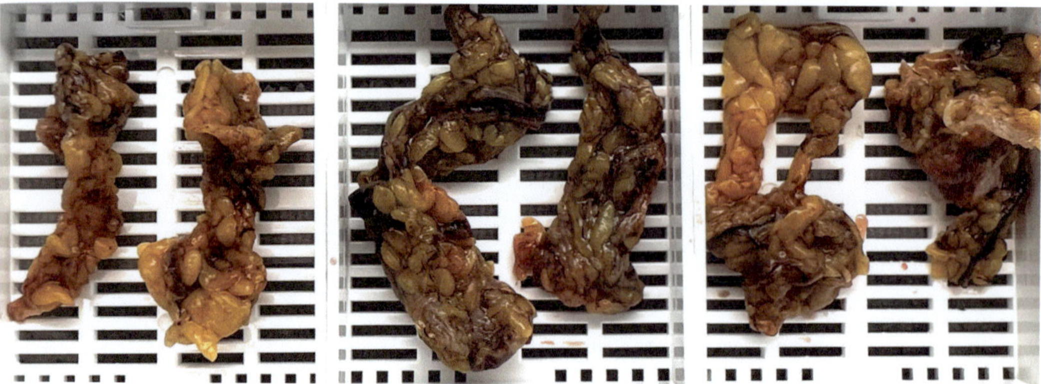

Fig. 5.43 Omentum Section submission

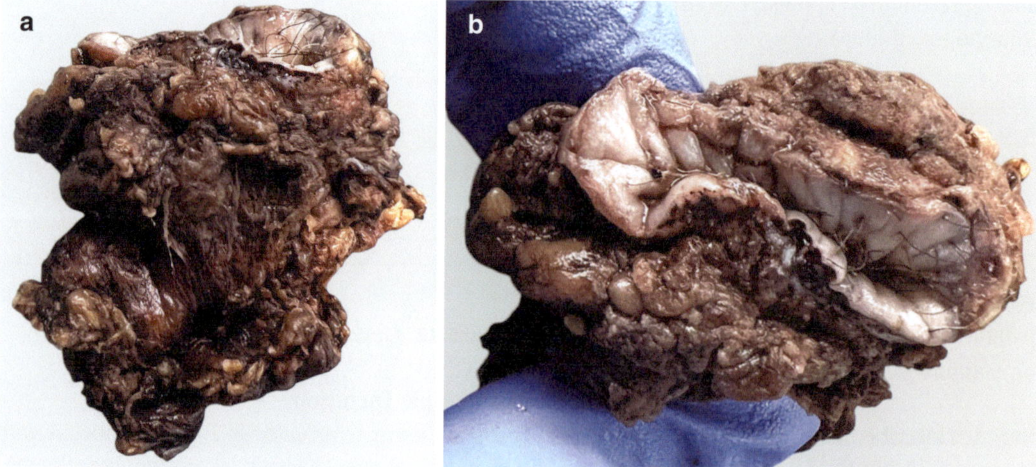

Fig. 5.44 (**a**) Ostomy; (**b**) external margin with skin

5.10   Colostomy Stoma:- Level III CPT 88304

A stoma is the end segment of the bowel that opens to the skin surface. During surgery for the removal of a segment of bowel, it is common for the surgeon to create an ostomy for the patient which will function while the patient heals from surgery. Once the patient is fully healed, the ostomy can be reversed, removing the stoma.

Step 1: Orient, describe, and measure the specimen. (Fig. 5.44a)

Step 2: Identify, describe, and measure the skin surface as shown in Fig. 5.44b. The skin is the external margin and is present in almost all ostomy specimens.

Step 3: Identify the mucosal margin as shown in Fig. 5.45a. The mucosal end is the internal margin.

Step 4: Shave and submit the internal margin en face as shown in Fig. 5.45b.

Step 5: Open the specimen from internal to external seen in Fig. 5.46.

Step 6: Describe the mucosa. (Fig. 5.47a)

Step 7: Take a perpendicular section of the mucosa in relation to the skin and submit on edge as seen in Fig. 5.47b.

Step 8: Submit the internal margin en face and a representative perpendicular section of the external margin with skin as shown in Fig. 5.48.

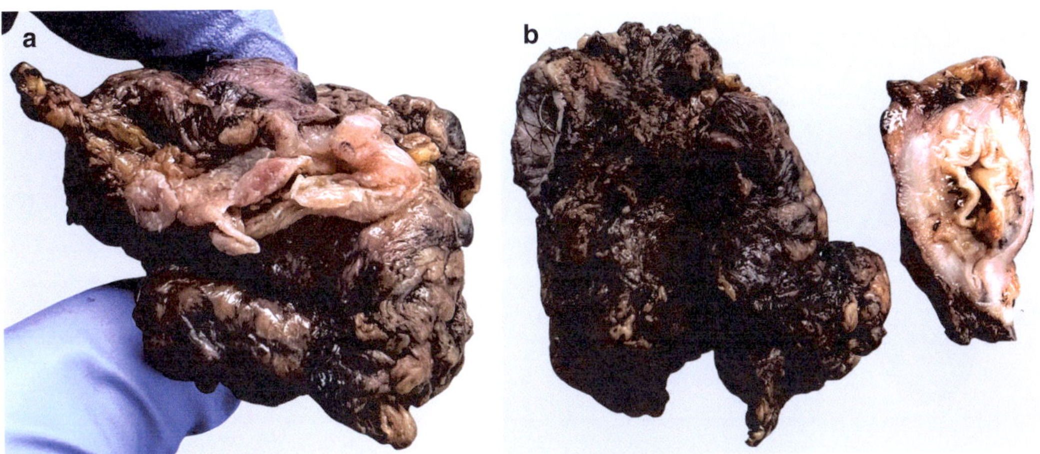

Fig. 5.45 (**a**) Internal end; (**b**) Internal margin en face

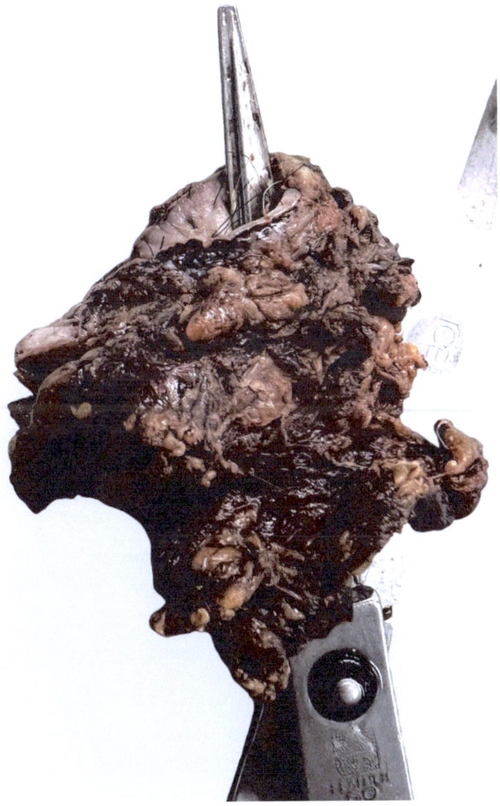

Fig. 5.46 Opening ostomy

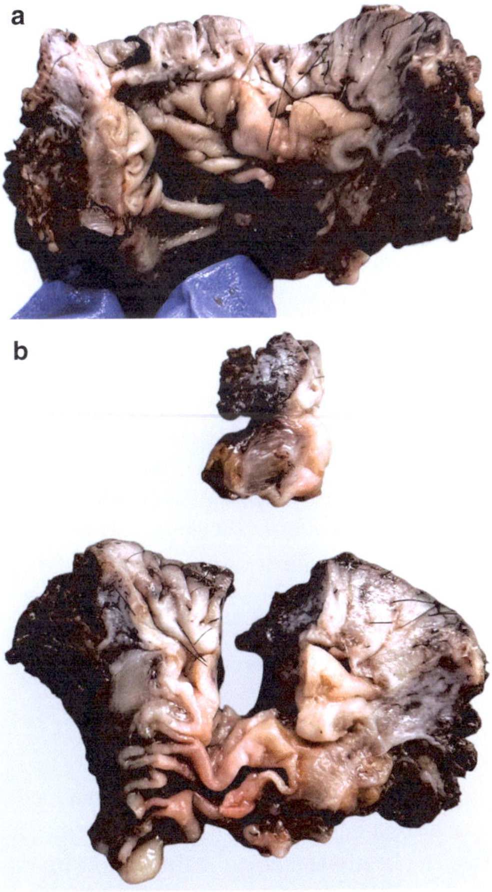

Fig. 5.47 (**a**) Ostomy opened; (**b**) Skin section perpendicular

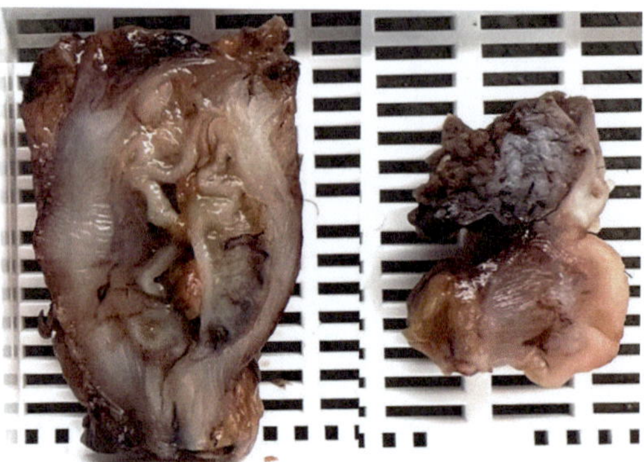

Fig. 5.48 Ostomy section submission

Example Dictation

Specimen A is received in formalin labeled with patient's name, medical record number, "ostomy" and consists of a segment of bowel (3.9 × 2.3 × 2.0 cm) extending to an ostomy site (3.1 × 1.0 cm) surrounded by tan-brown skin. The segment is opened to reveal tan, folded mucosa within.

Section code

    A1: Internal margin, en face

    A2: External margin, representative, perpendicular with skin

5.11 Small Bowel GSW:- Level V CPT 88307

Trauma such as gun-shot wound, stab wound, or motor vehicle accident can cause major damage to all organs but the bowel is very common as it spans the majority of the abdomen. These damaged segments are then resected.

Step 1: Describe and measure the segment of bowel. (Fig. 5.49)

Step 2: Submit the unoriented margins en face as shown in Fig. 5.50.

Step 3: Identify and describe the area of trauma. Figure 5.51a shows a defect from the external surface of the small bowel, and Fig. 5.51b shows the same defect from the mucosal surface of the bowel.

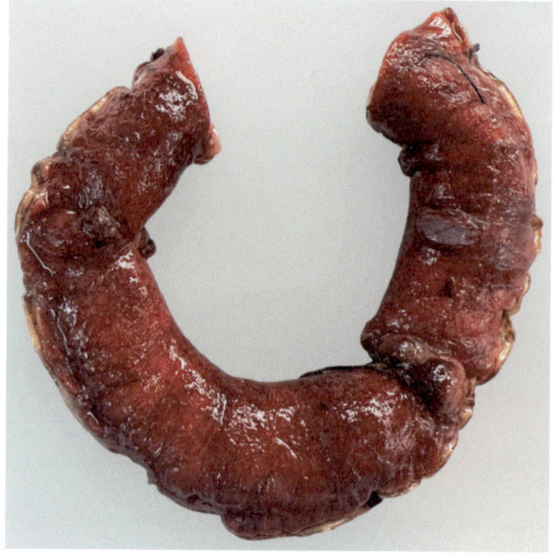

Fig. 5.49 Small bowel segment

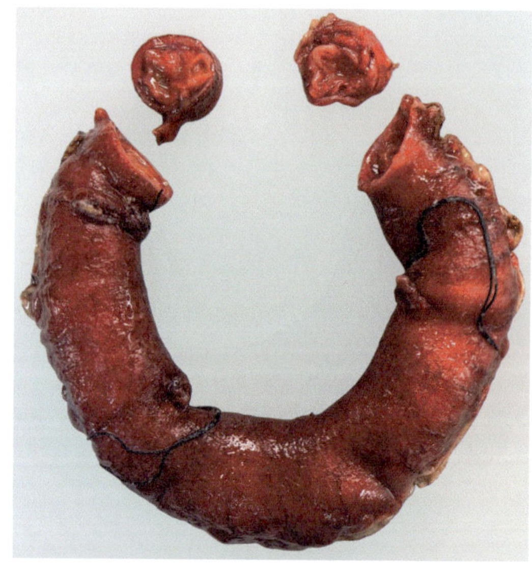

Fig. 5.50 Small bowel margins

Step 4: Count the number of defects and measure the range of size of the defects. Five or more defects can be described as multiple defects.

Step 5: Take representative sections of the defects as shown in Fig. 5.52.

Step 6: Assess the remainder of the small bowel for lesions.

Step 7: Submit sections. Sections submitted are the margins and representative sections of the defect as shown in Fig. 5.53.

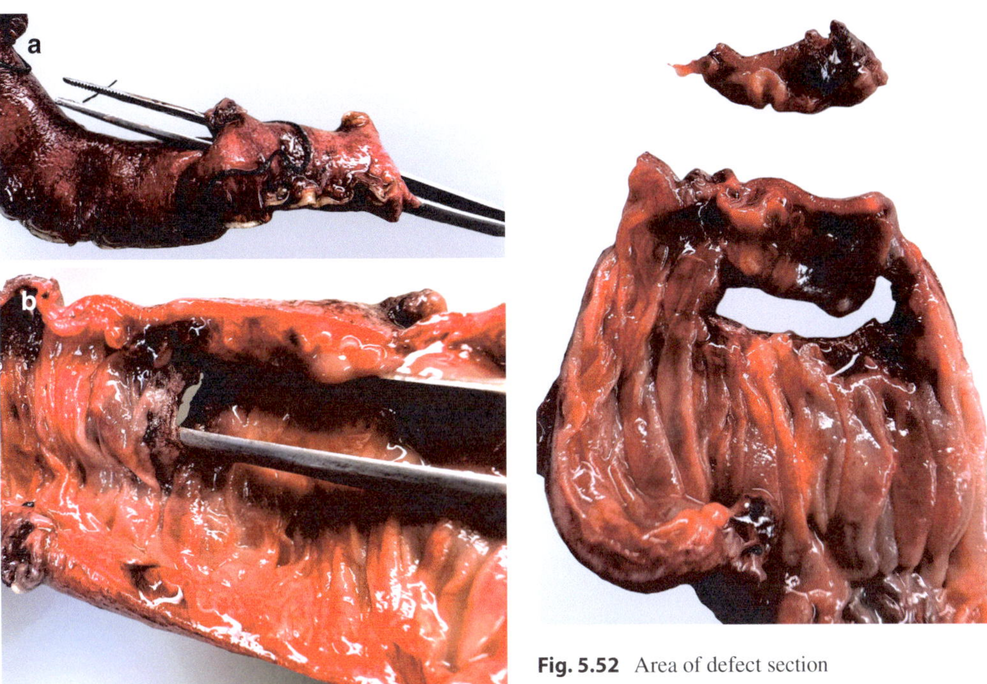

Fig. 5.52   Area of defect section

Fig. 5.51   (**a**) Small bowel defect external view; (**b**) small bowel defect internal view

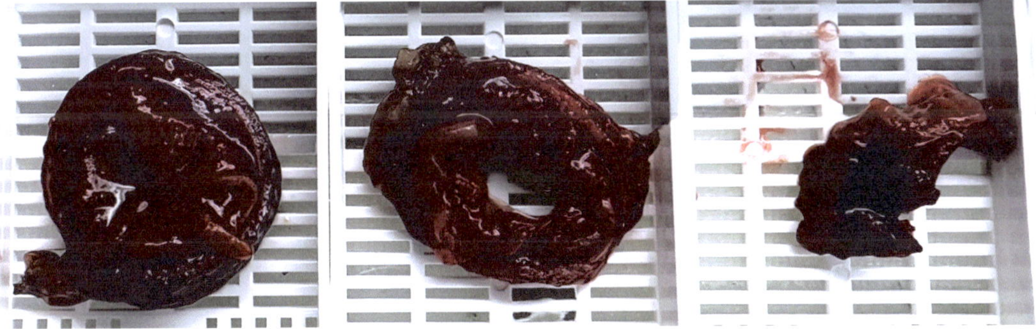

Fig. 5.53   Small bowel for trauma section submission

Example Dictation

Specimen A is received in formalin labeled with patient's name, medical record number, "small bowel" and consists of an unoriented segment of dusky small bowel (21.8 cm in length by 2.2 cm in diameter) with one transmural defect (1.3 cm in diameter) which comes within 2.9 cm of the closest unoriented margin. The bowel is opened to reveal tan, folded mucosa which is hemorrhagic surrounding the area of defect.

Section code

    A1-A2: Unoriented margins, en face

    A3: Area of defect, perpendicular, representative

5.12 Small Bowel for Stricture:- Level V CPT 88307

Stricture of the bowel can be caused by many reasons but often is due to chronic inflammation which causes the bowel wall to thicken in areas causing stricture of the bowel.

Step 1: Describe and measure the segment of the small bowel. (Fig. 5.54)

Step 2: Submit the margins en face as shown in Fig. 5.55.

Step 3: Open the small bowl along the antimesenteric border as shown in Fig. 5.56.

Step 4: Identify the area of stricture. In Fig. 5.57, the stricture is designated with a blue arrow.

Step 5: Measure the diameter of the stricture and how close it comes to each margin.

Step 6: Assess the remainder of the small bowel for defects or lesions.

Step 7: Sections submitted are the margins, area of stricture, and representative small bowel as shown in Fig. 5.58.

Example Dictation

Specimen A is received in formalin labeled with patient's name, medical record number, "small bowel stricture" and consists of an unoriented

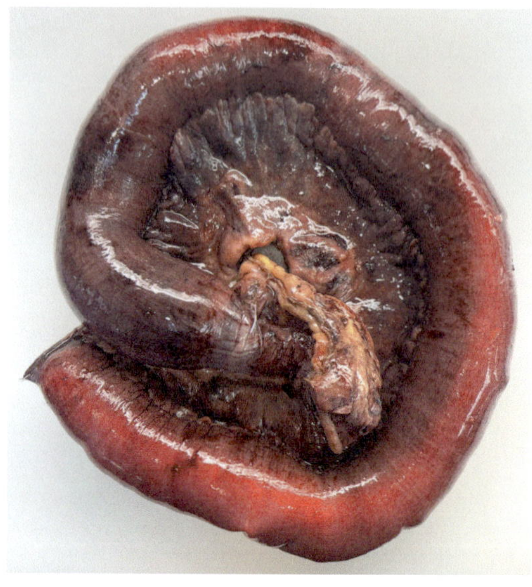

Fig. 5.54 Small bowel for stricture

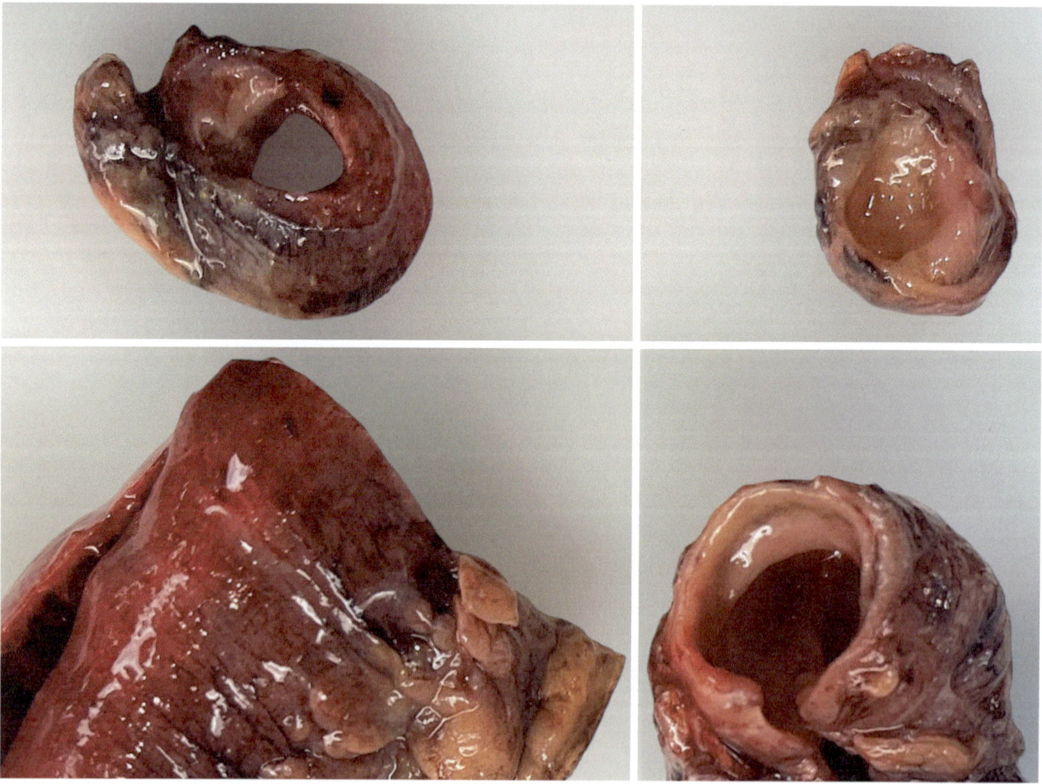

Fig. 5.55 Small bowel margins en face

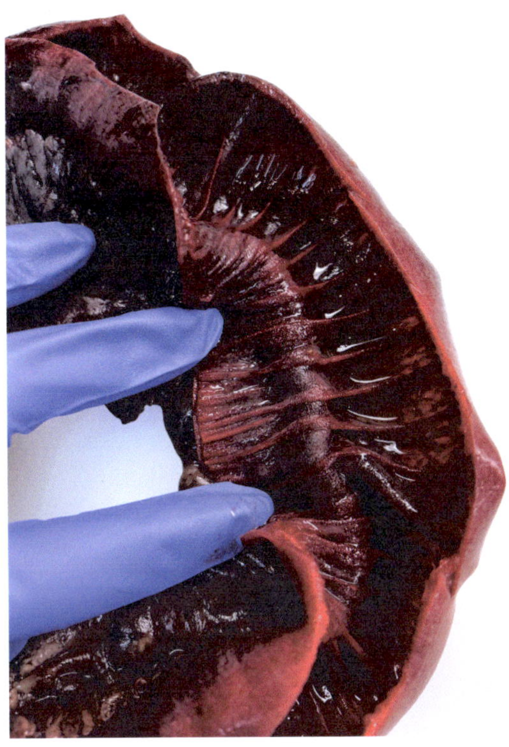

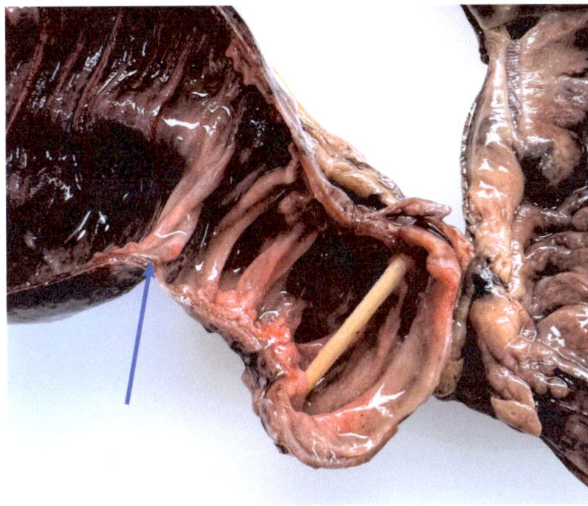

Fig. 5.57 Small bowel area of stricture

Fig. 5.56 Small bowel open

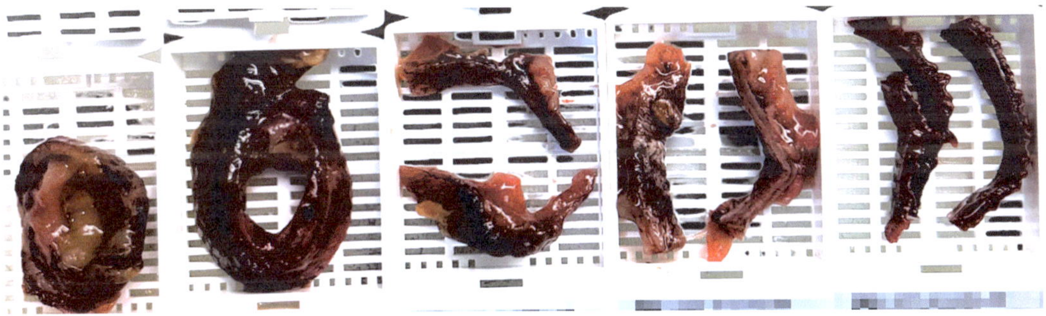

Fig. 5.58 Small bowel for stricture sections submission

segment of partially dusky small bowel (23.3 cm in length and ranging in diameter from 1.1 to 2.9 cm). The specimen is opened to reveal markedly dusky, flattened mucosa leading to a focal area of stricture (1.1 cm in diameter). The remaining mucosa is tan-pink and folded. No lesions or defects are identified.

Section code
A 1-A 2: Unoriented margins, en face
A3: Area of stricture, perpendicular, representative

A4: Tan, folded mucosa, representative
A5: Dusky, flattened mucosa, representative

5.13 Small Bowel for Crohn's or Ulcerative Colitis:- Level III CPT 88304

Crohn's and ulcerative colitis are both forms of inflammatory bowel disease that can often be confused due to their many similarities such as constipation, diarrhea, and cramps. The location can help differentiate. Crohn's disease causes irregular inflammation that can occur anywhere in the intestines. Ulcerative colitis occurs in the large intestine and is diffuse, continuous inflammation in the colon. Both types of inflammatory bowel disease are handled similarly in the gross room [6].

Step 1: Describe and measure the bowel segment. In Fig. 5.59, terminal ileum and cecum are present, and the appendix has previously been surgically removed.

Step 2: Describe the serosal surface and the mesenteric adipose tissue of the bowel.

Step 3: Shave and submit the proximal and distal margin. (Fig. 5.60)

Step 4: Open the bowel segment as shown in Fig. 5.60.

Step 5: Describe the mucosal surface of the bowel. In Fig. 5.61, the terminal ileum mucosa is intermittently flattened and granular (red arrow) with unremarkable mucosa between (blue arrow).

Step 6: Take representative sections of the flattened areas in relation to the unremarkable areas as seen in Fig. 5.62.

Step 7: Take representative sections of the cecum as seen in Fig. 5.63.

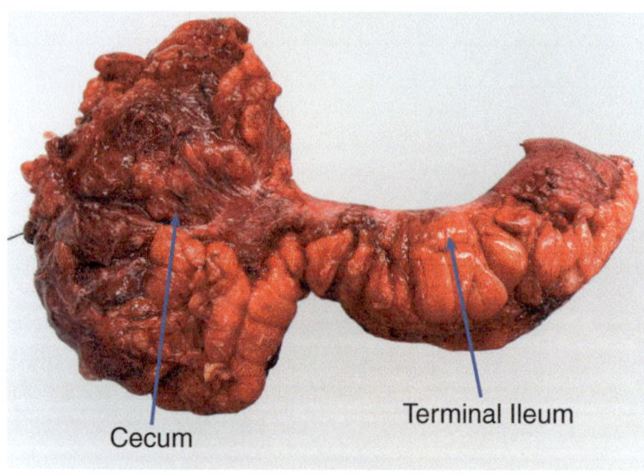

Fig. 5.59 Terminal ileum and cecum

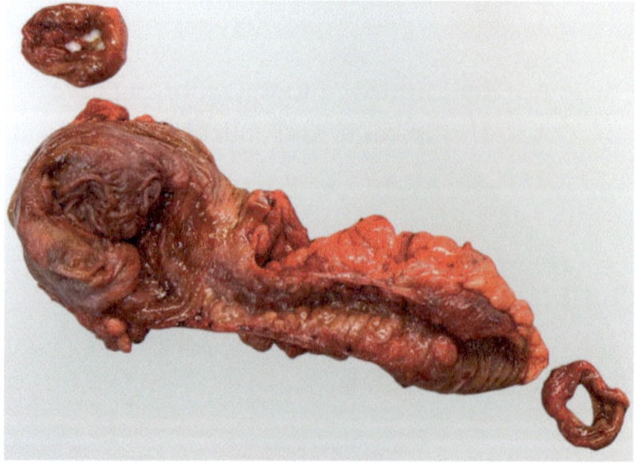

Fig. 5.60 Margins and bowel opened

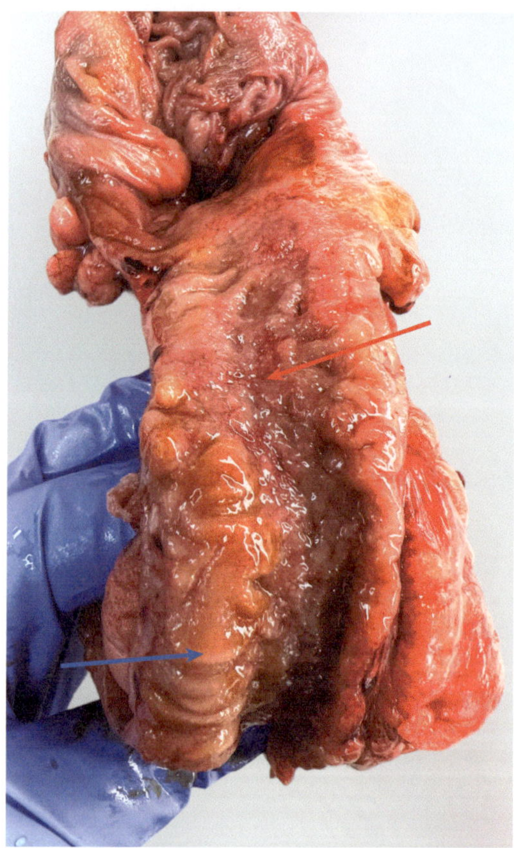

Fig. 5.61 Flat, granular mucosa and normal mucosa

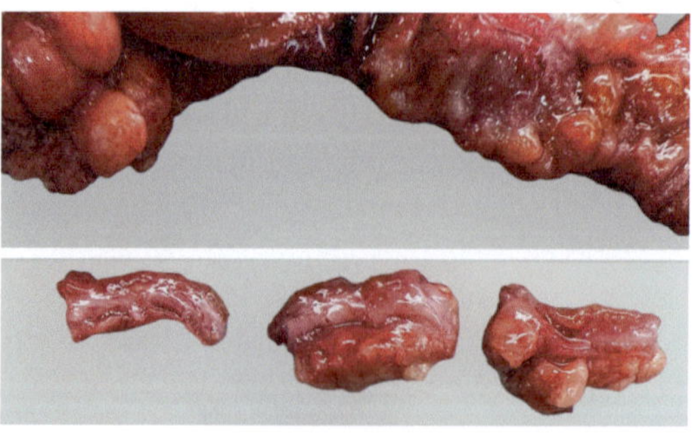

Fig. 5.62 Terminal ileum sections

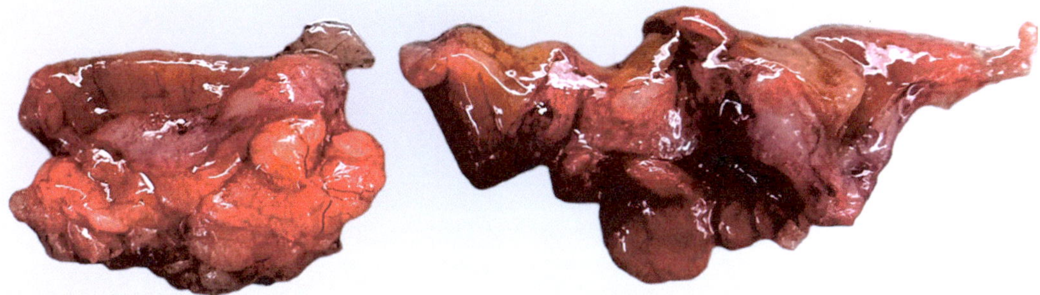

Fig. 5.63 Cecum sections

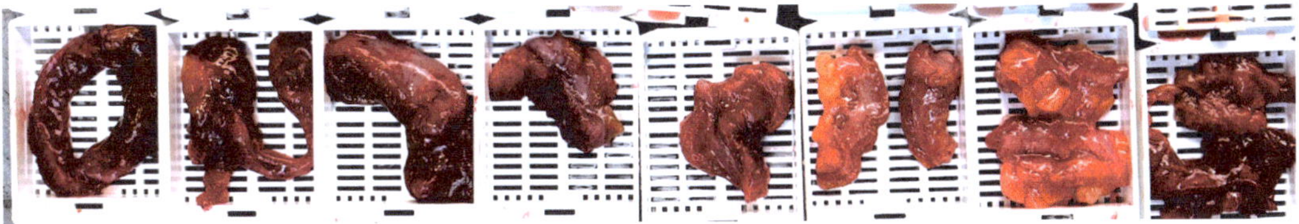

Fig. 5.64 Terminal ileum and cecum section submission

Step 8: Submit appendix, if present.

Step 9: Submit the margins and representative sections of the bowel as seen in Fig. 5.64.

Step 10: Submit lymph nodes. Lymph nodes are often slightly enlarged. Communicate with the pathologists concerning lymph nodes.

Example Dictation

Specimen A is received in formalin labeled with patient's name, medical record number, "small bowel and cecum" and consists of an unoriented segment of small bowel (18.2 cm in length by 2.4 cm in diameter) with attached cecum (7.8 × 4.6 × 4.0 cm) and no attached appendix. The bowel segment is opened to reveal granular, flattened mucosa irregularly spanning the terminal ileum, coming with-in 1.8 cm of the proximal margin and admixed with unremarkable mucosa. The cecum mucosa is tan-brown and folded. No masses or defects are identified.

Section code

A1: Unoriented margin, en face

A 2-A 3: Unoriented margins, bisected, en face

A4–A7: Granular, flattened mucosa of terminal ileum, representative

A8: Cecum, representative

5.14 Small Bowel for Intussusception: Level III CPT 88304

Intussusception occurs when a portion of the bowel folds inside itself. This causes obstruction of the bowel and can be dangerous to the patient. Intussusception is often caused secondary to a lesion within the bowel whether the lesion is cancer or a benign polyp, intussusception can occur.

Step 1: Describe and measure the bowel segment. (Fig. 5.65a)

Step 2: Identify the possible area of intussusception which is identified by the blue arrow in Fig. 5.65b. It is possible the area of intussusception cannot be identified. During surgery, the area can be pulled, and the folding of the bowel can be released.

Step 3: Shave and submit the margins en face as shown in Fig. 5.66.

Step 4: Open the bowl along the antimesenteric border exposing the area of intussusception as shown in Fig. 5.67.

Step 5: Identify, describe, and measure any mass within the area of intussusception.

Step 6: Measure how close the lesion comes to the margins.

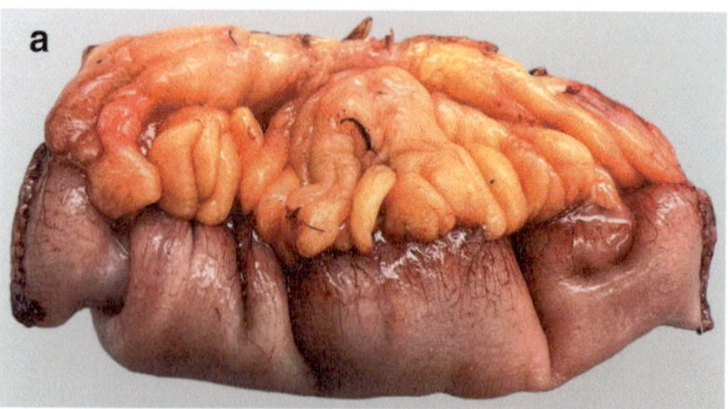

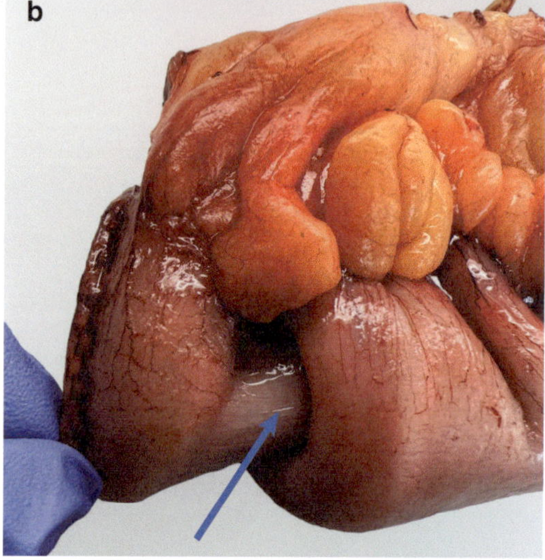

Fig. 5.65 (**a**) Unoriented small bowel segment; (**b**) area of intussusception

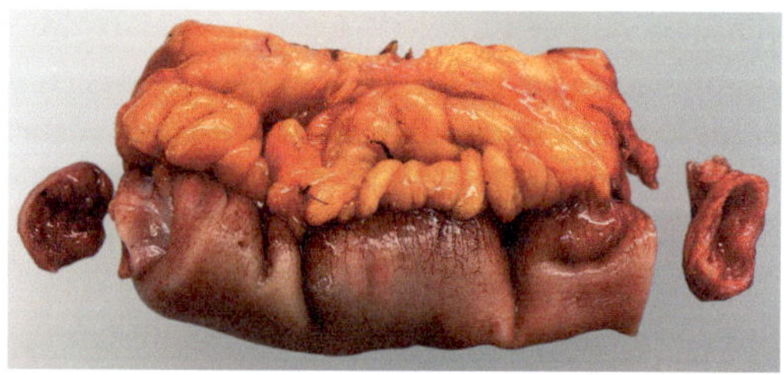

Fig. 5.66 Small bowel margins en face

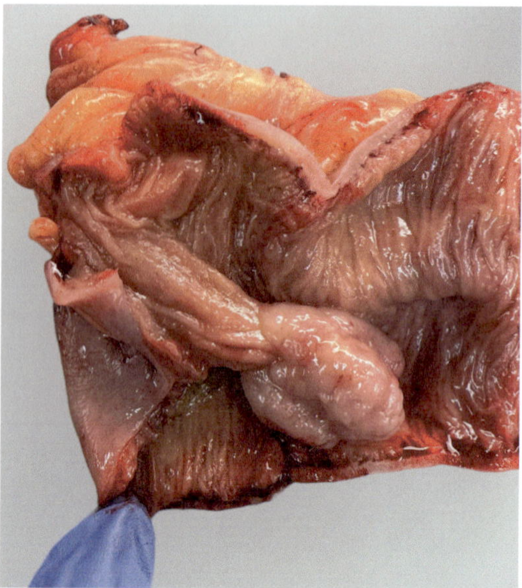

Fig. 5.67 Lesion within the area of intussusception

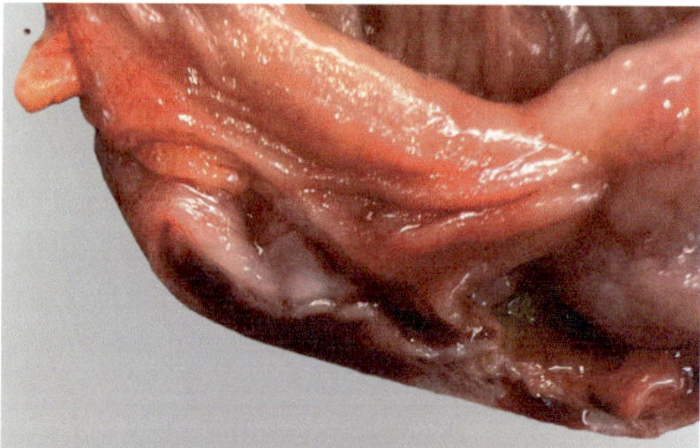

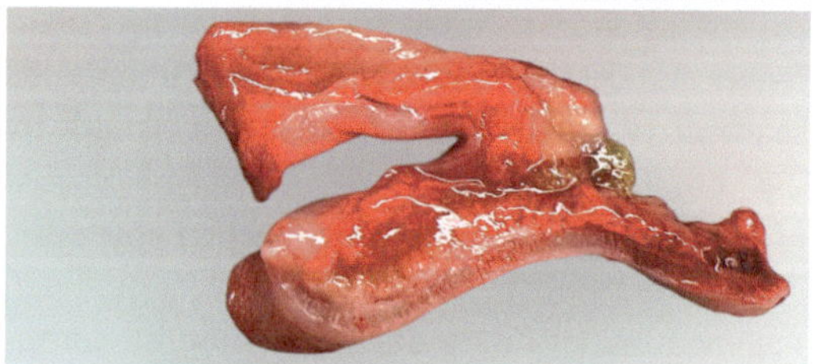

Fig. 5.68 Representative section of intussusception

Step 7: Submit a representative section of the area of intussusception as shown in Fig. 5.68.

Step 8: Take representative sections of the lesion. If the lesion is small, it can be submitted entirely as seen in Fig. 5.69a. In this example, the lesion can be bisected as shown in Fig. 5.69b and submitted entirely.

Step 9: Submit representative sections of the small bowel.

Step 10: Sections include margins, area of intussusception, the lesion, and representative unremarkable small bowel as shown in Fig. 5.70.

Example Dictation

Specimen A is received in formalin labeled with patient's name, medical record number, "small bowel resection and intra-abdominal mass" and

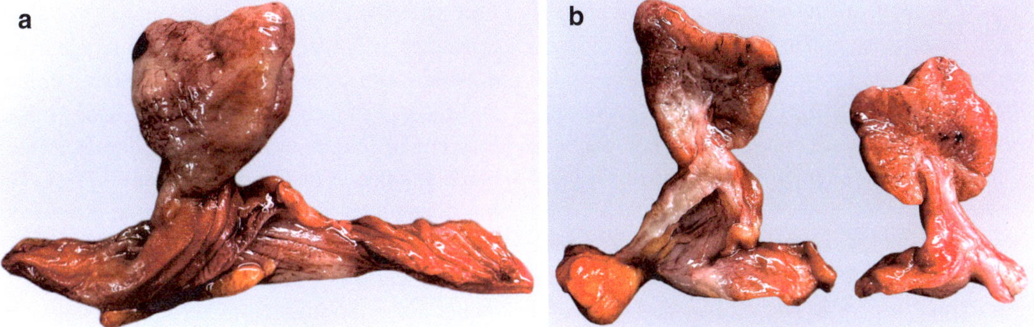

Fig. 5.69 (**a**) Lesion whole; (**b**) lesion bisected

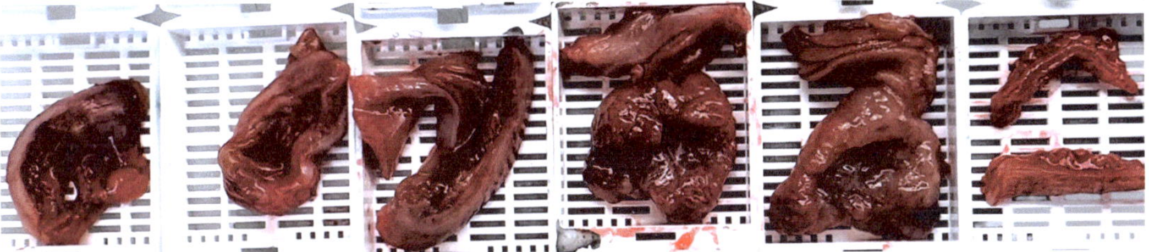

Fig. 5.70 Small bowel for intussusception section submission

consists of an unoriented segment of small bowel (11.5 cm in length by 2.2 cm in diameter) With an area of intussusception (2.0 cm in length) which comes with an 1.4 cm of the nearest unoriented margin. The bowel segment is opened to reveal a tan-pink, pedunculated polyp (2.6 × 2.5 × 1.9 cm) present within the area of intussusception. The polyp is sectioned to reveal tan cut surfaces. The remaining mucosa is tan-pink and folded.

Section code

    A 1-A 2: Unoriented margins, en face
    A3: Area of intussusception, representative
    A4-A5: Polyp, bisected
    A6: Unremarkable bowel, representative

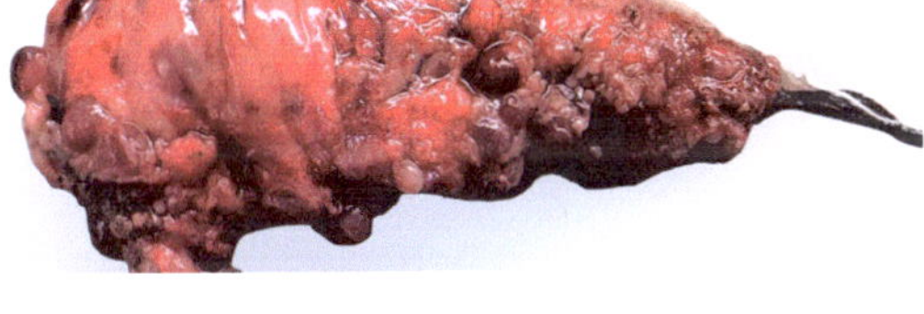

Fig. 5.71 Bowel for Hirschsprung's disease

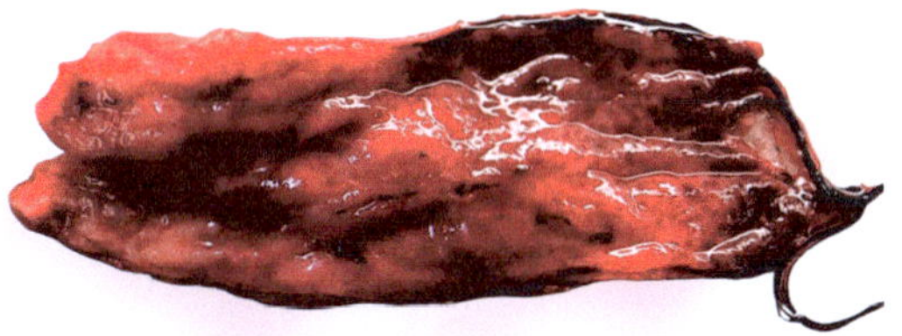

Fig. 5.72 Bowel opened

5.15   Hirschsprung's Resection

Hirschsprung's disease is the lack of ganglion cells present in the bowel. Without these cells, the bowel struggles to move stool and often becomes blocked. Typically, the lack of ganglion cells is segmental, and the portion of bowel lacking in these cells can be removed.

Step 1: Orient the segment of bowel. In Fig. 5.71, the black stitches designate the distal end.
Step 2: Describe and measure the segment of the bowel.
Step 3: Open the bowel segment as shown in Fig. 5.72.
Step 4: Describe the mucosal surface of the bowel.

Step 5: Remove a full-length, long thin strip of the bowel as shown in Fig. 5.73. Keep the strip oriented.

Step 6: Cut the strip of bowel into 1 cm segments as seen in Fig. 5.74. Use a ruler to measure 1 cm segments. Keep each segment oriented.

Step 7: Ink the proximal and distal end of each segment of the bowel strip. In Fig. 5.74, the proximal aspect is inked blue, and the distal aspect is inked black.

Step 8: Submit each segment of the strip per one cassette from proximal to distal as shown in Fig. 5.75. The first cassette will contain the true proximal margin and the last cassette will contain the true distal margin. Margins can also be submitted en face before the strip of colon is removed depending on the pathologist's preference.

Step 9: Palpate the attached adipose tissue for lymph nodes and submit all lymph nodes.

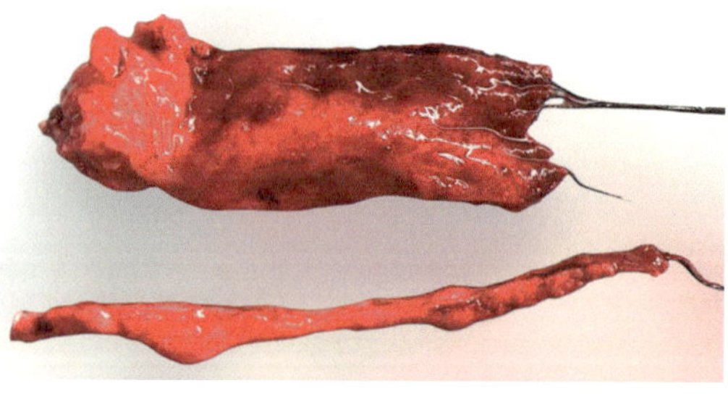

Fig. 5.73 Full-length strip of bowel removed

Example Dictation

Specimen A is received in formalin labeled with patient's name, medical record number, "colon" and consists of a segment of slightly dusky bowel (6.1 cm in length by 2.2 cm in diameter) with black stitches at one end designating distal. The bowel segment is opened to reveal hemorrhagic, markedly flattened mucosa. A longitudinal full-length section of bowel is divided into 1 cm segments and submitted from proximal to distal in A1–A6.

Ink code
  Blue: proximal of each segment
  Black: distal of each segment

5.16 Colon for Diverticulitis: Level III CPT 88304

Diverticulosis is the diagnosis of small bulging pouches present in the bowel. These pouches can become inflamed, leading to diverticulitis. Occasionally, if antibiotics fail or a diverticula ruptures, the bowel segment will need surgically removed.

Step 1: Describe and measure the specimen. (Fig. 5.76)
Step 2: Orient the specimen, if orientation is given.
Step 3: Shave the end margins and submit en face (Fig. 5.77)

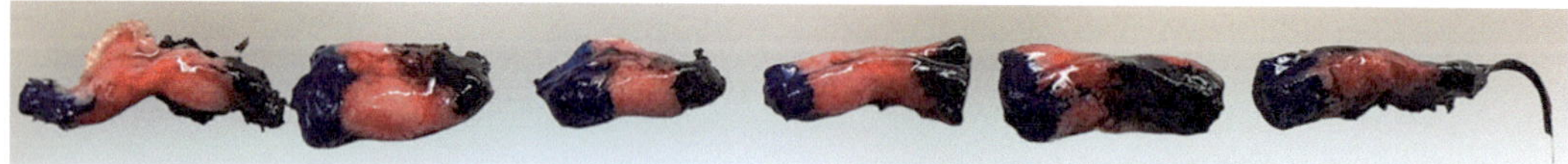

Fig. 5.74 Strip of bowel in 1 cm segments and inked

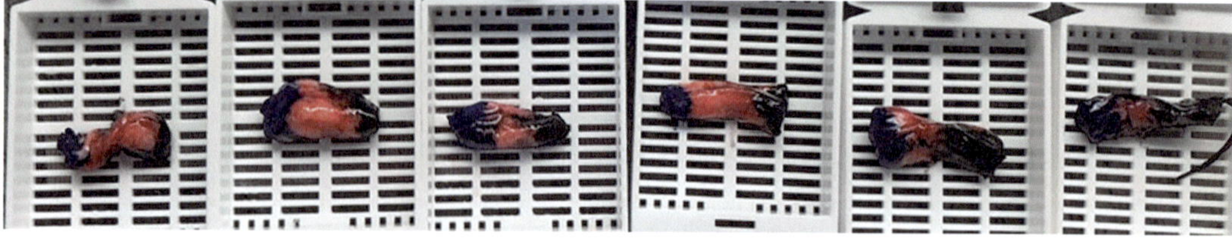

Fig. 5.75 Strip of bowel submitted from proximal to distal

Fig. 5.76 Colon segment

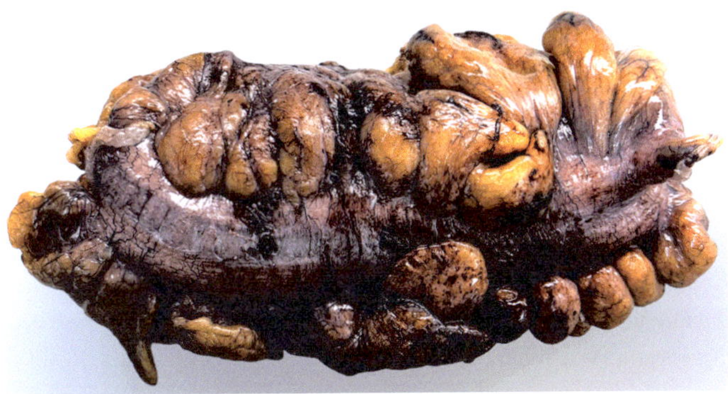

Fig. 5.77 Colon segment margins

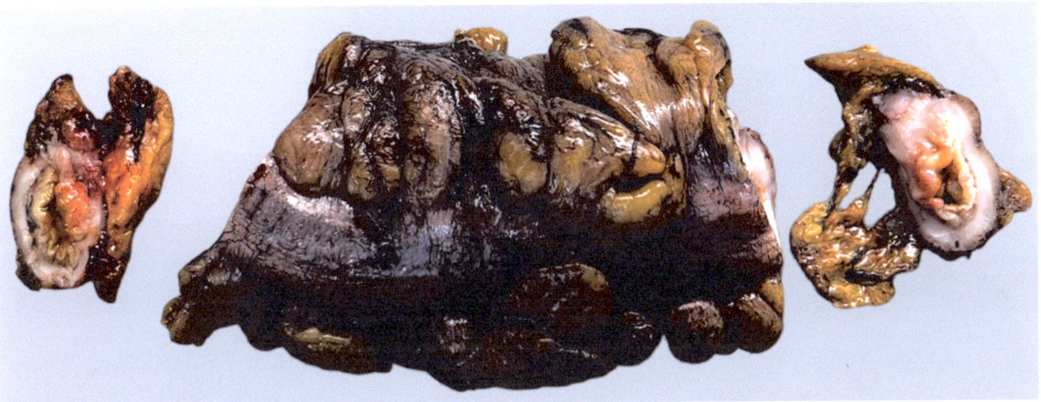

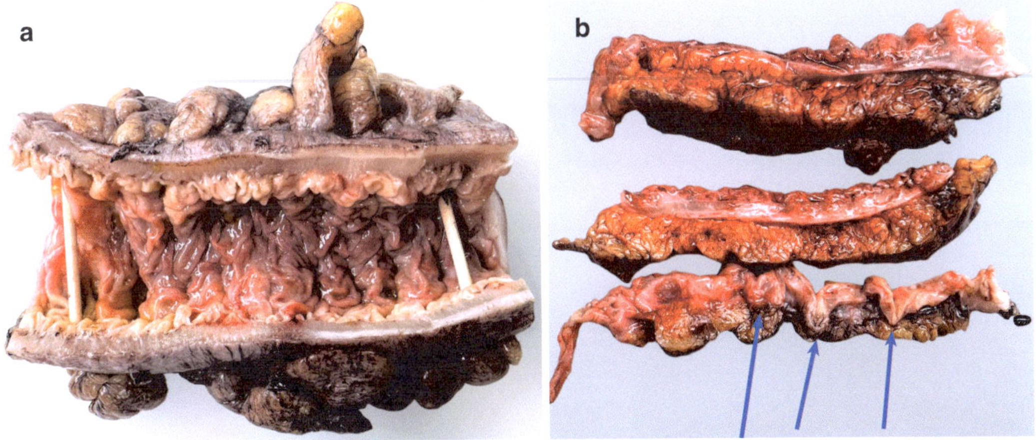

Fig. 5.78 (**a**) Colon segment opened; (**b**) colon longitudinally sectioned

Step 4: Open the colon segment along the antimesenteric border as shown in Fig. 5.78a.

Step 5: Longitudinally section the colon. Diverticula are best visualized after sectioning the colon. The blue arrows on Fig. 5.78b show diverticula after sectioning.

Step 6: Assess the diverticula for evidence of rupture. In Fig. 5.79a, the diverticula are intact.

Step 7: Take representative sections of diverticula as shown in Fig. 5.79b.

Step 8: Submit the resection margins and representative sections of the diverticula as shown in Fig. 5.80.

Step 9: Palpate the attached adipose tissue for lymph nodes.

Example Dictation

Specimen A is received in formalin labeled with patient's name, medical record number, "colon, sigmoid" and consists of an unoriented segment of colon (12.2 cm in length by 2.1 cm in diameter) which is opened to reveal tan mucosa. The bowel is longitudinally sectioned to reveal multiple intact diverticula spanning the length of the specimen, without grossly identifiable rupture. The surrounding adipose tissue is palpable for 2 lymph node candidates (0.2 and 0.3 cm in diameter).

Section code

    A 1-A 2: Unoriented margins, en face
    A3–A5: Diverticula, representative
    A6:2 Lymph node candidates, whole

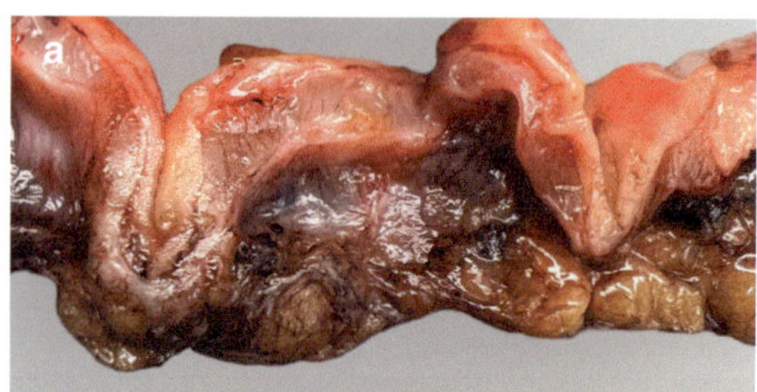

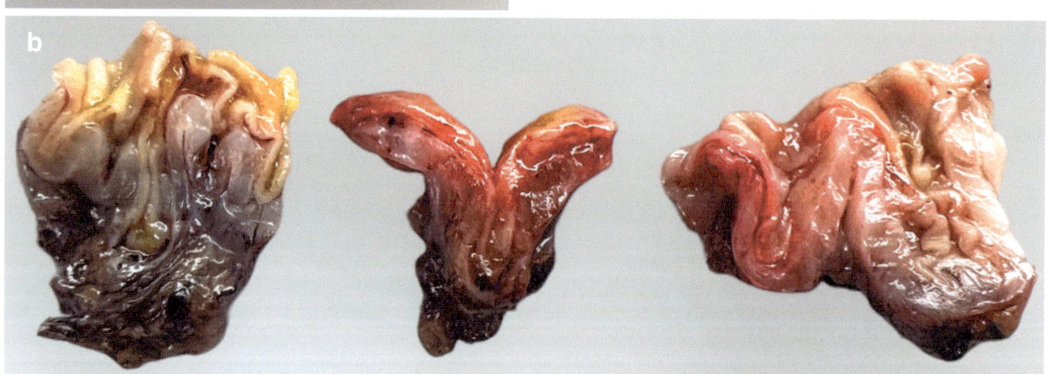

Fig. 5.79 (**a**) Colon diverticula; (**b**) diverticula sections

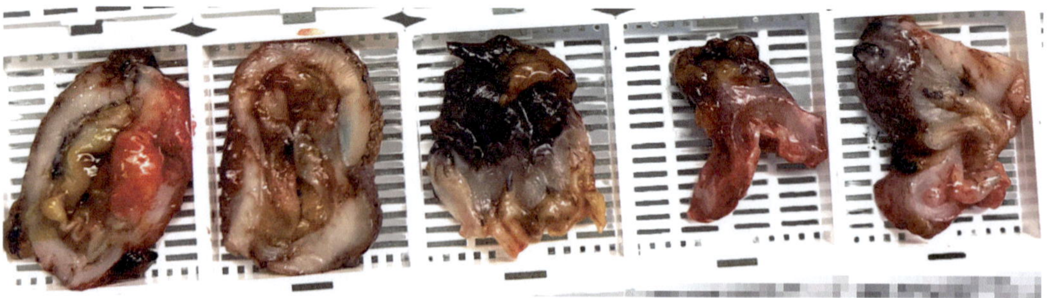

Fig. 5.80 Diverticulitis colon sections submitted

5.17 Right Hemicolectomy for Tumor: Level VI CPT 88309

Procedure (See Fig. 5.81 for Illustration of Procedures)

Right hemicolectomy: Removal of terminal ileum, cecum (with appendix), ascending colon, and possibly the hepatic flexure.

Transverse colectomy: Removal of transverse colon possibly with hepatic and/or splenic flexure.

Left hemicolectomy: Removal of distal transverse colon, splenic flexure, and descending colon.

Sigmoidectomy: Removal of entirety of the sigmoid with possible distal descending colon.

Low anterior resection: Removal of distal descending colon, sigmoid colon, and rectum.

Total abdominal resection: Removal of terminal ileum, cecum (with appendix), ascending colon, hepatic flexure, transverse colon, splenic flexure, descending colon, and sigmoid.

Abdominoperineal resection: Removal of distal descending colon, sigmoid colon, rectum, and anal skin [7]

Macroscopic Evaluation of Mesorectum The adipose tissue surrounding the rectum should be examined for completeness. The entire specimen is scored according to the worst area [7].

Incomplete
- Little bulk to the mesorectum
- Defects in the mesorectum down to the muscularis propria
- After transverse sectioning, the circumferential margin appears very irregular [7]

Nearly Complete
- Moderate bulk to the mesorectum
- Irregularity of the mesorectal surface with defects greater than 5 mm
- No visible areas of irregularity of the muscularis propria [7]

Complete
- Intact bulky mesorectum with a smooth surface

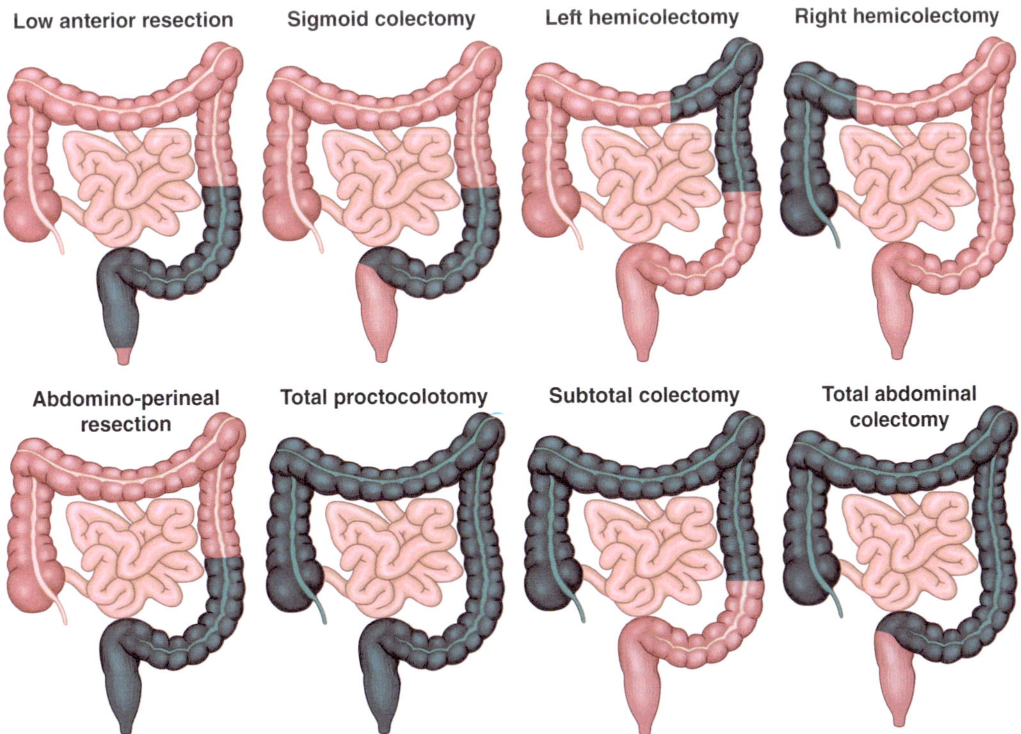

Fig. 5.81 Illustration of colectomy procedures

- Only minor irregularities of the mesorectal surface
- No surface defects greater than 5 mm in depth
- No coning toward the distal margin of the specimen
- After transverse sectioning, the circumferential margin appears smooth [7]

Tumor Site The protocol applies to all carcinomas arising in the colon and rectum. It excludes carcinomas of the vermiform appendix and low-grade neuroendocrine neoplasms (carcinoid tumors).

Describe the gross morphology of the tumor: exophytic/fungating, endophytic, ulcerated, and state its location. The right colon is subdivided into the cecum and the ascending colon. The left colon is subdivided into the transverse, descending colon, and sigmoid colon. The transition from sigmoid to rectum is marked by the fusion of the tenia coli of the sigmoid to form the circumferential longitudinal muscle of the rectal wall approximately 12 to 15 cm from the dentate line [7].

Tumor Size Measure the three-dimensional measurement of the tumor/mass.

Describe the tumor extent in terms of tumor involving the circumference of the lumen. State the distance of the tumor from the proximal, distal, and radial/circumferential margins [7].

Tumor Extent Measure the maximum depth of invasion (i.e., tumor invades through the muscularis propria into the pericolic fat but does not reach the serosa) [7.

Macroscopic Tumor Perforation Grossly identify if the lesion is perforating the bowel and/or is present on the outer surface of the specimen.

Margin Status Dictate how close the lesion comes to the proximal, distal, and radial margins of the specimen.

Describe Other Features Describe and measure all polyps identified. Describe any other structures or features (appendix, small bowel, diverticula).

Search for Lymph Nodes Search all pericolic adipose tissue for lymph nodes, lymph node candidates, and tumor deposits. Twelve lymph nodes are required, and additional adipose tissue should be submitted if 12 lymph nodes are not identified [7].

pT Designation
pT0: No evidence of primary tumor

pTis: Carcinoma in situ, intramucosal carcinoma

pT1: Tumor invades the submucosa

pT2: Tumor invades the muscularis propria

pT3: Tumor invades through the muscularis propria into pericolorectal tissues

pT4a: Tumor invades through the visceral peritoneum

pT4b: Tumor directly invades# or adheres to adjacent organs or structures [7]

The Radial Margin
The radial margin pT0: No evidence of primary tumor represents the adventitial soft tissue margin closest to the deepest penetration of tumor and is created surgically by blunt or sharp dissection of the retroperitoneal or subperitoneal aspect, respectively. Since the lower rectum is entirely extraperitoneal, the radial margin extends circumferentially and has been referred to as the circumferential radial margin or mesorectal envelope. Multivariate analysis has suggested that tumor involvement of the circumferential (radial) margin is the most critical factor in predicting local recurrence in rectal cancer. See Table 5.4 for radial margin descriptions [7].

Step 1: Describe and measure the specimen. A right hemicolectomy consists of terminal ileum (blue arrow), cecum (red arrow), a portion of ascending colon (yellow arrow), and appendix (green arrow) as shown in Fig. 5.82. Depending on the pathologist's preference, the bowel can be measured in segments (terminal ileum, cecum, ascending colon) or as one length.

Table 5.4 Radial margins [7]

Location	Area covered by peritoneum	Approximate length
Cecum	Almost entirely covered by peritoneum	5–9 cm in dimension
Ascending colon	Posterior surface lacks peritoneum	15–20 cm in length
Transverse colon	Intraperitoneal	Variable
Descending colon	Posterior surface lacks peritoneum	10–15 cm in length
Sigmoid colon	Intraperitoneal	Variable
Rectum	Upper 1/3: Lacks peritoneum on posterior and medial surface Middle 1/3: Lacks peritoneum on posterior, medial, and lateral surface Lower 1/3: Lacks peritoneum circumferentially	12 cm in length

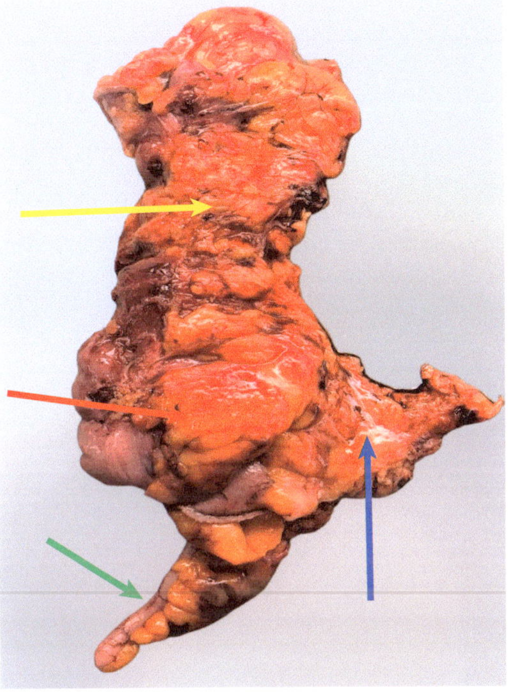

Fig. 5.82 Right hemicolectomy

Fig. 5.83 Right hemicolectomy margins and appendix removed

Step 2: Shave and submit the proximal and distal margins and submit en face. (Fig. 5.83)

Step 3: Amputate the appendix and set to the side.

Step 4: Identify and ink the radial margin. In Fig. 5.84, the radial margin is inked blue.

Step 5: Open the bowel along the antimesenteric border as shown in Fig. 5.85a. Palpate the bowel lumen as you cut to feel for the lesion without cutting through it.

Step 6: Identify the lesion, describe and measure as seen in Fig. 5.85b. Notice the dark color-

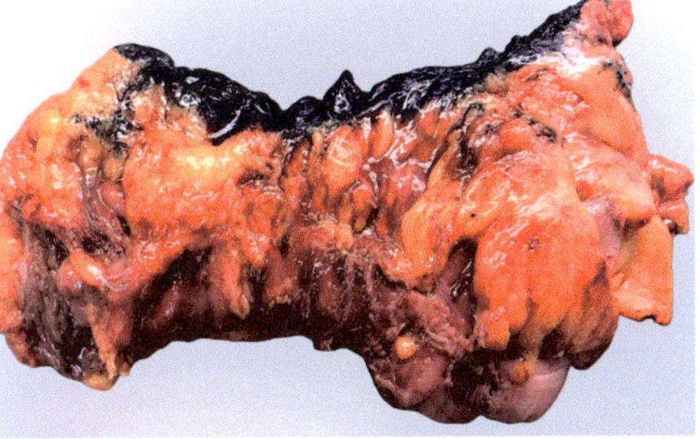

Fig. 5.84 Radial margin inked

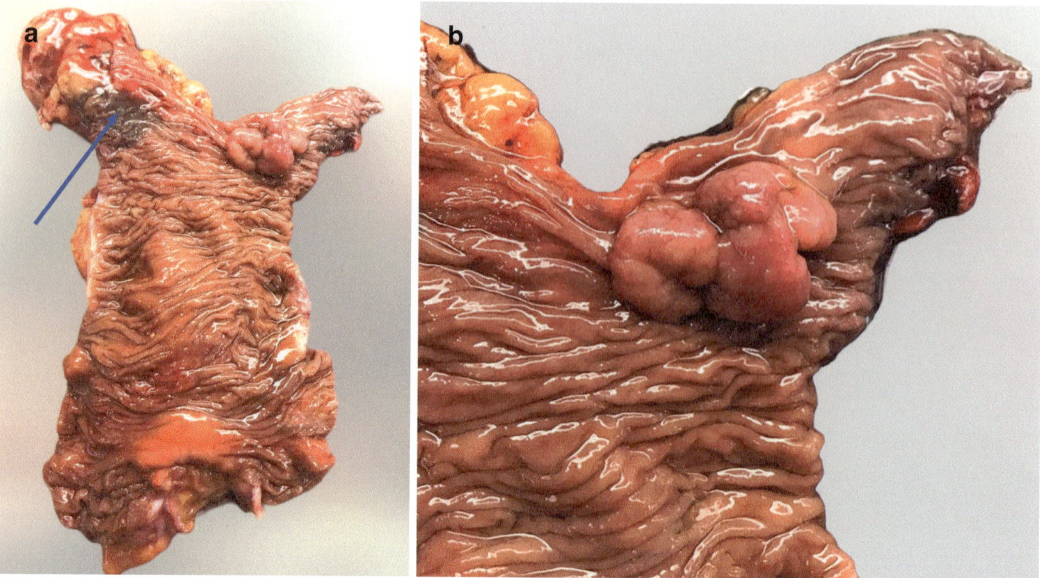

Fig. 5.85 (**a**) Right hemicolectomy opened; (**b**) lesion of right hemicolectomy

ation on the mucosal surface near the lesion in Fig. 5.85a designated with a blue arrow. The dark color is tattoo pigment and designates where a previous biopsy was taken.

Step 7: Measure the lesion to the proximal and distal margins.

Step 8: Ink the serosal surface under the lesion.

Step 9: Submit the radial margin. If the radial margin is far from the lesion, the margin can be shaved and submitted en face. If the lesion is within 1 cm, then perpendicular sections of the lesion in relation to the radial margin are submitted instead.

Step 10: Serially section the lesion as shown in Fig. 5.86.

Step 11: Dictate the greatest depth of invasion.

Step 12: Submit representative sections of the remaining aspects of the specimen. In Fig. 5.87, the terminal ileum, cecum, and ascending colon (away from the lesion) are submitted.

Step 13: Serially section the appendix and describe the lumen (Fig. 5.88)

Step 14: Submit representative sections of the appendix and the appendiceal tip, bisected.

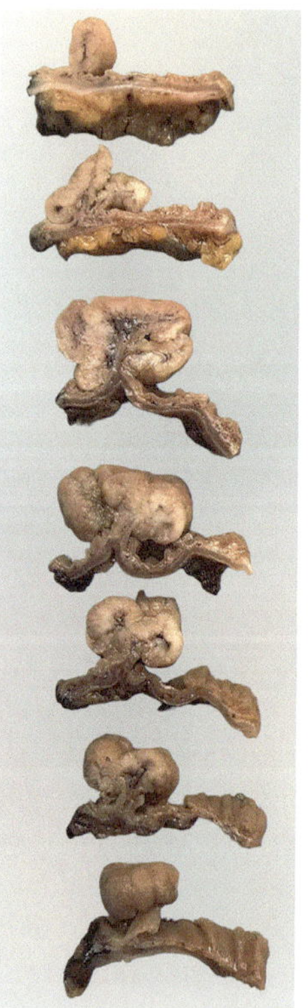

Fig. 5.86 Lesion serially sectioned

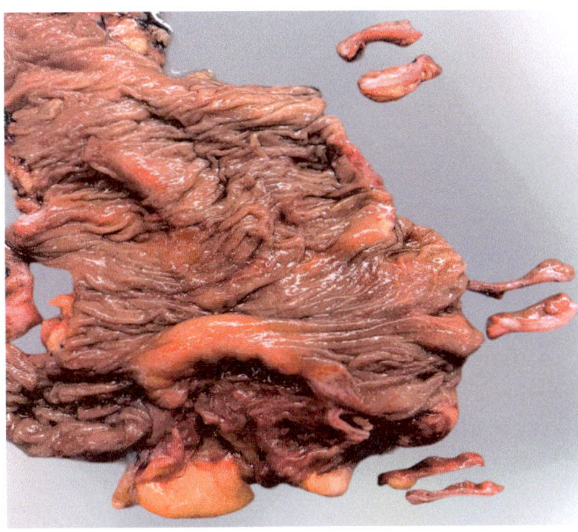

Fig. 5.87 Representative sections of right hemicolectomy

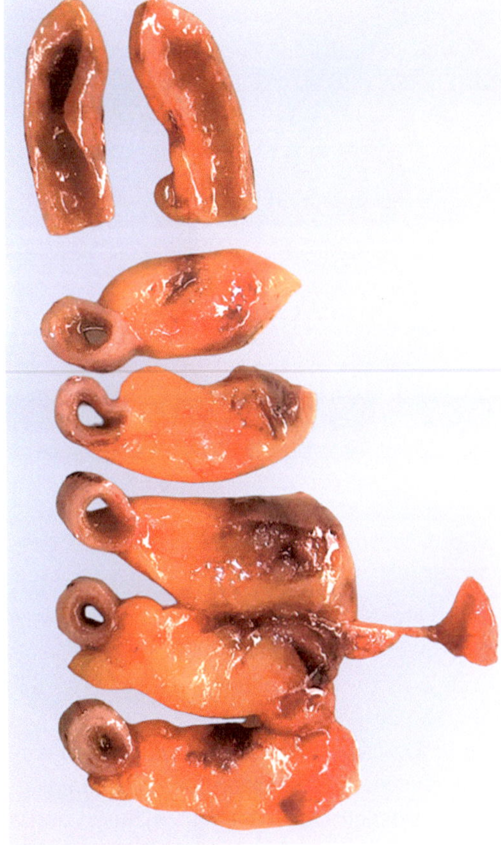

Fig. 5.88 Appendix

Step 15: Remove the remainder of the attached adipose tissue (Fig. 5.89a) and palpate for lymph nodes (Fig. 5.89b).

Step 16: Sections submitted are the proximal and distal margin, the radial margin, the lesion with the greatest depth of invasion, representative sections of remaining bowel, appendix, and all lymph nodes as shown in Fig. 5.90.

Example Dictation

Specimen A is received in formalin labeled with patient's name, medical record number, "right colon" and consists of a right hemicolectomy (28.2 cm in length and ranging in diameter from 1.9 to 3.4 cm) consisting of terminal ileum, cecum, ascending colon, and appendix ($5.9 \times 1.0 \times 0.9$ cm). The specimen is opened to reveal a single tan-pink, polypoid lesion ($2.1 \times 1.9 \times 0.8$ cm) present in the ascending colon, coming within 27.2 cm from the proximal margin and 1.1 cm from the distal margin, surrounded by black tattoo ink. The lesion is serially sectioned to reveal invasion confined to the submucosa with the lesion coming within 5.9 cm of the radial margin. The appendix is sectioned to reveal a tan lumen, and the surrounding adipose tissue is palpable for 14 lymph node candidates ranging from 0.2 to 0.9 cm.

Ink code
    Blue: radial margin
Section code
    A1: Proximal margin, en face
    A2-A3: Distal margin, bisected, en face
    A4-A5: Radial margin, en face
    A6–A10: Lesion, entirely
    A11: Terminal ileum, representative
    A12: Cecum, representative
    A13: Ascending colon, representative
    A14: Appendix, representative
    A16-A17: Four lymph node candidates per cassette, whole
    A18: Two lymph node candidates, whole

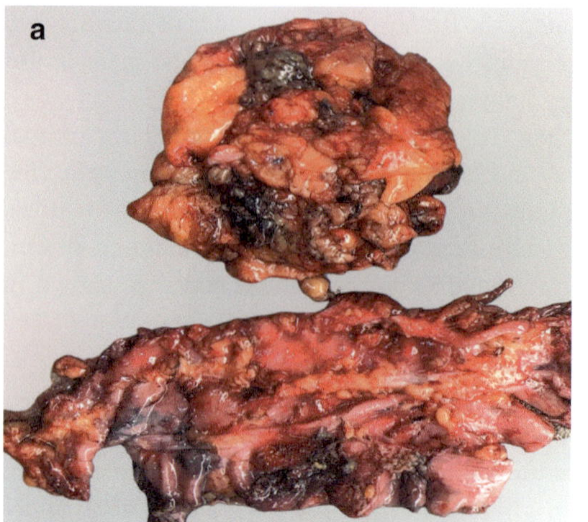

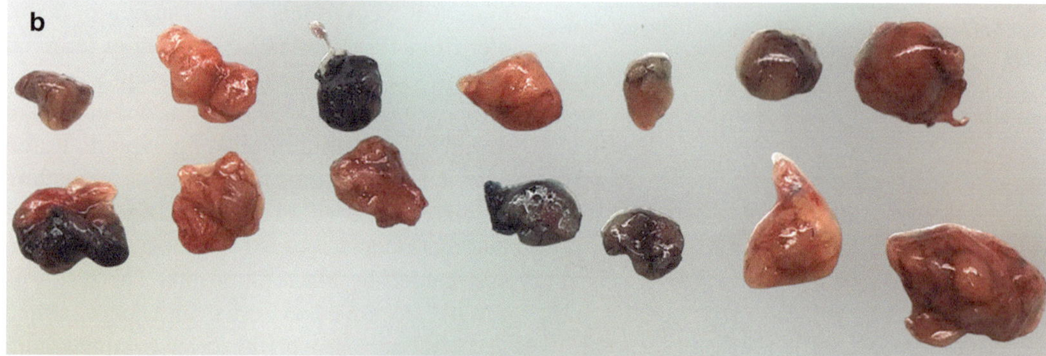

Fig. 5.89 (**a**) Adipose tissue; (**b**) lymph nodes

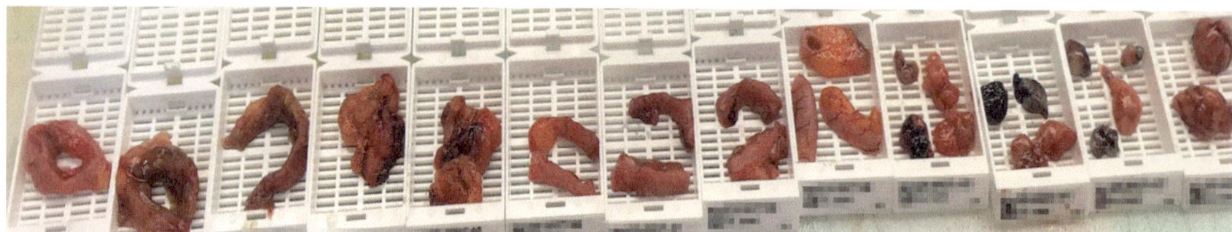

Fig. 5.90 Right hemicolectomy section submission

5.18 Rectosigmoid for Tumor: Level VI CPT 88309

Low anterior resection = for cancers in the proximal 2/3rds of the rectum.

Abdominoperineal resection = distal rectum + anal canal + perianal skin = for tumors of the distal 1/3rd of the rectum. See Fig. 5.91.

Step 1: Orient the specimen. The anterior aspect contains the tenia coli proximally as shown by the blue arrow in Fig. 5.92a while the posterior aspect is entirely radial margin as seen in Fig. 5.92b.

Step 2: Describe the radial margin in terms of completeness. The margin can be complete, near complete, or incomplete. In this example, the radial margin is complete.

Step 3: Ink the radial margin which is also referred to as the mesorectal envelope. In Fig. 5.93a, the anterior aspect of the radial margin is inked blue and in Fig. 5.93b, the

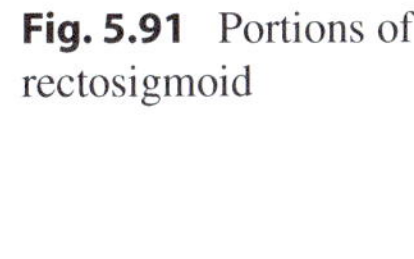

Fig. 5.91 Portions of rectosigmoid

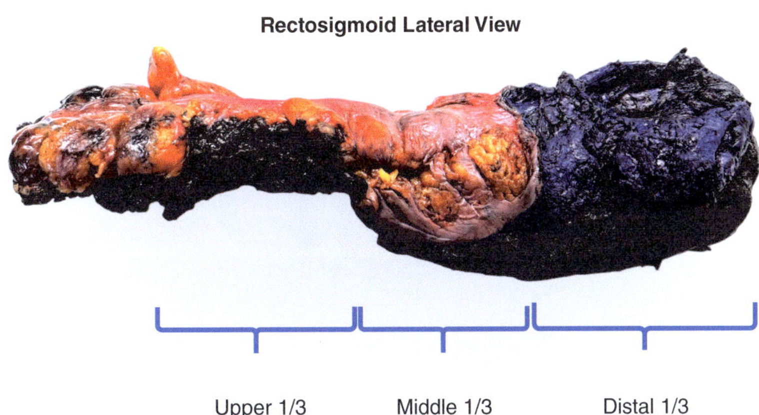

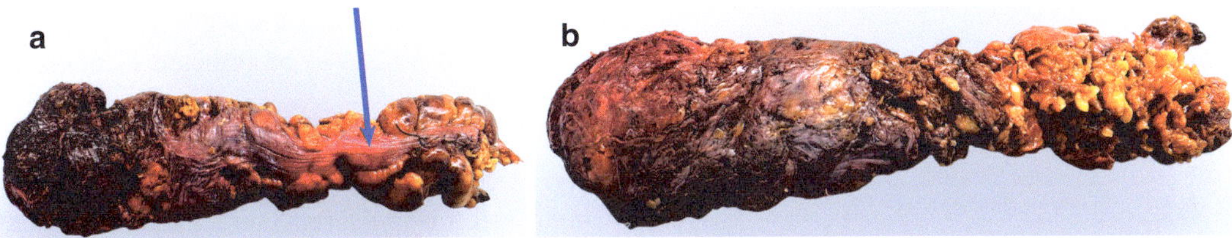

Fig. 5.92 (**a**) Anterior rectosigmoid; (**b**) posterior rectosigmoid

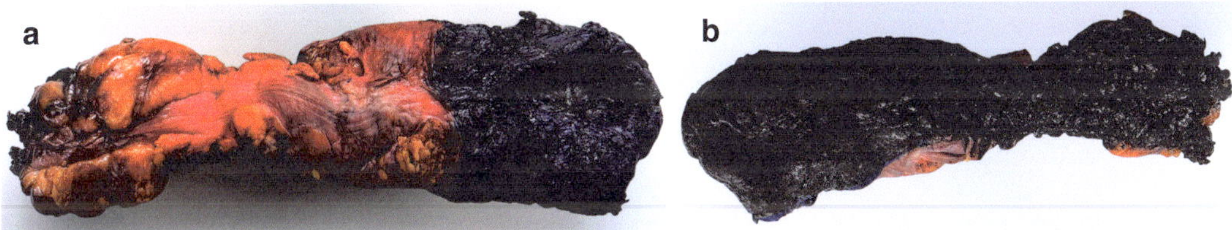

Fig. 5.93 (**a**) Anterior rectosigmoid inked. (**b**) Posterior rectosigmoid inked

posterior aspect of the radial margin is inked black.

Step 4: Shave and submit the proximal margin en face. In Fig. 5.94, surgical staples are present closing the proximal margin. Cut directly under the staples to remove them and then shave the proximal margin.

Step 5: Remove the staples from the distal margin (Fig. 5.95) but do not shave the margin.

Step 6: Open the bowel along the antimesenteric border as shown in Fig. 5.96. Palpate the length of the bowel so as to not cut through the lesion.

Step 7: Describe and measure the lesion as noted by the blue arrow in Fig. 5.97.

Step 8: Measure the lesion to the proximal and distal margin.

Step 9: If the lesion is 1 cm or greater from the distal margin, shave the distal margin and submit en face. If the margin is 1 cm or closer, perpendicular sections of the lesion in relation to the distal margins are submitted.

Step 10: Fix the specimen in formalin. If the specimen is soft, it needs to be fixed in formalin preferably overnight. If the specimen is firm and already fixed then grossing can continue.

Step 11: Pin the specimen to a wax board open and flat as shown in Fig. 5.98a.

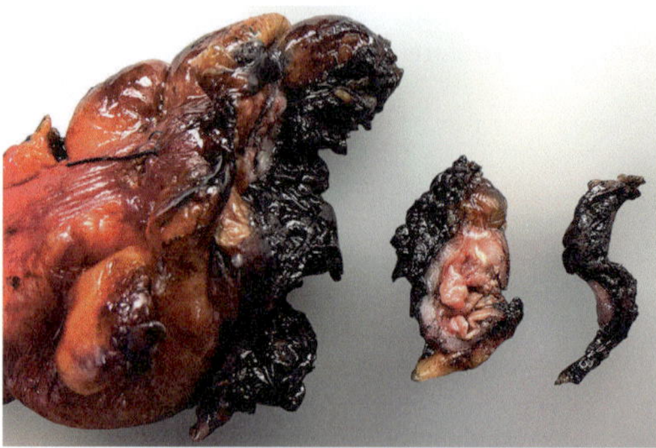

Fig. 5.94 Proximal margin of rectosigmoid

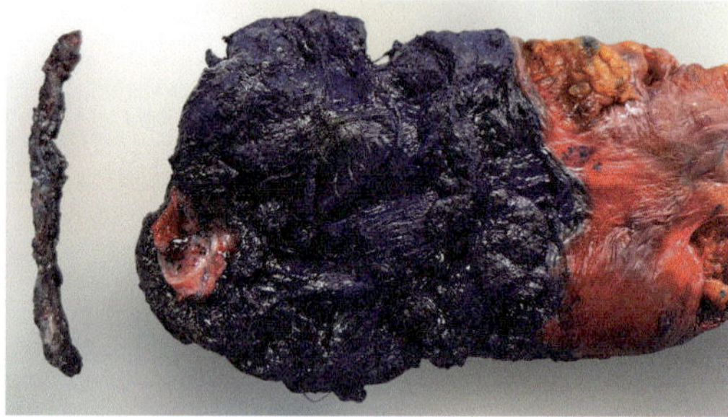

Fig. 5.95 Distal staples removed

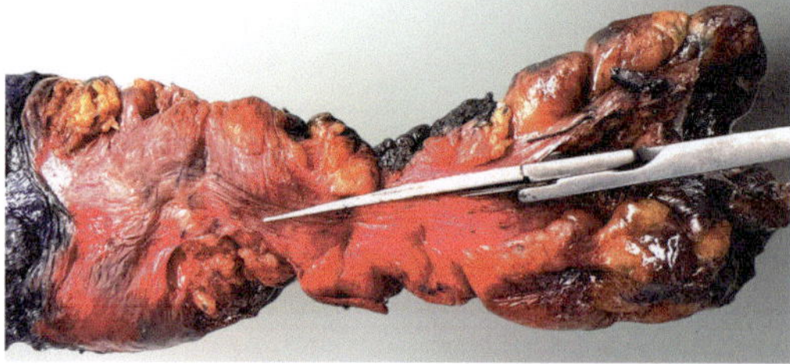

Fig. 5.96 Opening rectosigmoid

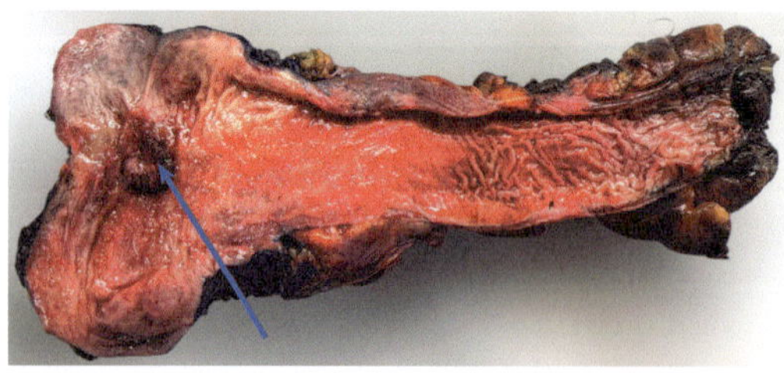

Fig. 5.97 Rectosigmoid with lesion

Step 12: Fill a large container with formalin and place the wax board upside-down as shown in Fig. 5.98b. The wax board will float keeping the tissue submerged in formalin without pressing the tissue to the bottom of the container. Continue grossing when fixed.

Step 13: Serially section the lesion perpendicular to the distal margin as shown in Fig. 5.99.

Step 14: Dictate the greatest depth of invasion of the lesion. Figure 5.100 shows a minimal depth of invasion (designated with blue arrows) without invasion into the radial soft tissue.

Step 15: Submit sections of the lesion with the greatest depth of invasion in relation to the closest distal and radial margin. In Fig. 5.101, the sections need to be bisected to fit in the cassettes.

Step 16: Submit representative bowel. (Fig. 5.102).

Step 17: Remove the remaining adipose tissue as shown in Fig. 5.103.

Step 18: Palpate and submit all lymph nodes. Twelve lymph nodes are required (Fig. 5.104)

Step 19: Submit sections. Sections submitted are proximal margin, lesion in relation to distal and radial margin, representative bowel and lymph nodes as shown in Fig. 5.105.

Example Dictation

Specimen A is received in formalin labeled with patient's name, medical record number, "lower anterior resection" and consists of a red-pink segment of colon (31.2 cm in length by 3.2 cm in diameter) with a complete surrounding radial margin. The specimen is opened to reveal an ulcerative, hemorrhagic lesion (2.1 × 2.0 cm) which comes within 27.5 cm of the proximal margin and 1.8 cm of the distal margin. The lesion is serially sectioned to reveal a greatest depth of invasion approximately 0.2 cm into the submucosa, without involvement of the serosal

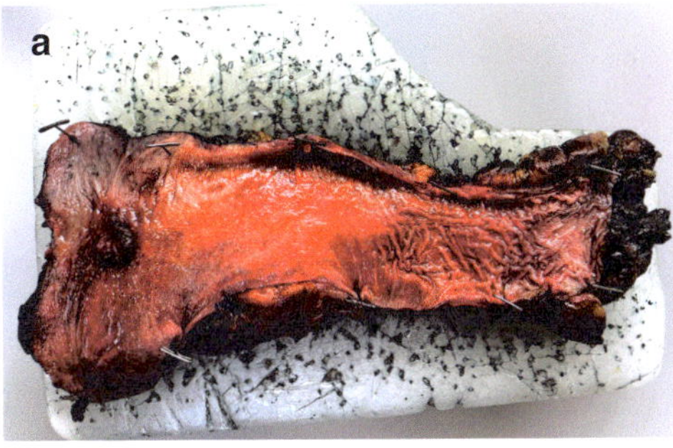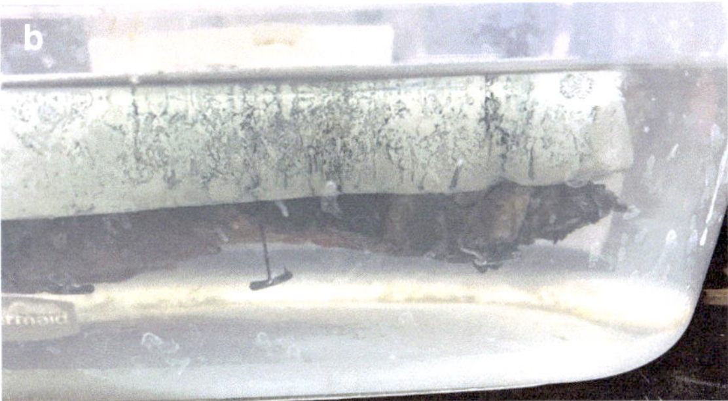

Fig. 5.98 (**a**) Rectosigmoid pinned to wax board; (**b**) rectosigmoid in formalin

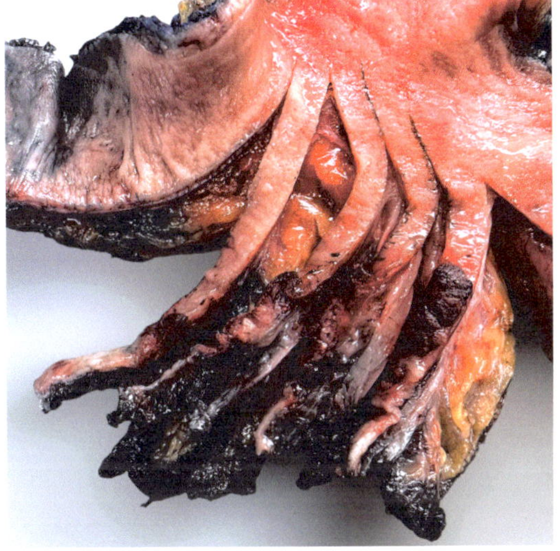

Fig. 5.99 Lesion serially sectioned perpendicular to distal margin

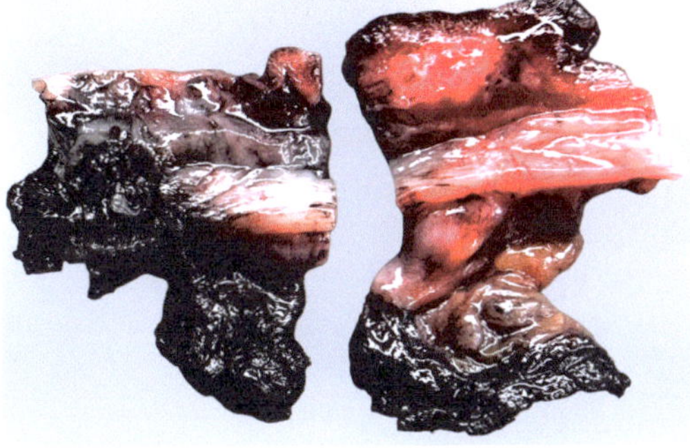

Fig. 5.101 Section of lesion in relation to distal and radial margins bisected

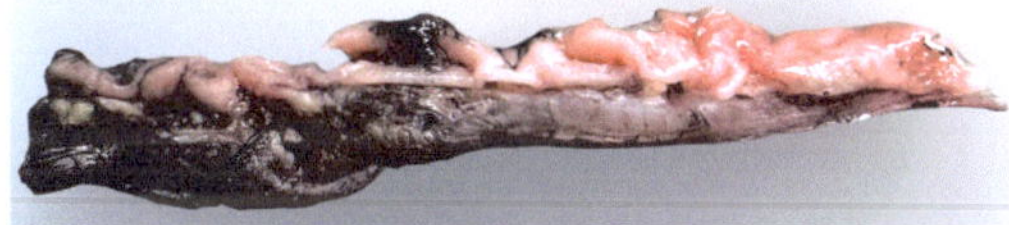

Fig. 5.102 Representative section of bowel

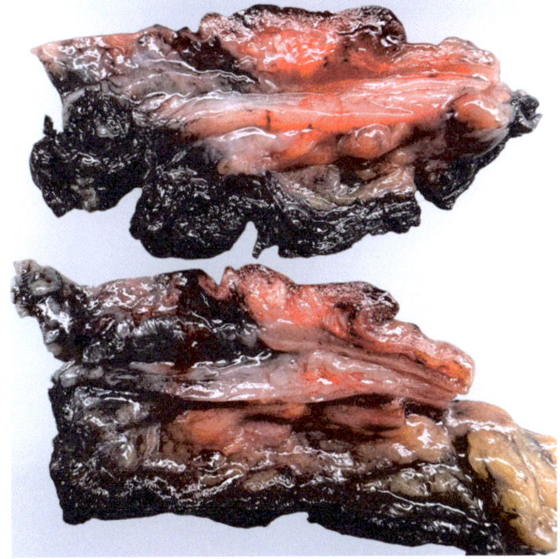

Fig. 5.100 Lesion with greatest depth of invasion

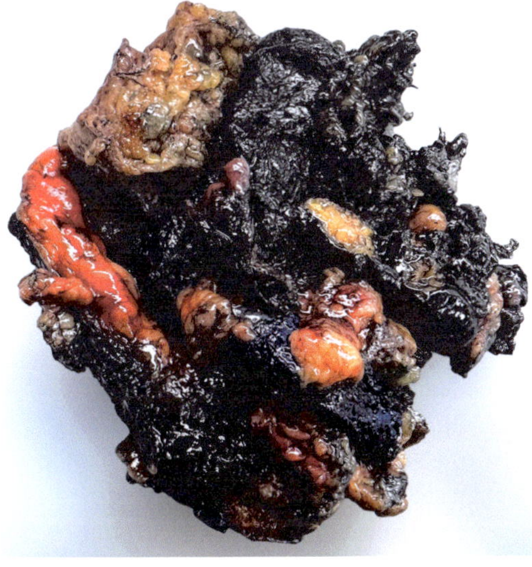

Fig. 5.103 Remainder of adipose tissue removed

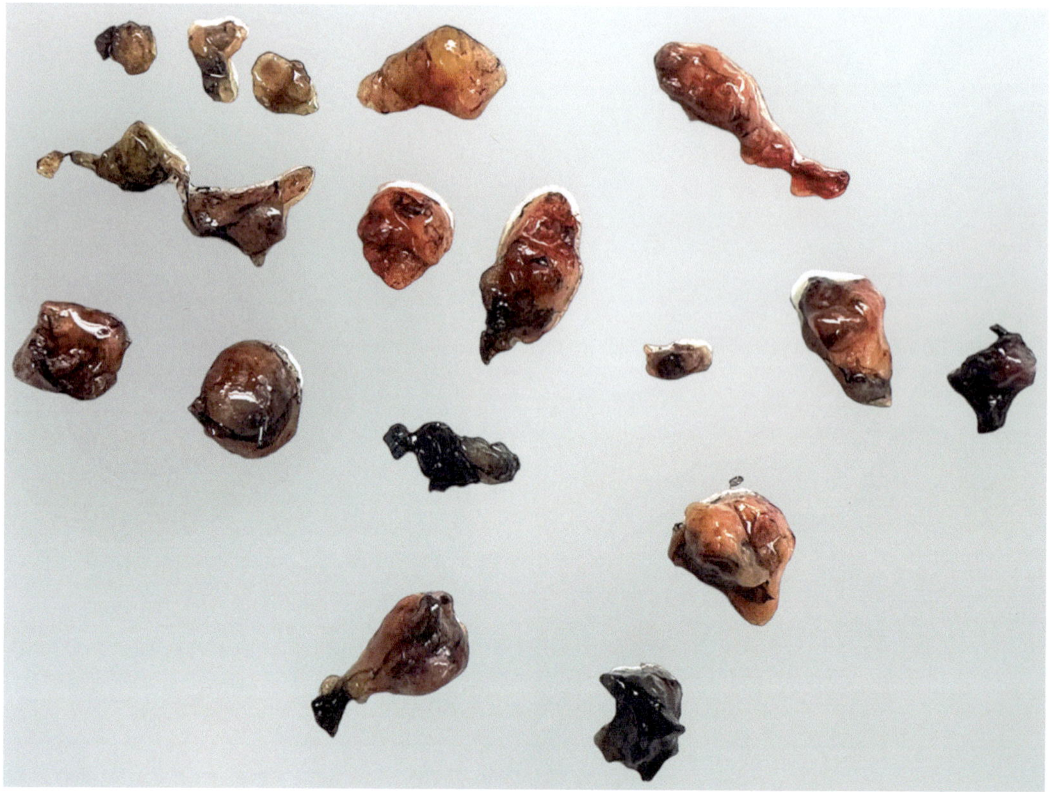

Fig. 5.104 Lymph nodes

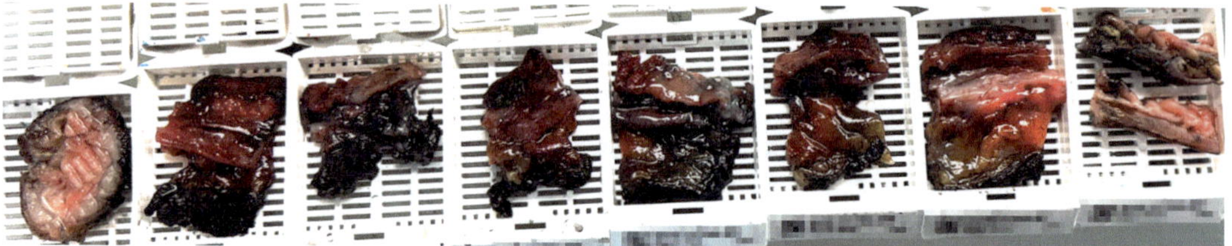

Fig. 5.105 Rectosigmoid section submission

surface and coming within 2.2 cm of the radial margin. The remaining mucosa is tan-pink and folded with no additional lesions identified. The surrounding adipose tissue is palpable for 18 lymph node candidates ranging from 0.1 to 0.7 cm.

Ink code

Blue: anterior radial margin

Black: posterior radial margin

Section code

A1: Proximal margin, en face

A2–A7: Lesion entirely in relation to distal end radial margin

A8: Representative bowel

A9–A12: Four lymph node candidates per cassette, whole

A 13: Two lymph node candidates, whole

Acknowledgments The author gratefully acknowledges Satyapal Chahar, MD, Hafiz A. Yahya, MD, and Muntha Chaudhari, MBBS, for their contribution to this chapter.

Quiz Questions

1. What is the T stage of the stomach cancer in Fig. 5.106?
   (a) T1
   (b) T2
   (c) T3
   (d) T4

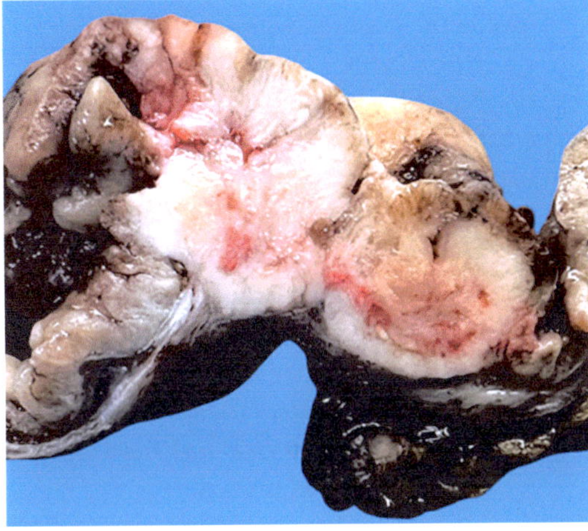

Fig. 5.106 Quiz question 1

2. What is the CPT code for the stomach resection that is not for tumor?
   (a) 88,309
   (b) 88,305
   (c) 88,307
   (d) 88,304

3. What is the standard for opening stomach in a gastrectomy specimen for stomach cancers?
   (a) Lesser curvature
   (b) Greater curvature
   (c) Radial margin

4. What is shown in Fig. 5.107?
   (a) Intussusception
   (b) Tumor
   (c) Polyp
   (d) Diverticulitis
   (e) Stricture

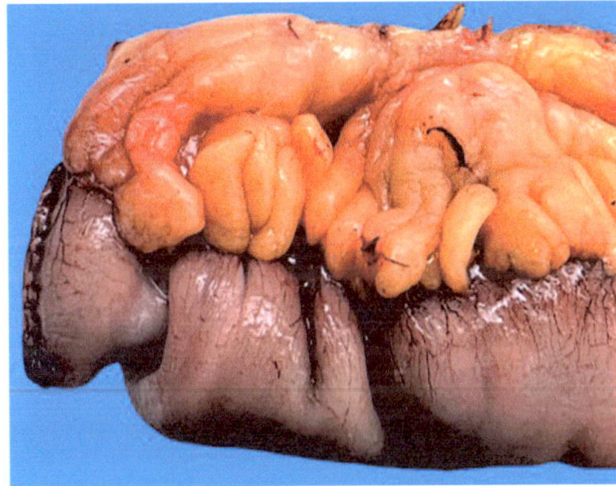

Fig. 5.107 Quiz question 4

5. What is the minimum number of lymph nodes you need to find for an esophagectomy specimen for esophageal adenocarcinoma?
   (a) 12
   (b) 15
   (c) 16
   (d) 18
6. What is the most common site of occurrence for the condition shown in Fig. 5.108?
   (a) Appendix
   (b) Jejunum
   (c) Rectum
   (d) Sigmoid colon

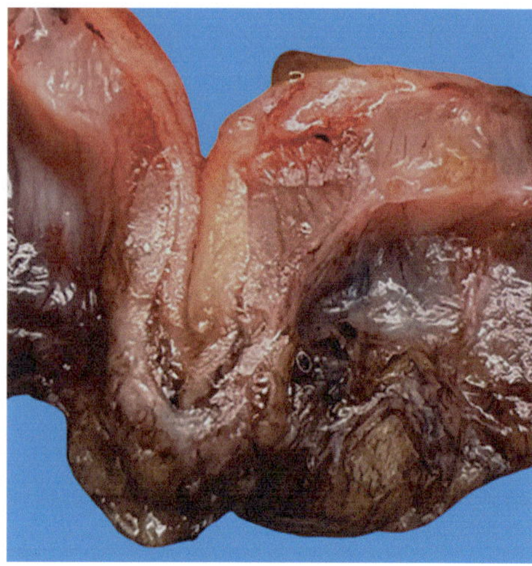

Fig. 5.108 Quiz question 6

7. What is not present in a low anterior resection?
   (a) Sigmoid colon
   (b) Anus
   (c) Rectum
   (d) Descending colon
8. An abdominoperineal resection is received with a 1.5 cm defect in the mesorectum exposing the serosa of the rectum. How should the mesorectum be evaluated?
   (a) Not present
   (b) Nearly Incomplete
   (c) Complete
   (d) Incomplete
9. An intact 1.0 cm polyp is received in the lab. The grossing person describes and measures the specimen. How to they proceeded?
   (a) Ink the polyp resection margin and bisect
   (b) Bisect without ink
   (c) Ink the polyp surface and the resection margin and submit whole
   (d) Ink the resection margin and submit whole
10. When grossing an appendix, how does the grossing person section the appendiceal tip?
   (a) Whole
   (b) Serially sectioned
   (c) En face
   (d) Longitudinally bisected

Answer Key

1. C- T3

   Explanation: The tumor invades the serosa in the gross image provided. So, the T stage of the tumor based on the gross examination is T3. If the tumor invades the adjacent structures, it becomes T4. If the tumor invades the muscularis propria without invading the serosa, it becomes T2.

2. C- 88307

   Explanation- The CPT code for the stomach resection that is not for tumor is 88,307. If the resection is for tumor, the CPT code is 88309.

3. B- Greater curvature

   Explanation: The standard is to open the stomach along the greater curvature due to most ulcers and lesions being present in the lesser curvature. If the majority of the lesion is present in the greater curvature, the stomach can be opened along the lesser curvature.

4. A-Intussusception

   Explanation: As shown in the picture, Intussusception is a condition in which one segment of intestine "telescopes" inside of another, causing an intestinal obstruction. It is most commonly seen in small intestine.

5. B-15

   Explanation: The minimum number of lymph nodes you need to find for an esophagectomy specimen for esophageal adenocarcinoma is 15. But we should not submit as many as we could find.

6. D-Sigmoid colon

   Explanation: The condition illustrated in the picture is called diverticulosis. Diverticulosis occurs most commonly in sigmoid colon in 90% of cases.

7. B-Anus

   Explanation: A low anterior resection is a resection of the distal descending colon, sigmoid colon, and rectum. Therefore, B is correct. If anal skin is present, it is referred to as an abdominoperineal resection.

8. D- Incomplete

   Explanation: An incomplete mesorectum is described as minimal adipose tissue bulk or defects reaching to the muscularis propria. D is the correct answer because there is a defect in the mesorectum. Nearly complete mesorectum contains moderate adipose tissue bulk with irregularities in the adipose tissue but no defects are identified. Complete mesorectum contains intact adipose tissue bulk with only minor irregularities.

9. D- Ink the resection margin and bisect.

   Explanation: The resection margin of any polyp needs to be inked. This allows for microscopic visualization of any invasive tumor in relation to the resection margin. Since the polyp is 1.0 cm, the specimen will not fit in the cassette whole and will need to be bisected to fit appropriately. Therefore, A is the correct answer.

10. D- Longitudinally bisected

   Explanation: The appendiceal tip is always bisected longitudinally to microscopically assess the distal lumen of the appendix, so answer D is correct. En face and whole will only reveal serosa on the slide and serially sectioned will not microscopically show the distal curve of the tip.

References

1. FirstPath. 2009–2023. [Online]. Available: https://www.firstpathlab.com/cpt-codes/. Accessed 2 Jun 2023.
2. UChicago Medicine. 2023. [Online]. Available: https://www.uchicagomedicine.org/conditions-services/interventional-endoscopy/procedures-services/endoscopic-submucosal-dissection-esd. Accessed 7 Sept 2023.
3. Protocol for the examination of specimens from patients with. CAP; 2022.
4. Protocol for the examination of biopsy specimens from patients. College of American Pathologists; 2022.
5. Protocol for the examination of specimens from patients with. College of American Pathologists; 2023.
6. Crohn's disease vs. ulcerative colitis. Temple Health; 2023. [Online]. Available: https://www.templehealth.org/services/conditions/crohns-disease-versus-ulcerative-colitis. Accessed 1 Sept 2023.
7. Protocol for the examination of resection specimens from. College of American Pathologists; 2023.

Grossing of Genitourinary Specimens

6

Contents

Genitourinary gross specimens should be handled with care, as they are an essential part of providing excellent care to patients who have undergone genitourinary procedures. Obtaining an accurate microscopic diagnosis requires correct description and submission of genitourinary specimens/tissue sections for histologic evaluation. Managing these specimens is often a daunting task, especially for trainees; however, by understanding a few fundamental principles, one can develop a framework for approaching these cases. Presented is a stepwise approach to handling genitourinary gross specimens.

See Table 6.1 for CPT codes [1].

© The Author(s), under exclusive license to Springer Nature Switzerland AG 2024

A. Illingworth, *Manual of Pathologic Grossing*, https://doi.org/10.1007/978-3-031-72694-1_6

Table 6.1 CPT codes [1]

Kidney biopsy	88305
Kidney partial or total nephrectomy	88307
Adrenal gland resection	88307
Prostate needle biopsy	88305
Prostate transurethral resection (TURP)	88305
Prostate except radical resection/TURP/needle biopsy	88307
Prostate radical resection	88309
Bladder biopsy	88305
Bladder, transurethral resection of bladder tumor (TURBT)	88307
Bladder partial or total resection	88309

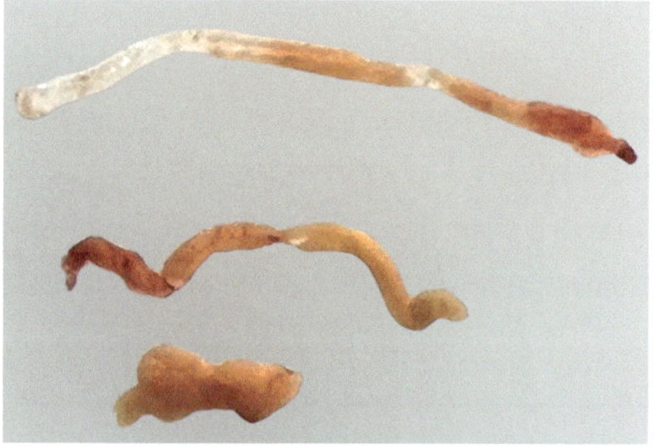

Fig. 6.1 Kidney biopsy for a mass, three biopsy cores

6.1 Kidney Biopsy for a Mass: Level IV CPT 88305

An image-guided percutaneous core needle biopsy is performed to diagnose unresectable renal tumors, small renal tumors (typically less than 3.0 cm prior to ablation) and suspected benign renal neoplasms (to avoid unnecessary surgical resections). A guide needle (16G to 19G) is used to perform the biopsy, and it yields linear strips of tissue which are sent to the laboratory in formalin. The biopsy should be submitted fresh if lymphoma is suspected, with the case flagged for lymphoma workup.

Step 1: Describe, count, and measure the core lengths (if multiple cores are submitted, a range may be provided). (Fig. 6.1)

Step 2: Submit the specimen entirely in a biopsy bag. (Fig. 6.2)

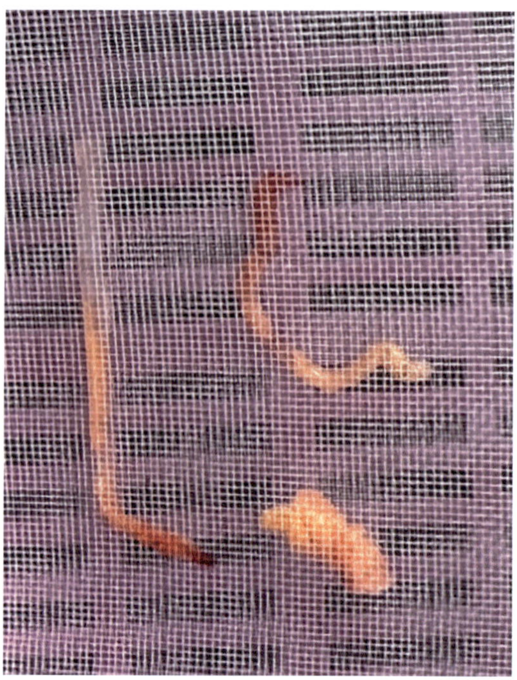

Fig. 6.2 Kidney biopsy for a mass section submission

Example Dictation

Specimen A is received in formalin labeled with the patient's name, medical record number, "kidney mass biopsy" and consists of 3 tan-yellow cores ranging from 0.6 cm to 2.1 cm. The specimen is submitted entirely in a biopsy bag in A1.

6.2 Kidney Biopsy for a Systemic Disease: Level IV CPT 88305

As with a renal biopsy for a suspicious lesions, a kidney biopsy for a systemic disease such as renal failure or transplant rejection is performed similarly. These biopsies are typically sent to the lab immediately to be assessed under the microscope while the patient is still on the procedure table. The glomeruli in the biopsy specimens are counted and deemed adequate or inadequate for subsequent analysis. If the biopsy is inadequate, the physician has the option to retrieve more tissue for an adequate sample.

Step 1: Place cores on a glass slide with a drop of saline (Fig. 6.3).

Step 2: Assess the cores microscopically on low power and count the glomeruli (Fig. 6.4).

Step 3: Divide the cores for light microscopy, electron microscopy, and immunohistochemistry containing appropriate glomeruli for each and place in appropriate fixatives. The cores can be cut with a scalpel blade, if necessary (Fig. 6.5).

Glomerular count is approximate and should be divided as follows:

> Light microscopy 12+ glomeruli, formalin
> Electron microscopy 1–3 glomeruli, glutaraldehyde
> Immunohistochemistry 7–10 glomeruli, Michel's fixative

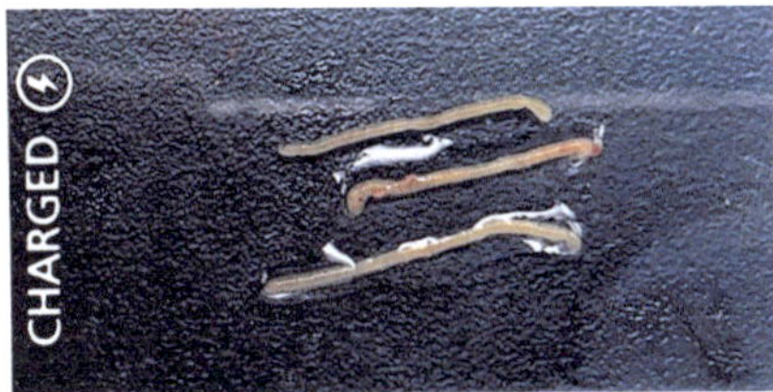

Fig. 6.3 Kidney biopsy for a systemic disease, three biopsy cores on slide

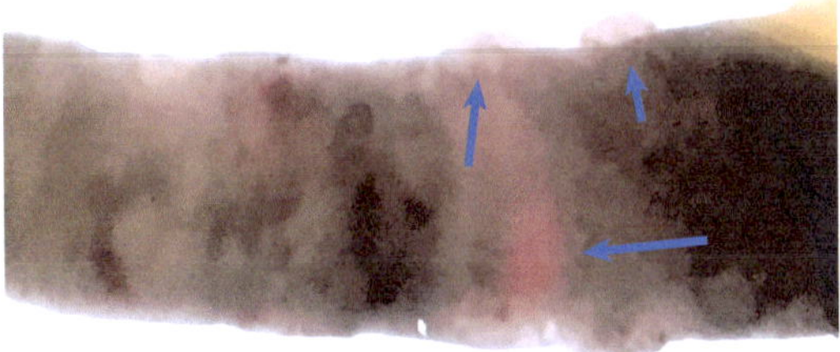

Fig. 6.4 Kidney biopsy for a systemic disease microscopic assessment of renal cores, arrows indicate glomeruli

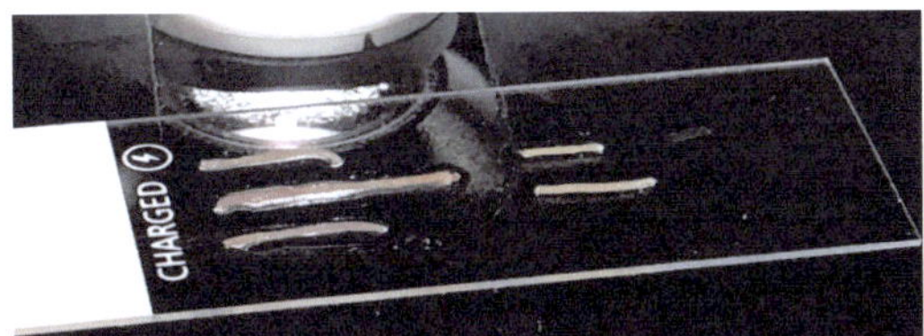

Fig. 6.5 Kidney biopsy for a systemic disease, divided renal cores

Example Dictation

Specimen A is received in formalin labeled with the patient's name, medical record number, "transplant left kidney" and consists of 3 tan-yellow cores ranging from 2.1 cm to 2.5 cm. The cores are assessed microscopically to reveal adequate glomeruli present. The cores are divided, and portions are submitted for electron microscopy and immunofluorescence. The remaining tissue is submitted in A1–A3 for light microscopy.

6.3 Partial Nephrectomy: Level V CPT 88307

Kidney wedge resections are performed for lesions in the periphery of the kidney. The surgeon removes the lesion and a small perimeter of unremarkable kidney, leaving the remaining functioning kidney in place.

A partial nephrectomy is also called a kidney-sparing surgery and is used for a clinically localized renal mass (clinically T1a and T1b when technically feasible) with the goal of sparing the unremarkable kidney.

Step 1: Measure and weigh the kidney wedge specimen. (Fig. 6.6).

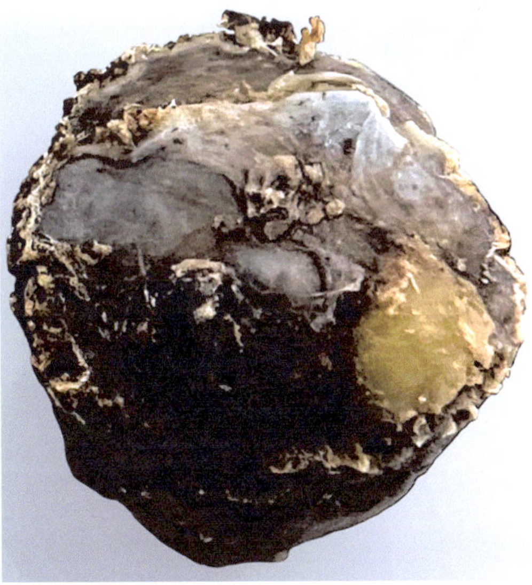

Fig. 6.6 Partial nephrectomy showing the capsular surface

Step 2: Identify the renal capsule and resection margin. (Fig. 6.7).

Step 3: Ink both the resection margin and the renal capsule in separate colors. (Fig. 6.8)

Step 4: Serially section the specimen perpendicular to the resection margin so both ink colors can be seen in each slice. (Fig. 6.9)

Step 5: This specimen is small and can be submitted entirely (Fig. 6.10). If the specimen is greater than 6–7 cm, representative sections of the mass in relation to the capsule and to the margin are acceptable. Submit 1 section per 1 cm of mass.

Example Dictation

Specimen A is received in formalin labeled with the patient's name, medical record number, "right kidney wedge" and consists of a portion of tan-brown kidney (3.7 × 3.2 × 3.1 cm, 5 g) which is serially sectioned to reveal an irregular, red-

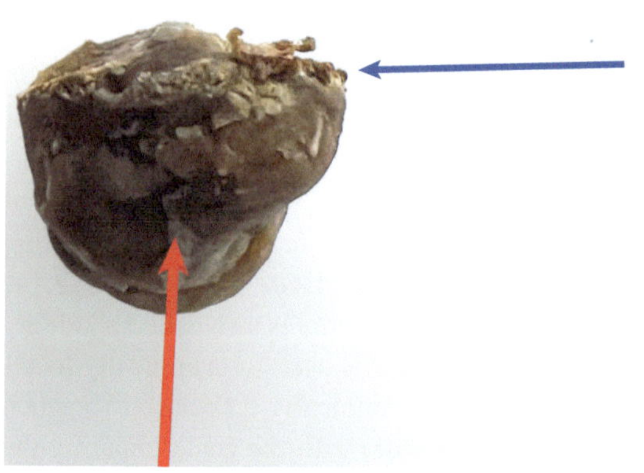

Fig. 6.7 Partial nephrectomy side view, showing the edge of the renal capsule (blue arrow) and the resection margin (red arrow)

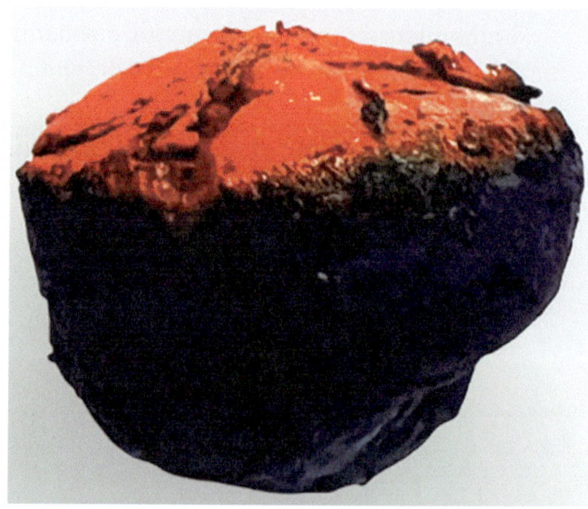

Fig. 6.8 Partial nephrectomy inked resection margin (blue) and renal capsule (orange)

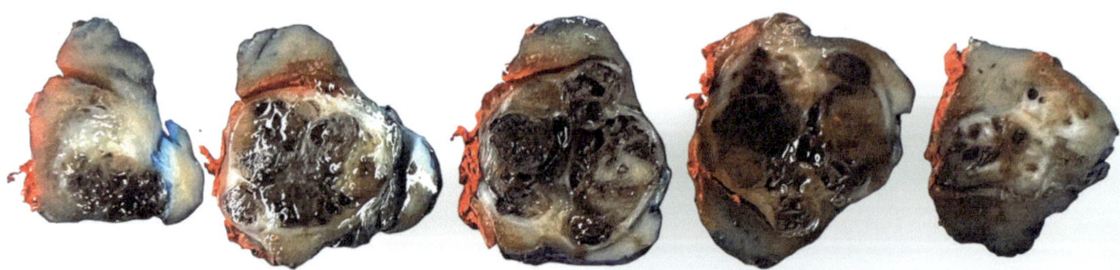

Fig. 6.9 Partial nephrectomy serially sectioned

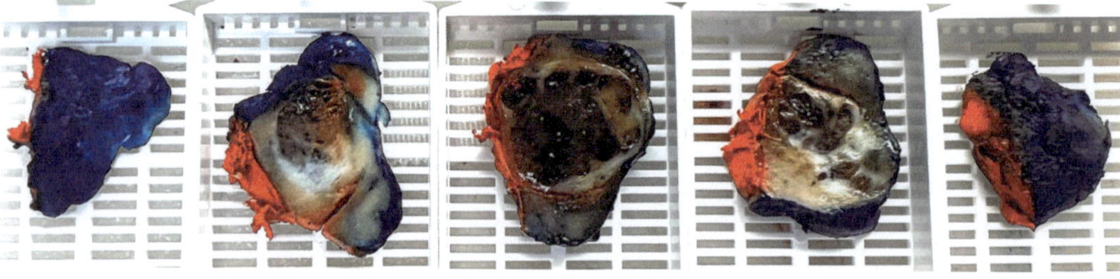

Fig. 6.10 Partial nephrectomy section submission

yellow hemorrhagic mass (3.5 × 3.3 × 3.3 cm) coming less than 0.1 cm from the resection margin and abuts the overlying renal capsule without invasion through the capsule. The specimen is sequentially submitted, entirely in A1–A5.

Ink code
> Blue: resection margin
> Orange: renal capsule

6.4 Nephroureterectomy for Urothelial Tumor: Level V CPT 88307

Nephroureterectomy is the standard of care for invasive upper tract urothelial carcinoma arising in the renal pelvis and/or ureter. The specimen is composed of the kidney, ureter, and possibly bladder cuff.

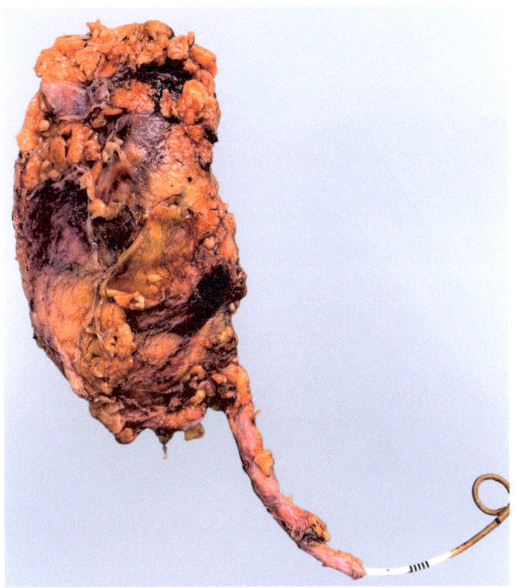

Fig. 6.11 Nephroureterectomy for urothelial tumor

Step 1: Weigh and measure the overall dimensions of the specimen. Ink the surface of kidney/Gerota's fascia or perinephric fat. Measure the length and diameter of the ureter and the bladder cuff. Describe the external surface of the ureter and palpate for a tumor in the ureter. A review of the imaging and previous biopsy for tumor location is recommended before the grossing begins (Fig. 6.11).

Step 2: The hilar vessels are often clipped or stapled closed. Remove the staples and clips (Fig. 6.12).

Step 3: When the renal vein and artery are visualized (See Fig. 6.13).

Step 4: If a bladder cuff is present, amputate and radially section through the ureteral orifice, and submitted entirely. If bladder cuff is not present, shave the ureter margin (blue arrow) and submit en face. Additionally, shave and submit the renal vein (green arrow) and renal artery (red arrow) and submit en face (Fig. 6.14).

Step 5: Ink the anterior and posterior aspects of the kidney. Figure 6.15a shows anterior blue

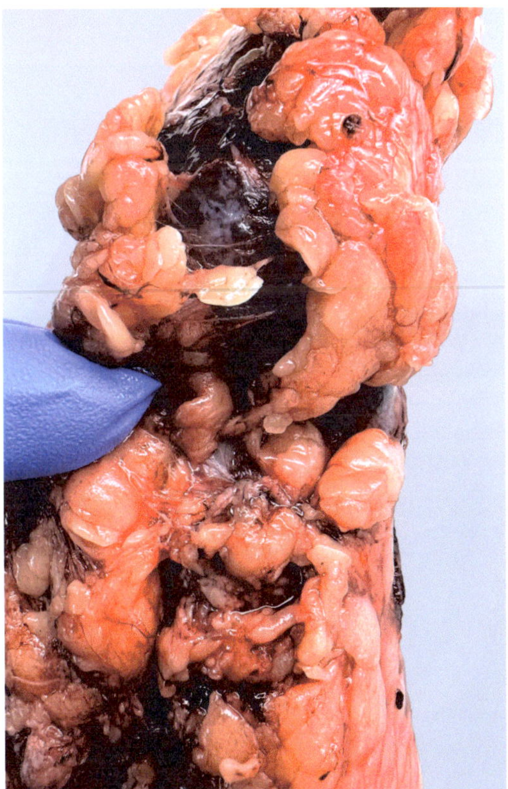

Fig. 6.12 Nephroureterectomy renal hilum

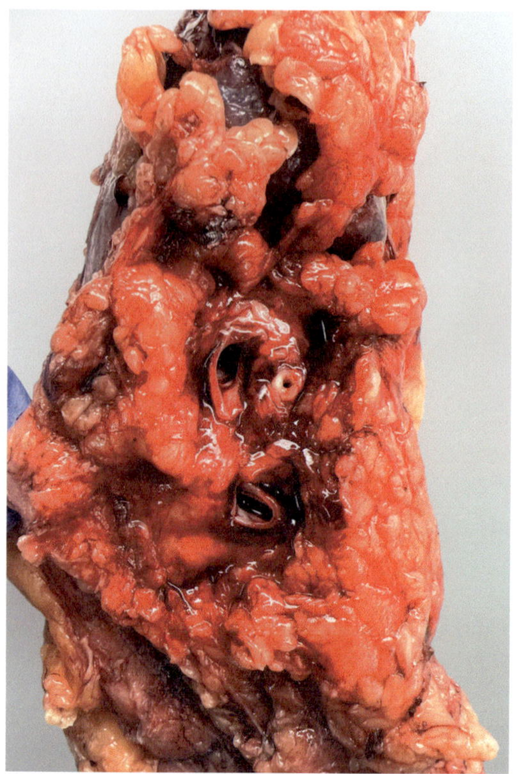

Fig. 6.13 Nephroureterectomy renal hilum vessels

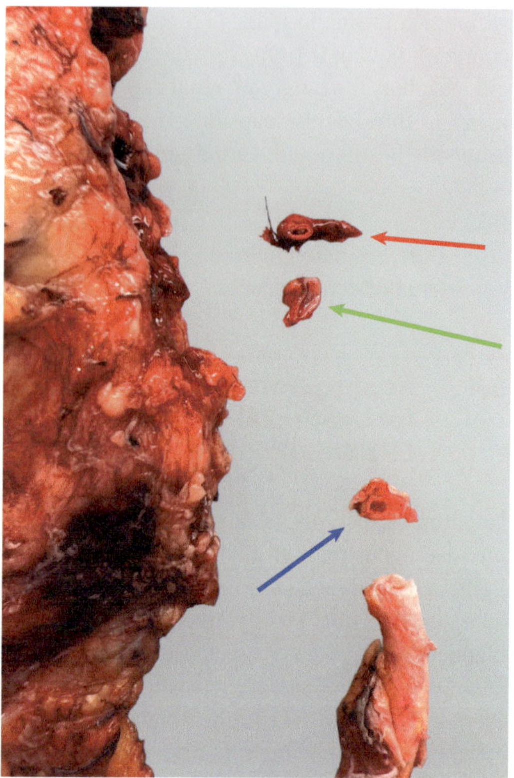

Fig. 6.14 Kidney margins shaved

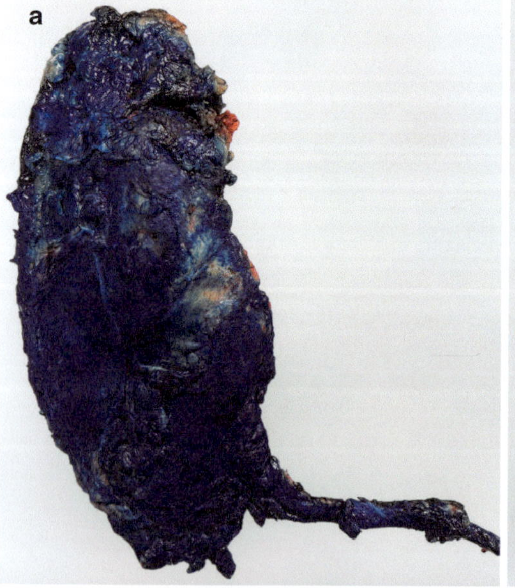

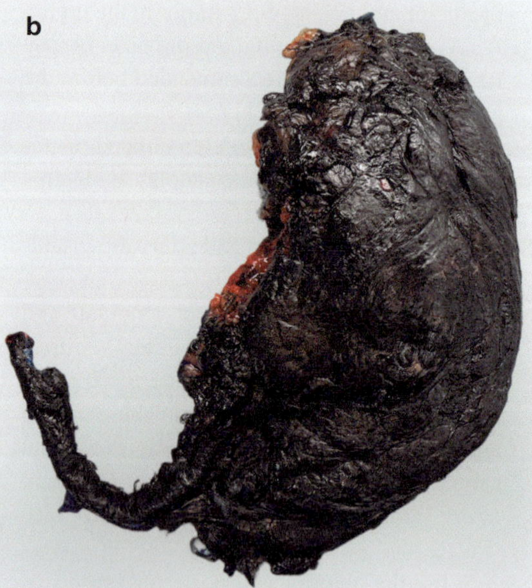

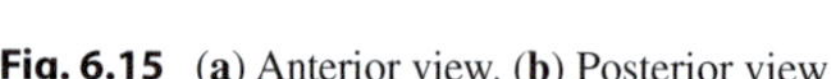

Fig. 6.15 (**a**) Anterior view. (**b**) Posterior view

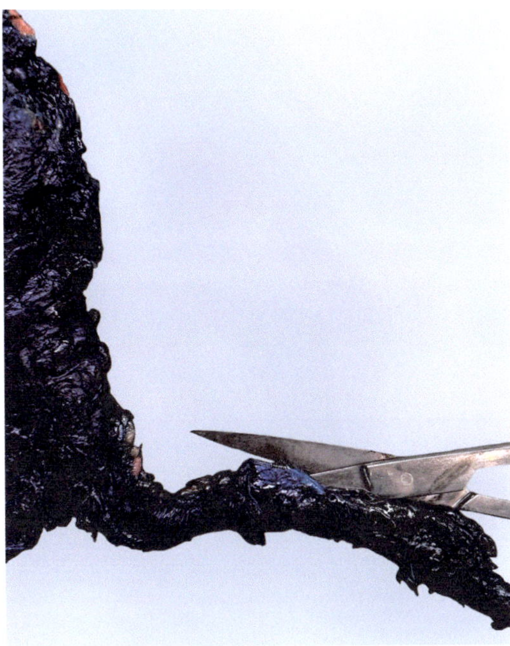

Fig. 6.16 Nephroureterectomy for urothelial tumor, opening the ureter

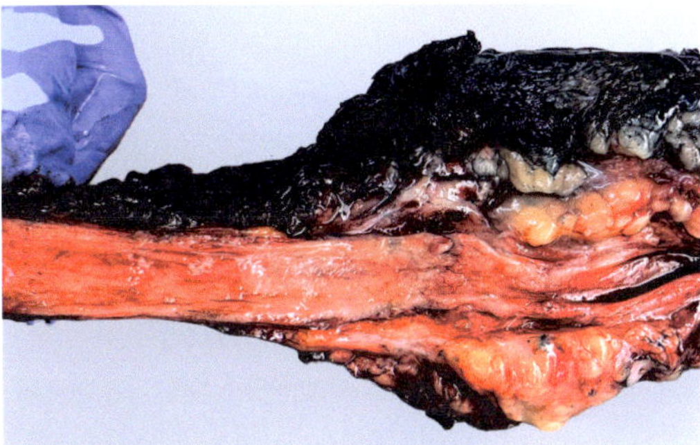

Fig. 6.17 Nephroureterectomy for urothelial tumor, ureter lesion

ink, and Fig. 6.15b shows posterior black ink of the kidney.

Step 6: Using small scissors, open the ureter from distal to proximal (Fig. 6.16).

Step 7: Carefully examine the mucosal surface of the ureter for tumor. Describe the number, shape, and location of the tumor(s). Urothelial carcinomas can be multifocal. Handle the ureter with care since urothelial carcinomas are very soft and friable. Rubbing the lumen of the ureter could damage the lesion.

Step 8: Measure the lesion in three dimensions. The lesion is identified by the blue arrow (Fig. 6.17)

Step 9: Bivalve the kidney. Move the ureter to the posterior side and place forceps within the renal pelvis as shown in Fig. 6.18a. Using a blade, slice the kidney into anterior and posterior halves. Assess the cut surface of the kidney. Examine the pelvis and renal calyces for lesions or tumors and/or for extension of the lesion into the renal pelvis or calyxes shown in Fig. 6.18b

Step 10: Measure the distance of the lesion from the distal ureter margin and the pelvicalyceal junction.

Step 11: Serially section the ureter distal to the lesion and submit representative sections. Take transverse sections of the ureter (Fig. 6.19).

Step 12: Serially section the area of the lesion (Fig. 6.20).

Step 13: Assess the slices of the lesion for invasion outside the ureter. Describe extent of invasion, measure depth of invasion and distance to circumferential/deep margin. In this example, the lesion is confined to the ureter (Fig. 6.21).

Step 14: Submit the entire area of the lesion proximal to distal sequentially.

Step 15: Serially section the ureter proximal to the lesion and submit representative sections.

Step 16: Serially section the anterior and posterior halves of the kidney (Fig. 6.22). Assess for any additional lesions or cysts.

Step 17: Palpate the renal hilum for lymph nodes.

Step 18: Confirm the presence or absence of the adrenal gland.

Step 19: Submit sections. Sections should include the vein, artery and ureter margin, representative ureter proximal and distal to the lesion, the lesion, renal pelvis, and renal parenchyma (Fig. 6.23).

Example Dictation

Specimen A is received in formalin labeled with patient's name, medical record number, "right kidney with right ureter" and consists of a tan kidney (11.2 × 6.5 × 5.2 cm, 659 g) with attached surrounding perinephric adipose tissue ranging from 0.1 to 5.6 cm, and attached segment of ureter

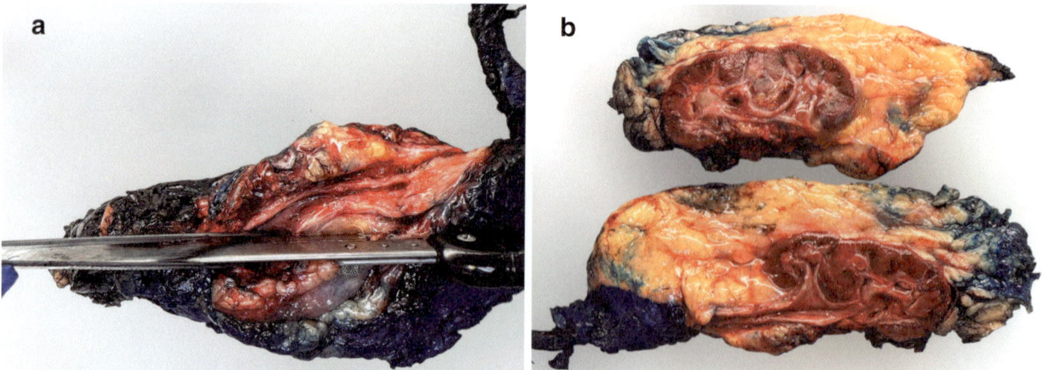

Fig. 6.18 (a) Bivalving kidney using forceps in renal pelvis. (b) Kidney bivalved

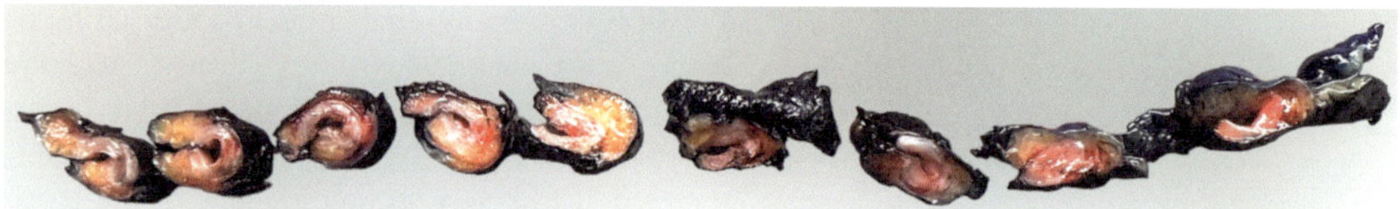

Fig. 6.19 Ureter serially sectioned

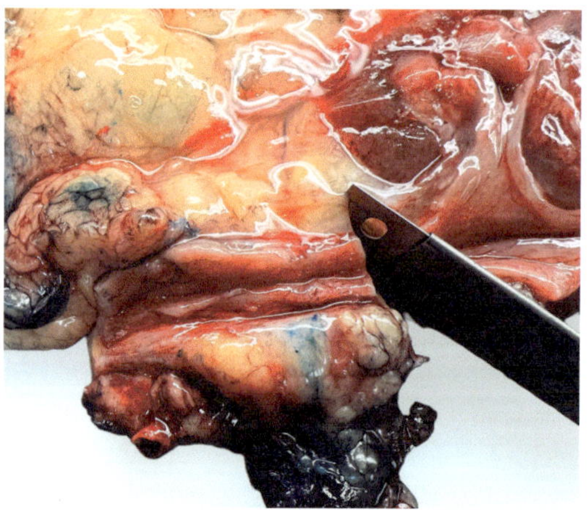

Fig. 6.20 Section of ureter with entire lesion

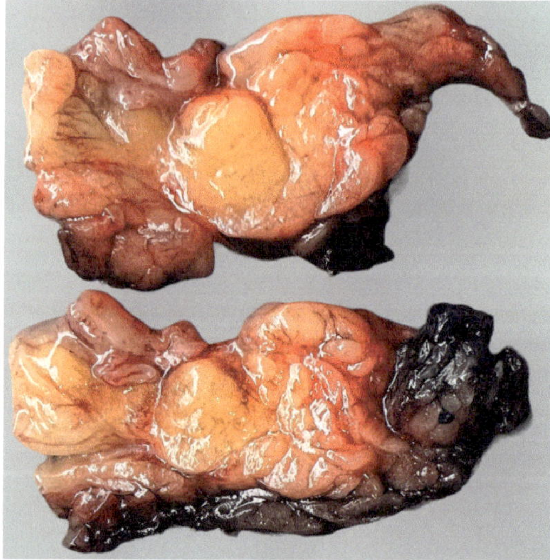

Fig. 6.21 Sections of ureter with lesion

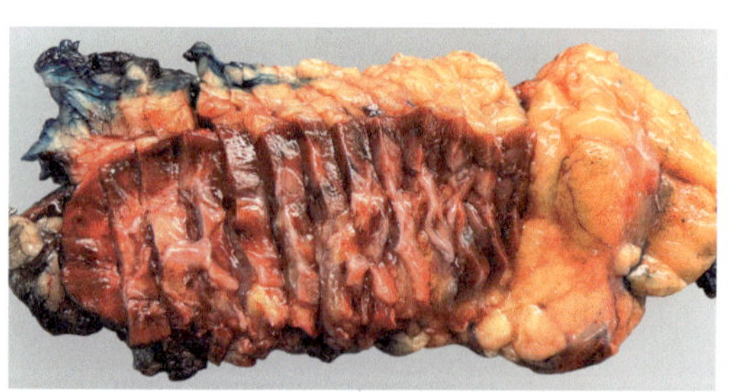

Fig. 6.22 Nephroureterectomy for urothelial tumor, kidney serially sectioned

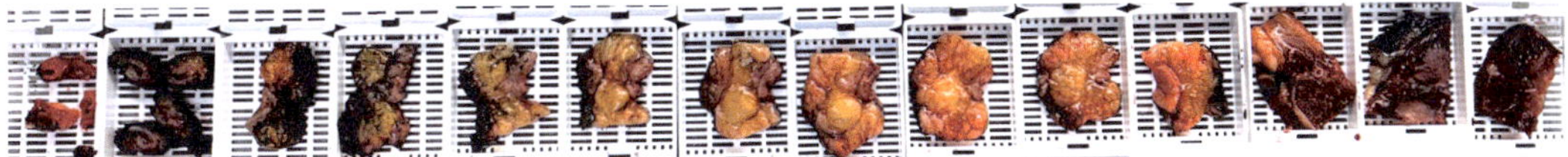

Fig. 6.23 Nephroureterectomy for urothelial tumor section submission

(24.1 cm in length by 0.4 cm in diameter). The ureter is opened to reveal tan-pink, flattened mucosa with a focal slightly lobulated and ill-defined lesion (2.0 × 0.6 cm) which is present proximally and 75% circumferential and is present 5.5 cm from the renal pelvis and 16.8 cm from the ureter resection margin. The kidney is bivalved to reveal a dilated renal pelvis and renal calyces with slightly dusky renal parenchyma and a renal cortex ranging from 0.2 to 0.7 cm. The area of the ureter lesion is serially sectioned to reveal no invasion through the ureter wall. The surrounding adipose tissue at the area of lesion is markedly dense and slightly scarred. The remainder of the kidney is serially sectioned to reveal no additional lesions or cysts present within. No adrenal gland is present.

Ink code

    Blue: anterior

    Black: posterior

Section code

    A1 Ureter and vasculature margins, en face

    A 2 Ureter distal to lesion

    A3–A10 Ureter lesion, entirely from distal to proximal

    A11 Ureter proximal to lesion

    A 12 Renal pelvis, representative

    A 13-A 14 Dusky renal parenchyma, representative

6.5 Kidney Resection for a Mass: Level V CPT 88307

A nephrectomy involves the removal of the kidney, either laparoscopically or through an abdominal incision. In this procedure, the kidney, proximal ureter segment, and sometimes the adrenal gland are removed.

Cancer Protocol Breakdown Relative to Grossing Nephrectomy

Procedure: Partial nephrectomy:- The excision of a portion of the kidney

Total nephrectomy:- The removal of the entire kidney with surrounding fatty tissue and some proximal ureter

Radical nephrectomy:- The removal of the entire kidney with surrounding adipose tissue, length of the proximal ureter, adrenal gland, and lymph nodes

Laterality: Dictate the laterality of the kidney and correlate with the orientation of the specimen

Tumor focality: Dictate if the tumor within the kidney is unifocal or multifocal

Tumor site: Dictate where the tumor is located within the kidney (i.e. superior pole, middle, lower pole, or interpolar)

Tumor size: Measure the tumor in three dimensions

Tumor extent: Dictate what anatomical aspects are involved in the tumor. The tumor can be limited to the kidney parenchyma or extend into the perinephric or sinus adipose tissue. Additionally, the mass can extend into the Gerota's fascia, major vessels, renal calyx, or outside the kidney into the adjacent structures.

Tumor necrosis: Dictate the amount of grossly identifiable necrosis present within the tumor (this can be stated in percentage).

Margin status: Perinephric adipose tissue, sinus adipose tissue, Gerota's fascia, renal vein, and ureter, all are included while looking for the margin status.

pT Categories [2]

pT0 No evidence of primary tumor

pT1a Tumor less than or equal to 4 cm in greatest dimension, limited to the kidney pT1b Tumor greater than 4 cm but less than or equal to 7 cm in greatest dimension limited to the kidney

pT2a Tumor greater than 7 cm but less than or equal to 10 cm in greatest dimension, limited to the kidney

pT2b Tumor greater than 10 cm, limited to the kidney

pT3a Tumor extends into the renal vein or its segmental branches, or invades the pelvicalyceal system, or invades perirenal and/or renal sinus fat but not beyond Gerota's fascia

pT3b Tumor extends into the vena cava below the diaphragm

pT3c Tumor extends into the vena cava above the diaphragm or invades the wall of the vena cava

pT4 Tumor invades beyond Gerota's fascia

Gross appearance of kidney tumors is described in Table 6.2.

Step 1: Measure and weigh the specimen. (Fig. 6.24)

Step 2: Identify the renal hilum. (Fig. 6.25)

Step 3: The hilar vessels are often clipped or stapled shut. Remove the staples and clips. (Fig. 6.26)

Step 4: When the renal vein and artery are visualized (Fig. 6.27), shave the margins and submit en face.

Step 5: Identify the ureter and measure the length and diameter. (Fig. 6.28)

Step 6: Shave the ureter margin and submit en face.(Fig. 6.29)

Step 7: Submit the vessels and ureter margins in 1 cassette. (Fig. 6.30)

Step 8: The specimen can now be oriented using the ureter and vessels. The renal vein is anterior, and the ureter is posterior with the artery in between.

Table 6.2 Gross appearance of kidney tumors [3]

Renal tumors	Gross appearance
Renal cell tumors	*Renal papillary adenoma:* Well circumscribed, usually subcapsular, often wedge-shaped grayish-white to yellow nodule *Oncocytoma of the kidney:* Well-circumscribed mahogany-brown tumor with a central stellate scar *Clear cell renal cell carcinoma:* A well-circumscribed (pseudo-capsulated) golden yellow tumor that commonly has hemorrhage, necrosis, calcification, and cystic change; sarcomatous area may not look that yellow *Multilocular cystic renal cell neoplasm of low malignant potential:* Well-demarcated tumor with a fibrous pseudocapsule, composed entirely of variably sized cysts filled with serous or hemorrhagic fluid; no solid areas *Papillary renal cell carcinoma:* Encapsulated tan-brown tumor; the intracystic papillary growth may mimic extensive necrosis *Chromophobe renal cell carcinoma:* Well-circumscribed solitary tumor with a homogeneous gray to brown-cut surface, typically devoid of hemorrhage or necrosis *Tubulocystic carcinoma:* Well-circumscribed (usually not capsulated) tumor with spongy/bubble wrap cut surface *Collecting duct carcinoma:* Gray-white and firm tumor with hemorrhage and necrosis; have an irregular, poorly defined contour or are multinodular *Acquired cystic disease-associated renal cell carcinoma:* Identified in acquired cysts (in patients with end-stage kidney disease) either as an intracystic mass or not in association with the cysts; has a brown to yellow-tan cut surface, sometimes with hemorrhage or necrosis; background kidney with numerous cysts *Succinate dehydrogenase deficient renal cell carcinoma:* Well-circumscribed and solid tumor with red/brown cut surface, variable multicystic change, and generally with no necrosis
Metanephric adenoma	Unicentric, well-circumscribed and solid gray-white tumor; mean diameter 50–60 mm (can reach 150 mm)
Classic angiomyolipoma	Well-demarcated (but not encapsulated) and solid mass with yellow to white firm cut surface
Nephroblastoma	Well-delineated and fleshy tumor with small yellow areas of necrosis. A multinodular internal structure is typical

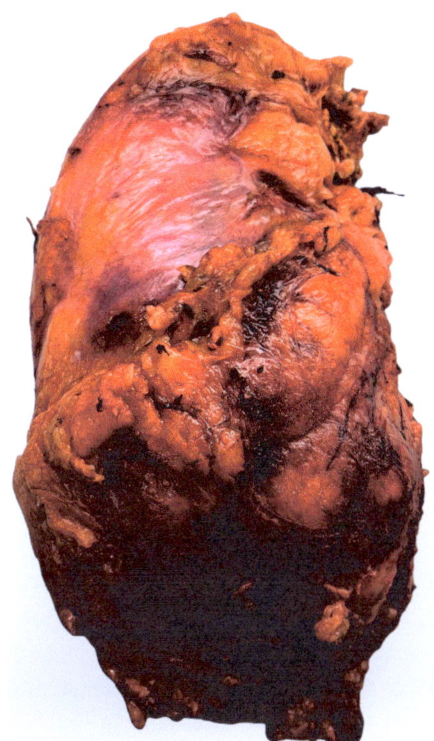

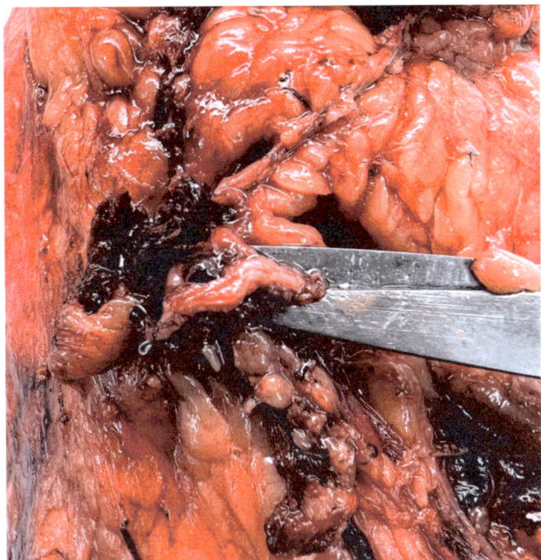

Fig. 6.26 Kidney hilum vessel margin

Fig. 6.24 Kidney resection for a mass

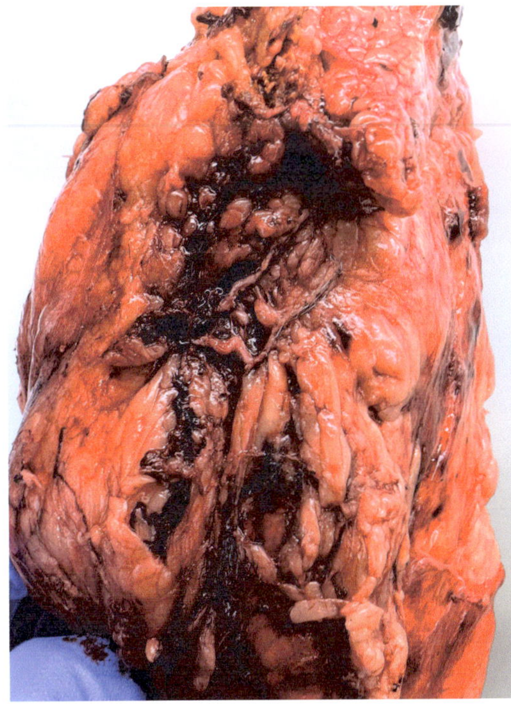

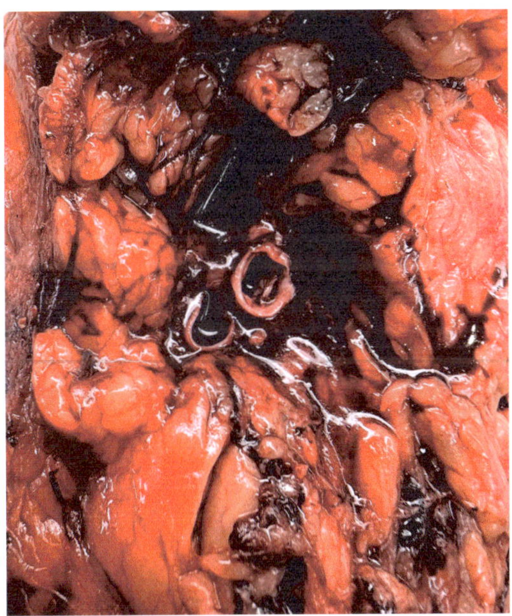

Fig. 6.27 Kidney hilar vessels opened

Step 9: Ink the anterior (Fig. 6.31a) and posterior (Fig. 6.31b) aspects of the kidney.

Step 10: Using small scissors, open the length of the ureter. (Fig. 6.32)

Step 11: Assess the length of the ureter for lesions (Fig. 6.33). Be very careful not to rub or scrape the ureter mucosa. Lesions or tumor deposits are easily brushed off.

Fig. 6.25 Kidney hilum

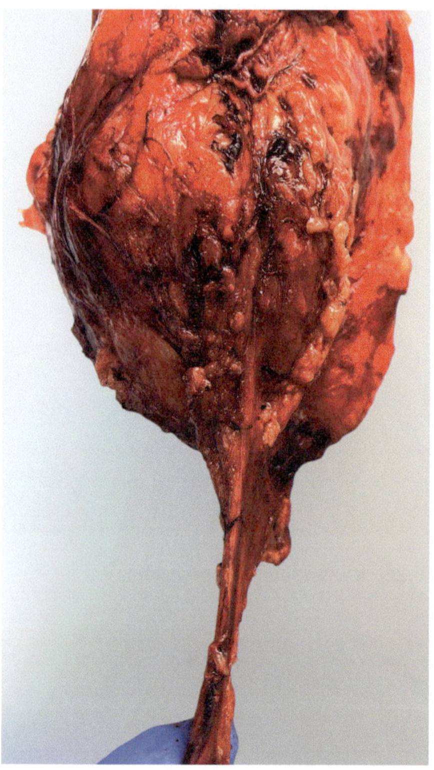

Fig. 6.28 Kidney resection for a mass segment of ureter

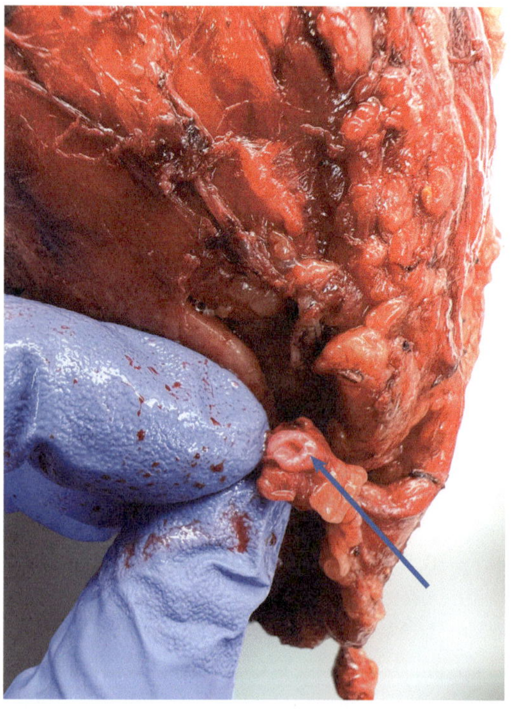

Fig. 6.29 Kidney resection for a mass ureter margin (blue arrow)

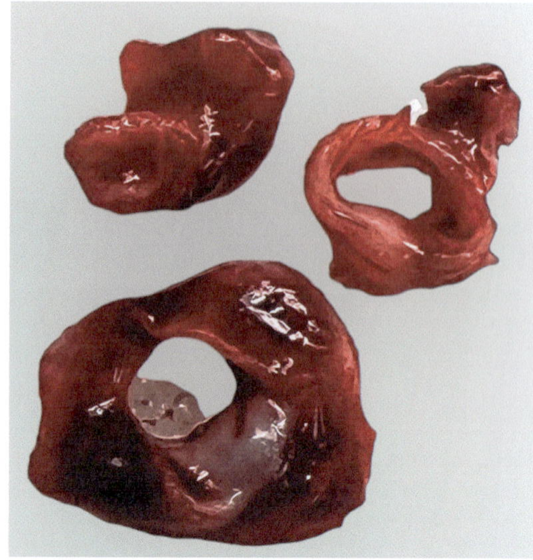

Fig. 6.30 Kidney resection for a mass, ureter, vein, and artery margin

Step 12: Assess the lumen of the renal vein for tumor thrombus or extension. In Fig. 6.34, a small extension of the tumor is protruding into the renal vein.

Step 13: Take a section of the extension of tumor into the renal vein, if applicable. (Fig. 6.35)

Step 14: Place forceps in the renal pelvis (Fig. 6.36). Also note the hemostat clipped to the renal vein. The vessels margins can easily be lost once inked. The hemostat is clipped to the renal vein to find it easily after specimen inking.

Step 15: Place the blade between the forceps to accurately bivalve the kidney. (Fig. 6.37)

Step 16: Describe the mass, circumscription, color, necrosis (quantify as a %), and fleshy areas (quantify as a %) (Fig. 6.38).

Step 17: Dictate where the mass is located and how close the mass comes to the renal pelvis, sinus adipose tissue, and hilar adipose tissue.

Step 18: Serially section both halves of the kidney. Once sectioned, a three-dimensional measurement of the mass can be obtained (Fig. 6.39).

Step 19: Assess how close the mass comes to the renal capsule, perinephric adipose tissue, and renal pelvis (Fig. 6.40)

Step 20: Describe and measure the adrenal gland (Fig. 6.41)

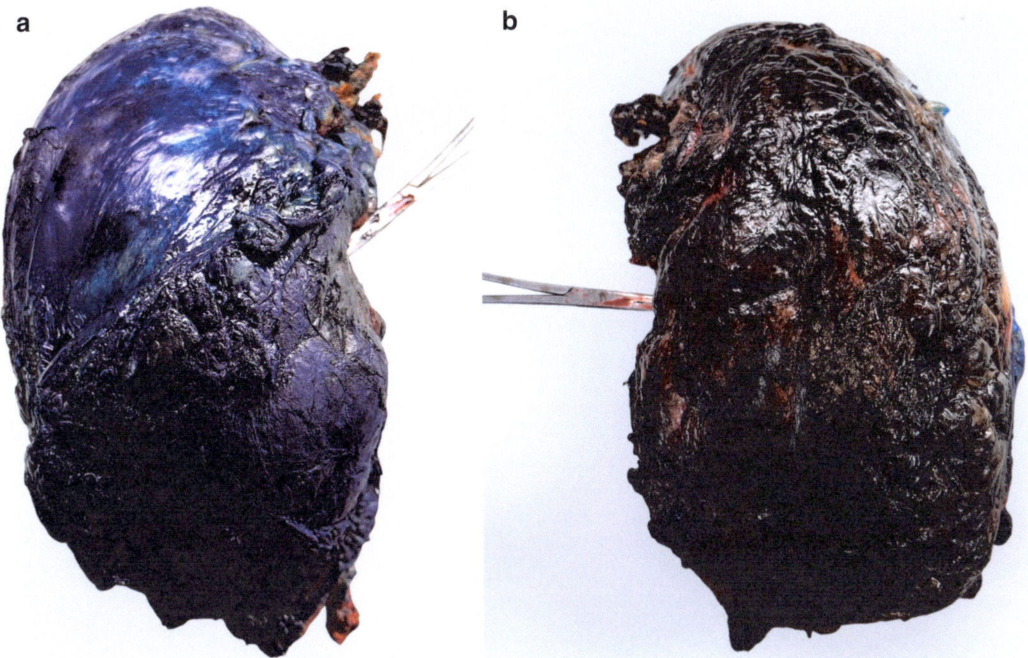

Fig. 6.31 (**a**) Anterior view. (**b**) Posterior view

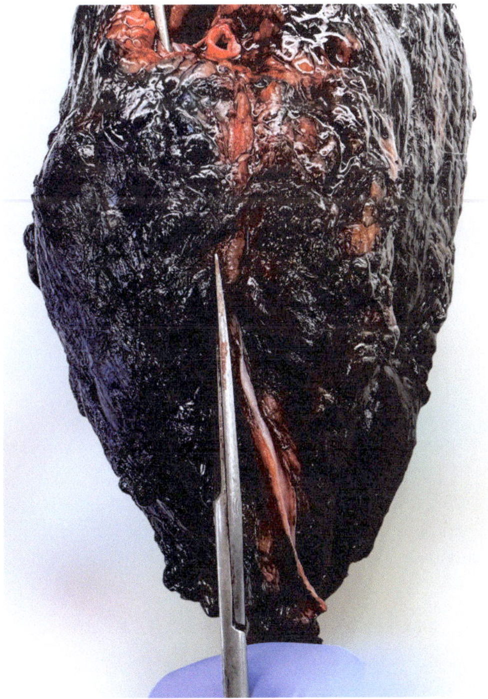

Fig. 6.32 Kidney resection for a mass, opening the ureter

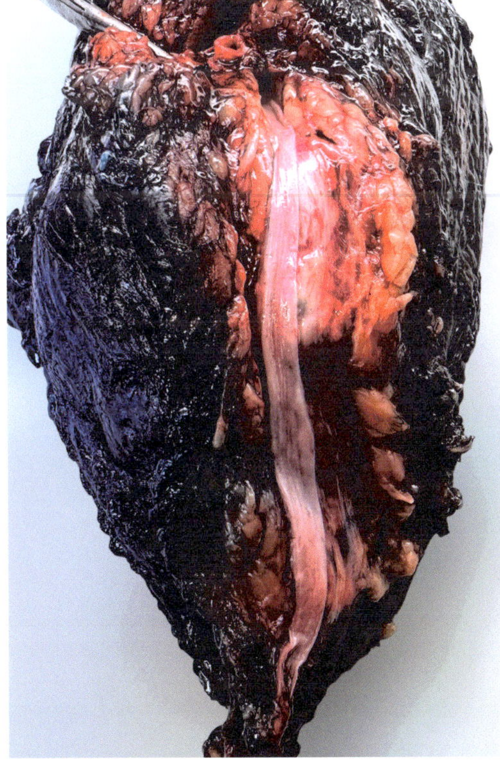

Fig. 6.33 Kidney resection for a mass, ureter opened

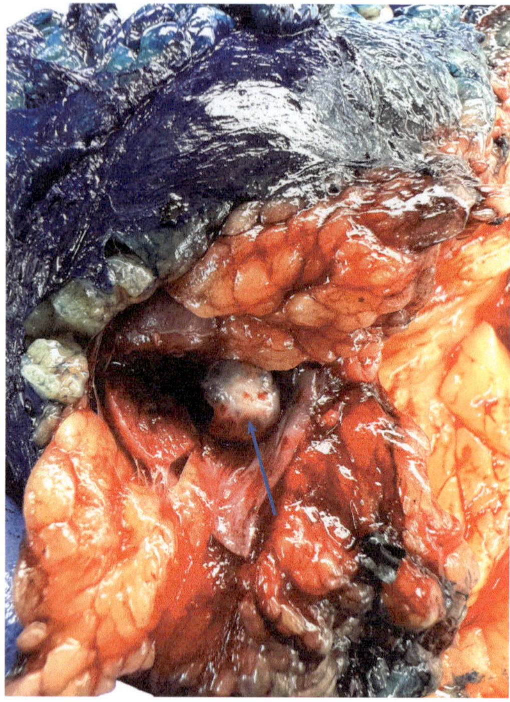

Fig. 6.34 Renal vein with tumor extension (blue arrow)

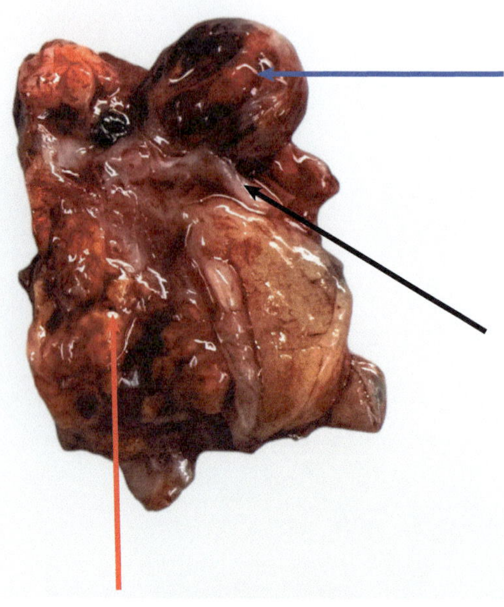

Fig. 6.35 Section of tumor extension. The main mass (red arrow) with the extension of tumor (blue arrow) into the renal vein (black arrow)

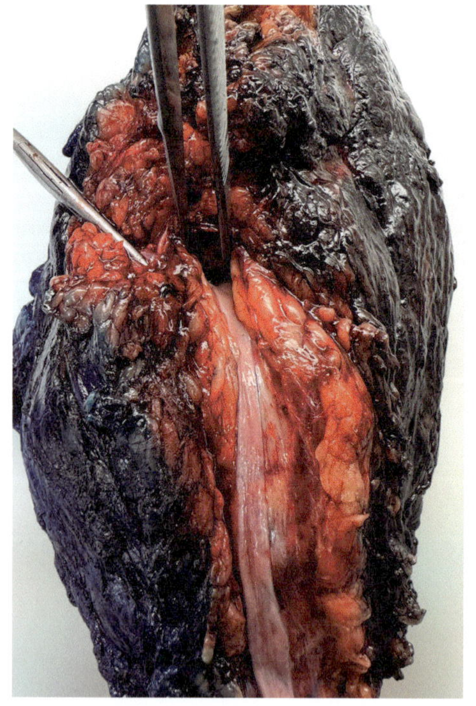

Fig. 6.36 Kidney resection for a mass, kidney with forceps placed in renal pelvis

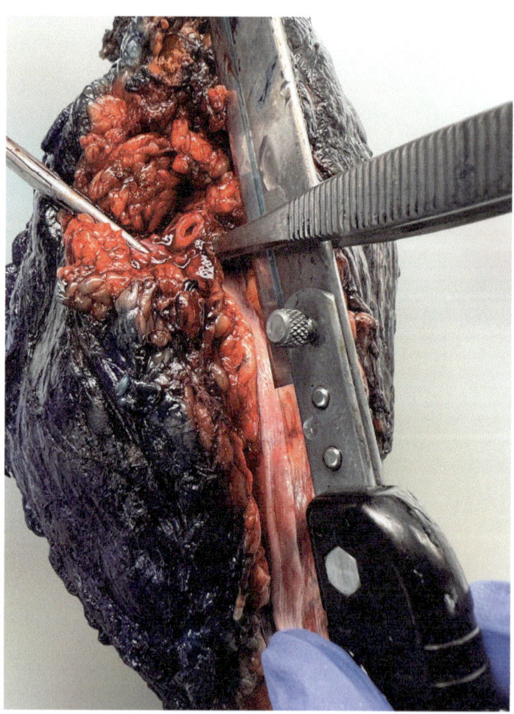

Fig. 6.37 Kidney resection for a mass, using forceps to bivalve kidney

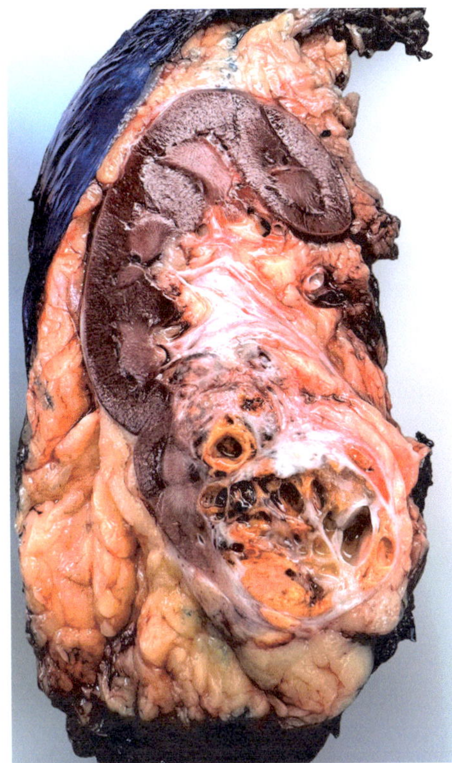

Fig. 6.38 Kidney resection for a mass

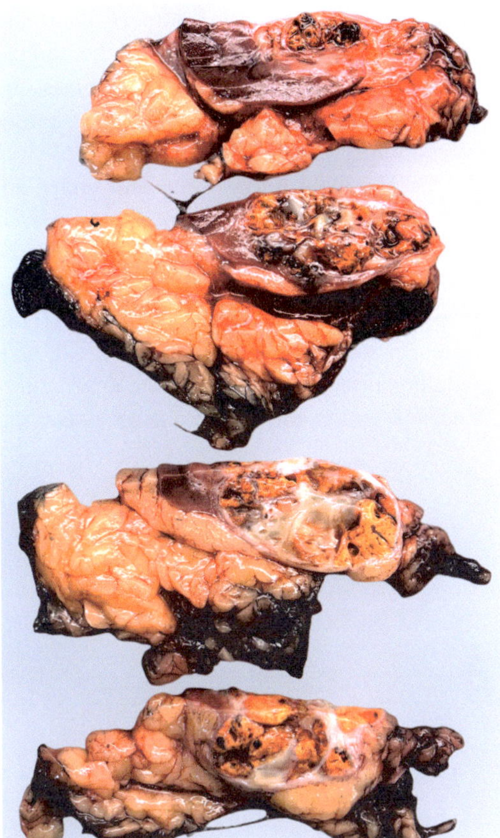

Fig. 6.40 Mass in relation to renal capsule

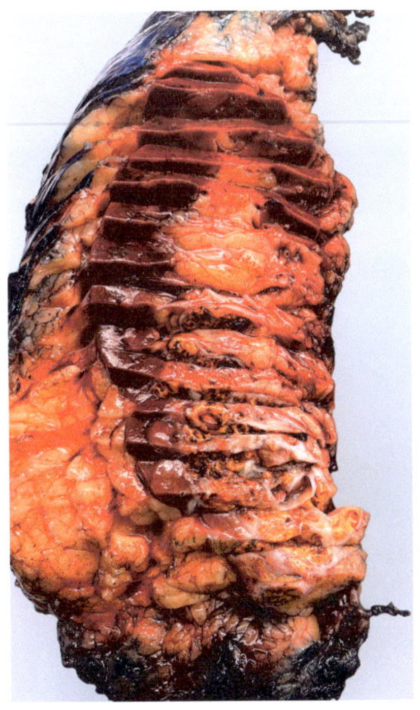

Fig. 6.39 Kidney serially sectioned

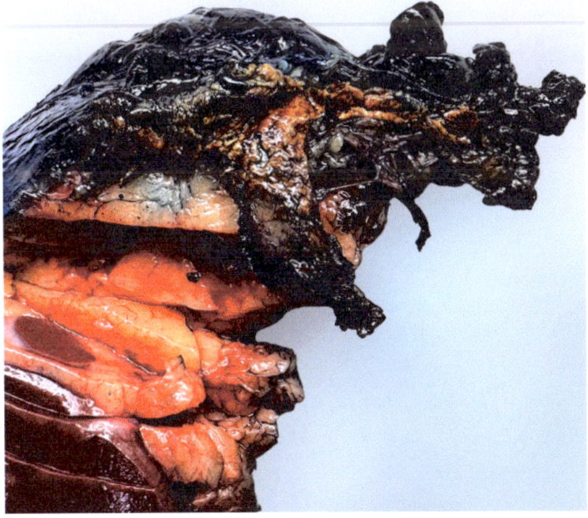

Fig. 6.41 Adrenal gland present with kidney

Step 21: Serially section the adrenal gland and assess for nodules (Fig. 6.42). If the adrenal gland is not involved by the renal mass, the adrenal gland can be removed before sectioning.

Step 22: The renal artery, vein, and ureter are submitted en face. A representative section of tumor extension within renal vein is submitted. Mass in relation to sinus, hilar, and perinephric adipose tissue is submitted. If the tumor is too close to the hilar/pelvic fat, take additional sections or sample the entire interface of tumor and pelvic fat to assess the involvement of hilar/pelvic fat. If the tumor is far from hilar fat, one section in relationship to sinus/hilar fat is adequate. A section of mass in relation to the renal pelvis and unremarkable renal tissue is also submitted. One or two sections of the adrenal gland are submitted if unremarkable (Fig. 6.43)

Note: One way to simplify cassette submission is to map the specimen (Fig. 6.44)

Example Dictation

Specimen A is received in formalin labeled with patient's name, medical record number, "kidney, right" and consists of a tan-brown kidney ($13.4 \times 7.5 \times 6.2$ cm, 844 g) with attached length of ureter (11.5 cm in length by 0.2 cm in diameter),

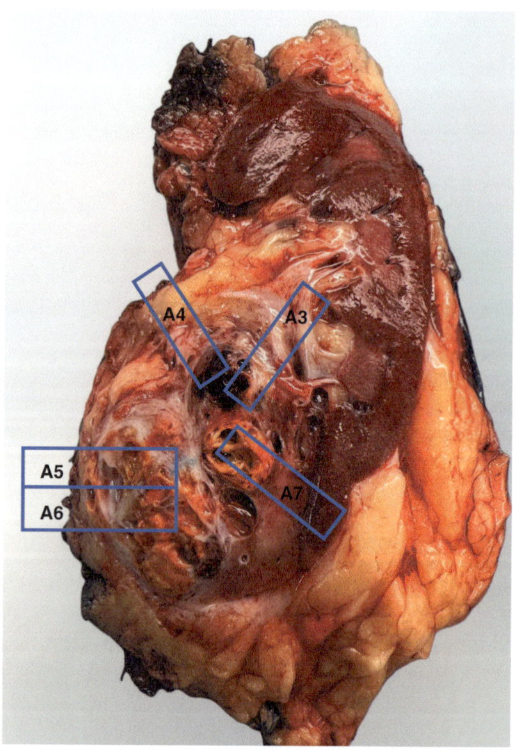

Fig. 6.44 Kidney resection mass mapping

Fig. 6.42 Adrenal gland serially sectioned

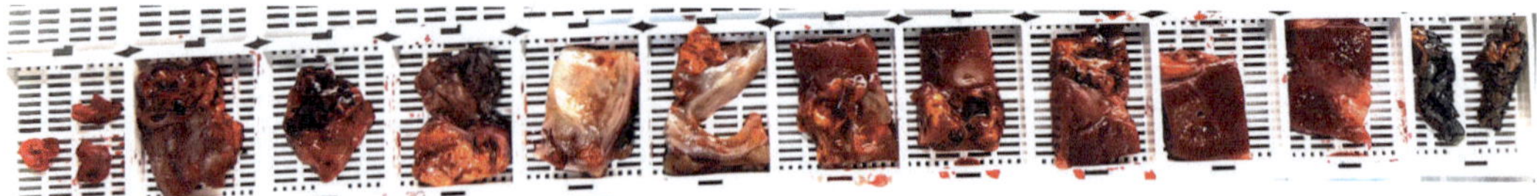

Fig. 6.43 Kidney resection for a mass section submission

surrounding perinephric adipose tissue ranging from 0.5 cm to 5.4 cm and an attached, markedly ragged, fragmented adrenal gland (4.2 × 1.6 × 1.5 cm). The ureter is opened to reveal a tan-pink, stellate lumen. The kidney is bivalved to reveal a multiloculated bright-yellow, hemorrhagic, solid, and cystic mass (6.5 × 5.5 × 5.0 cm) present in the inferior pole, abutting the hilar adipose tissue, invading the sinus adipose tissue, and coming within 0.3 cm of the renal pelvis. The renal vein is opened to reveal tumor extension into the vein, coming within 1.9 cm of the vein margin. Both halves are serially sectioned to reveal capsulated mass abutting the renal capsule posteriorly, without invasion through the renal capsule. The remaining renal parenchyma is red-brown with no additional lesions or cysts identified. The renal cortex ranges from 0.6 to 0.8 cm. The ragged adrenal gland is sectioned to reveal ragged, friable cut surfaces. No nodules are identified within. The renal hilum is palpable for 0 lymph node candidates.

1. Ink code
     Blue: anterior
     Black: posterior
2. Section code
     A1 Ureter, artery and vein margins, en face
     A 2 Mass extension into renal vein
     A3 Mass extension into sinus adipose tissue
     A4 Mass in relation to hilar adipose tissue
     A5-A6 Mass to closest renal capsule, representative.
     A7–A10 Mass in relation to renal parenchyma
     A11 Unremarkable renal parenchyma, representative
     A12 Adrenal gland, representative

6.6   Adrenal Gland: Level V CPT 88307

The adrenal gland is removed for lesions or for increased hormone levels. The gland is often removed with its surrounding adipose tissue and may or may not be oriented.

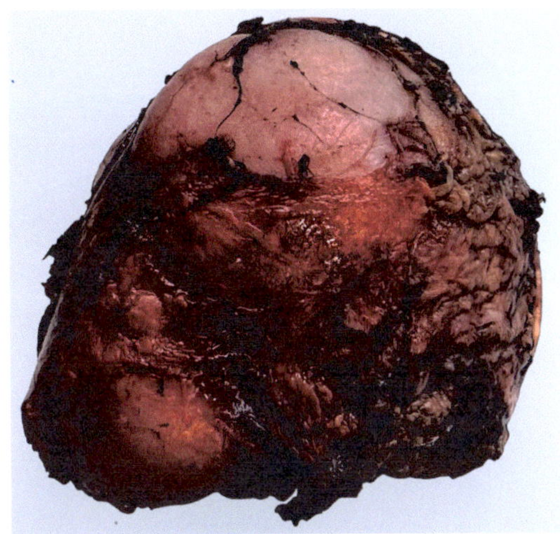

Fig. 6.45 Adrenal gland

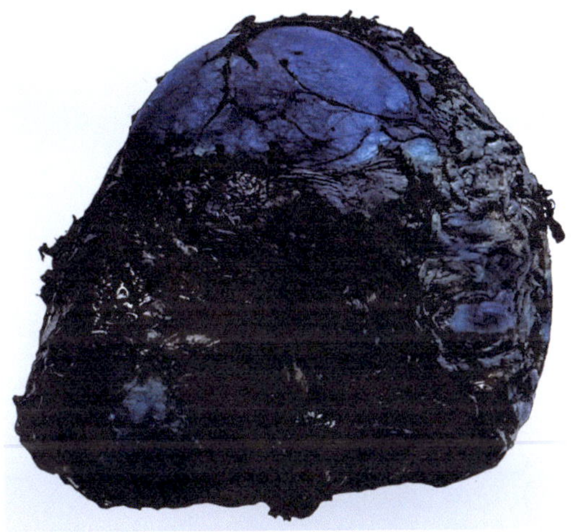

Fig. 6.46 Adrenal gland inked

Step 1: Measure and weigh the adrenal gland. (Fig. 6.45)
Step 2: Often the adrenal gland comes unoriented. However, orient the gland if orientation instructions are given.
Step 3: Ink the adrenal gland one color, if unoriented. (Fig. 6.46)
Step 4: Serially section the adrenal gland. (Fig. 6.47)
Step 5: Describe and measure the mass. (Fig. 6.48)
Step 6: Measure how close the mass comes to the closest margin.

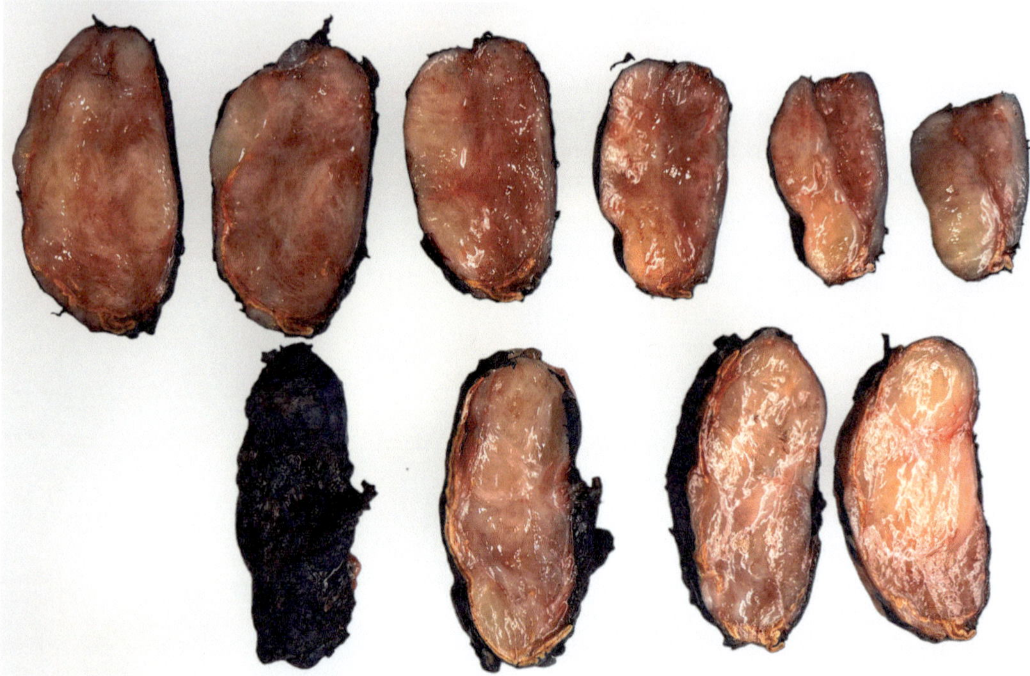

Fig. 6.47 Adrenal gland serially sectioned

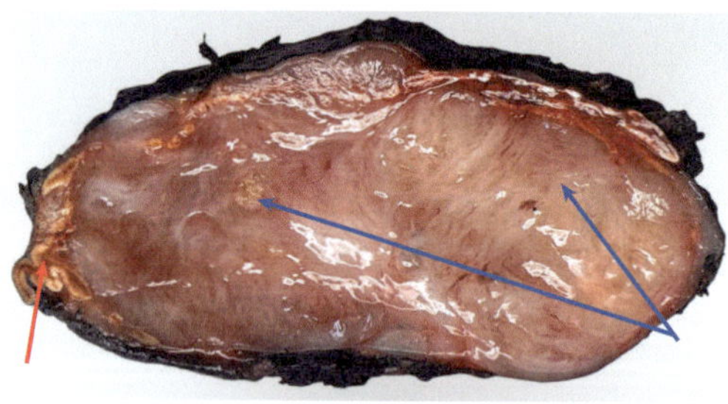

Fig. 6.48 Adrenal gland. Unremarkable adrenal gland (red arrow) with mass (blue arrows)

Step 7: Dictate if any unremarkable adrenal gland is present. (Fig. 6.48)
Step 8: Submit representative sections of the adrenal gland is large. A full cross section of adrenal gland with mass is divided to be submitted in Fig. 6.49.

Step 9: Submit representative sections (one section per 1.0 cm). (Fig. 6.50)

Example Dictation

Specimen A is received in formalin labeled with patient's name, medical record number, "adrenal, left" and consists of an unoriented, tan-brown, enlarged adrenal gland (11.2 × 7.6 × 7.1 cm, 123 g) which is entirely inked blue and serially sectioned to reveal a solid, tan-white, trabeculated mass (11.0 × 7.4 × 7.0 cm) extending to within 0.1 cm of the closest unoriented margin with identifiable bright yellow adrenal gland present at the periphery. Representative sections are submitted in A1–A6.

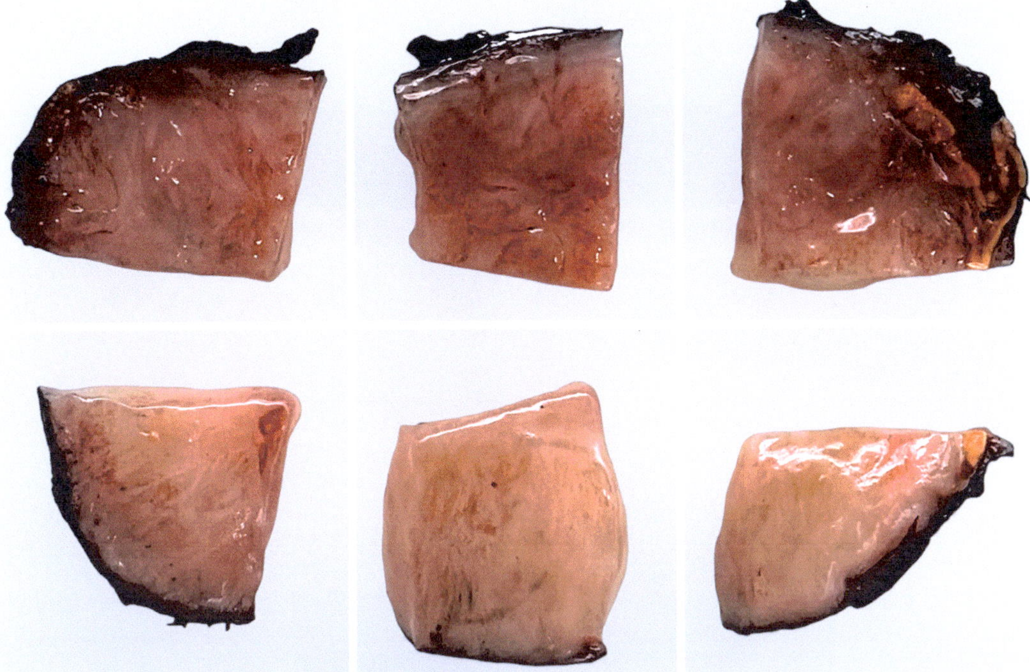

Fig. 6.49 Adrenal gland full cross section of adrenal gland with mass

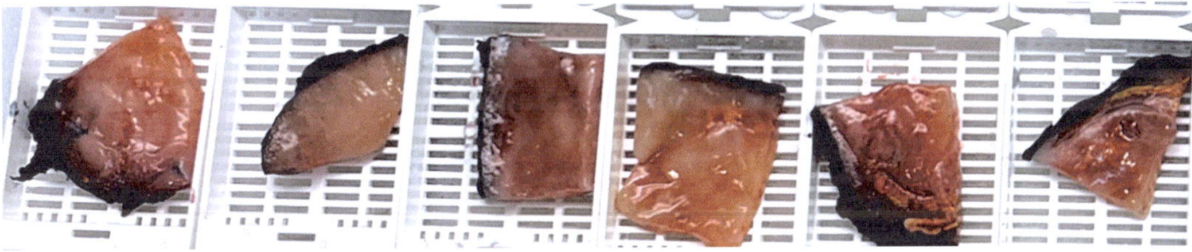

Fig. 6.50 Adrenal gland section submission

6.7 Prostate Biopsy: Level IV CPT 88305

Prostate biopsies are performed for palpable lesions or increased PSA levels. A biopsy needle is used to retrieve these specimens and often come oriented by the anatomic area of the prostate.

Step 1: Count, describe, and measure the prostate cores. (Fig. 6.51)

Step 2: Lightly ink the prostate cores (Fig. 6.52). Prostate cores are difficult for the histology staff to visualize once embedded in paraffin wax. Inking the cores can help histology staff when sectioning but it is otherwise not necessary. Communicate with pathologists concerning inking the prostate biopsies.

Step 3: Submit the prostate cores in a biopsy bag (Fig. 6.53). Communicate with the pathologist concerning how many cores should be placed in a single cassette.

Example Dictation

Specimen A is received in formalin labeled with patient's name, medical record number, "right base" and consists of 2 tan-white cores (2.0 cm and 2.2 cm in length) which are inked blue and submitted entirely in A1.

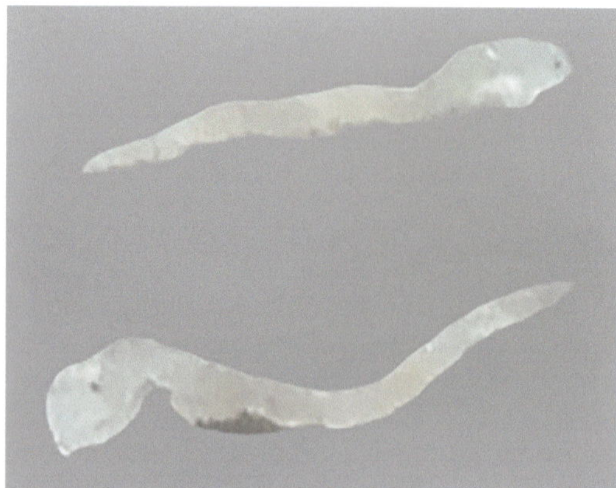

Fig. 6.51 Prostate biopsy cores

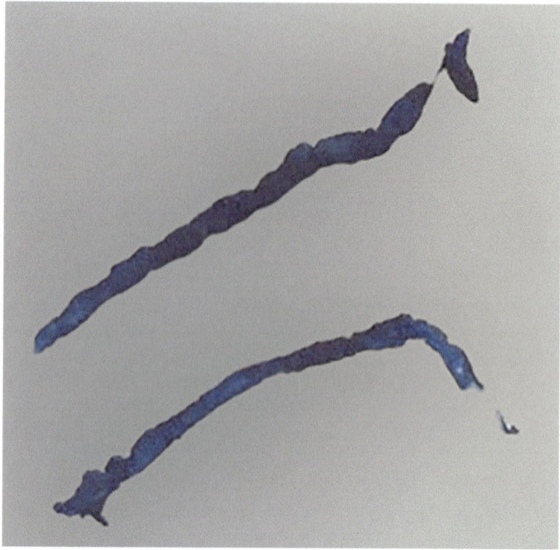

Fig. 6.52 Prostate biopsy cores inked

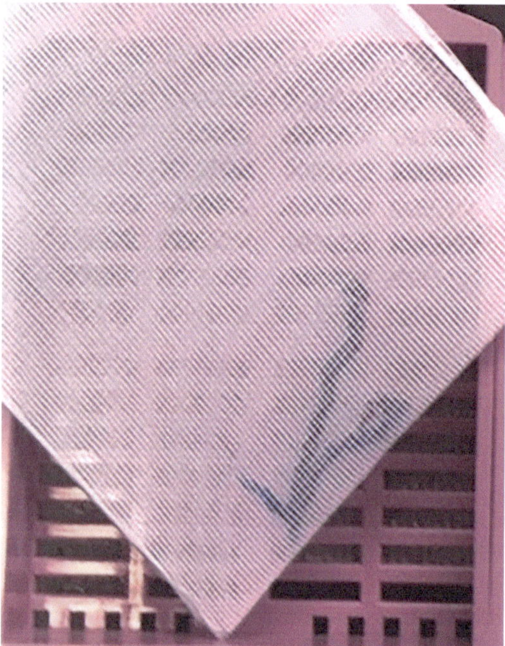

Fig. 6.53 Prostate biopsy cassette submission

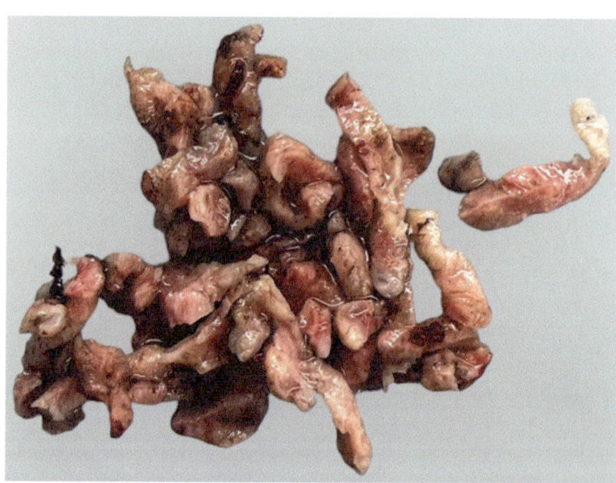

Fig. 6.54 Transurethral Resection of the Prostate (TURP), prostate chips

6.8 Transurethral Resection of the Prostate (TURP): Level IV CPT 88305

TURP procedures are typically performed for benign prostatic hyperplasia. The prostatic tissue is removed using electrocautery or sharp dissection to remove the area in fragments.

Step 1: Describe, measure, and weigh the aggregate. (Fig. 6.54)

Step 2: Submit sections. The standard rule is to submit 30 g of tissue entirely. For every 5 g of tissue over the initial 30 g, one cassette of prostate chips is submitted. For example, if 45 g of prostate chips is received, 30 g is submitted entirely, and 3 additional cassettes are submitted. Make sure that the fragments are not overlapping in the cassette. (Fig. 6.55)

Example Dictation

Specimen A is received in formalin labeled with patient's name, medical record number, "prostate TURP" and consists of an aggregate of tan-pink

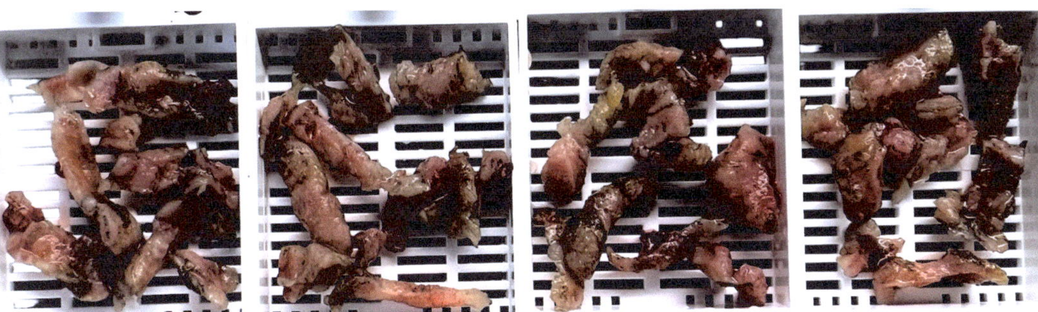

Fig. 6.55 Transurethral Resection of the Prostate (TURP) section submission

tissue fragments (4.1 × 3.9 × 1.8 cm, 6 g) which is submitted entirely in A1–A4.

6.9 Prostatectomy: Level VI CPT 88309

The removal of the prostate (prostatectomy) is performed for malignancy or benign prostatic hyperplasia. The entire prostate is dissected along with the seminal vesicles and a length of the vas deferens.

Cancer Protocol Breakdown Relative to Grossing Prostate

Procedure: A radical prostatectomy is the removal of the entire prostate with bilateral seminal vesicles and a length of the bilateral vas deferens.

Size: Dictate a three-dimensional measurement of the prostate and its weight in grams.

pT categories [2]

No T1 classification for prostatectomy

pT2 Organ confined

pT3a Extraprostatic extension or microscopic invasion of bladder neck

pT3 Subcategory cannot be determined

pT3b Tumor invades seminal vesicle

pT4 Tumor is fixed or invades adjacent structures other than seminal vesicles such as external sphincter, rectum, bladder, levator muscles, and/or pelvic wall

Gross appearance of prostate tumors is described in Table 6.3 [2]

Table 6.3 Gross appearance of prostate lesions [2]

Prostate lesions	Gross appearance
Benign prostatic hyperplasia	Variously sized nodules of gray to yellow color and a granular appearance projecting above the cut surface
Prostatic adenocarcinoma	Often not visible grossly; solid, firm, and poorly circumscribed (if visible)

Step 1: Orient the prostate. Placing a probe in the prostatic urethra is a good way to identify the apex and base of the prostate as shown in Fig. 6.56a. The vas deferens and the seminal vesicles are present on the posterior-superior aspect of the prostate (Fig. 6.56b), and the posterior prostate is often flat in appearance (Fig. 6.56c).

Step 2: Measure and weigh the prostate. Measure the bilateral vas deferens and seminal vesicles. (Fig. 6.57)

Step 3: Ink the right and left prostate. (Fig. 6.58)

Step 4: Shave the bilateral vas deferens margins and submit en face. (Fig. 6.59)

Step 5: Amputate the vas deferens and seminal vesicles at the insertion point. Take representative sections of the seminal vesicles at the insertion point, this is periprostatic seminal vesicle section. (Fig. 6.60)

Step 6: The first slice of the prostate at the apex is the apex margin. Remove the apex margin. (Fig. 6.61)

Step 7: Radially section the apex margin using the urethra as the focal point. (Fig. 6.62)

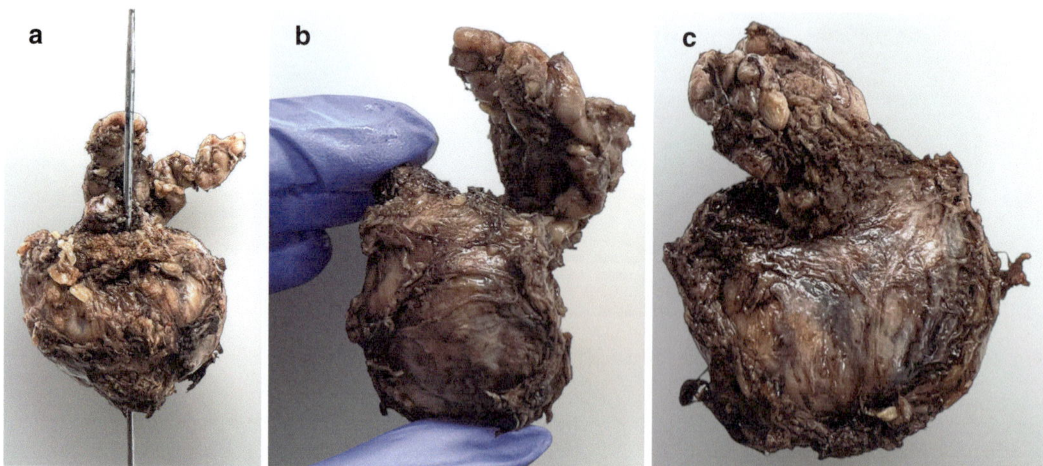

Fig. 6.56 (**a**) Anterior view. (**b**) Lateral view. (**c**) Posterior view

Fig. 6.57 Prostatectomy orientation

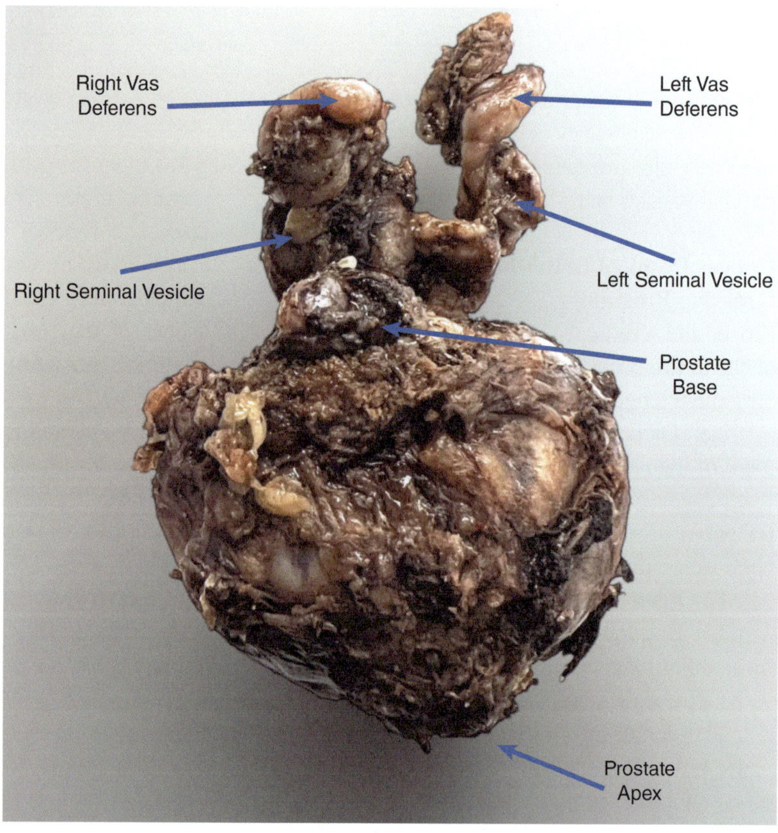

Step 8: The last slice of the prostate will include the prostate base margin. Radially section the base margin using the urethra as the focal point and submit on edge. (Fig. 6.63)

Step 9: Serially section the remaining prostate from apex to base. Make sure that every slice has ink surrounding the periphery. (Fig. 6.64)

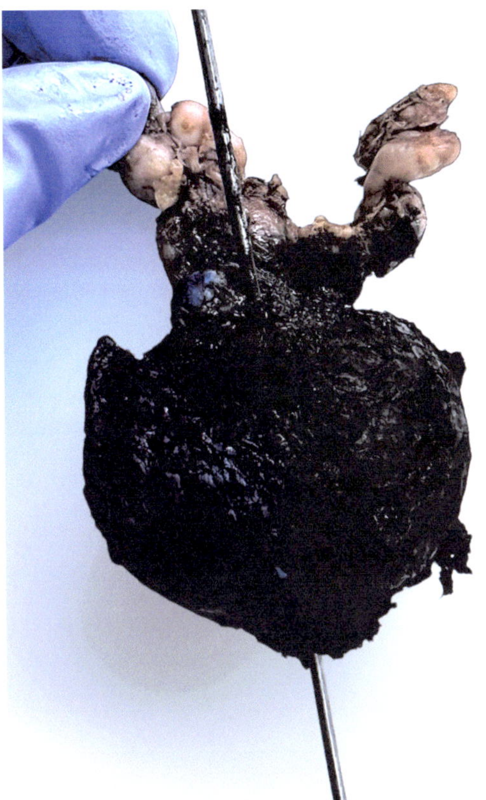

Fig. 6.58   Prostate inked

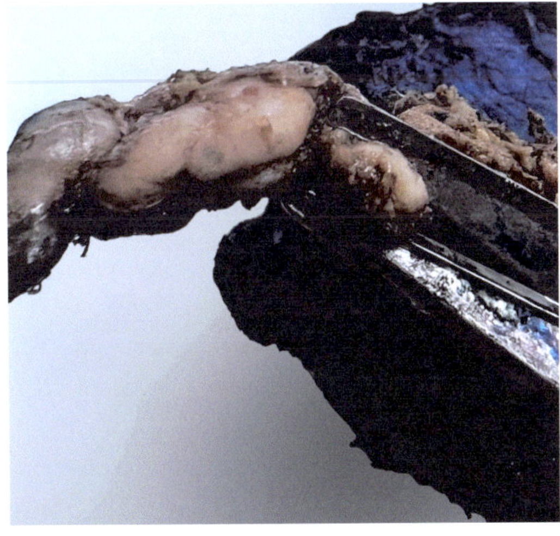

Fig. 6.59   Prostate vas deferens margin

Step 10: Assess the slices for lesions. Often prostate cancer is difficult to identify with the eye. In Fig. 6.65, a solid white area is noted on the posterior-left aspect.

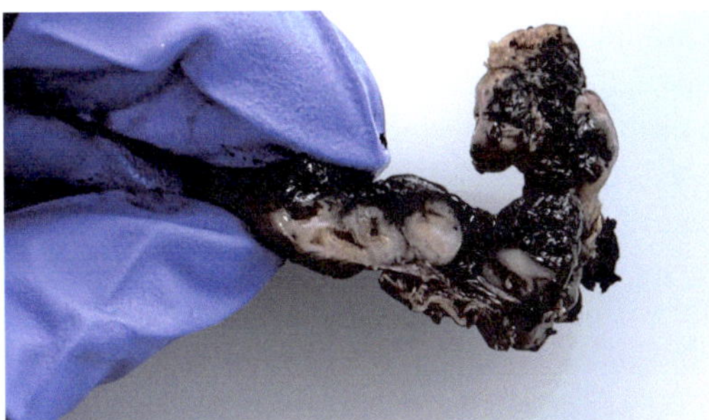

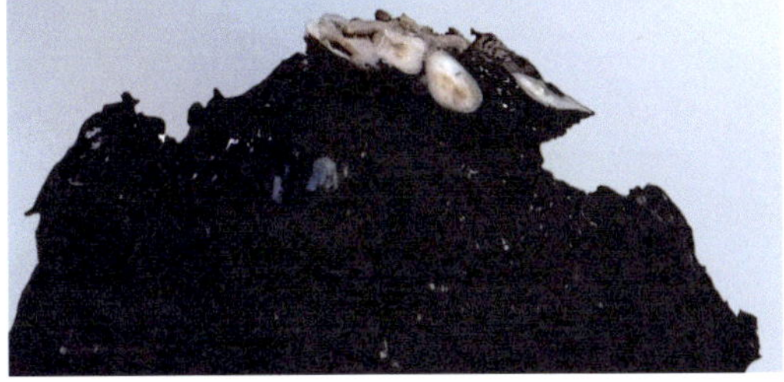

Fig. 6.60   Prostate seminal vesicles

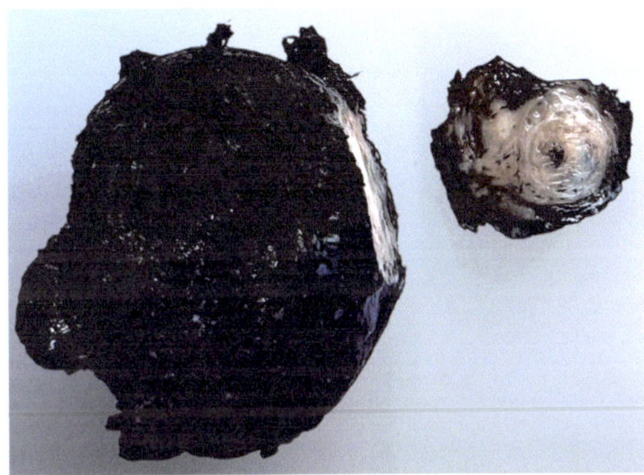

Fig. 6.61   Prostate apex section

Step 11: Measure the lesion in three dimensions and measure how close the lesion comes to the closest margin.

Step 12: Each prostate slice is quadrisected and submitted oriented. Fig. 6.66 shows how the slices are section into quadrants.

Step 13: The remaining sections are submitted entirely, oriented into quadrants and submitted from apex to base. If the prostate is large, communicate with the pathologists for changes in cassette submission. (Figs. 6.67 and 6.68)

Step 14: The prostate can also be submitted with a map to streamline communication. (Fig. 6.69)

Example Dictation

Specimen A is received in formalin labeled with patient's name, medical record number, "prostate" and consists of a slightly ragged, tan prostate (5.2 × 4.5 × 4.3 cm, 53 g) with attached bilateral vas deferens (right 2.5 cm in length, left 1.9 cm in length) with tan lumens and attached bilateral seminal vesicles (right 4.4 × 1.5 × 0.5 cm, left 4.2 × 1.5 × 0.6 cm) with unremarkable cut surfaces. The specimen is serially sectioned to reveal a slightly lobulated central zone with small nodules ranging from 0.1 to 0.7 cm. The peripheral zone contains an ill-defined tan-white area (1.9 × 1.8 × 1.3 cm) present at the left apical aspect coming within 0.3 cm of the left peripheral margin. The remainder of the periph-

eral zone contains multiple irregular pale areas ranging from 0.3 to 0.5 cm, spanning both the right and left aspect.

3. Ink code:
   Blue-right
   Black-left
4. Section code:
   A 1 Right vas deferens margin and representative section of right periprostatic seminal vesicle
   A 2 Left vas deferens margin representative section of left periprostatic seminal vesicle
   A 3 Right apex, radially sectioned
   A 4 Left apex, radially sectioned

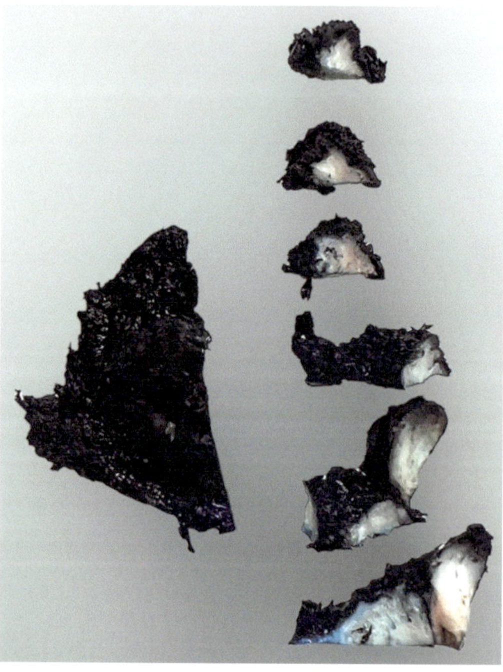

Fig. 6.62 Prostate apex radially sectioned

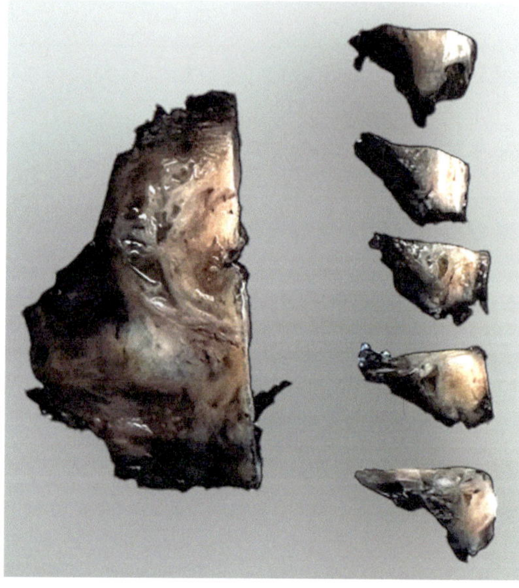

Fig. 6.63 Prostate base radially sectioned

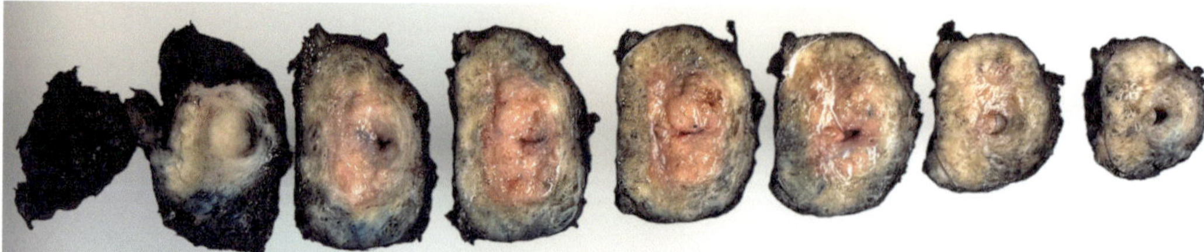

Fig. 6.64 Prostate serially sectioned

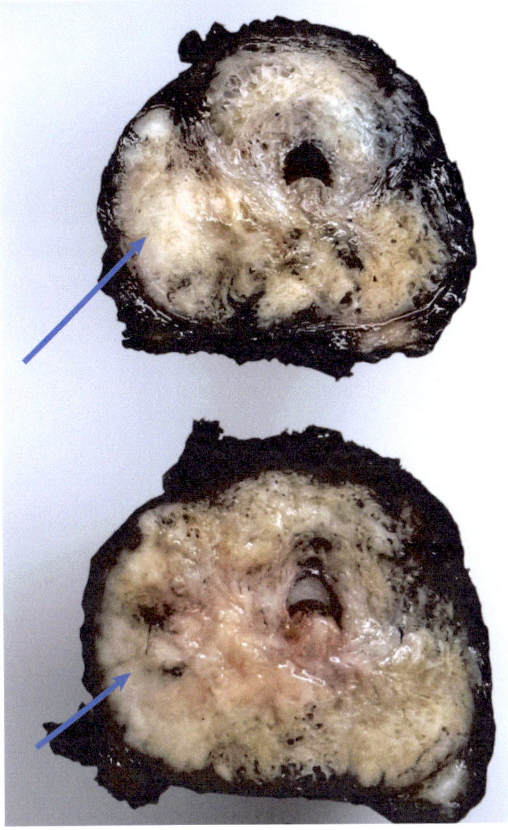

A 5 Right base, radially sectioned

A 6 Left base, radially sectioned

A 7–A 34 prostate entirely from apex to base, 1 slice per 4 cassettes quadrisected as follows: anterior right, posterior right, anterior left, posterior left, respectively.

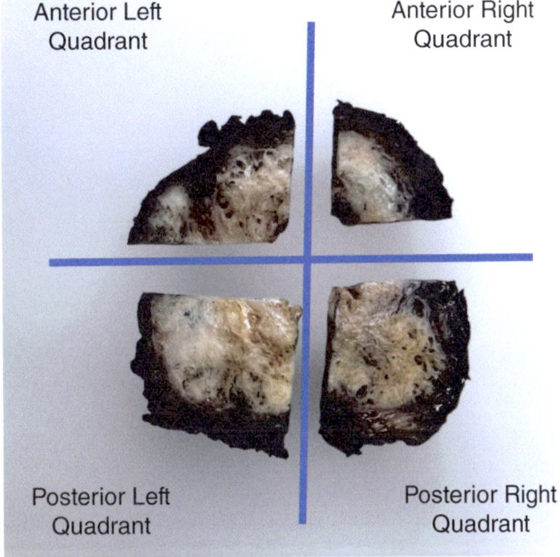

Fig. 6.65 Prostatectomy. Prostate lesion area (indicated by blue arrow)

Fig. 6.66 Prostatectomy. Prostate quadrisected

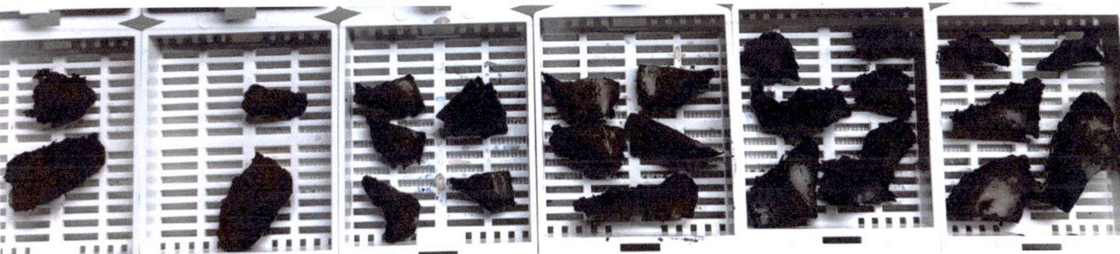

Fig. 6.67 Prostate margin sections

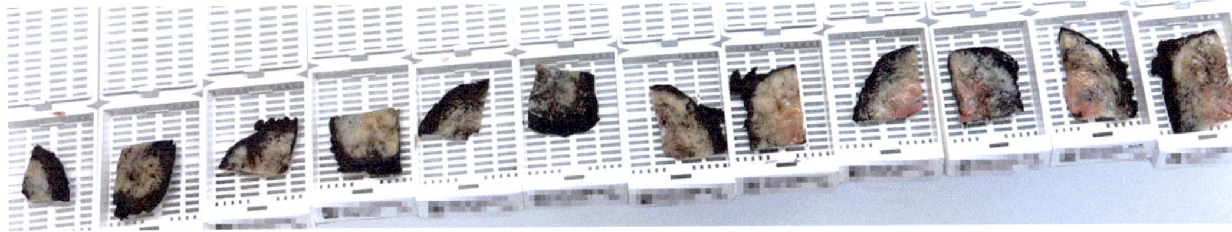

Fig. 6.68 Prostate cross sections quadrisected

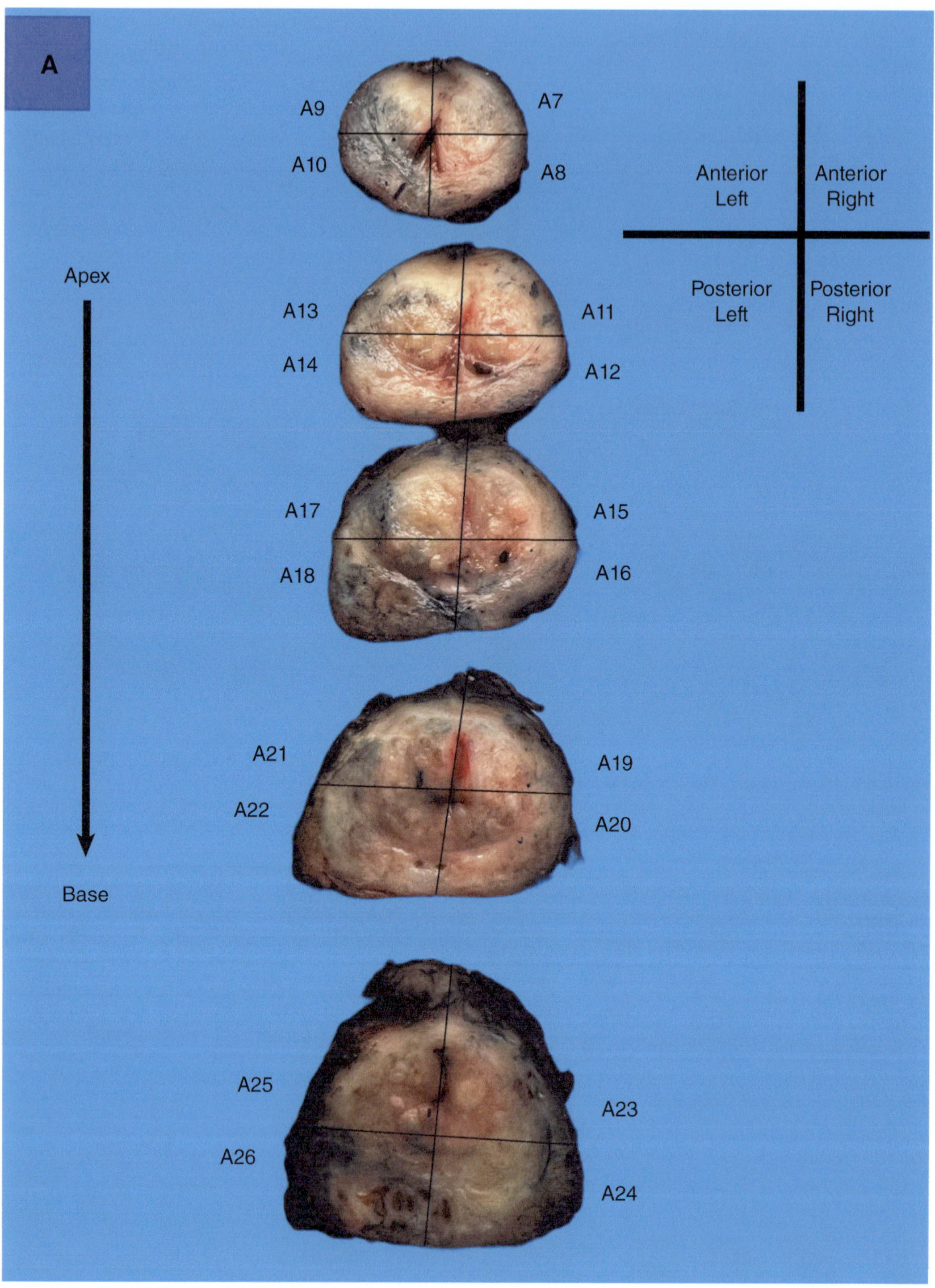

Fig. 6.69 Prostate mapping

6.10   Bladder Transurethral Resection of Bladder Tumor (TURBT): Level V CPT 88307

A TURBT is performed to remove suspected bladder cancer using electrocautery or sharp dissection. The fragments are then assessed microscopically for muscular invasion. If invasion is identified, the bladder may be surgically removed entirely.

Step 1: Describe and measure the specimen. (Fig. 6.70).

Step 2: Submit the specimen. In Fig. 6.71, the specimen is submitted entirely. If the aggregate is large, communicate with the pathologist for cassette submission.

Example Dictation

Specimen A is received in formalin labeled with patient's name, medical record number, "bladder" and consists of an aggregate of brown-pink, ragged tissue fragments (3.9 × 2.4 × 0.4 cm) which is divided and submitted entirely in A1-A2.

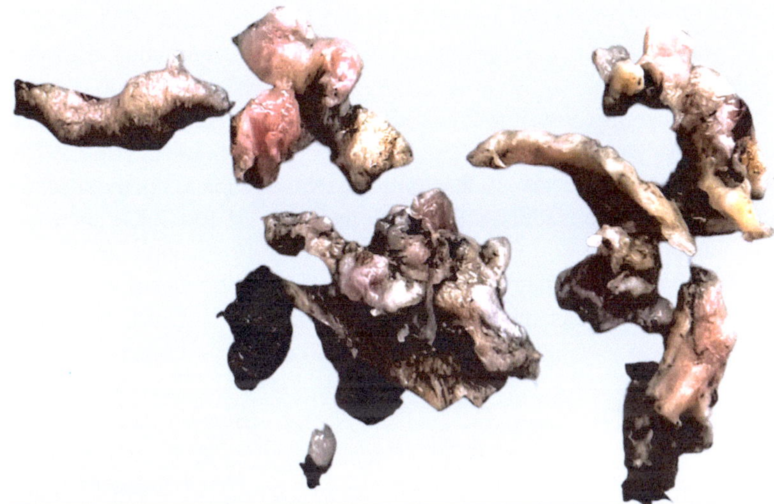

Fig. 6.70 Bladder transurethral resection of bladder tumor (TURBT)

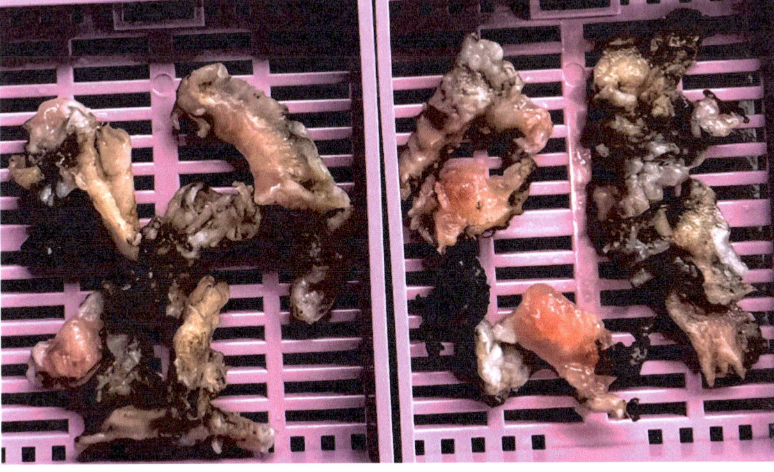

Fig. 6.71 Bladder transurethral resection of bladder tumor section submission

6.11 Bladder with Prostate: Level VI CPT 88309

A cystoprostatectomy is the surgical removal of the bladder and the prostate in male patients who have biopsy proven cancer with muscular invasion.

Cancer Protocol Breakdown Relative to Grossing Bladder.

Procedure: Dictate if the specimen is a partial resection, a radical cystectomy or a radical cystoprostatectomy.

Tumor site: Dictate all the anatomical structures involved by the tumor. This can include the trigone, right lateral wall, left lateral wall, anterior wall, posterior wall, and bladder dome.

Tumor size: Measure the tumor size in three dimensions.

Tumor extent: Dictate if the tumor extends into or through the bladder wall or into the surrounding organs.

Margin status: Dictate how close the tumor comes from the ureter margins and the ureteral margin.

pT Categories [2]

pT0 No evidence of primary tumor

pTis Urothelial carcinoma in situ

pT1 Tumor invades lamina propria

pT2 Tumor invades superficial muscularis

pT3 Tumor invades perivesical soft tissue

pT4 Extravesical tumor invades directly into prostatic stroma, uterus, vagina, pelvic, or abdominal wall

Gross appearance of prostate tumors is described in Table 6.4 [2]

Table 6.4 Gross appearance of bladder lesions [2]

Bladder lesions	Gross appearance
Endometriosis of bladder	Multiple small red nodules protrude from the bladder surface
Invasive urothelial carcinoma	Variety of gross appearances including papillary, sessile, polypoid, nodular, and ulcerative; can be unifocal or multifocal; concurrent CIS can have a flat erythematous appearance

Step 1: Identify and measure the bladder and prostate. The anterior aspect is more ragged as seen in Fig. 6.72a, and the posterior aspect is flatter in appearance as seen in Fig. 6.72b. The posterior aspect will also contain the seminal vesicle and vas deferens.

Step 2: Measure the bilateral vas deferens and bilateral seminal vesicles. (Fig. 6.73)

Step 3: Identify and measure the bilateral ureters. The ureters insert posterior-laterally towards the inferior aspect of the bladder. Fig. 6.74a, b show the ureters on each side of the bladder.

Step 4: The right ureter margin, right vas deferens margin, and right seminal vesicle can be submitted in 1 cassette and the left ureter margin, left vas deferens margin, and left seminal vesicle can be submitted in a separate single cassette. (Fig. 6.75)

Step 5: Ink the specimen four colors. Note that all four inks converge at the prostate apex. In this example, the ink code is as follows:

Blue- anterior (Fig. 6.76a)

Black- posterior r(Fig. 6.76b)

Orange- right (Fig. 6.76a)

Green- left (Fig. 6.76a)

Step 6: Shave the prostate apex margin approximately 0.5 cm thick. (Fig. 6.77)

Step 7: Radially section the prostate apex margin and submit on edge. (Fig. 6.78)

Step 8: Serially section the remainder of the prostate up to the area of the prostate base as shown in Fig. 6.79a.

Step 9: Quadrisect and submit the prostate entirely (or representative-communicate with the pathologist) in an oriented manner as shown in Fig. 6.79b.

Step 10: Place scissors in the urethra and cut along the anterior-left aspect up to the bladder dome (Fig. 6.80a) and make a second cut along the anterior-right aspect up to the bladder dome. This will create a flap of the anterior bladder wall to open the bladder. (Fig. 6.80b)

Step 11: Identify the right (Fig. 6.81a) and left (Fig. 6.81b)ureteral orifice as identified by blue arrows. The ureteral orifices are difficult to identify and may take practice to recognize.

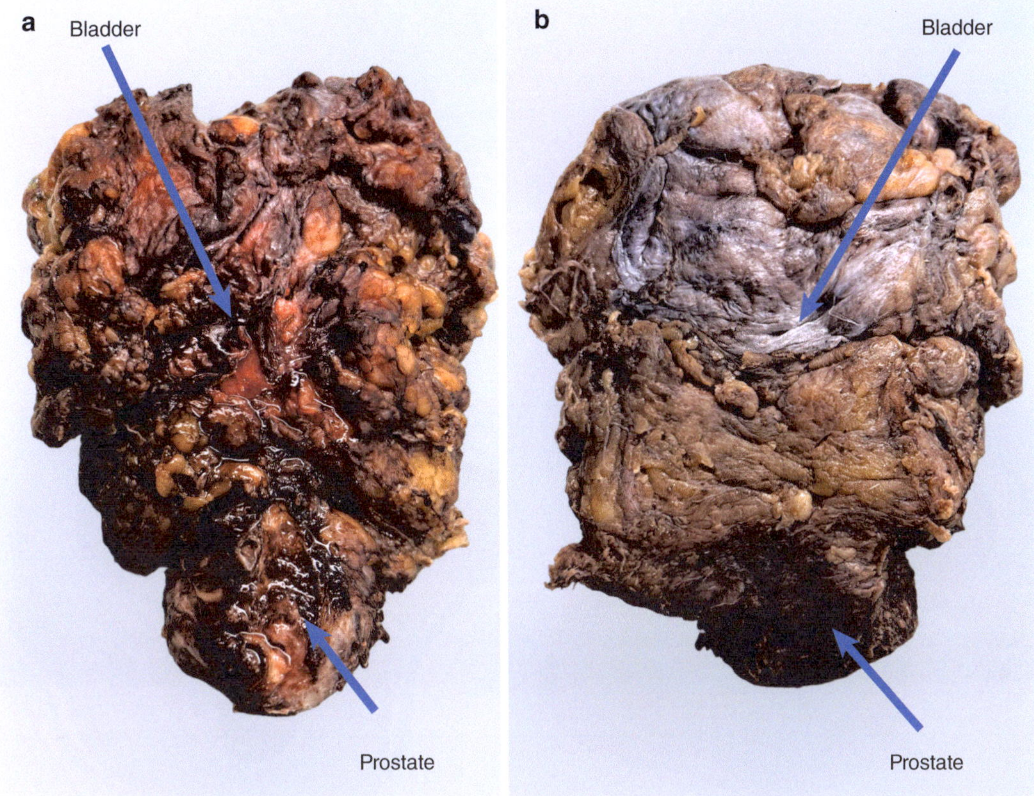

Fig. 6.72 (**a**) Cystoprostatectomy anterior view. (**b**) Cystoprostatectomy posterior view

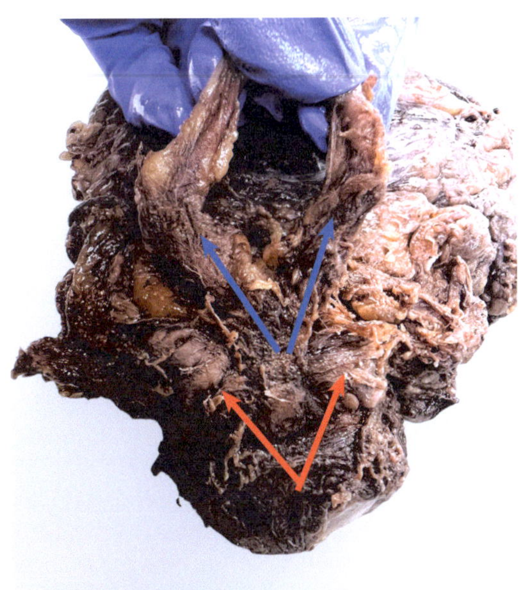

Fig. 6.73 Vas deferens (blue arrows) and seminal vesicles (red arrows)

Step 12: Place probes into the ureteral orifices, extending through the ureter margins.

Step 13: Pin the bladder open onto a wax board as flat as possible (Fig. 6.82). Submerge the bladder in formalin to fix. Wax will float so flip the wax board upside-down allowing the specimen to be totally submerged in formalin. The specimen can be fixed for a few hours or overnight.

Step 14: After fixation, remove the bladder from the wax board but leave the probes in place.

Step 15: Describe and measure the lesion identified by the blue arrow in Fig. 6.83. Describe where the lesion is present and how close the lesion comes to the remaining bladder wall aspects, bilateral ureteral orifices, and the urethral margin. In Fig. 6.83, the lesion is present in the bladder dome, extending onto the anterior, posterior, and left bladder walls.

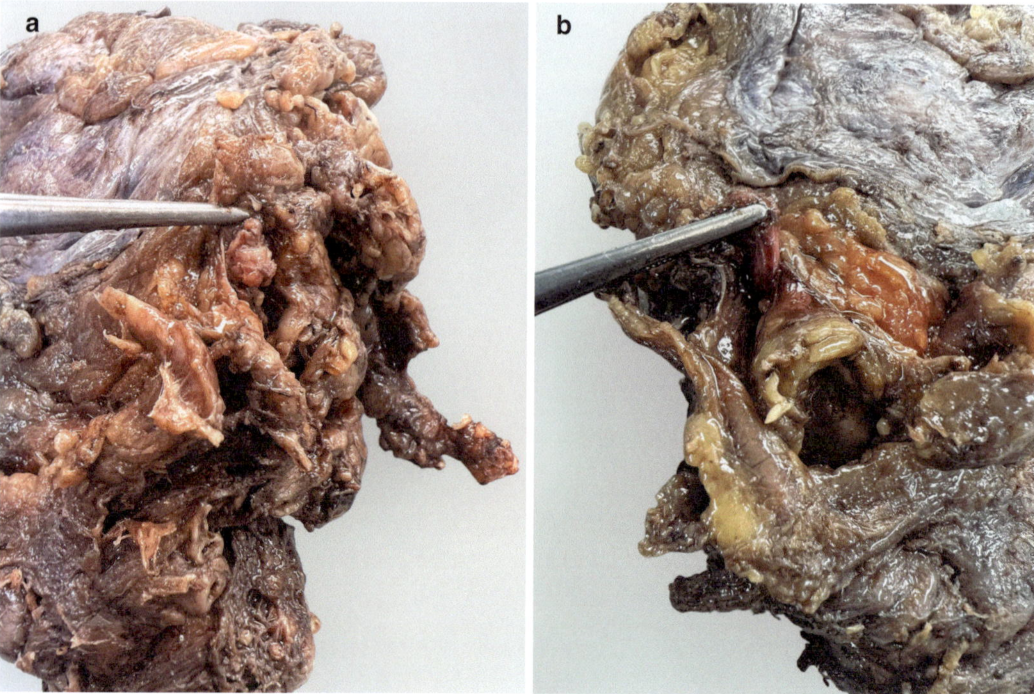

Fig. 6.74 (**a**) Right ureter. (**b**) Left ureter

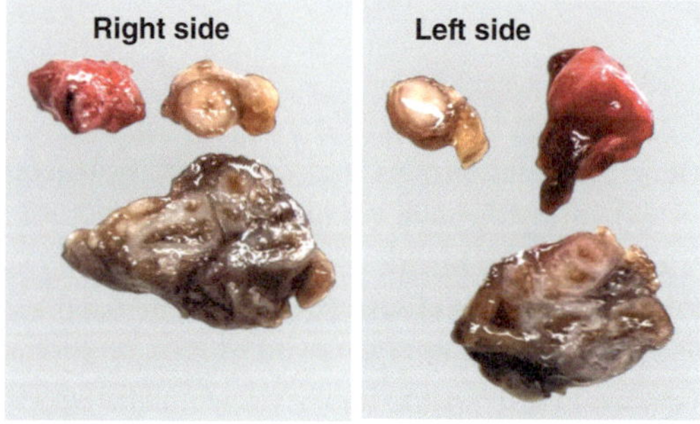

Fig. 6.75 Bilateral ureter margins, bilateral vas deferens margins and representative bilateral seminal vesicles

Step 16: Amputate the bladder trigone which is the junction of the bladder and prostate base (Fig. 6.84)

Step 17: Take a perpendicular section of the bladder trigone (Fig. 6.85). This section shows the relationship between the bladder and the prostate.

Step 18: Using the probes as guides, bivalve the ureters (Fig. 6.86a). This can be done with both probes together or each probe separately to expose the lumen of each ureter. (Fig. 6.86b)

Step 19: Serially section the remainder of the bladder and lay each slice flat for optimal visualization. (Fig. 6.87)

Step 20: Identify and measure the greatest depth of lesion invasion and state if the lesion invades through the bladder wall or into the surrounding adipose tissue. (Fig. 6.88)

Step 21: If the lesion has not been previously treated with therapy and is clearly extending into the bladder wall or invading the surrounding adipose tissue, representative sections of the greatest depth of invasion are sufficient. If the lesion has been treated with therapy and only a scar remains, then the entire lesion should be submitted to identify any residual cancer cells present. (Fig. 6.89)

Step 22: Palpate the surrounding adipose tissue for lymph node candidates.

Example Dictation

Specimen A is received in formalin labeled with patient's name, medical record number, "urinary bladder" and consists of a tan-brown bladder (7.6 × 6.5 × 3.5 cm) with attached short length of

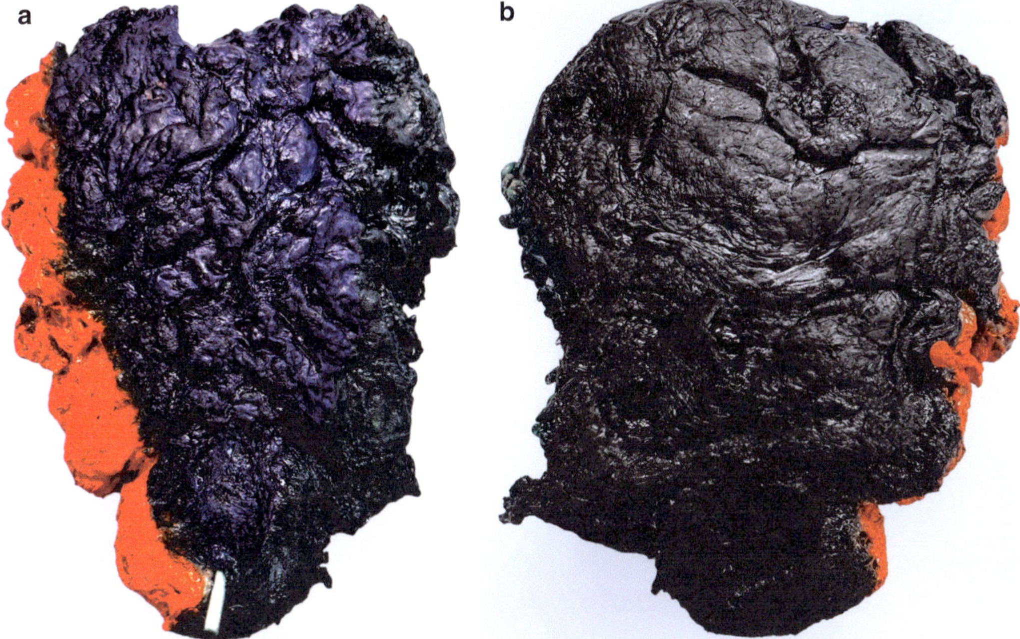

Fig. 6.76 (**a**) Anterior ink view. (**b**) Posterior ink view

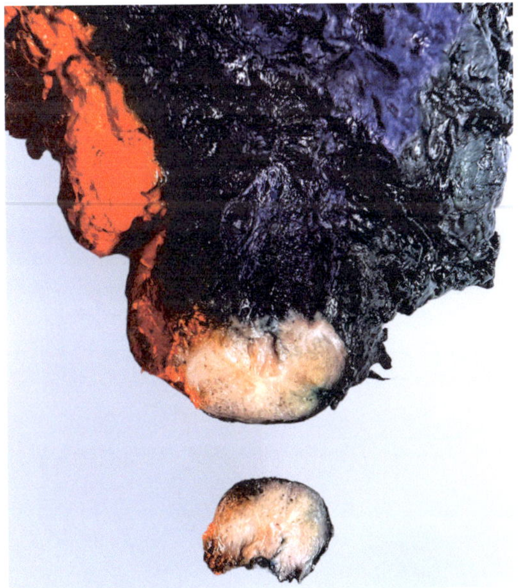

Fig. 6.77 Cystoprostatectomy, prostate apex margin

bilateral ureters (right 1.6 cm in length by 0.3 cm in diameter, left 2.1 cm in length by 0.4 cm in diameter), prostate (4.2 × 3.5 × 3.2 cm) with attached bilateral vas deferens (right 5.2 × 0.3 cm, left 5.9 × 0.3 cm), and attached bilateral seminal

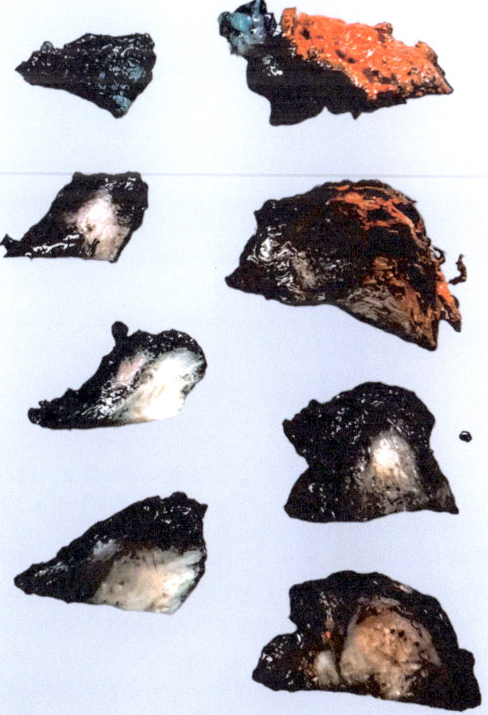

Fig. 6.78 Cystoprostatectomy, prostate apex margin radially sectioned

Fig. 6.79 (**a**) Prostate serially sectioned. (**b**) Prostate slice quadrisected

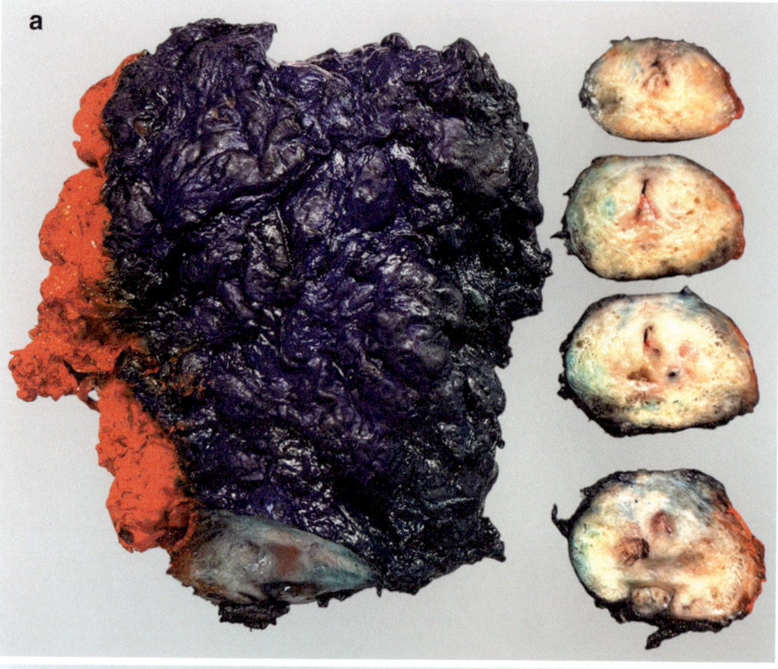

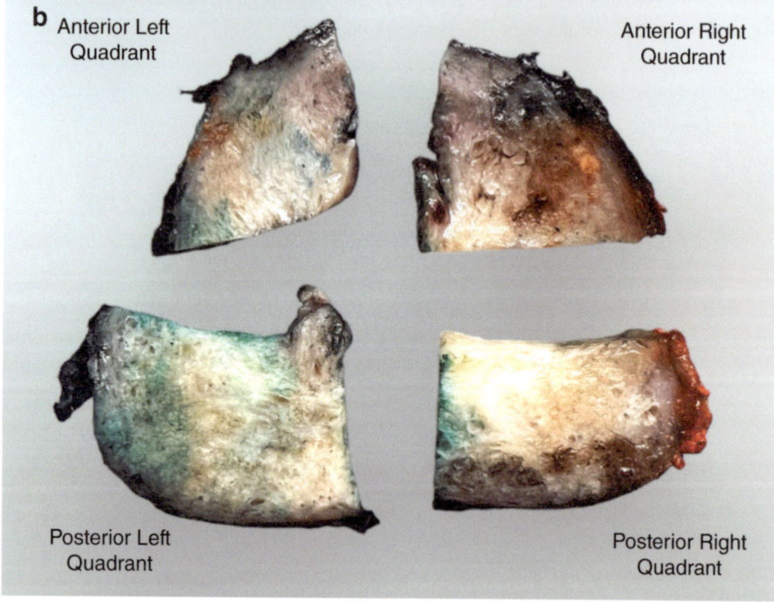

vesicles (right 2.0 × 1.3 × 1.0 cm, left 2.8 × 1.5 × 0.9 cm). The prostate is serially sectioned to reveal tan, fibrous, slightly cystic cut surfaces. The bladder is opened to reveal a scarred, ill-defined lesion (4.1 × 2.1 × 0.5 cm) present at the left aspect of the bladder dome, extending onto the left posterior-lateral wall approximately 1.1 cm and onto the left anterior wall approximately 2.0 cm. Additionally, the mass comes within 2.7 cm of the left ureteral orifice, 3.9 cm from the right ureteral orifice, and 7.2 cm from the prostate apex margin. The mass is serially sectioned to reveal a greatest depth of invasion approximately 0.2 cm, without invasion through the bladder wall or into the surrounding adipose tissue, surrounded by scarring of the bladder wall. The surrounding adipose tissue is palpable for 0 lymph node candidates.

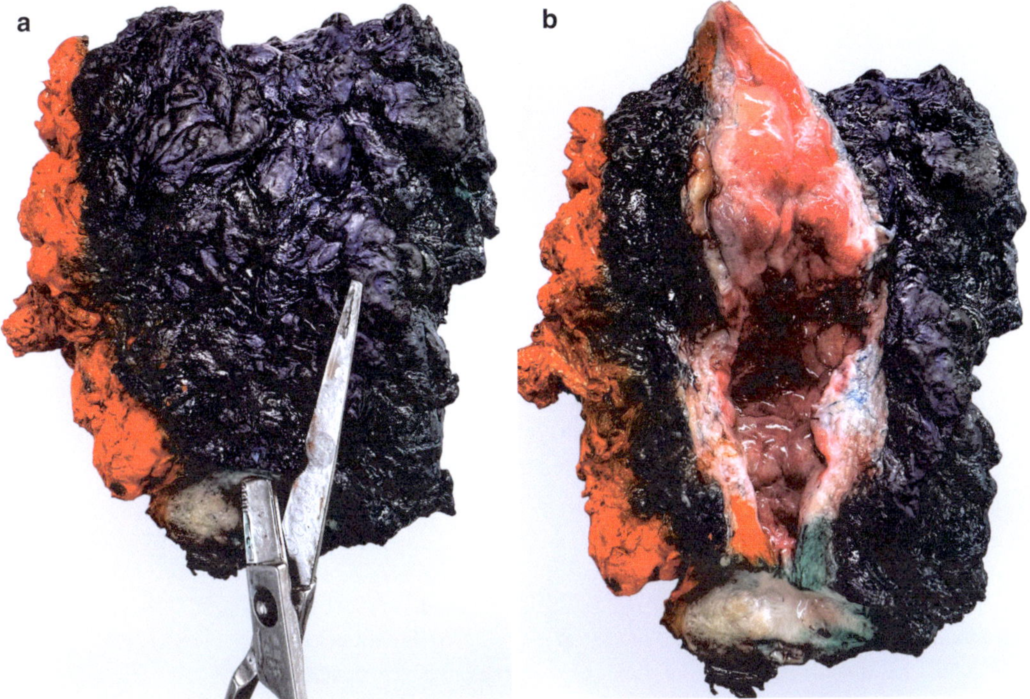

Fig. 6.80 (**a**) Cystoprostatectomy opening. (**b**) Cystoprostatectomy anterior flap open

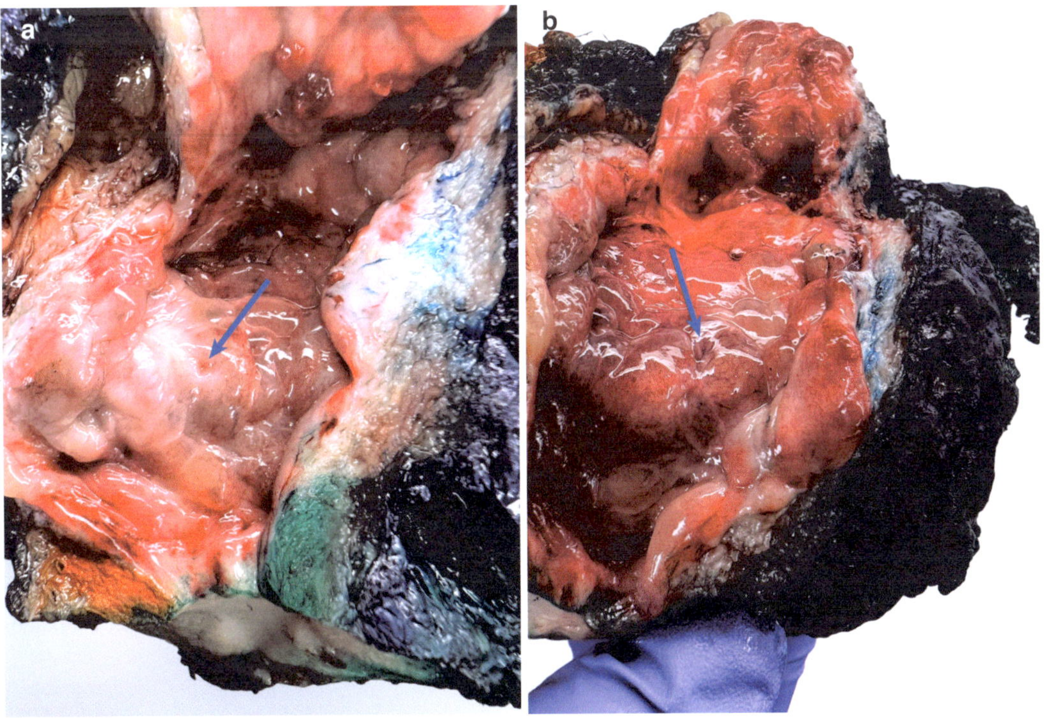

Fig. 6.81 (**a**) Right ureteral orifice. (**b**) Left ureteral orifice

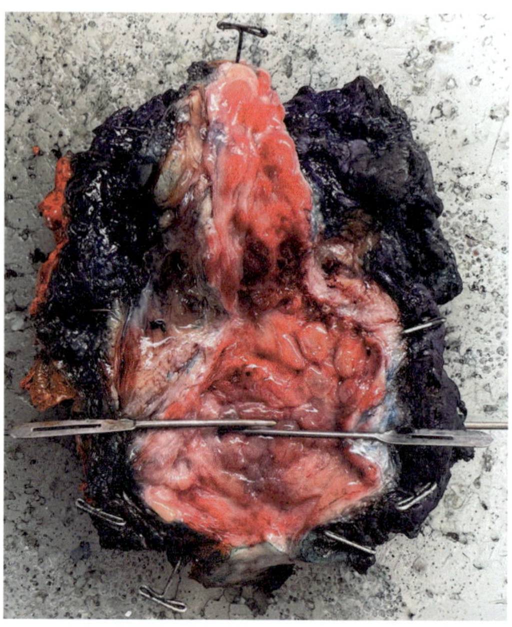

Fig. 6.82 Cystoprostatectomy pinned

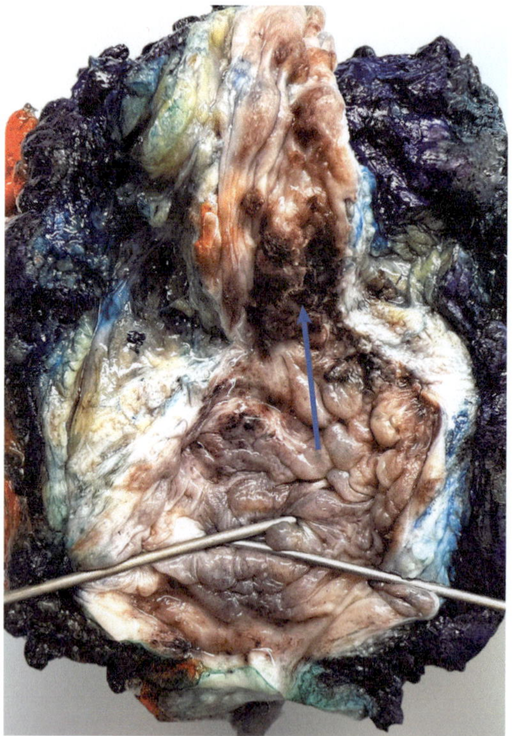

Fig. 6.83 Cystoprostatectomy post-fixation

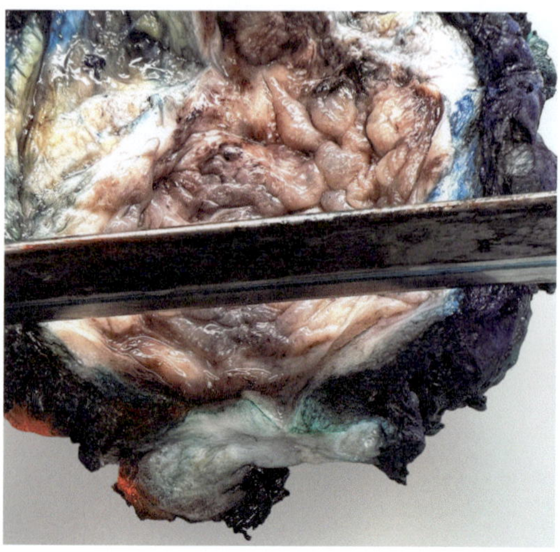

Fig. 6.84 Cystoprostatectomy trigone

Ink code:

 Blue-anterior
 Black-posterior
 Orange-right
 Green-left

Section code:

A1 Right ureter margin, right vas deferens margin and representative section of right seminal vesicle

A2 Left ureter margin, left vas deferens margin and representative section of left seminal vesicle

A3 Right prostate apex, radially sectioned

A4 Left prostate apex, radially sectioned

A5–A20 Prostate entirely from apex to base, 1 slice per 4 cassettes quadrisected as follows: Anterior right, posterior right, anterior left, posterior left, respectively

A21 Bladder trigone, representative, perpendicular

A22 Right ureteral orifice, representative

A23 Left ureteral orifice, representative

A24–A33 Mass entirely from posterior bladder wall to anterior bladder wall (29 and 30 Bladder dome)

A34 Unremarkable right lateral bladder wall, representative

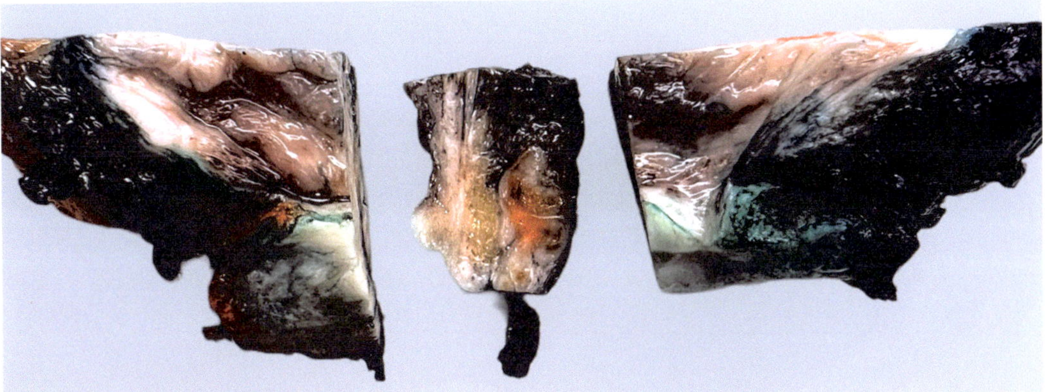

Fig. 6.85 Cystoprostatectomy trigone section

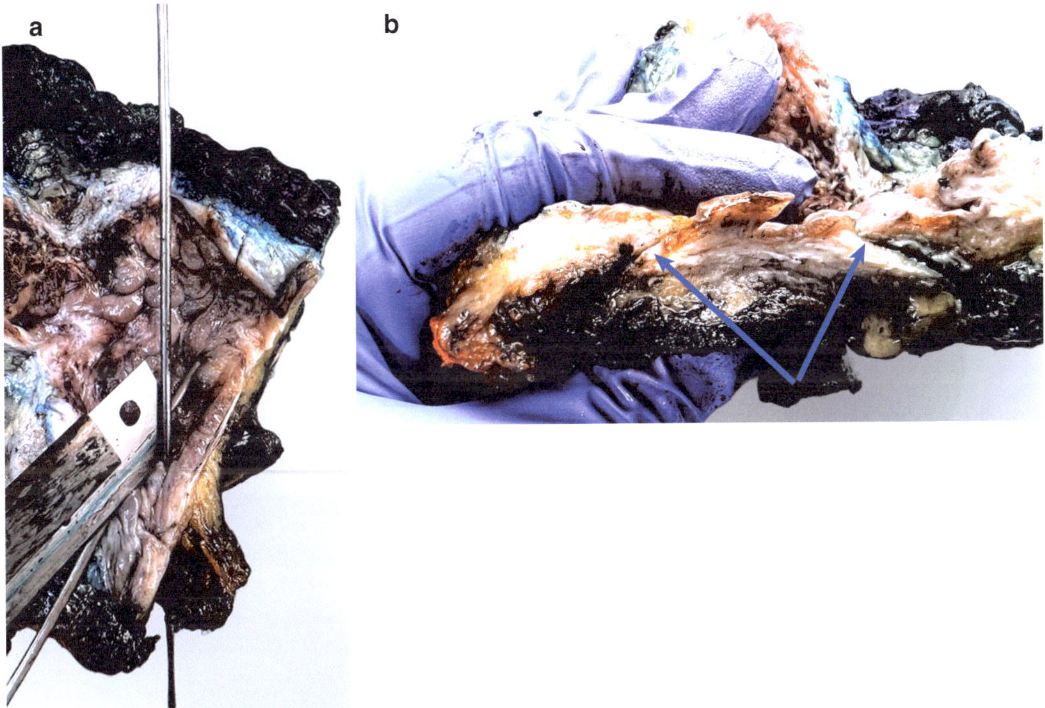

Fig. 6.86 (**a**) Sectioning ureteral orifice. (**b**) bilateral longitudinal ureters

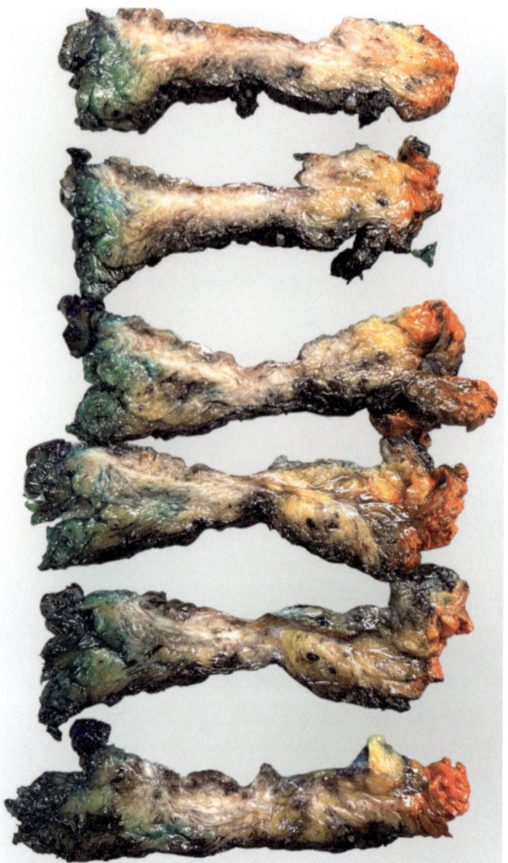

Fig. 6.87 Cystoprostatectomy serially sectioned

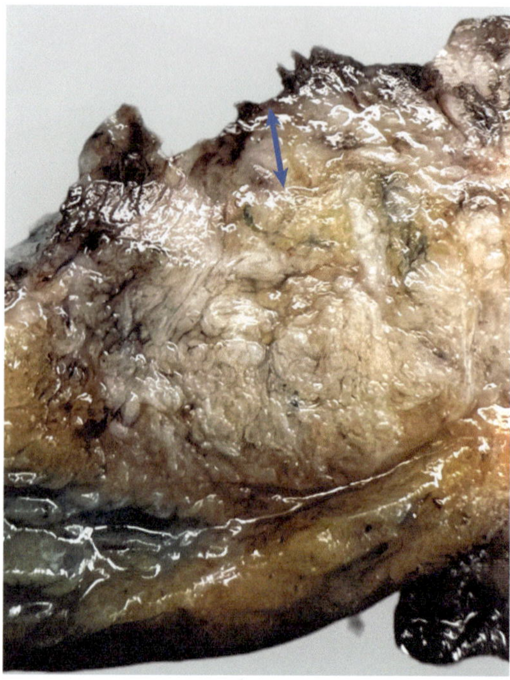

Fig. 6.88 Bladder wall with the greatest depth (identified by the blue arrow)

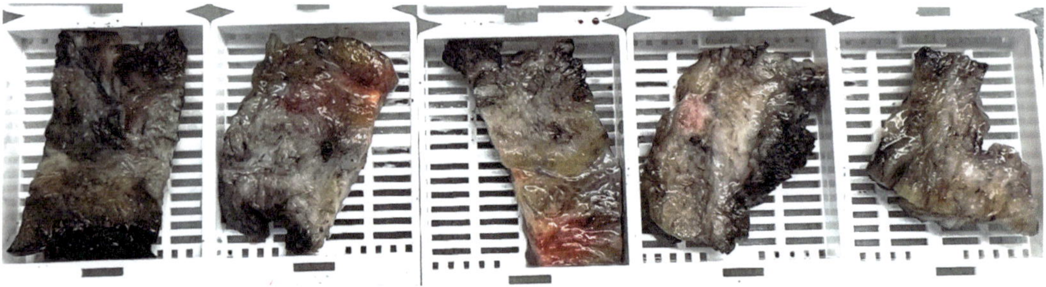

Fig. 6.89 Cystoprostatectomy section submission

6.12 Female Bladder: Level VI CPT 88309

A radical cystectomy with a uterus is the surgical removal of the bladder with the attached anterior aspect of the vaginal canal present on the posterior aspect of the bladder. The uterus is often present if it hasn't been previously resected due to a prior surgery.

Step 1: Identify and measure the bladder and urethra. Figure 6.90 shows the anterior and the posterior aspect. Blue arrow indicates urethra.

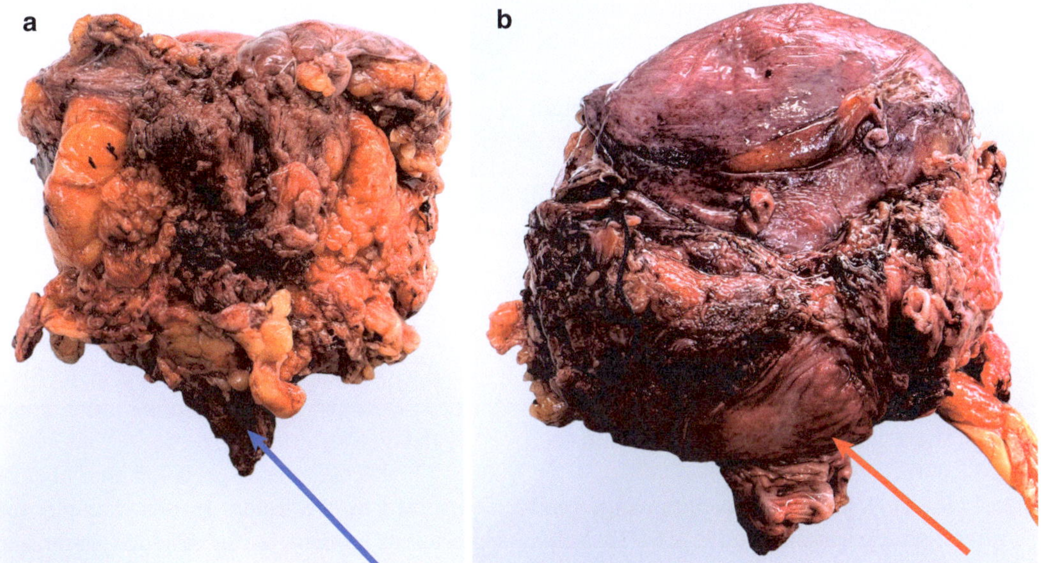

Fig. 6.90 (**a**) Female bladder anterior view. (**b**) Female bladder posterior view

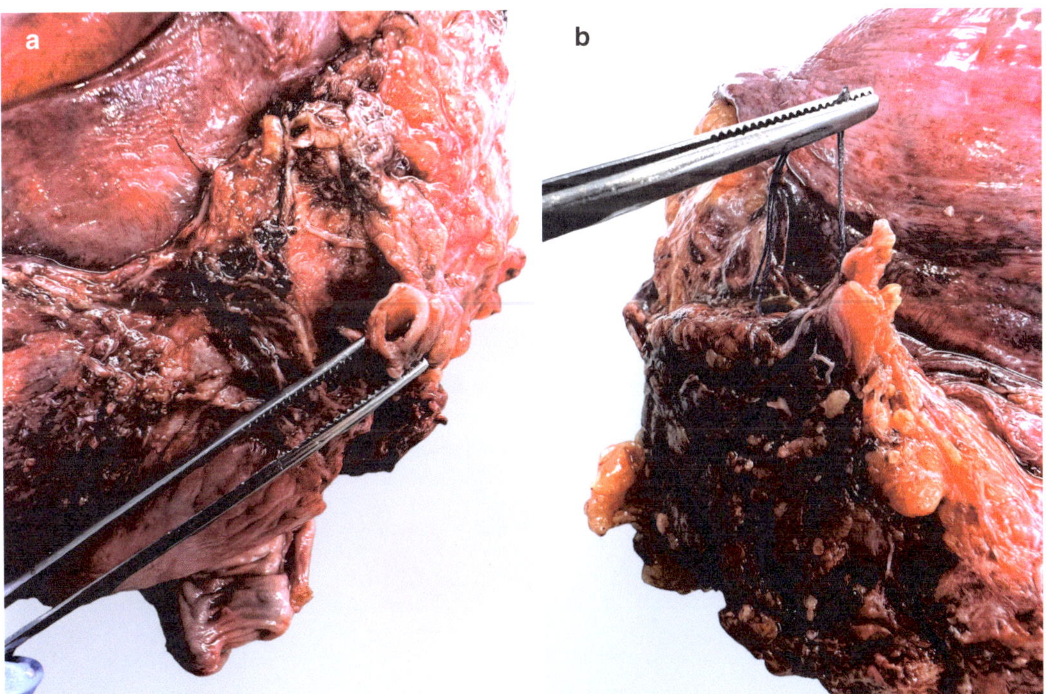

Fig. 6.91 (**a**) Female bladder right ureter. (**b**) Female bladder left ureter

Step 2: Describe and measure the vaginal canal shown by the red arrow in Fig. 6.91. If the uterus is present, it can be described and measured. See Chap. 8 for grossing of uterus.

Step 3: Identify and measure the bilateral ureters. The ureters insert posterolaterally into the inferior aspect of the bladder. Figure 6.91 show the ureters on each side of the bladder.

Step 4: Shave and submit the ureter margins en face. They can be placed in separate cassettes or inked individually and placed in the same cassette. For example, A1 right ureter (inked red) and left ureter (inked blue), en face.

Step 5: Ink the specimen four colors. Note that all four inks converge at the distal urethra. In this example, the ink code is as follows:

Blue- anterior (Fig. 6.92a)
Black- posterior (Fig. 6.92b)
Orange- right (Fig. 6.92a)
Green- left (Fig. 6.92a)

Step 6: Shave the urethra margin approximately 0.5 cm thick. (Fig. 6.93a)

Step 7: Radially section the urethra margin and submit on edge as shown in Fig. 6.93b. Some pathologists may prefer the urethra margin submitted en face, communicate for further instruction.

Step 8: Take additional cross sections of urethra. If the lesion is noted in the chart to be present in the urethra, the urethra should be serially sectioned and submitted entirely. Assess the patient's chart and communicate with the pathologists for instruction.

Step 9: Shave the peripheral vaginal canal margins and submit en face (Fig. 6.94). In this example, the superior right margin, inferior right margin, superior left margin, and inferior left margin are shaved and submitted en face in separate cassettes.

Step 10: Place scissors in the urethra and cut along the anterior-left aspect up to the bladder dome and make a second cut along the anterior-right aspect up to the bladder dome. This will create a flap of the anterior bladder wall to open the bladder shown. (Fig. 6.95)

Step 11: Describe and measure the lesion noted by the blue arrow in Fig. 6.95.

Step 12: Dictate the aspects of the bladder involved by the lesion. In this example, the lesion is present in the bladder dome and extends on to the right, left, anterior, and posterior bladder walls.

Step 13: Measure the distance of the lesion to the right and left ureteral orifice and the urethral margin.

Step 14: Place probes in the right and left ureteral orifices as shown in Fig. 6.96a.

Step 15: Fix the specimen. It is common to fix the specimen in formalin for a few hours to over-

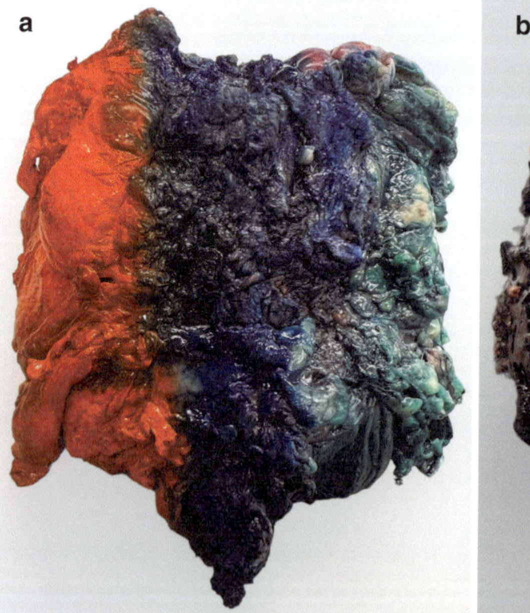
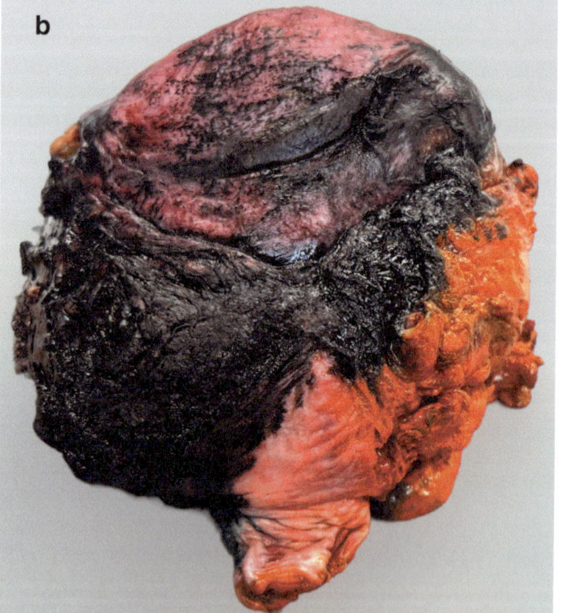

Fig. 6.92 (**a**) Female bladder anterior ink. (**b**) Female bladder posterior ink

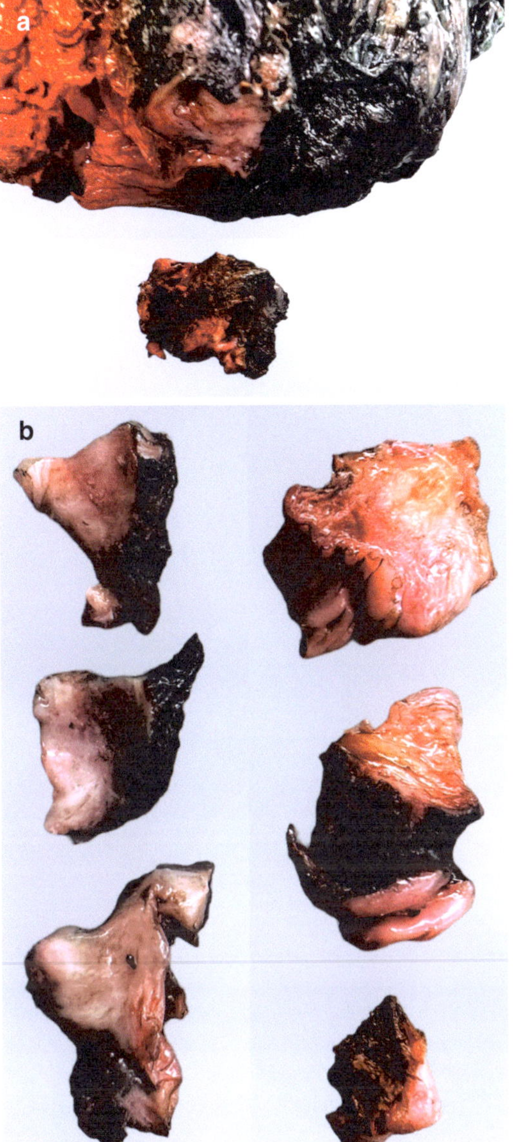

Fig. 6.93 (**a**) Urethral margin shaved. (**b**) Urethral margin radially sectioned

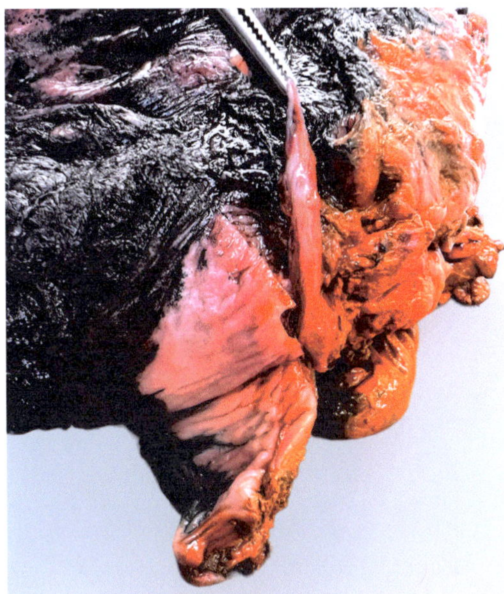

Fig. 6.94 Female bladder vaginal canal margins

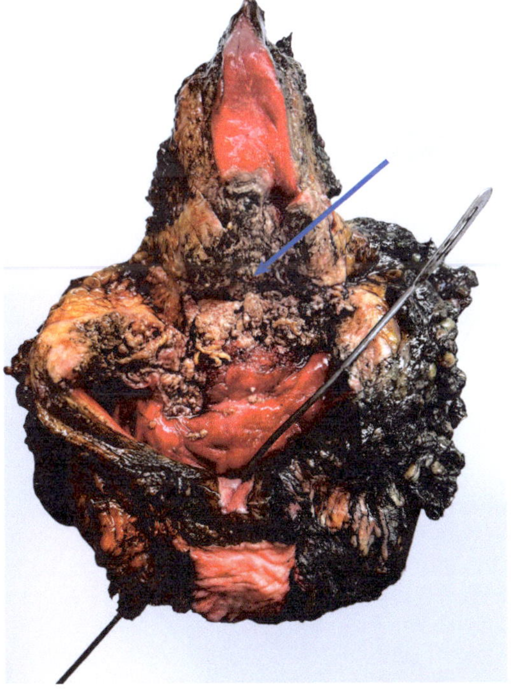

Fig. 6.95 Female bladder opened with right ureteral orifice probe inserted

night. Review Figs. 6.82 and 6.83 for additional instruction.

Step 16: Amputate the bladder trigone. (Fig. 6.96b)

Step 17: Take a perpendicular section of the bladder trigone shown in Fig. 6.96b. This section shows the relationship between the bladder and the vaginal canal.

Step 18: Using the probes as guides, bivalve the ureters as shown in Fig. 6.97b. This can be done with both probes together or each probe separately to expose the lumen of each ureter as shown by the blue arrows in Fig. 6.97a.

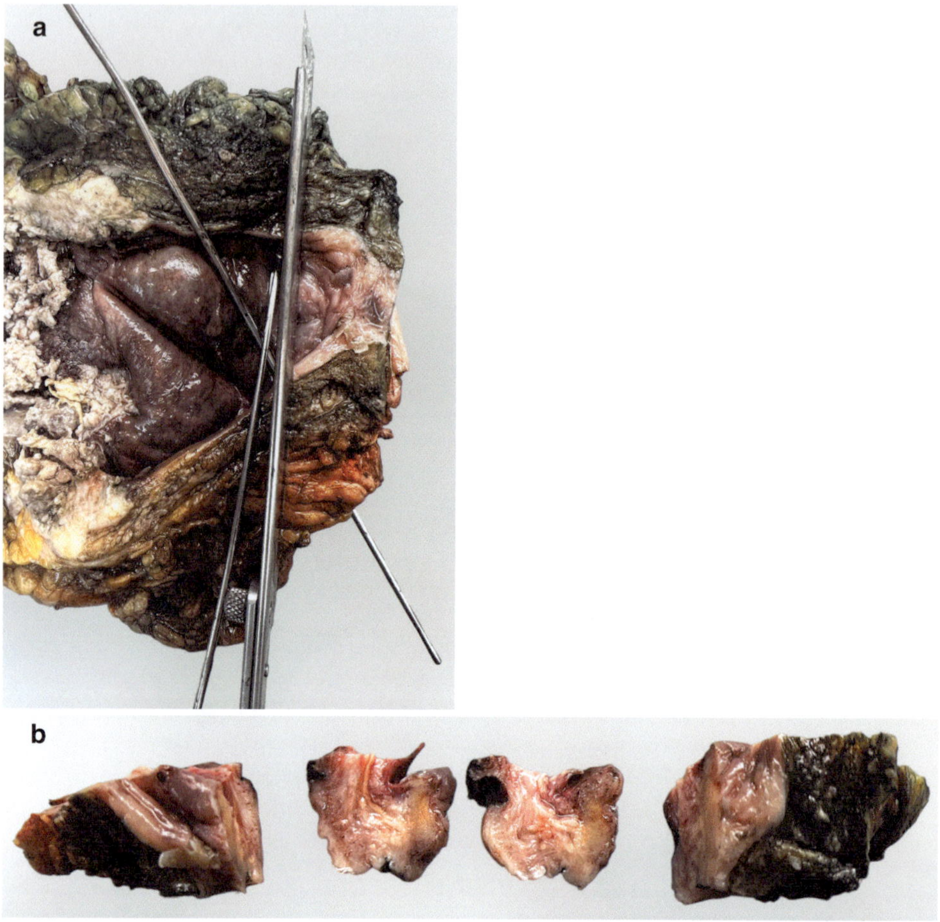

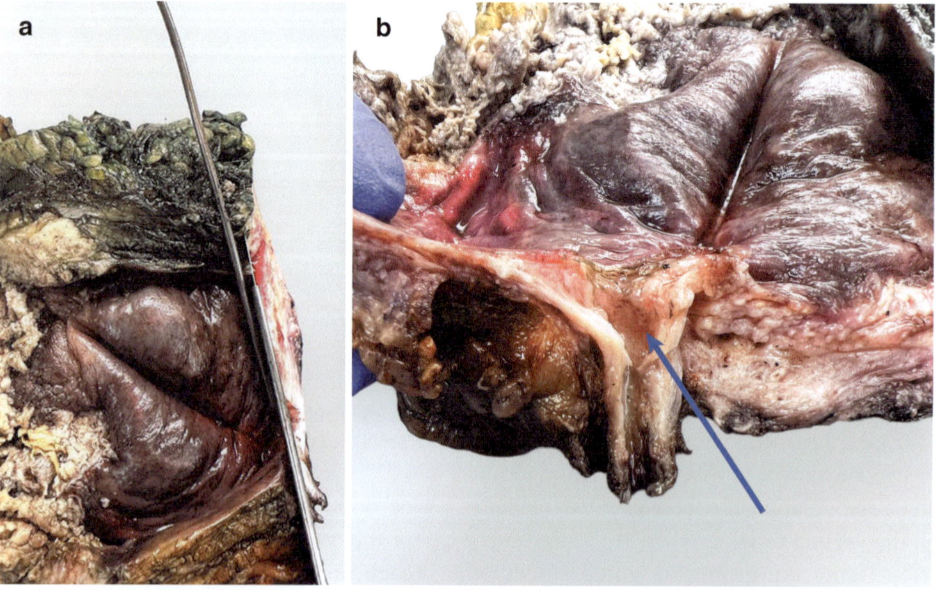

Fig. 6.96 (**a**) Ureteral orifice probes. (**b**) Longitudinal bladder trigone section

Fig. 6.97 (**a**) Ureteral orifice sectioning. (**b**) Ureter longitudinally sectioned

Step 19: Serially section the remainder of the bladder and lay each slice flat for optimal visualization. (Fig. 6.98)

Step 20: Identify and measure the greatest depth of lesion invasion and state if the lesion invades through the bladder wall, the surrounding adipose tissue, or the vaginal canal mucosa. In Fig. 6.99, the depth of invasion is identified by the blue arrows. In this example, the lesion invades through the entirety of the bladder wall and into the surrounding adipose tissue.

Step 21: If the lesion has not been previously treated with therapy and is clearly extending into the bladder wall or invading the surrounding adipose tissue, representative sections of the greatest depth of invasion are sufficient. If the lesion has been treated with therapy and only a scar remains, then the entire lesion should be submitted to identify any residual cancer cells present.

Step 22: If the uterus is present, submit a section demonstrating if the lesion invades into the uterus. Then submit sections of the uterus. See Chap. 8 for further instruction.

Step 23: Palpate the surrounding adipose tissue for lymph node candidates.

Example Dictation

Specimen A is received in formalin labeled with patient's name, medical record number, "bladder and vaginal canal" and consists of a tan bladder (9.9 × 9.2 × 5.2 cm) with attached length of urethra (4.2 cm in length by 0.4 cm in diameter), attached bilateral ureters (right 2.5 cm in length by 0.4 cm in diameter, left 2.2 cm in length by 0.2 cm in diameter), and attached anterior vaginal canal (7.5 × 3.5 cm) present on the posterior aspect of the bladder and urethra. The bladder is opened to reveal an irregular, necrotic tan-brown mass (8.2 × 7.1 × 0.9 cm) present in the bladder dome which comes within 9.2 cm of the urethral margin, 4.5 cm from the right ureteral orifice, and 7.1 cm from the area of left ureteral orifice. The mass extends onto the right and left bladder wall approximately 4.2 cm and 4.4 cm, respectively, extends onto the posterior bladder wall approximately 2.2 cm and the anterior bladder wall approximately 3.4 cm. The right and left ureteral orifices are probe patent. The mass is serially sectioned to reveal a greatest depth of invasion approximately 2.4 cm, extending through the bladder wall and into the surrounding adipose tissue coming within less than 0.1 cm of the bladder dome margin. Mass extension is present through the right and left lateral walls, bladder dome, and anterior bladder wall. No involvement of the vaginal canal mucosa is identified. The remaining mucosa is flattened, dusky and slightly edematous with marked underlying calcifications present within the bladder wall and vessels. The surrounding adipose tissue is palpable for 0 lymph node candidates.

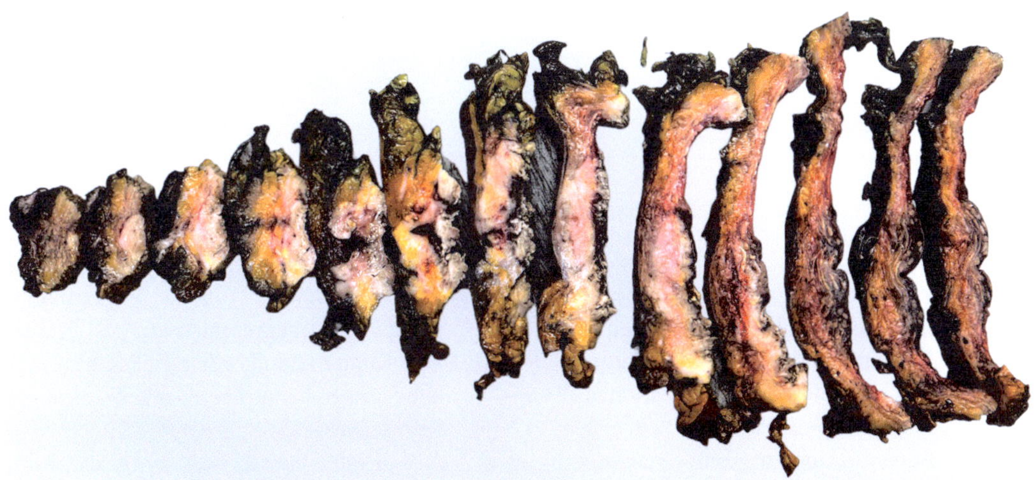

Fig. 6.98   Female bladder serially sectioned

Fig. 6.99 Female bladder slices with greatest depth of invasion

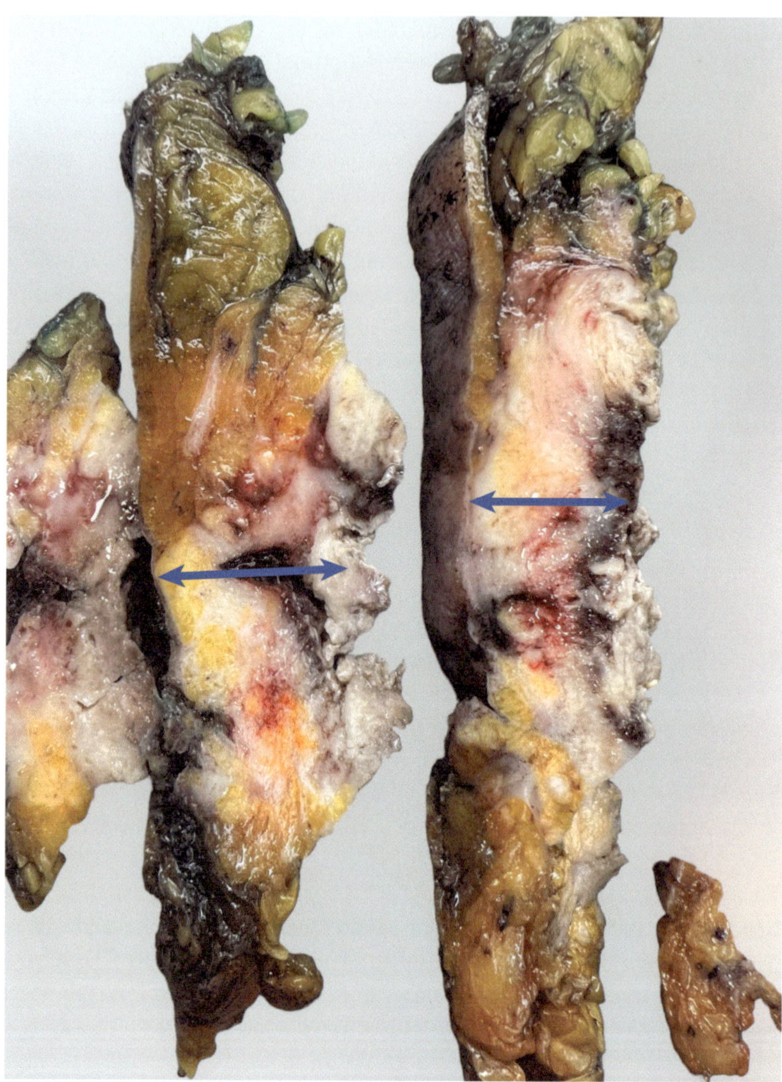

Ink code:

 Blue-anterior

 Orange-right

 Green-left

 Black-posterior

Section code:

 A1 Right ureter margin (inked blue) and left ureter margin (inked orange), en face

 A2-A3 Right urethra, radially sectioned

 A4-A5 Left urethra, radially sectioned

 A6 Urethra, representative

 A7 Superior right vaginal canal margin, shave, en face

A8 Inferior right vaginal canal margin, shave, en face

A9 Superior left vaginal canal margin, shave, en face

A10 Inferior left vaginal canal margin, shave, en face

A11-A12 Bladder trigone in relation to vaginal canal, representative

A13 Right ureteral orifice (inked blue) and left ureteral orifice (inked orange), representative

A14 Right lateral wall with extension through the bladder wall, representative

A15 Posterior wall with extension through the bladder wall, representative

A16-A17 Bladder dome with greatest depth of invasion and extension through bladder wall, representative, bisected

A18 Anterior bladder wall with extension through the bladder wall, representative

A19 Left lateral wall with extension through the bladder wall, representative

A20 The posterior inferior dusky bladder wall with calcified areas, representative

6.13   Distal Penis: Level V CPT 88307

A distal penectomy is surgical removal of a small portion of the distal end of the penis. This is often performed for skin lesions surrounding the glans of the penis.

Cancer Protocol Breakdown Relative to Grossing Penis

Procedure: Dictate the type of resection that is present. This can be an incisional or excisional specimen, a partial penectomy, or a total penectomy.

Presence/absence of foreskin: Dictate the presence or absence of foreskin.

Tumor focality: Dictate if the mass is unifocal or multifocal.

Tumor site: Dictate the anatomic structures of the mass involved. This can be the glans, foreskin, coronal sulcus, skin of the shaft, or penile urethra.

Macroscopic features: Describe the gross features of the mass.

Tumor size: Measure the mass in centimeters.

Tumor thickness: The thickness is also the greatest depth of invasion of the mass.

Tumor extent: Dictate all the internal anatomic structures involved by the mass. This can include the corpus spongiosum, corpus cavernosum, tunica albuginea, urethra, and regional skin.

Margin status: Measure how close the mass comes from the proximal skin and soft tissue margins.

pT Categories [2]

pT0 No evidence of primary tumor

pTis Carcinoma in situ

pTa Noninvasive localized squamous cell carcinoma

pT1a Tumor is without lymphovascular invasion or perineural invasion and is not high grade

pT1b Tumor exhibits lymphovascular invasion and/or perineural invasion or is high grade

pT2 Tumor invades into corpus spongiosum (either glans or ventral shaft) with or without urethral invasion

pT3 Tumor invades into corpora cavernosum (including tunica albuginea) with or without urethral invasion

pT4 Tumor invades into adjacent structures

Gross appearance of selected penile lesions is described in Table 6.4 [3].

Step 1: Describe and measure the specimen noting all anatomic structures present. (Fig. 6.100)

Step 2: Orient the specimen. The two corpus cavernosum designate the dorsal aspect, and the corpus spongiosum designate, the ventral aspect (Fig. 6.101). The corpus spongiosum also contains the urethra.

Step 3: Describe, measure and dictate the location of the lesion. (Fig. 6.102)

Step 4: Dictate how close the lesion comes to the skin margin.

Step 5: Ink the proximal resection margin. The margin is inked to designate ventral, dorsal, right, and left. The margins can be inked one or multiple colors for designation. Communicate with the pathologists for suggestions. (Fig. 6.103)

Step 6: A short segment of distal penis is easily radially sectioned. Start by placing a probe in the urethra and quadrisecting the specimen. (Fig. 6.104)

Step 7: Radially section each quadrant keeping each quadrant oriented. (Fig. 6.105)

Step 8: This specimen is small and is submitted entirely in an oriented manner (see Fig. 6.106). Communicate with the pathologist for instructions.

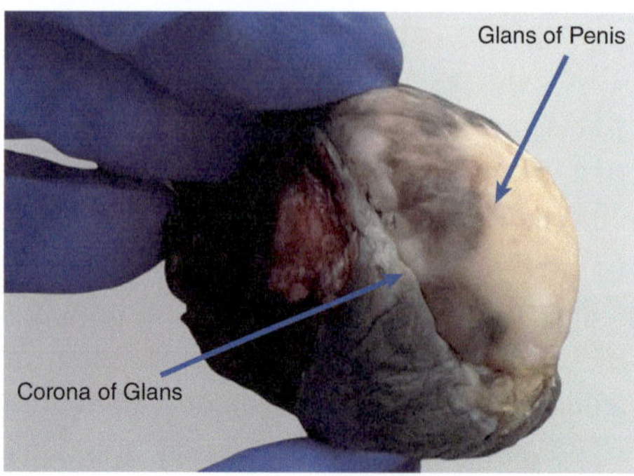

Fig. 6.100 Distal penis. The glans and the corona are indicated by blue arrows

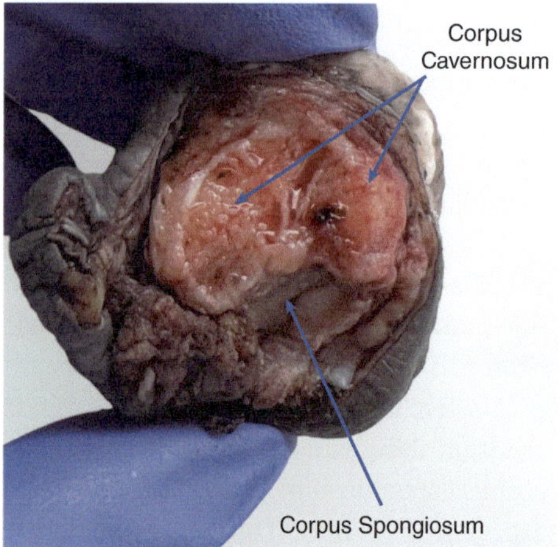

Fig. 6.101 Distal penis resection margin. The two corpus cavernosum designate the dorsal aspect and the corpus spongiosum designate the ventral aspect

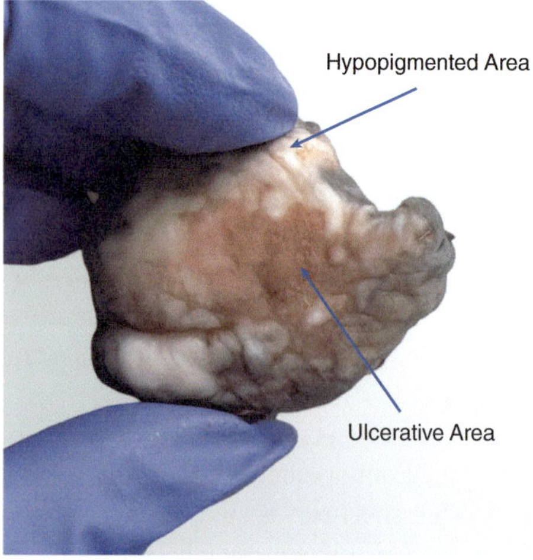

Fig. 6.102 Distal penis lesion. There is a slightly ulcerative lesion surrounded by hypopigmentation

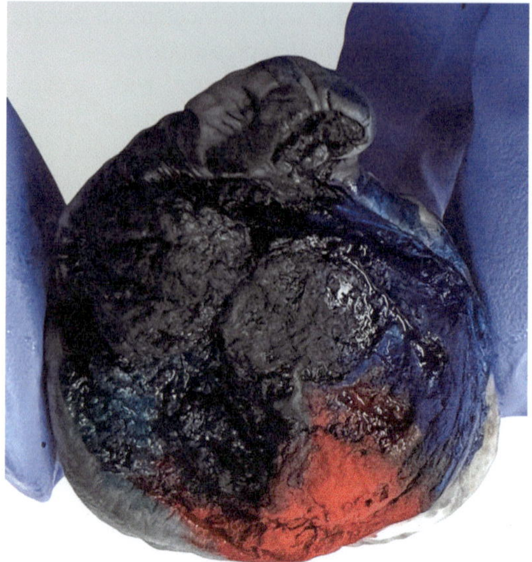

Fig. 6.103 Distal penis

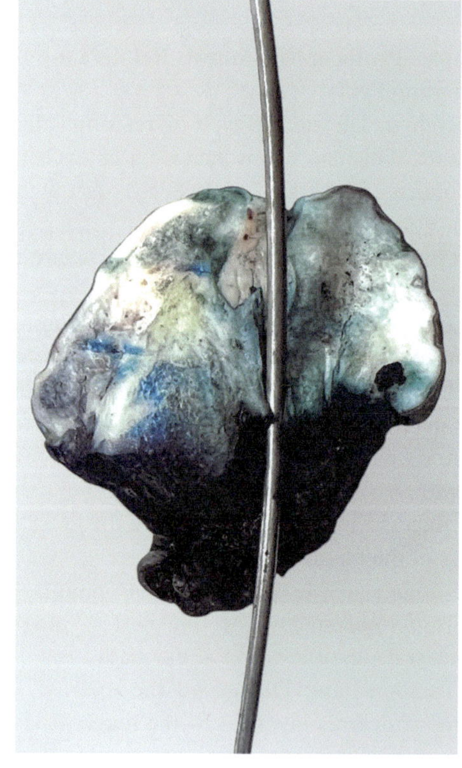

Fig. 6.104 Distal penis bisected through urethra

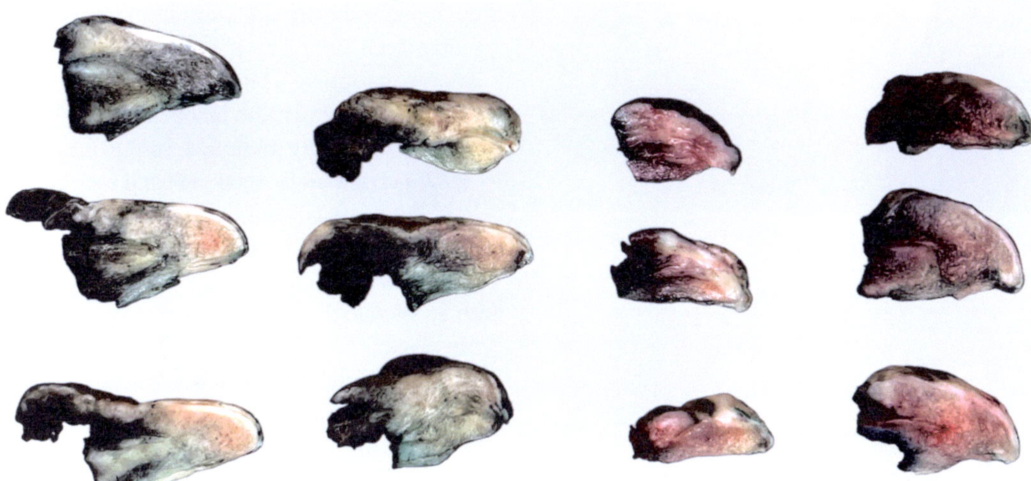

Fig. 6.105 Distal penis radially sectioned through urethra

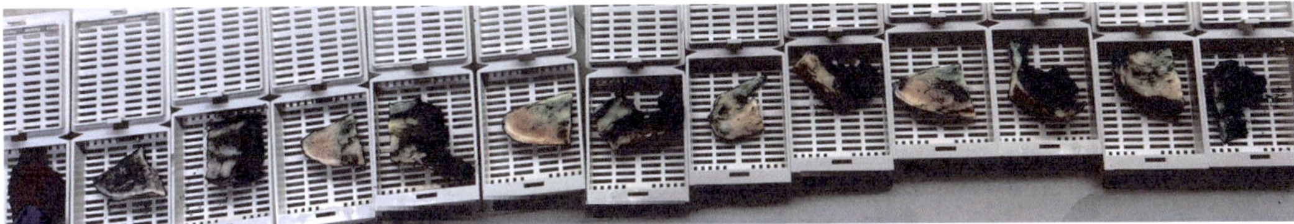

Fig. 6.106 Distal penis section submission

Example Dictation

Specimen A is received in formalin labeled with patient's name, medical record number, "glans penis" and consists of resection of the distal penis (3.5 × 3.0 × 2.8 cm) with tan-brown skin and a markedly ill-defined, tan-brown, slightly ulcerative lesion (3.5 × 2.9 cm) on the left aspect, coming within 0.2 cm of the ventral skin margin. The specimen is radially sectioned around the urethra to reveal a greatest depth of invasion approximately 0.4 cm, coming within 0.3 cm the resection margin on the left soft tissue margin and does not extend to the urethra. The remainder of the skin surface is tan-brown with large areas of hypopigmentation ranging from 0.5 to 2.5 cm.

Ink code:

> Blue-dorsal resection margin
> Green-ventral resection margin
> Red-right resection margin
> Black- left resection margin

Section code:

> A 1–A 6 Right side radially sectioned from dorsal to ventralw
> A 7–A 18 Left side radially sectioned from dorsal to ventral (1 slice per 2 cassettes, bisected)

6.14   Penis: Level V CPT 88307

In penectomy, the majority of the length of the penis is surgically removed. This is performed for penile skin lesions or urethral cancers.

Step 1: Describe and measure the specimen. The distal aspect of penis is skin covered, and the proximal aspect of penis does not contain skin. (Fig. 6.107)

Step 2: Orient the specimen. The corpus cavernosum is dorsal, and the corpus spongiosum is ventral. (Fig. 6.108)

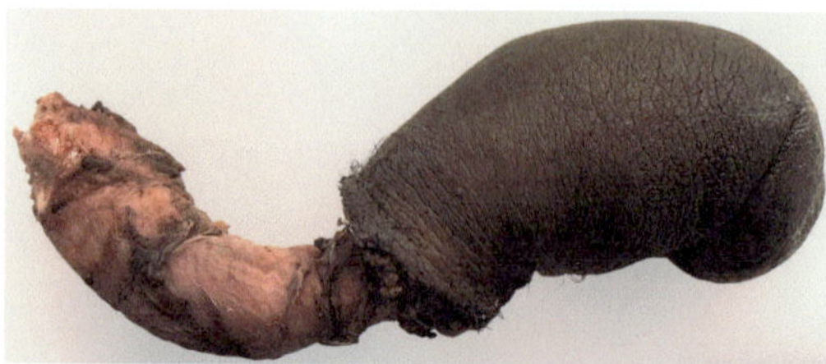

Fig. 6.107   Penectomy

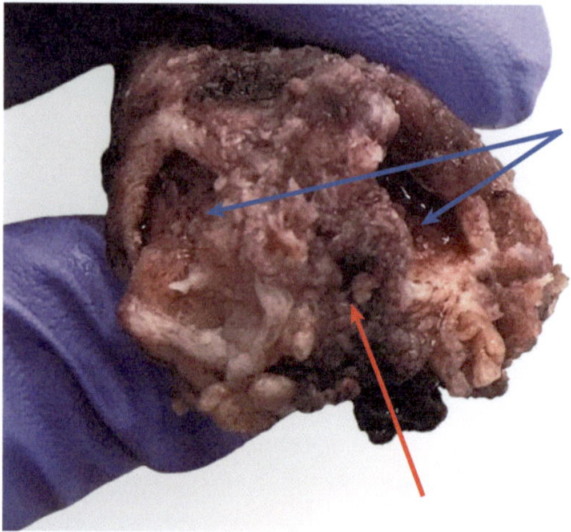

Fig. 6.108   Penectomy margin. The corpus cavernosum (blue arrows) is dorsal, and the corpus spongiosum (red arrow) is ventral

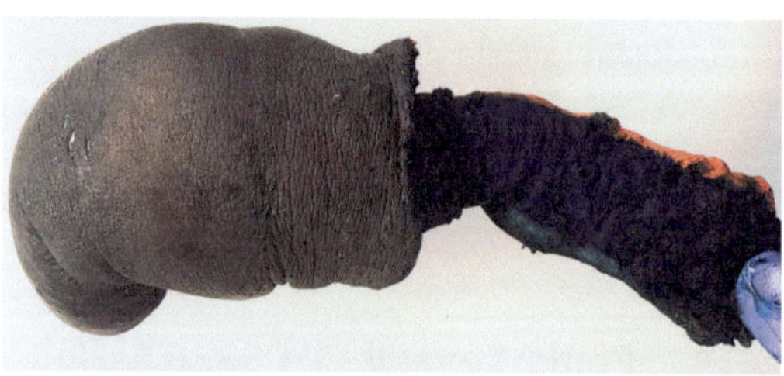

Fig. 6.109   Penis margins inked

Step 3: Ink the margins. Communicate with the pathologist for inking instructions. In Fig. 6.109, the dorsal, ventral, right, and left aspects are inked.

Step 4: Shave the skin margins and submit en face. In Fig. 6.110, the dorsal, ventral, right, and left skin margins are submitted en face. If the lesion is close to the margin then perpendicular sections of lesion in relation to the margin is best.

Step 5: Shave the proximal soft tissue margin and submit en face or submit perpendicular if more appropriate. (Fig. 6.111)

Step 6: The specimen can be opened through the urethra or serially sectioned. In Fig. 6.112, the specimen is serially sectioned and each slice is laid flat to visualize the mass.

Step 7: Measure the mass and measure how close the mass comes from the margins.

Step 8: Dictate the anatomic structures the mass involves.

Step 9: The distal glans can be bivalved longitudinally to visualize how close the mass comes from the distal end. (Fig. 6.113)

Example Dictation

Specimen A is received in formalin labeled with patient's name, medical record number, "penis" and consists of a total resection of the penis (17.9 × 3.9 × 3.8 cm cm) with tan-brown skin extending the distal 9.2 cm. The specimen is serially sectioned to reveal a well-circumscribed, solid tan-white, homogenous mass (4.1 × 3.7 × 3.6 cm) encompassing the entirety of the corpus cavernosa, corpus spongiosum and abutting the peripheral dermis circumferentially without invasion through the skin surface. The mass extends into the glans penis, coming within 0.7 cm from the urethral orifice, 3.9 cm from the proximal skin margin, and 11.6 from the proximal soft tissue margin.

Ink code:

    Blue-dorsal resection margin
    Green-ventral resection margin
    Red-right resection margin
    Black- left resection margin

Section code:

    A1 Dorsal skin margin, en face
    A2 Ventral skin margin, en face
    A3 Right skin margin, en face
    A4 Left skin margin, en face
    A5 Proximal urethral and soft tissue margin, en face
    A6–A9 Full face section of mass, bisected per 2 cassettes
    A10 Mass in relation to urethral orifice, perpendicular

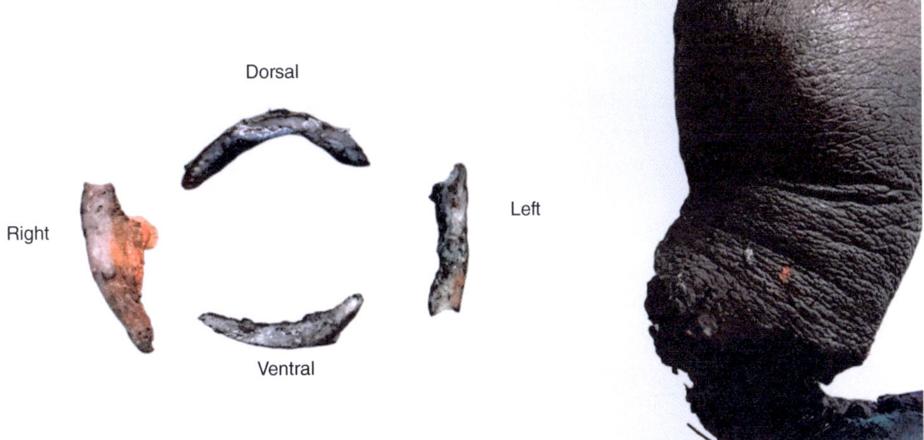

Fig. 6.110   Penectomy skin has margins

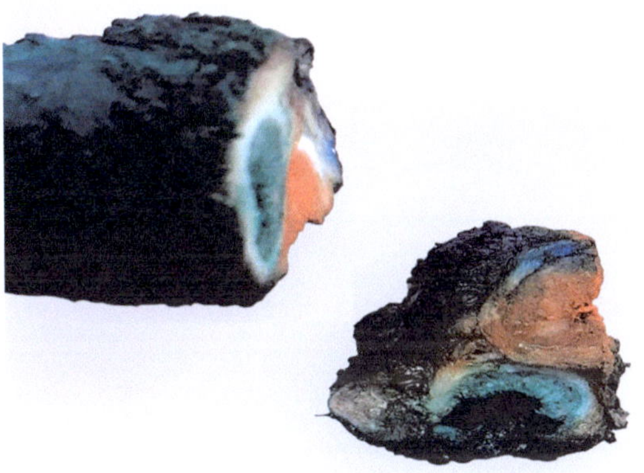

Fig. 6.111   Penis proximal resection margin shaved

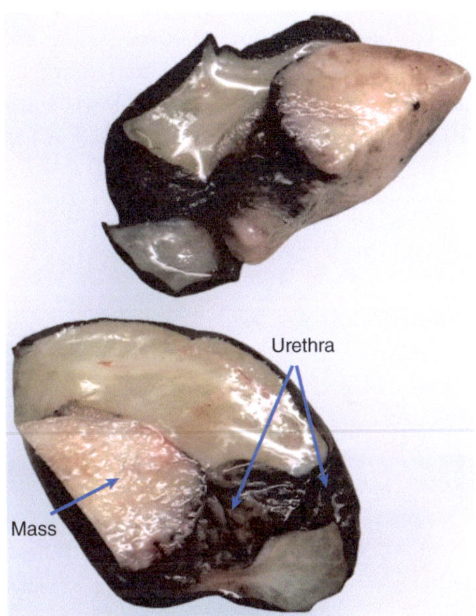

Fig. 6.113   Bivalved penile tip showing the mass in relation to the urethra

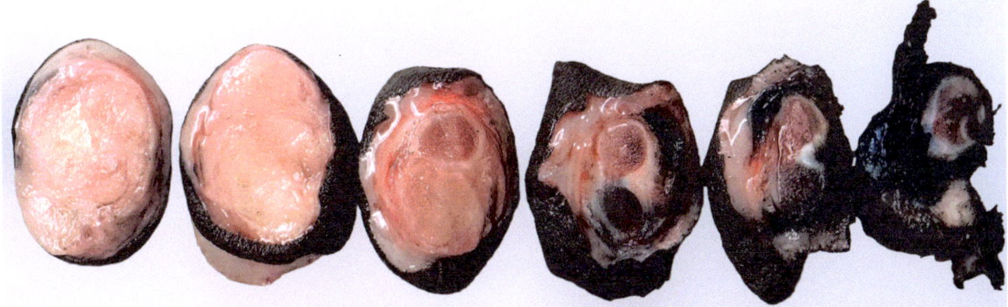

Fig. 6.112   Penis serially sectioned

6.15 Testis for Torsion: Level IV CPT 88305

Torsion occurs when the testis is twisted within the scrotal sac. Torsion can be caused by trauma or by tumors enlarging within the testis.

Step 1: Describe and measure the specimen. Figure 6.114 shows the testis with epididymis and a short length of spermatic cord.

Step 2: Shave the spermatic cord margin and submit en face.

Step 3: Bivalve the testis into medial and lateral halves (Fig. 6.115). The epididymis is present on the posterior aspect of the testis.

Step 4: Describe the cut surface.

Step 5: Serially section each half. Assess for any lesions present within the testis. (Fig. 6.116)

Step 6: Submit the spermatic cord margin (en face), representative sections of testis and testis in relation to the epididymis. (Fig. 6.117)

Example Dictation

Specimen A is received in formalin labeled with patient's name, medical record number, "left Testis" and consists of a diffusely dusky, intact testis (3.8 × 3.0 × 2.9 cm, 13 g) with attached epididymis (3.9 × 1.0 × 0.9 cm) and short length of spermatic cord (1.7 cm in length). The testis is bivalved to reveal diffusely hemorrhagic seminiferous tubules and epididymis. No lesions are identified within

Section code:
  A1 Spermatic cord margin, en face
  A2 Testis in relation to epididymis
  A3 Testis, representative

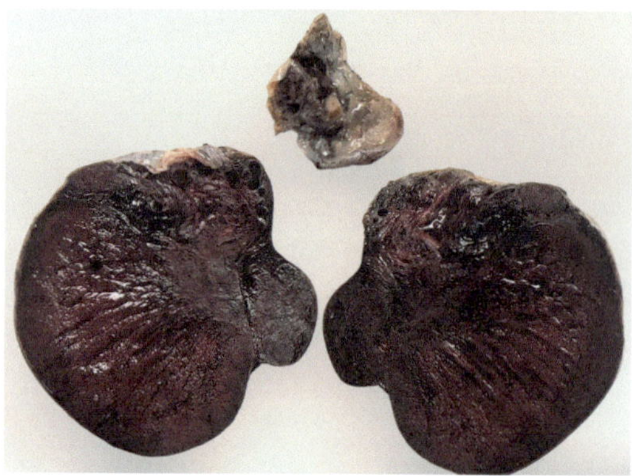

Fig. 6.115 Testis bivalved

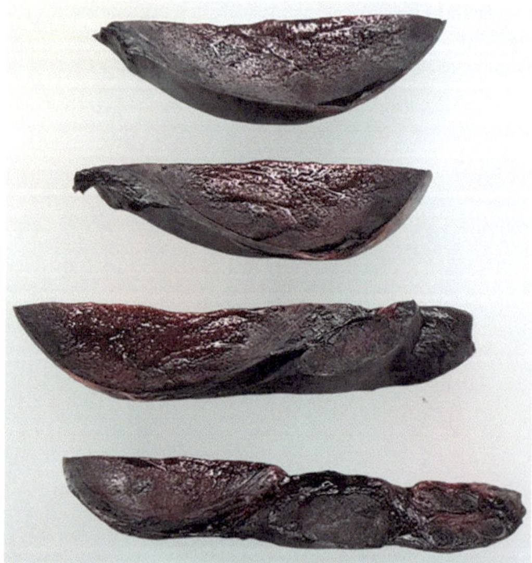

Fig. 6.116 Testis serially sectioned

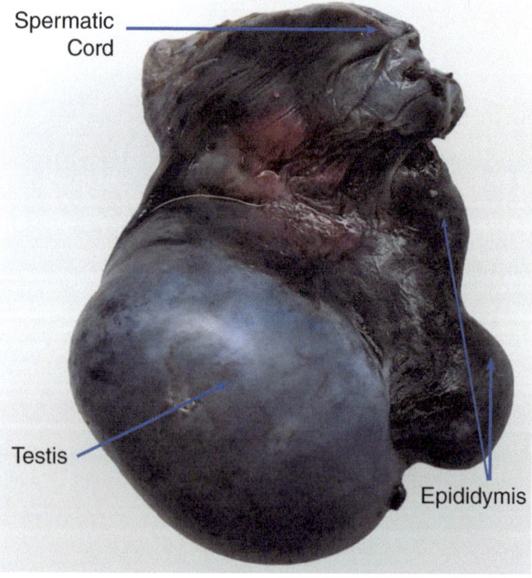

Fig. 6.114 Testis for torsion

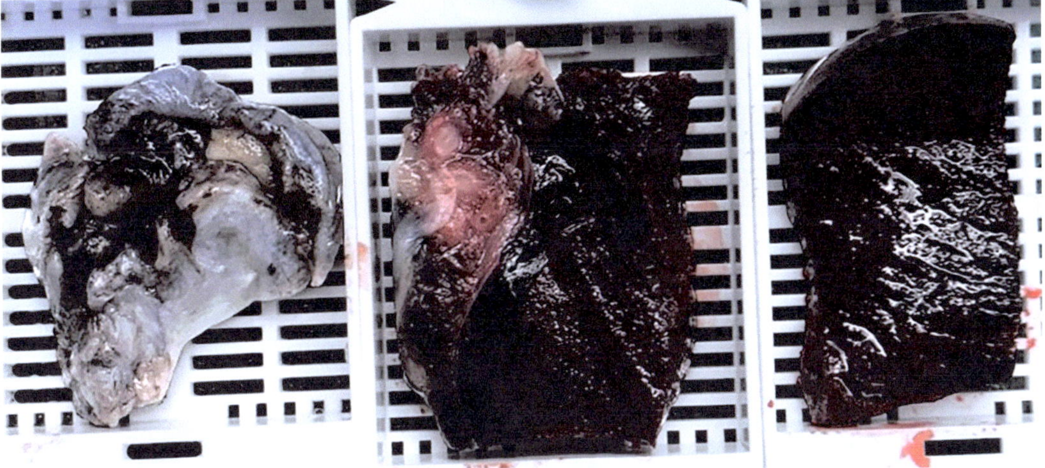

Fig. 6.117 Testis section submission

6.16   Testis for a Mass: Level VI CPT 88309

An orchiectomy is the removal of the testis for torsion, mass or prostate cancer in an advanced stage.

Cancer Protocol Breakdown Relative to Grossing Testis.

Laterality: Dictate the laterality of the testis.

Tumor focality: Dictate if the mass is unifocal or multifocal.

Tumor size: Measure the mass in three dimensions.

Tumor extent: Dictate if the mass is confined to the testis or if it extends into the rete testis, surrounding soft tissue, epididymis, tunica albuginea, tunica vaginalis, spermatic cord, or scrotum.

Margin status: Dictate if the mass is present at the spermatic cord margin.

pT Categories [2]

pT0 No evidence of primary tumor

pTis Germ cell neoplasia *in situ*

pT1a Tumor smaller than 3 cm

pT1b Tumor 3 cm or larger

pT2 Tumor limited to testis with lymphovascular invasion, or tumor invading hilar soft tissue or epididymis or penetrating visceral mesothelial layer covering the external surface of tunica albuginea with or without lymphovascular invasion

pT3 Tumor directly invades spermatic cord soft tissue with or without lymphovascular invasion

pT4 Tumor invades scrotum with or without lymphovascular invasion

Gross appearance of selected testicular tumors is described in Table 6.5 [3]

Table 6.5 Gross appearance of testicular tumors [3]

Germ cell tumors derived from germ cell neoplasia in situ	*Gonadoblastoma:* Soft to firm; brown, yellow, or gray in appearance; can reach 80 mm in size; often show multifocal calcification *Seminoma:* Solid, lobulated to multinodular, relatively homogeneous tumor; often cream-colored to tan, or pale yellow to pink; on sectioning, bulge above the surrounding normal parenchyma; mean size 50 mm *Embryonal carcinoma:* Variegated appearance; ranging from solid and white or tan in color to showing cysts, hemorrhage, and/or necrosis *Yolk sac tumor, post pubertal-type:* Solid to partially cystic, with a grayish white to tan cut surface that may have a myxoid appearance *Choriocarcinoma:* Smaller size; the cut surface appears nodular with extensive hemorrhage and necrotic areas *Teratoma, post pubertal-type:* Firm and nodular; the cut sections show heterogeneity and usually appear solid and cystic; the solid areas are firm to soft to myxoid; the cysts are filled with serous, mucoid, or keratinous material; cartilage, bone, and pigmented areas may be identified
Germ cell tumors unrelated to germ cell neoplasia in situ	*Spermatocytic tumor:* Solid and lobular to multinodular; the cut surface varies from grayish white to hemorrhagic and from fleshy to myxoid; sarcomatous foci may be appreciated as fleshy, sometimes firm, nodular areas with necrosis and hemorrhage *Yolk sac tumor, prepubertal-type:* Solid gray to yellow tumor with occasional small cysts and a myxoid surface on sectioning *Teratoma, prepubertal-type:* Solid or have a variably prominent cystic component filled with keratinaceous or mucoid material; may also show calcification or bone formation; grossly identifiable hair may be present in the *dermoid subtype*
Sex cord stromal tumors of the testis	*Leydig cell tumor:* Small, solid, well-circumscribed mass with a maximum diameter ranging from 5 to 50 mm; yellow, homogeneous, and soft; may show gross hemorrhage, necrosis, hyalinization, and calcification *Sertoli cell tumor:* Well-circumscribed, firm, lobulated, tan-white, and usually 5–40 mm in size; show occasional cystic changes and hemorrhage *Adult granulosa cell tumor:* Well circumscribed and solid (although cysts may be seen); the cut surface is lobulated and tan-white to yellowish *Juvenile granulosa cell tumor:* Partly cystic tumor containing watery or mucoid fluid, with tan-white/yellow solid areas *Tumors in the fibroma thecoma group:* Well-circumscribed tan-white or red lesions

Step 1: Describe, measure (testis, epididymis, and spermatic cord seperatly), and weight the specimen. (Fig. 6.118)

Step 2: Orient the specimen. The epididymis is present on the posterior aspect of the testis.

Step 3: Ink the specimen. In Fig. 6.119, the testis is inked medial and lateral. Communicate with the pathologist for inking suggestions.

Step 4: Shave the spermatic cord margin and submit en face.

Step 5: Serially section the remainder of the spermatic cord and submit representative sections. (Fig. 6.120)

Step 6: Bivalve the testis into medial and lateral halves. (Fig. 6.121)

Step 7: Describe and measure the mass in three dimensions.

Step 8: Describe where the mass is located, and how close the mass comes to the epididymis and spermatic cord margin. In Fig. 6.122, the mass is present in the testis and comes close to the epididymis.

Step 9: Take a fullface section of the testis with mass. If the entire tumor can be submitted in 10 cassettes, submit the tumor entirely. If not, submit 1 section per 1.0 cm (make sure to include all the areas that look different).

Step 10: Serially section the remainder of the medial and lateral aspects to visualize areas where the mass is closest to the surrounding tunica. (Fig. 6.123)

Step 11: Submit sections from the areas where the mass is closest to the surrounding ink.

Step 12: Submit sections from the junction of the spermatic cord and testis.

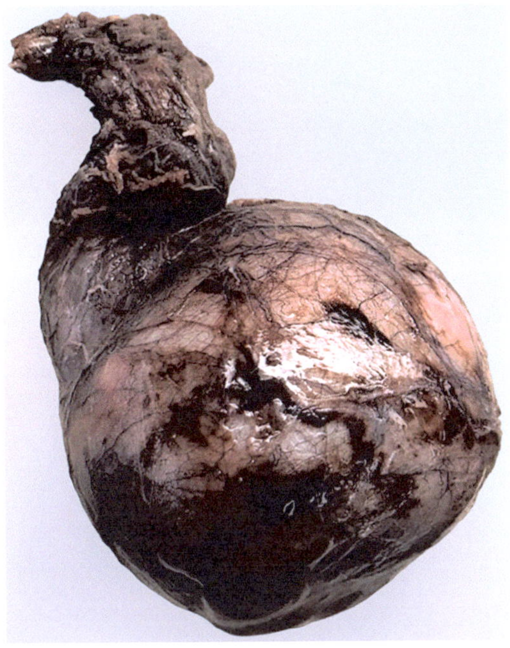

Fig. 6.118 Testis with a mass

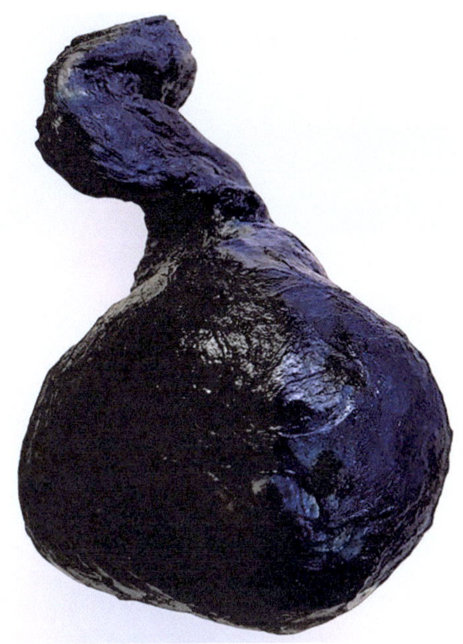

Fig. 6.119 Testis with mass, inked

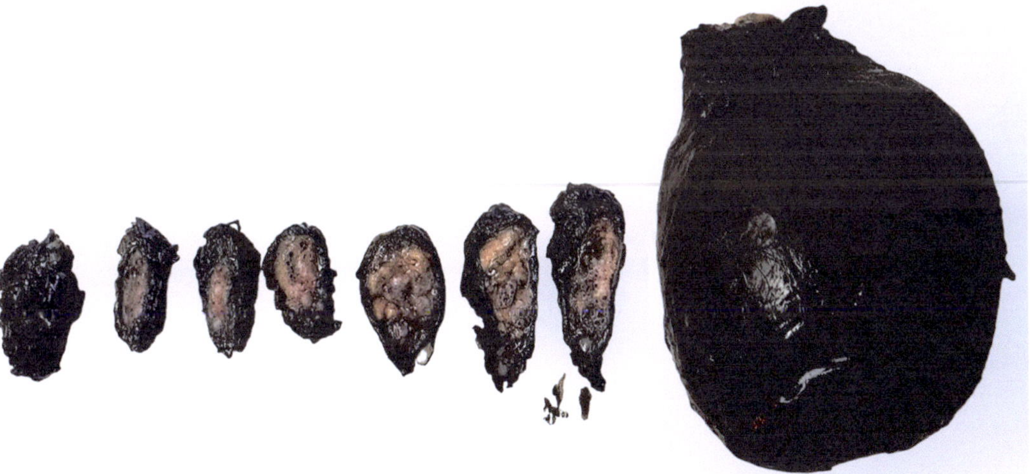

Fig. 6.120 Spermatic cord, serially sectioned

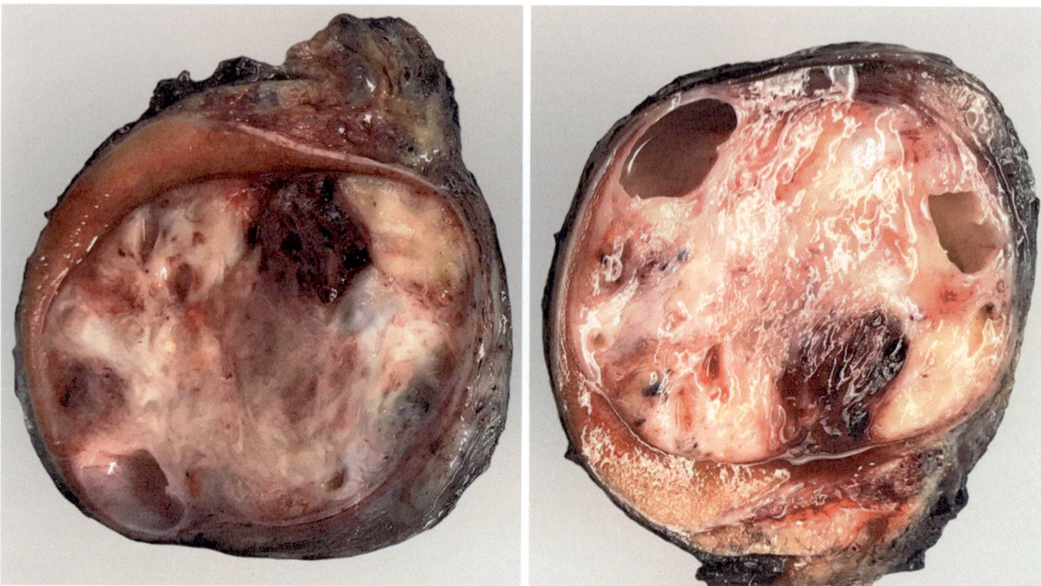

Fig. 6.121   Testis with mass, bivalved

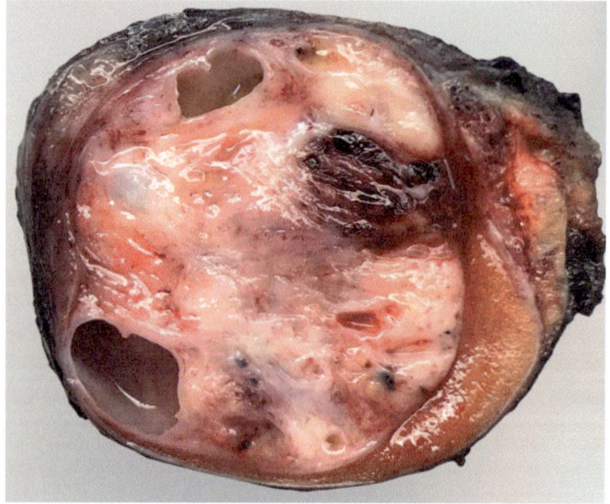

Fig. 6.122   Testis with mass, full cross section

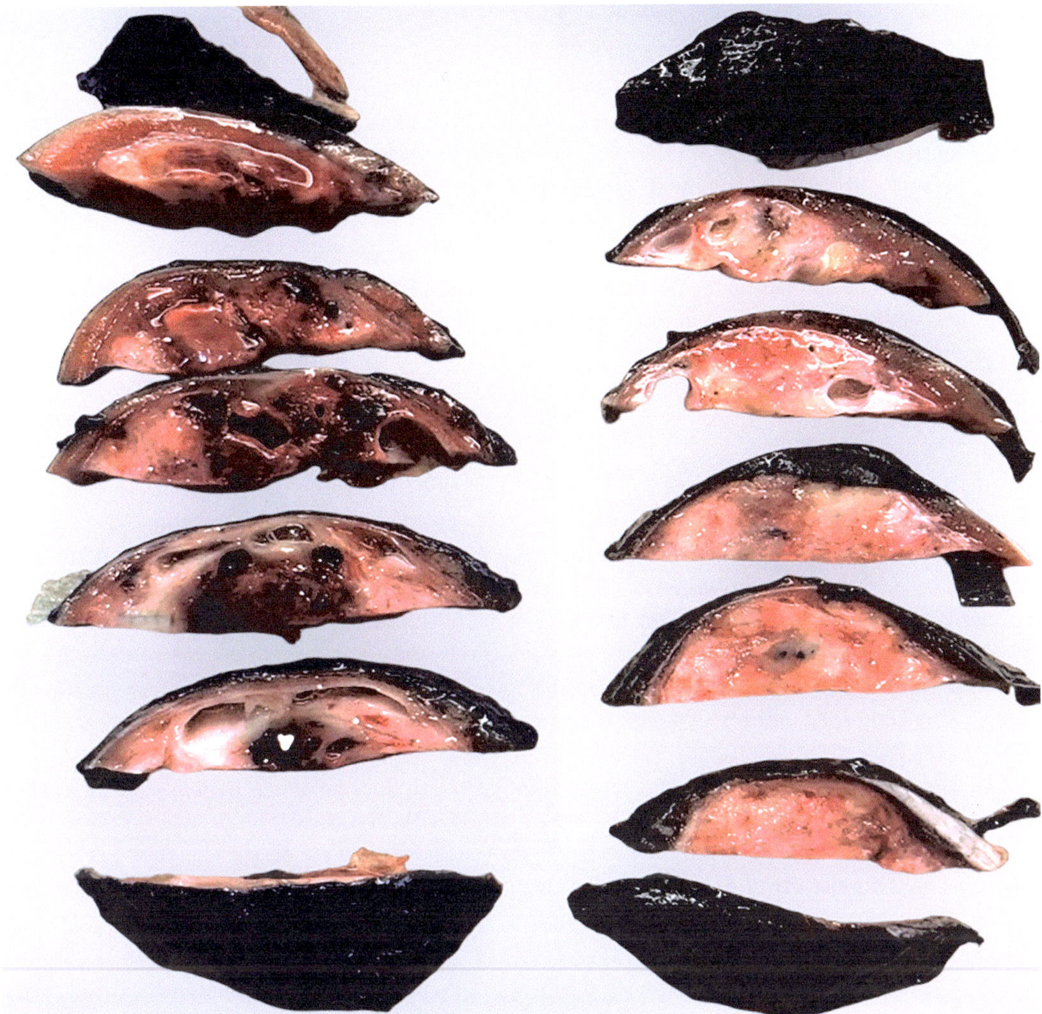

Fig. 6.123 Testis with the remainder of mass serially sectioned

Example Dictation

Specimen A is received in formalin labeled with patient's name, medical record number, "left Testis" and consists of an enlarged, intact testis (7.1 × 6.5 × 6.1 cm, 51 g) with attached flattened epididymis (7.5 × 1.0 × 0.3 cm) and length of spermatic cord (6.7 cm in length). The testis is bivalved to reveal a tan-white, well-circumscribed, focally cystic and hemorrhagic mass (6.1 × 5.9 × 5.5 cm) present within the seminiferous tubules. The mass comes within 1.2 cm from the epididymis and 8.2 cm from the spermatic cord margin without invasion through the tunica albuginea. Unremarkable testicular parenchyma is identified in the posterior aspect.

Section code

    A1 Spermatic cord margin, en face

    A2 Additional representative sections of spermatic cord (including one mid and one at the base of the spermatic cord)

    A3–A8 Fullface section of testis with mass in relation to epididymis

    A9 Mass in relation to medial aspect

    A10 Mass in relation to lateral aspect

Acknowledgments The author gratefully ackno wledges Varsha Manucha, MD, and Varsha Prakash, MD, MD, for their contribution to this chapter.

Quiz Questions

1. A 38-year-old male presents with a painless mass in the right testis. On gross examina-tion, a 5.5 cm well-circumscribed, lobulated, homogeneous, and tan tumor is noted which bulges above the surrounding normal parenchyma.

   What is the most likely diagnosis based on the gross description?
   A. Choriocarcinoma
   B. Seminoma
   C. Teratoma, post-pubertal type
   D. Leydig cell tumor

2. Which of the following statement(s) best describe multilocular cystic renal cell neo-plasm of low malignant potential?
   A. It has a prominent fibrous pseudocapsule
   B. It is composed entirely of variably sized cysts
   C. Presence of expansile, solid areas is incompatible with its diagnosis
   D. All of the above

3. What is the most likely diagnosis based on the gross appearance? (Fig. 6.124 Quiz Question)
   A. Clear cell renal cell carcinoma
   B. Oncocytoma of the kidney
   C. Acquired cystic disease-associated renal cell carcinoma
   D. Collecting duct carcinoma

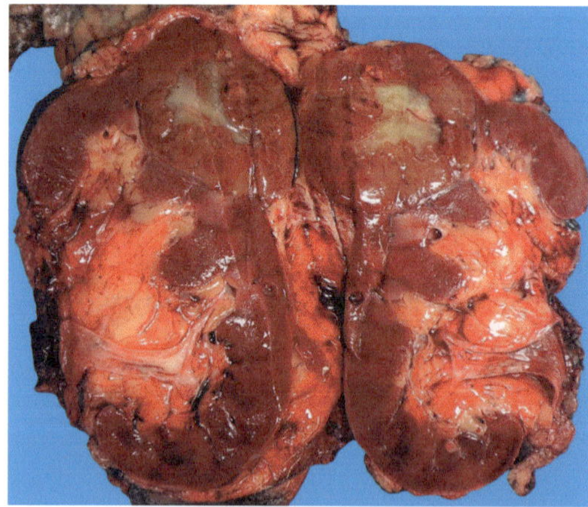

Fig. 6.124 Quiz question

4. Which statement best describes a Leydig cell tumor?
   A. Solid, well-circumscribed, soft yellow mass which shows gross hemorrhage, necrosis, hyalinization, and calcification
   B. Small tumor having a nodular surface with extensive hemorrhage and necrotic areas
   C. Partly cystic tumor containing a mucoid fluid with yellow solid areas
   D. Nodular tumor with myxoid solid areas and keratinous material in the cystic areas

5. Which of the following statement(s) is (are) true regarding acquired cystic disease-associated renal cell carcinoma?
   A. It is among the most common subtypes of renal cell carcinoma in end-stage kidneys
   B. It is important to pay attention to the cys-tic areas during gross examination of end-stage kidneys as, many a times, this tumor appear to arise within a cyst
   C. It does not occur in end-stage kidneys
   D. Both A & B
   E. None of the above

6. Which of the following renal tumor has a spongy/bubble wrap surface on cut sections?
   A. Oncocytoma of the kidney
   B. Nephroblastoma
   C. Tubulocystic renal cell carcinoma
   D. Renal papillary adenoma

7. Which of the following is a subtype of HPV-associated squamous cell carcinoma of penis?
   A. Lymphoepithelioma-like carcinoma
   B. Basaloid squamous cell carcinoma
   C. Clear cell squamous cell carcinoma
   D. All of the above

8. Which of the following statement is true regarding prostatic adenocarcinoma?
   A. It is often not visible grossly
   B. If visible, it is solid, firm, and poorly circumscribed
   C. Grossly, it usually shows variably sized yellow nodules that project above the cut surface
   D. Both A & B

9. Which of the following statement best match the gross description of teratoma, post pubertal-type, of testis?

    A. A heterogenous tumor with firm solid areas and mucous and hair-containing cystic areas

    B. A tan solid, lobulated homogeneous nodule that bulges above the normal parenchyma

    C. A myxoid partially cystic tumor with tan cut surfaces

    D. Small, predominantly hemorrhagic and necrotic tumor

10. What is the most likely diagnosis based on the gross appearance? (Fig. 6.125 Quiz question)

    A. Oncocytoma of the kidney

    B. Clear cell renal cell carcinoma

    C. Tubulocystic renal cell carcinoma

    D. Metanephric adenoma

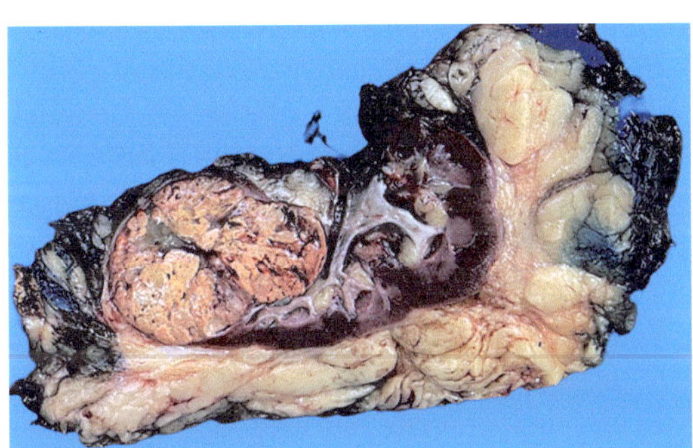

Fig. 6.125 Quiz question

Answer Key

1. B—Seminoma

    Explanation On sectioning, seminomas are usually solid, lobulated to multinodular, relatively homogeneous nodules that are cream-colored to tan or pale yellow to pink, and bulge above the normal parenchyma. Tumor size varies greatly, with a mean of around 50 mm. Choriocarcinoma is frequently small, predominantly hemorrhagic tumor. Teratoma, postpubertal type, is a firm and nodular tumor. Its cut section shows a tremendous heterogeneity due to the pres-

ence of several types of tissues, and it is usually solid and cystic in nature. In solid areas, the color varies from whitish-tan to translucent and the texture varies from firm to soft to myxoid. Cysts may contain serous, mucoid, or keratinous material. Leydig cell tumor is typically small, solid, and well-circumscribed mass. It is soft in consistency and yellow in color.

2. D—All of the above

    Explanation Multilocular cystic renal neoplasm of low malignant potential is a well-demarcated tumor with a fibrous pseudocapsule and is composed entirely of variably sized cysts filled with clear, gelatinous, serous, or hemorrhagic fluid. The cysts have thin septa and do not contain expansile, solid areas. Presence of expansile, solid areas is incompatible with its diagnosis.

3. B—Oncocytoma of the kidney

    Explanation Oncocytomas of the kidney are usually well-circumscribed mahogany-brown tumors with central stellate scar. Clear cell renal cell carcinomas are usually well circumscribed (pseudo-capsulated) golden yellow tumors that mostly have hemorrhage, necrosis, calcification, and cystic changes. Acquired cystic disease-associated renal cell carcinoma is identified in acquired cysts, either as an intracystic mass or not in association with the cysts. It has a brown to yellow-tan cut surface, sometimes with hemorrhage or necrosis. Background kidney will usually have numerous cysts. Collecting duct carcinomas are gray-white and firm tumors with hemorrhage and necrosis. They have an irregular, poorly defined contour.

4. A—Solid, well-circumscribed, soft yellow mass which shows gross hemorrhage, necrosis, hyalinization, and calcification

    Explanation Leydig cell tumors are usually small, solid, well-circumscribed tumors with a diameter ranging from 5 to 50 mm. They are yellow, homogeneous, and soft and may show gross hemorrhage, necrosis, hyalinization, and calcification. Choriocarcinomas are small in size and have nodular cut surfaces with extensive hemorrhage. Juvenile granulosa cell tumors are partly cystic tumors containing watery or mucoid fluid, with tan-white/yellow solid areas. Teratoma, postpubertal-type, is firm and nodular tumor. Their cut sections show heterogeneity and usually have solid and cystic areas. The solid areas are firm to soft and may be myxoid. The cysts are filled with serous, mucoid, or keratinous material. Cartilage, bone, and pigmented areas may also be identified.

5. **D—Both A & B**

   Explanation Acquired cystic disease-associated renal cell carcinoma is among the most common renal cell carcinomas in end-stage kidneys. It is identified in acquired cysts (either as an intracystic mass or not in association with the cysts). These tumors have a brown to yellow-tan cut surface, sometimes with hemorrhage or necrosis. Background kidney will usually have numerous cysts. It is important to pay attention to the cystic areas during gross examination of end-stage kidneys as, many a times, this tumor appear to arise within a cyst.

6. **C—Tubulocystic Renal Cell Carcinoma**

   Explanation Tubulocystic renal cell carcinomas are usually well circumscribed, solitary tumors, with a spongy or bubble wrap-like appearance. The cut surface consists of small white cysts containing clear fluid. No hemorrhage or necrosis is observed. Oncocytomas of the kidney are usually well-circumscribed mahogany-brown tumors with central stellate scar. Nephroblastomas are well delineated and fleshy tumor with small yellow areas of necrosis. A multinodular internal structure is typical for nephroblastomas. Renal papillary adenomas are usually well circumscribed, subcapsular, often wedge-shaped grayish-white to yellow nodules.

7. **D—All of the above**

   Explanation There are four subtypes of HPV-associated squamous cell carcinoma (SCC) of penis. The gross description of each subtype is described below:

   1. Basaloid SCC large, ulcerated, non-exophytic mass

   2. Warty carcinoma cauliflower-like, exophytic, white to gray mass

   3. Clear cell SCC large white-gray mass measuring 25–55 mm and sometimes replacing the distal penis

   4. Lymphoepithelioma-like carcinoma exophytic, well- to poorly circumscribed white-gray mass

8. **D—Both A & B**

   Explanation Prostatic adenocarcinoma is often not visible grossly. If visible, it is solid, firm, and poorly circumscribed. Benign prostatic hyperplasia is grossly composed of variously sized nodules which are gray to yellow in color and project above the cut surfaces.

9. **A—A heterogenous tumor with firm solid areas, and mucous and hair-containing cystic areas**

   Explanation Teratoma, post pubertal-type, is a firm and nodular tumor. Its cut sections show heterogeneity due to the presence of several types of tissues, and it is usually solid and cystic in nature. Cysts may contain serous, mucoid, or keratinous material. Seminomas are usually solid, lobulated to multinodular, homogeneous nodules that are tan or pale yellow to pink, and bulge above the normal parenchyma. Yolk sac tumor, post pubertal-type, is a solid to partially cystic tumor with a grayish white to tan cut surface that may have a myxoid appearance. Choriocarcinoma is frequently small, predominantly hemorrhagic and necrotic tumor.

10. **B—Clear Cell Renal Cell Carcinoma**

    Explanation Clear cell renal cell carcinomas are usually well circumscribed (pseudo-capsulated) golden yellow tumors that commonly have hemorrhage, necrosis, calcification, and cystic change. Oncocytomas of the kidney are usually well-circumscribed mahogany-brown tumors with central stellate scar. Tubulocystic renal cell carcinomas are usually well circumscribed, solitary tumors, with a spongy or bubble wrap-like appearance. Metanephric adenomas are usually unicentric, well-circumscribed and solid gray-white tumors.

References

1. UMHS DEPARTMENT OF PATHOLOGY: specimen to charge code radip finder list. 8 April 2011. [Online]. Available: https://www.uslegalforms.com/jsfiller-desk14/?mode=cors&requestHash=659dcb29097b509499ee51bf7ee3b40e29ab0b416312f299042d2943f2b3335a&lang=en&ref=https://www.uslegalforms.com&projectId=1334581953&loader=tips&MEDIUM_PDFJS=true&PAGE_REARRANGE_V2_MVP=true&isP. Accessed 28 Aug 2023.

2. College of American Pathologists. June 2021. [Online]. Available: https://www.cap.org/protocols--and-guidelines/cancer-reporting-tools/cancer-protocol-templates. Accessed 15 Jun 2023.

Gross Examination Only Specimens

7

Contents

Specimens for gross examination only are some of the most trying specimens to dictate. Choosing words to describe these objects is often difficult. Documentation of these specimens is important even though no tissue is being examined microscopically. If a patient has a chemotherapy port removed, dictation of the appropriate brand and serial number is necessary. If that chemotherapy port happens to be associated with a class action lawsuit, the correct serial number is important and must be correct in the dictation. Remember, gross only specimens have no other documentation in pathology, other than the gross description. These descriptions must be detailed and accurate.

Gross examination only specimens is a list of specimens derived by each institution to be designated as gross examination only, where micro-

Table 7.1 CPT Code

Gross examination only	88300

scopic evaluation is not applicable. This list can change from hospital to hospital, but the final decision as to whether sections are taken for a given specimen is reserved for the pathologist. If a surgeon submits tissue for gross examination only, communicate with the pathologist. If the pathologist feels that histologic examination is necessary, then samples of the specimen should be submitted. See Table 7.1 for CPT code.

7.1 Chemotherapy Port ("chemoport"): Level I CPT 88300

A chemoport is a medical device implanted, often in the chest, to give patients intravenous medications. The tube from the chemo port is placed in a vein. Once treatment is completed, the chemo port is removed. This is an example of a medical device that contains an identification number. Identification information should be put in quotation in the gross description or somehow designated as the identification information for the specific device.

Step 1: Describe and measure the chemo port. (Fig. 7.1)
Step 2: Describe and measure the tube extending from the port.
Step 3: Dictate exactly how the identification information reads on the device (Fig. 7.2). This example has been de-identified.

Example Dictation
Specimen A is received in formalin labeled with the patient's name, medical record number, and "chemo port," and consists of a purple chemo port (2.9 x 2.9 x 1.1 cm) which bears the inscription, "chemo port identification information," with a segment of white tubing (22.5 cm in length) extending from one aspect. The specimen is for gross examination only and no sections are submitted.

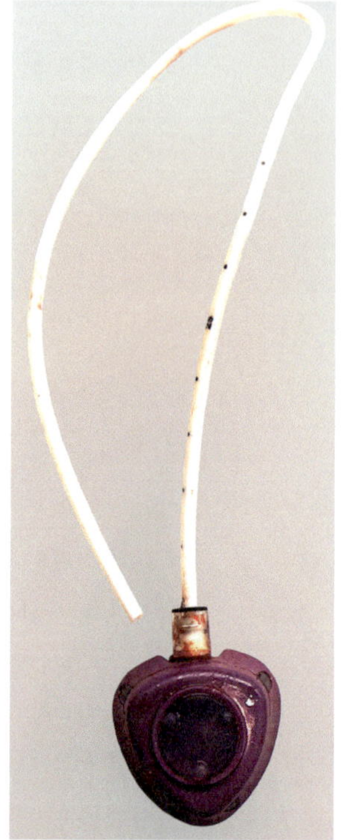

Fig. 7.1 Chemo port, anterior

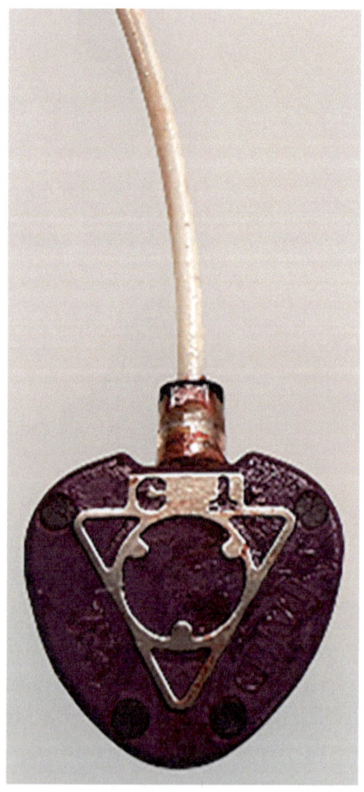

Fig. 7.2 Chemo port, posterior

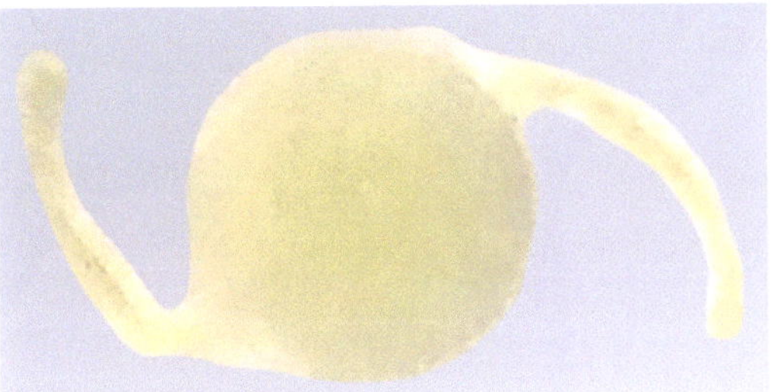

Fig. 7.3 Intraocular lens

7.2 Intraocular Lens: Level I CPT 88300

An intraocular lens (IOL) is an artificial implant meant to replace the native eye lens to help restore vision. An intraocular lens is a disc-shaped plastic foreign object placed in the eye. Some IOLs are yellow in color, and some are translucent. There are 2 extensions on opposite sides called "haptics."

Step 1: Dictate the size and color of the lens. (Fig. 7.3)
Step 2: Dictate if the haptics are present attached to the IOL or present separately in the container and if there are any cracks in the lens.
Step 3: If any part of the IOL is broken or missing, dictate what parts are broken or missing.

Example Dictation

Specimen A is received in formalin labeled with the patient's name, medical record number, "IOL, right," and consists of a yellow-translucent intraocular lens (0.8 cm in diameter) with two yellow translucent haptics on opposing aspects. The specimen bears no description. The specimen is for gross examination only and no sections are submitted.

7.3 Intrauterine Device: Level I CPT 88300

An intrauterine device (IUD) is a form of birth control. The device is placed inside the uterus where it can remain for years, until it is either necessary to remove or the patient wishes to become pregnant.

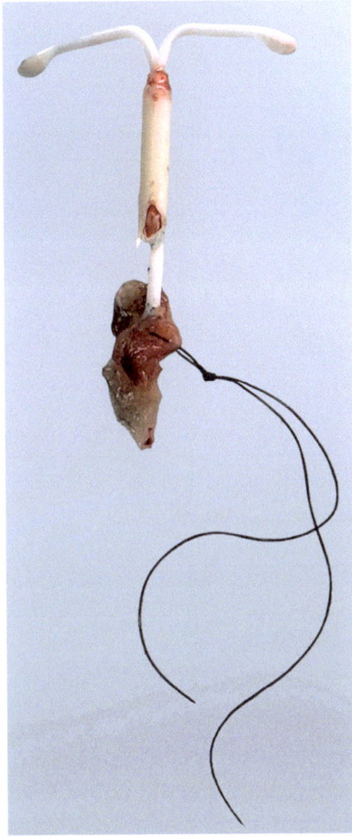

Fig. 7.4 Intrauterine device

Step 1: Describe and measure the IUD.
Step 2: Describe if the IUD is intact or broken. In Fig. 7.4, the IUD is fractured but all parts of the IUD are present.

Example Dictation

Specimen A is received in formalin labeled with the patient's name, medical record number, and "IUD" and consists of an intrauterine device (3.0 x 3.0 x 0.3 cm) with an intact string present, and a single fracture site present inferiorly. The specimen bears no inscription. The specimen is for gross examination only and no sections are submitted.

7.4 Inferior Vena Cava Filter (IVC Filter): Level I CPT 88300

The purpose of an IVC filter is to retrieve thrombi as they travel from the large veins in the legs to the heart. They are typically metal, umbrella-

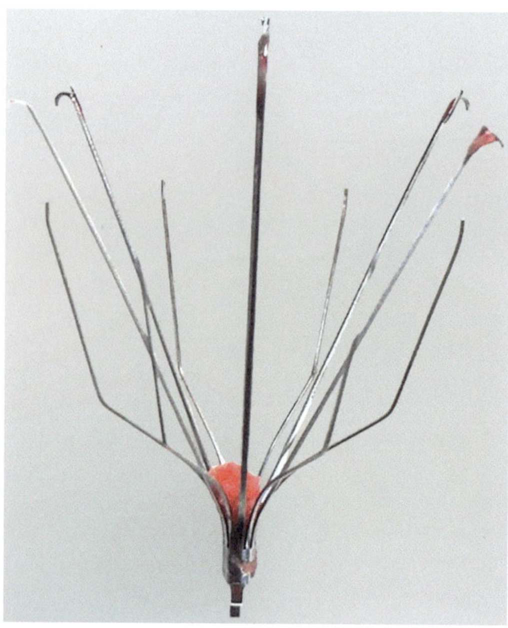

Fig. 7.5 IVC filter

shaped devices placed in the inferior vena cava. It is important to have a general knowledge of the different brands of filters to help identify if these filters are received intact or broken.

Step 1: Dictate and measure the IVC filter. (Fig. 7.5)
Step 2: Assess and dictate if the filter is intact or broken. Dictate if portions of the IVC filter are broken or missing. Check the container for those broken portions.

Example Dictation
Specimen A is received in formalin labeled with the patient's name, medical record number, and "IVC filter" and consists of an intact, silver-metallic IVC filter (5.5 x 2.7 x 2.5 cm) with a scant amount of adhered tan-pink soft tissue. The specimen is for gross only and no sections are submitted.

7.5 Mandibular Plate: Level I CPT 88300

Mandibular plates are used to hold the mandible in the correct position after a fracture or surgery. Plates can then be removed later for reasons such as pain, infection, or plate exposure.

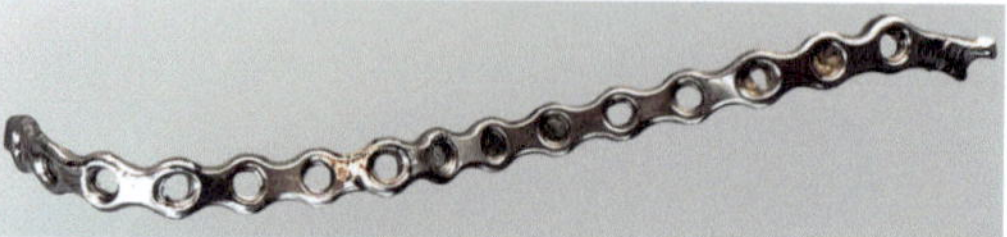

Fig. 7.6 Mandibular plate

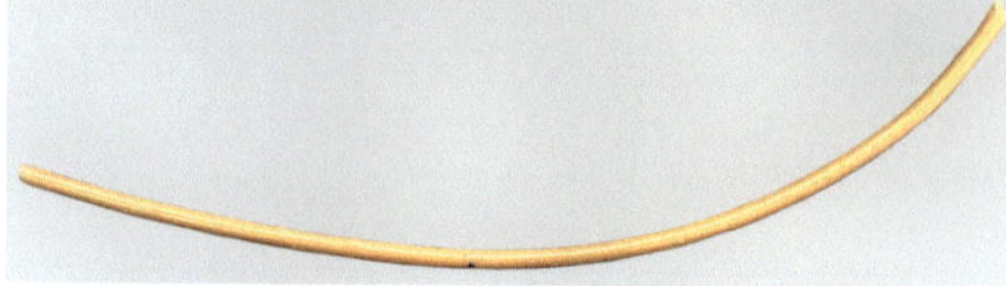

Fig. 7.7 Stent

Step 1: Describe and measure the segment mandibular plate. (Fig. 7.6)
Step 2: Dictate the inscription, if any.

Specimen A is received in formalin labeled with the patient's name, medical record number, and "mandibular plate" and consists of a segment of a silver-metallic segment of the surgical mandibular plate (12.2 x 0.5 x 0.3 cm) which bears no inscription. The specimen is for gross only and no sections are submitted.

7.6 Stent: Level I CPT 88300

Stents are medical devices meant to keep anatomic structures open such as vessels, ureters, etc., and can be temporary or permanent.

Step 1: Describe and measure the segment of tubing. (Fig. 7.7)
Step 2: Dictate the inscription, if any.

Specimen A is received in formalin labeled with the patient's name, medical record number, and "stent" and consists of a segment of tan-yellow, rubber tubing (6.0 x 0.2 cm in diameter) which bears no inscription. The specimen is for gross only, and no sections are submitted.

7.7   Implantable Cardioverter Defibrillator: Level I CPT 88300

An implantable cardioverter defibrillator (ICD) is a device that is implanted to detect and correct cardiac arrhythmias. It is implanted in the chest with leads extending to the heart. This device is commonly removed due to infection that can happen around the device, pericardium, or in the heart.

Step 1: Describe and measure the ICD.
Step 2: Describe and measure the leads.
Step 3: Dictate exactly how the identification information reads on the device (Fig. 7.8). This example has been de-identified.

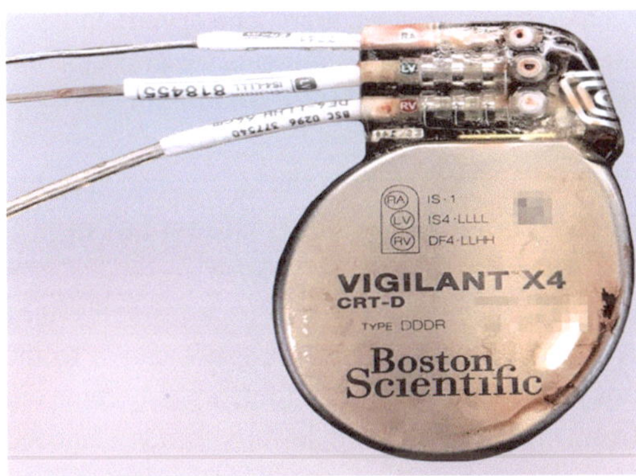

Fig. 7.8 Implantable cardioverter defibrillator

Example Dictation
Specimen A is received in formalin labeled with the patient's name, medical record number, "IDC" and consists of a silver-metallic implantable cardioverter defibrillator (4.8 x 3.5 x 1.0 cm) which bears the inscription, "VIGILANT X4, CRT-D, Type, model number, serial number, Boston Scientific." The device has 3 leads (12.2 cm, 7.5 cm, and 5.9 cm in length) extending from one side. The specimen is for gross only and no sections are submitted.

7.8   Heart Valve: Level I CPT 88300

Prosthetic heart valves are implanted when the native valves no longer function. However, a prosthetic valve can also become nonfunctional or infected over time and is therefore replaced.

Step 1: Describe and measure the valve.
Step 2: Describe the prosthetic leaflets. In Fig. 7.9, there are 3 leaflets that are intact, but contain adhered calcification.

Example Dictation
Specimen A is received in formalin labeled with the patient's name, medical record number, and "prosthetic aortic valve" and consists of an intact prosthetic valve (2.5 cm in diameter x 1.5 cm)

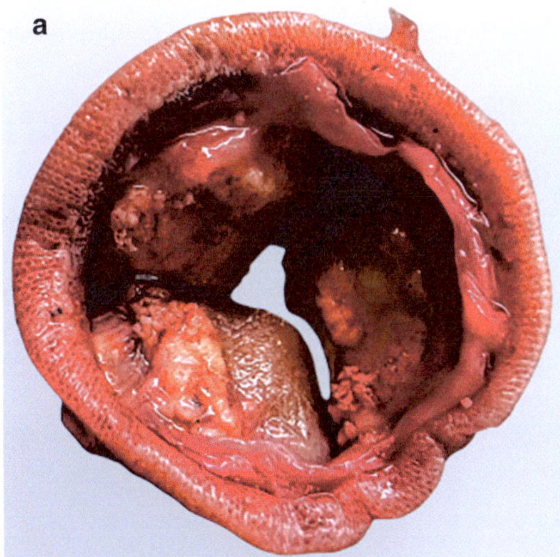
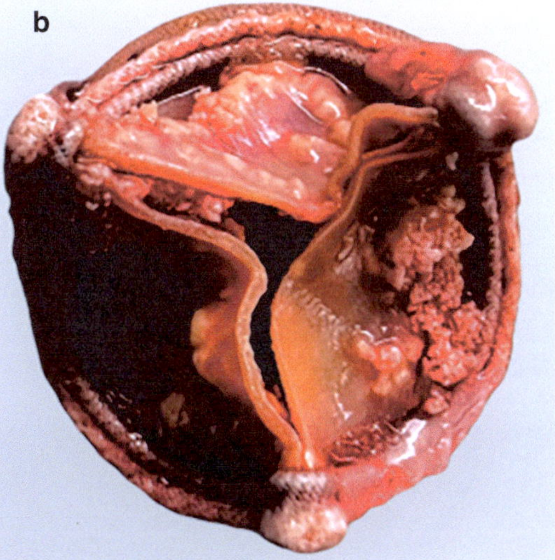

Fig. 7.9 (**a**) Prosthetic heart valve, superior; (**b**) prosthetic heart valve, inferior

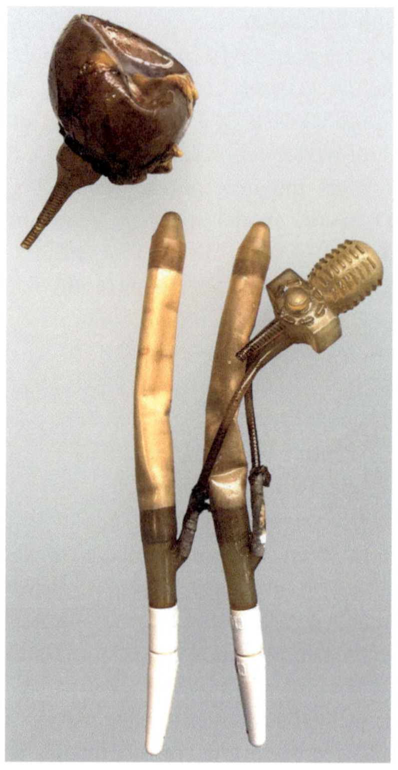

Fig. 7.10 Penile implant

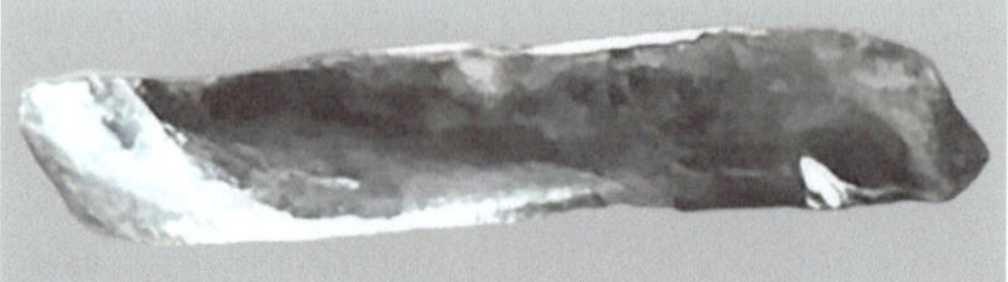

Fig. 7.11 Glass fragment

Step 3: Dictate if there are any words or serial numbers on the implant.

Example Dictation
Specimen A is received in formalin labeled with the patient's name, medical record number, and "penile implant" and consists of a complete penile implant of 2 cylinders (12.5 x 1.3 cm in diameter and 12.7 x 1.3 cm in diameter) with an attached reservoir (3.5 x 1.4 x 1.0 cm) and a separate pump (6.2 x 4.5 x 4.5 cm) all containing a scant amount of clear fluid. The specimen bears no description. The specimen is for gross examination only and no sections are submitted.

7.10 Foreign Object, Glass: Level I CPT 88300

A foreign object is something not native to the body. Glass pulled from a foot, a penny removed from the stomach, and jewelry beads removed from the nose are all examples of foreign objects. These are received and dictated in the gross room to document the removal of the foreign object.

Step 1: Describe and measure the foreign object. Explain in detail what the object looks like. (Fig. 7.11)

Example Dictation
Specimen A is received in formalin labeled with the patient's name, medical record number, and "foreign object" and consists of a sharply demarcated fragment of translucent glass (0.9 x 0.3 x 0.3 cm). The specimen is for gross only and no sections are submitted.

with marked adhered calcification on the leaflets. The specimen is for gross only and no sections are submitted.

7.9 Penile Implant: Level I CPT 88300

A penile implant is a medical device that is used in cases of impotency. It consists of 2 cylinders that are inserted into the penis, a pump inserted behind the testes, and a reservoir implanted in the abdomen.

Step 1: Identify, describe, and measure all the parts. (Fig. 7.10)
Step 2: If any parts are missing, dictate what parts are not present.

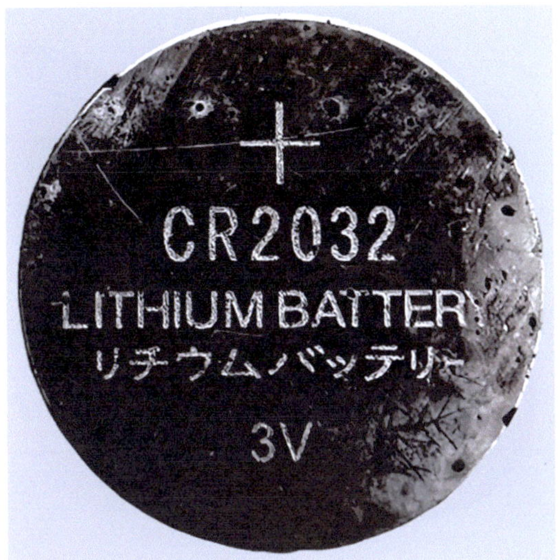

Fig. 7.12 Battery

7.11 Foreign Object, Battery: Level I CPT 88300

Patients can accidentally or intentionally swallow objects that can get stuck anywhere within the GI tract. A battery is an excellent example.

Step 1: Describe and measure the foreign object as seen in Fig. 7.12. Explain in detail what the object looks like.

Step 2: Dictate the inscription of the object, if any.

Example Dictation

Specimen A is received in formalin labeled with the patient's name, medical record number, "battery" and consists of a single, flat, silver-metallic battery (2.0 cm in diameter) which bears the inscription, "CR2032, LITHIUM BATTERY." The specimen is for gross only and no sections are submitted.

7.12 Tonsils: Level I CPT 88300

Tonsils for gross only often have an age range to be gross only specimens. This varies by institution. Typically, the tonsils of an 11-year-old patient or younger can be gross examination only.

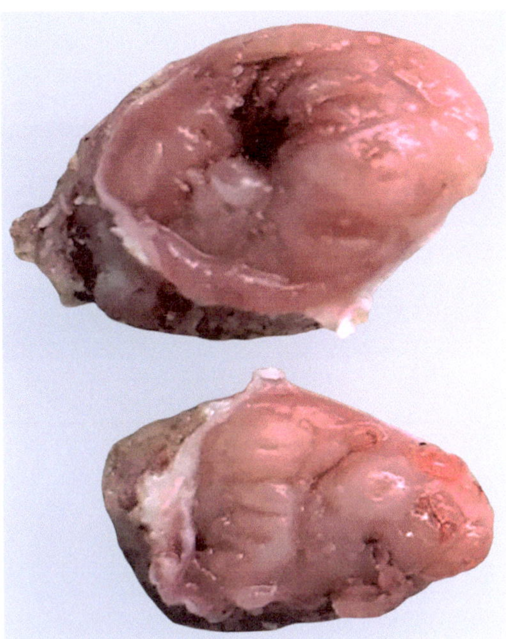

Fig. 7.13 Tonsils, intact

Any patient, 12 years or older may have representative sections submitted. Always pay attention to the pre-operative diagnosis. If the diagnosis includes malignancy, the tonsils need to be grossed in an entirely different manner, including inking of margins or other studies. Significant size asymmetry between the tonsils could indicate pathology. Communicate with the pathologists if there is a need to analyze a gross only tonsil microscopically.

Step 1: Dictate if the tonsils are unoriented (right/ left). (Fig. 7.13)
Step 2: Measure and describe the tonsils.
Step 3: Serially section each tonsil as shown in Fig. 7.14.
Step 4: Identify any lesions, ulcers, or caseous material. Tonsils naturally have crypt architecture where the tonsils fold, creating small crypts.

Example Dictation

Specimen A is received in formalin labeled with the patient's name, medical record number, and "tonsils" and consists of two unoriented tonsils (2.4 x 1.5 x 1.0 cm, 1.9 x 1.4 x 1.0 cm) which are

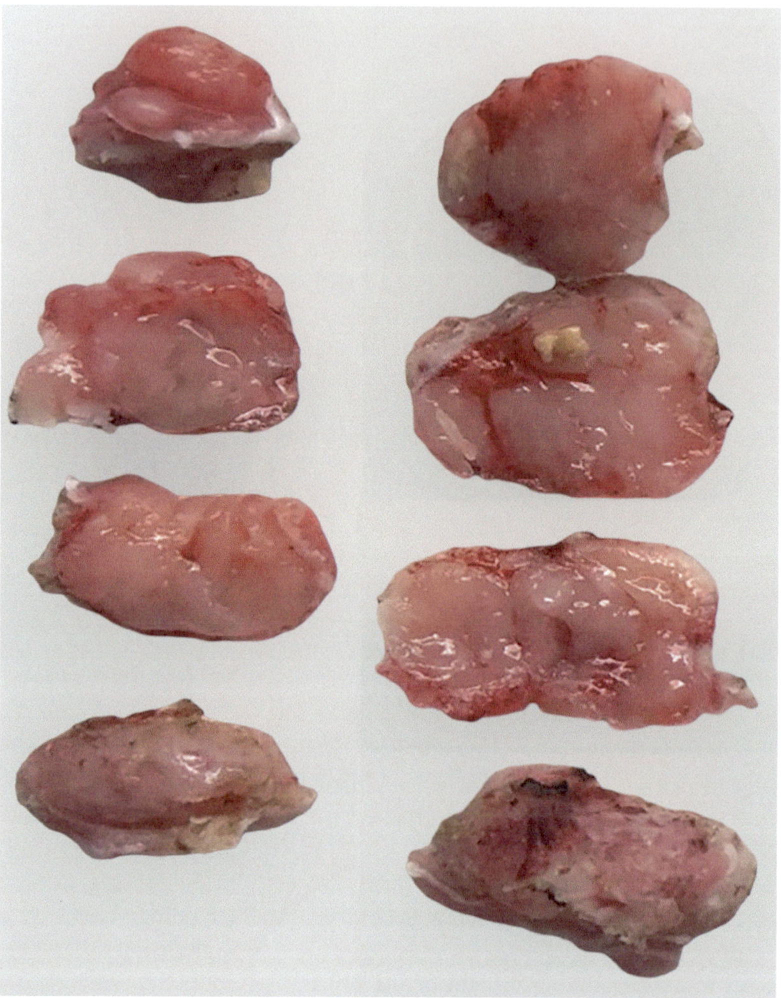

Fig. 7.14 Tonsils serially sectioned

serially sectioned to reveal tan-pink cut surfaces with crypt architecture and a scant amount of caseous material. The specimen is for gross examination only and no sections are submitted.

7.13 Extra Digit: Level I CPT 88300

Polydactyly is a common congenital condition where a baby is born with extra digits. This condition accounts for one or multiple extra digits on the hands or feet. Most often, these extra digits do not function and are frequently removed.

Step 1: Describe the skin color and the presence or absence of bone and nails. (Fig. 7.15)

Step 2: Measure the specimen.

Example Dictation

Specimen A is received in formalin labeled with the patient's name, medical record number, and "extra digit" and consists of a single, disarticulated, tan-pink, nail-bearing digit (4.2 x 1.4 x 1.1 cm) with an identifiable nail and bone within. The specimen is for gross examination only and no sections are submitted.

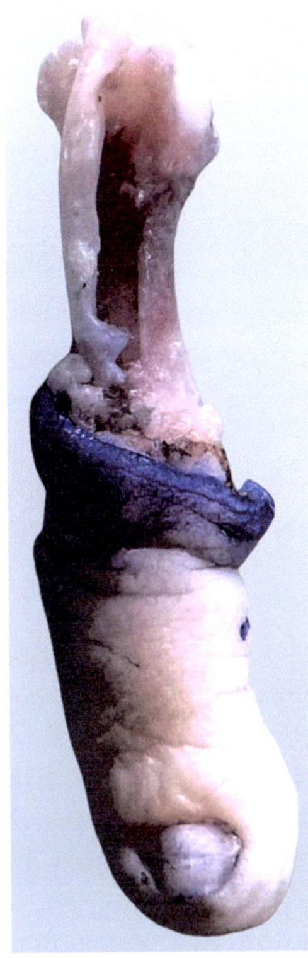

Fig. 7.15 Digit

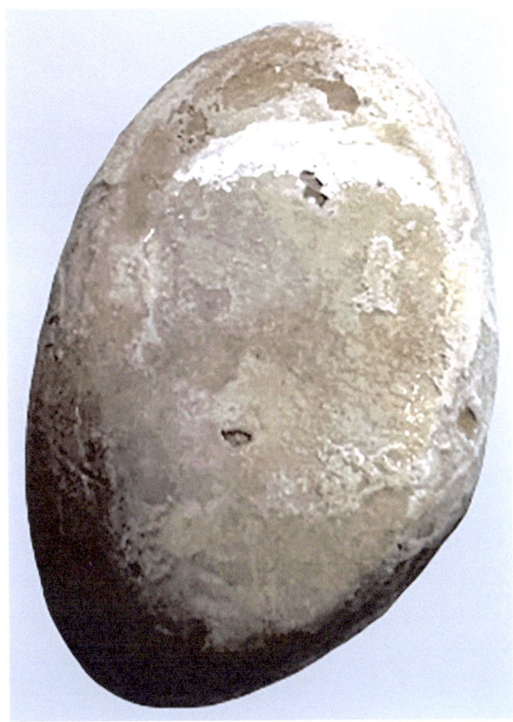

Fig. 7.16 Stone

7.14   Stones: Level I CPT 88300

Stones can form in many organs of the body, but they are all grossed in the same manner. In some cases, as per protocol or at the physician's request, stones are submitted for analysis to identify chemical composition. At the end of these gross descriptions, "the specimen is for gross examination only and no sections are submitted" will be replaced with a statement indicating the stone is submitted for stone analysis. For example, "the specimen is sent to University Hospital for further analysis."

Step 1: Dictate and measure the stone or stones. If the stone is large, a weight may be necessary. (Fig. 7.16).

Example Dictation

Specimen A is received in formalin labeled with the patient's name, medical record number, and "bladder stone" and consists of a single, tan-yellow, smooth stone (4.2 x 3.1 x 1.9 cm, 23 grams). The specimen is for gross examination only and no sections are submitted.

7.15   Teeth: Level I CPT 88300

Teeth are extracted for various reasons, but in a hospital setting, they are often removed to clear a specific area for surgery. Teeth can be decalcified and submitted to histology, if necessary.

Step 1: Dictate and measure the tooth or teeth. (Fig. 7.17)
Step 2: Assess for any fractures of the tooth.

Example Dictation

Specimen A is received in formalin labeled with the patient's name, medical record number, and "tooth" and consists of a tan, fractured tooth (1.1 x 1.0 x 1.0 cm) with a separate fractured root fragment (0.9 x 0.4 x 0.4 cm) present in the container. The specimen is for gross examination only and no sections are submitted.

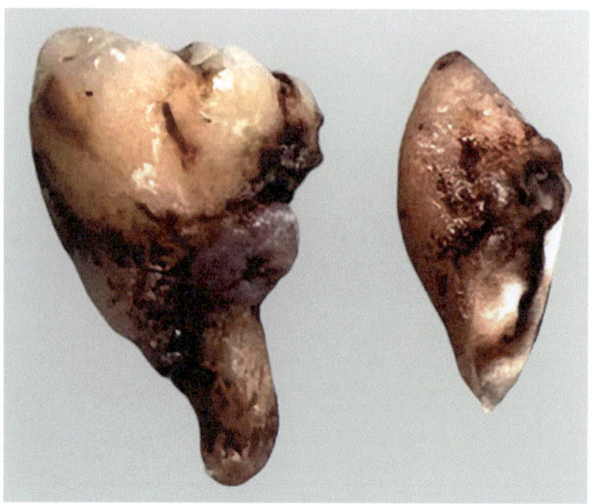

Fig. 7.17 Tooth

Acknowledgments The author gratefully acknowledges William P. Daley, MD, and Ritica Chaudhary, MD, for their contribution to this chapter.

Quiz Questions

1. If a gross identification only specimen contains writing on it, which of the following is the correct procedure?
    a. Dictate "the specimen contains writing on it"
    b. Dictate the exact writing that is on the specimen using quotes
    c. Submit representative sections of the specimen
    d. Ignore the writing altogether
2. Which of the following is not appropriate for a gross examination only specimen?
    a. Chemo port from a 65-year-old male
    b. A single gallstone
    c. A rib was removed to access a certain part of the lung
    d. Fallopian tubes for sterilization
3. What is the purpose of a gross examination specimen?
    a. To give the grossing person more work
    b. To document how much time it took for the surgeon to remove the specimen
    c. To document a pattern of removed specimens
    d. To document what type of specimen the surgeon removed from the patient

Answer Key

1. B—Dictate the exact writing that is on the specimen using quotes.

    Explanation- Serial numbers and other inscriptions are ways to identify the specimen. The serial number on an implant is directly associated with that specific patient. Dictating exactly what is written on the specimen documents the removal of the appropriate item.
2. D—Fallopian tubes for sterilization.

    Explanation: All gross only specimen needs to be approved by the pathologists first, but in this case, fallopian tubes are to be analyzed microscopically to ensure that the specimen is indeed fallopian tube, and that the tube has been transected, so "D" is the correct option. All other options do not require microscopic examination for identification.
3. D—To document what type of specimen the surgeon removed from the patient.

    Explanation: A complete gross description documenting the specimen allows secondary confirmation that the specimen matches that of the surgical record. As an example, what if four ingested magnets appear on imaging, but only three magnets are received in the gross room? The grossing individual dictates that three magnets are present, indicating a discrepancy that must be resolved.

Reference

1. FirstPath. 2009–2023. [Online]. Available: https://www.firstpathlab.com/cpt-codes/. Accessed Aug 2023.

Grossing of Gynecologic and Perinatal Specimens

8

Contents

Table 8.1 CPT codes

Abortion, induced	88304
Abortion, spontaneous/missed	88305
Cervix, biopsy	88305
Cervix, conization	88307
Endocervix, biopsy	88305
Endometrium, curettings/biopsy	88305
Fallopian tube, biopsy	88305
Fallopian tube, ectopic pregnancy	88305
Fallopian tube, sterilization	88302
Fetus w/dissection	88309
Ovary, biopsy/wedge resection	88305
Ovary, w/or w/o tube, non-neoplastic	88305
Ovary, w/or w/o tubes, neoplastic	88307
Placenta, 1st/second trimester	88305
Placenta, third trimester	88307
Polyp, cervical/endometrial	88305
Uterus, w/or w/o tubes and ovaries, neoplastic	88309
Uterus, w/or w/o tubes and ovaries, other than tumor or prolapse	88307
Uterus, w/or w/o tubes and ovaries, prolapse	88305
Vagina, biopsy	88305
Vaginal mucosa, incidental	88302
Vulva, total/subtotal resection	88309
Vulva/labia biopsy	88305

Gynecologic and perinatal specimens are common specimens seen in all pathology labs. Solid knowledge of the anatomy is required for the grossing person to maintain proper grossing techniques and organization of these complex specimens. Assess the CPT codes in Table 8.1 for basic knowledge of the charge codes [1].

8.1 Vaginal Biopsy: Level IV CPT 88305

The purpose of a vulvar or vaginal/cervical biopsy is to sample and microscopically examine the specimen due to complaints of itching, redness, rash, and potential cancerous cells.

Step 1: Describe the tissue, count the number of fragments, and give a three-dimensional mea-

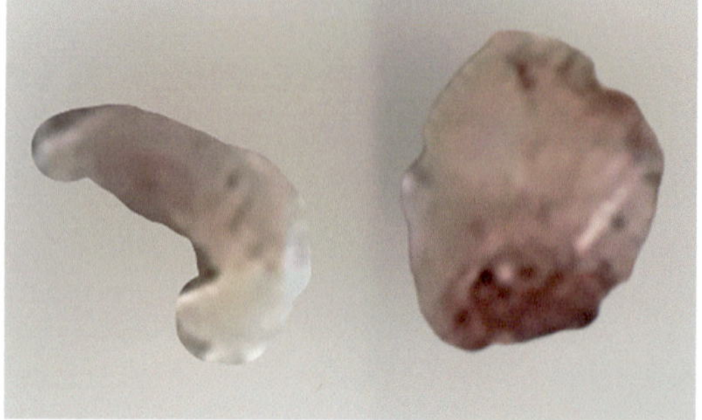

Fig. 8.1 Cervical biopsies

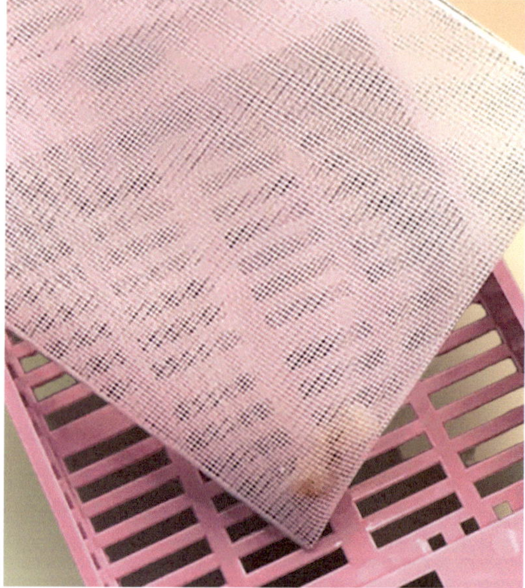

Fig. 8.2 Cervical biopsies in a biopsy bag

surement. If the number of fragments is greater than 3, the specimen can be dictated as an aggregate (Fig. 8.1).

Step 2: State how the biopsy is submitted in cassettes (Fig. 8.2).

Example Dictation

Specimen A is received in formalin labeled with patient's name, medical record number, "vaginal bx" and consists of 2 tan-pink, hemorrhagic tissue fragments ($0.7 \times 0.4 \times 0.4$ cm) which are submitted in toto in a biopsy bag in A 1.

8.2   Vulvar Excision: Level V CPT 88309

The purpose of a vulvar excision is to remove the area of abnormal or malignant cells. This is typically diagnosed on biopsy and then the excision is performed, if necessary.

Cancer Protocol Breakdown Relative to Grossing Vulva Specimens.

Procedure: Excision of the vulva can produce a range of specimens from a small ellipse of skin to a total vulvectomy. Identify what type of excision is present.

Tumor focality: On the skin surface, identify if the lesion is unifocal or multifocal.

Tumor site: For larger excision that may include bilateral vulva and/or clitoris, identify at which anatomical sites the lesion is located.

Tumor size: Measure the lesion in three dimensions. Also, measure how close the lesion comes from all surrounding skin margins, oriented or unoriented.

Depth of tumor invasion: Once the specimen is sliced, identify and measure the greatest depth of tumor invasion. Also, measure how close the tumor comes from the deep margin. [2].

Step 1: Orient the excision and measure in three dimensions. In this example, the stitch is at the 12 o'clock tip (Fig. 8.3).

Step 2: Identify the lesion and measure in three dimensions.

Step 3: Measure the lesion to the 12 o'clock tip, 3 o'clock margin, 6 o'clock tip, and 9 o'clock margin.

Step 4: All margins must be inked (Fig. 8.4). In the above photo, the ink code is as follows:

    Orange: 3 o'clock margin

    Blue: 9 o'clock margin

    Black: deep margin

Step 5: Serially section the excision along the long axis, keeping the specimen slices in order (Fig. 8.5).

Step 6: Measure the greatest depth of invasion and how close the lesion comes to the deep margin.

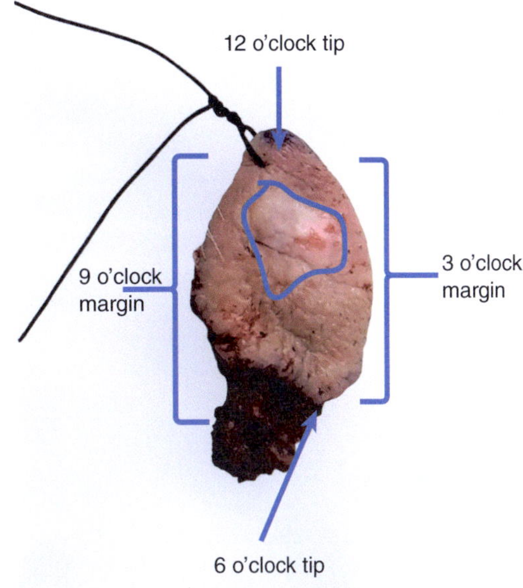

Fig. 8.3 Vulvar excision with orientation

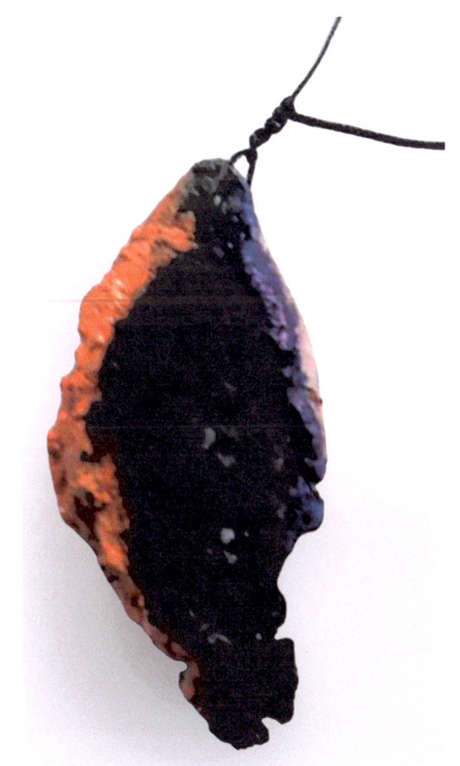

Fig. 8.4 Vulvar excision with ink for orientation

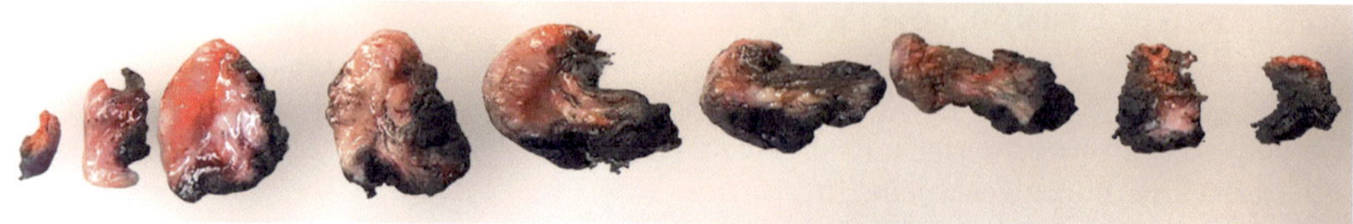

Fig. 8.5 Vulvar excision, serially sectioned

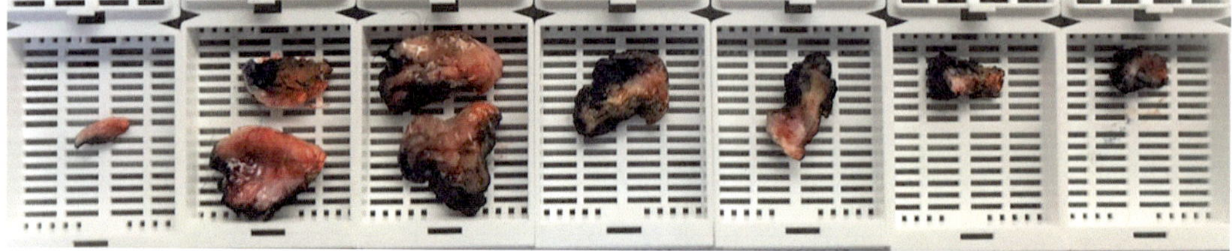

Fig. 8.6 Vulva, cassette submission

Step 7: Submit the specimen entirely from the 12 o'clock tip to the 6 o'clock tip. Always place the oriented tips in a cassette alone. The remainder of the body of the excision can have multiple sections per cassette as long as the slices stay in order (Fig. 8.6).

Example Dictation

Specimen A is received in formalin labeled with patient's name, medical record number, "left vulvar lesion" and consists of a tan ellipse of skin (3.6 × 2.1 × 0.9 cm) with a stitch designating the 12 o'clock tip. The skin surface contains a tan-white, slightly ulcerated lesion (1.0 × 0.7 cm) which comes within 0.4 cm of the 12 o'clock tip, 1.4 cm from the 6 o'clock tip, 0.3 cm from the 3 o'clock margin, and 0.2 cm from the 9 o'clock margin. The specimen is serially sectioned to reveal tan cut surfaces with the greatest depth of invasion of approximately 0.3 cm, coming within 1.1 cm of the underlying deep margin.

Ink code:

    Orange: 3 o'clock margin

    Blue: 9 o'clock margin

    Black: deep margin

Section code:

    A 1: 12 o'clock tip, en face

A 2-A 6: Body of the specimen, entirely from 12-6 o'clock

A 7: 6 o'clock tip, en face

8.3 Cervical Polyp: Level IV CPT 88305

The purpose of a cervical polypectomy is to remove and microscopically examine the polyp for malignancy. With any polyp, it is best to ink the resection margin where the clinician cut to remove the specimen. This way if the polyp is cancerous, then the final report can state if the malignancy is present at the true margin.

Step 1: Measure the specimen in three dimensions and grossly identify the stalk resection margin.

Step 2: Ink resection margin. The polyp can be bisected if it is too large to fit in the cassette (see blue dotted line) (Fig. 8.7).

Step 3: Dictate how the specimen is submitted in cassettes.

Example Dictation

Specimen A is received in formalin labeled with the patient's name, medical record number, "polyp" and consists of an intact, tan-pink polyp (1.9 × 0.8 × 0.6 cm). The resection margin is inked blue, and the specimen is submitted in toto in A1.

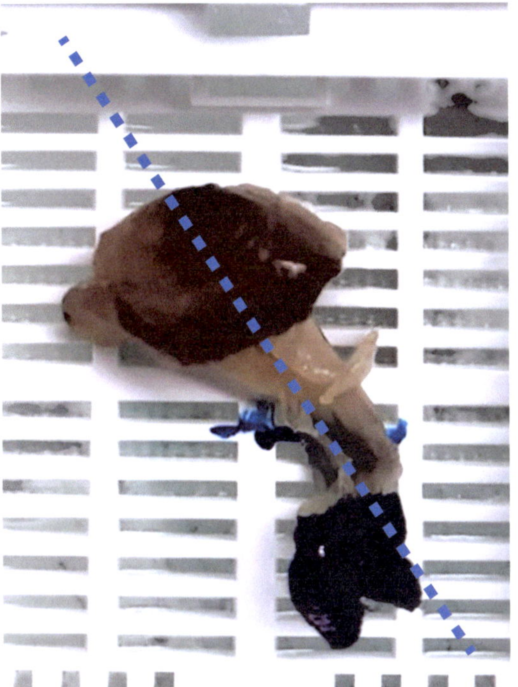

Fig. 8.7 Cervical polyp with inked margin

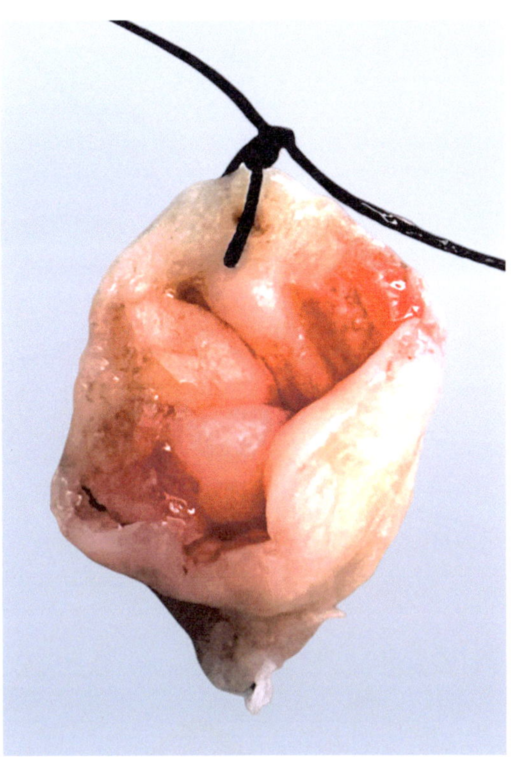

Fig. 8.8 Cervix oriented

8.4   Cervical Excision: Level V CPT 88307

The purpose of a cervical excision is to remove the area of abnormal or malignant cells of the cervical mucosa which then allows healthy cells to regrow.

Cancer Protocol Breakdown Relative to Grossing Cervix.

Procedure: Cervix excisions are normally performed by two slightly different methods: conization and LEEP (loop electrosurgical excision procedure). Conization is typically an inpatient procedure where a blade is used to remove a small cone-shaped portion of the cervix. LEEP procedure utilizes an electrified wire to excise abnormal tissue in the cervix and cervical stroma. It is possible to have a conization biopsy and then LEEP to remove additional tissue.

Tumor site: A cervical specimen is often oriented in a clock fashion. The cancer protocol report requires cancer/dysplasia to be identified per quadrant of the clock (i.e., 12-3 o'clock quad-rant, 3-6 o'clock quadrant, 6-9 o'clock quadrant, and 9-12 o'clock quadrant).

Tumor size: Often it is difficult to grossly identify a lesion on the cervical mucosa. However, grossly or microscopically, the greatest dimension of tumor size is needed. [2].

Step 1: Describe the specimen and dictate a three-dimensional measurement (Fig. 8.8).

Step 2: Ink the edge of the endocervical canal margin (seen in orange). Ink the remaining stromal margin (seen in blue) (Fig. 8.9).

Step 3: Divide the cervix into quadrants using the os as the center point (Fig. 8.10a). Radially section each quadrant like a pie as seen by the blue lines in Fig. 8.10b.

Step 4: Each quadrant can be submitted in one or more cassette, on edge (Fig. 8.11).

Cervical Cone, Unoriented:

Specimen A is received in formalin labeled with patient's name, medical record number, "cer-

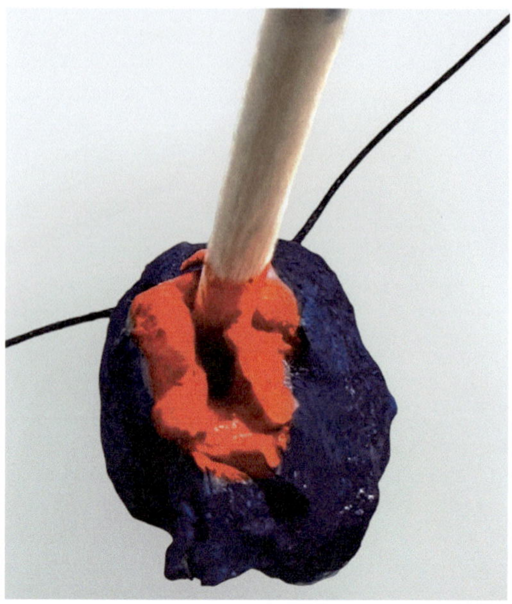

Fig. 8.9 Cervix with inked margins

vix" and consists of an intact, unoriented cervical cone (2.4 × 1.9 × 0.9 cm) with tan-pink ectocervical mucosa on the one side. A flat, tan-white lesion (0.4 × 0.3 cm) is identified. The specimen is radially sectioned to reveal tan-brown cut surfaces. One unoriented quadrant is submitted, per cassette, in A1-A4 (A1-quadrant with the lesion).

Ink code

>Orange: endocervical canal margin
>Blue: stroma

Cervical cone, oriented:

Specimen A is received in formalin labeled with patient's name, medical record number, "cervix" and consists of an intact cervical cone (2.4 × 1.9 × 0.9 cm) with a stitch designating 12 o'clock. A flat, tan-white lesion (0.4 × 0.3 cm) is

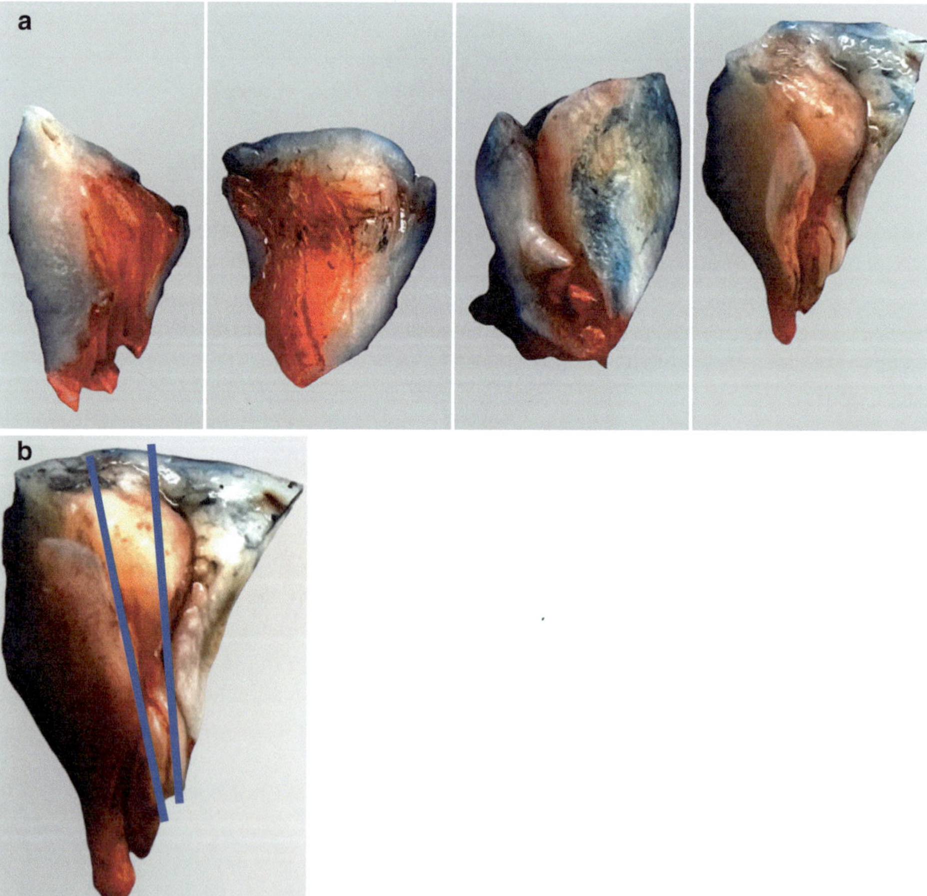

Fig. 8.10 (**a**) Quadrants of cervix. (**b**) Cervix, radial section

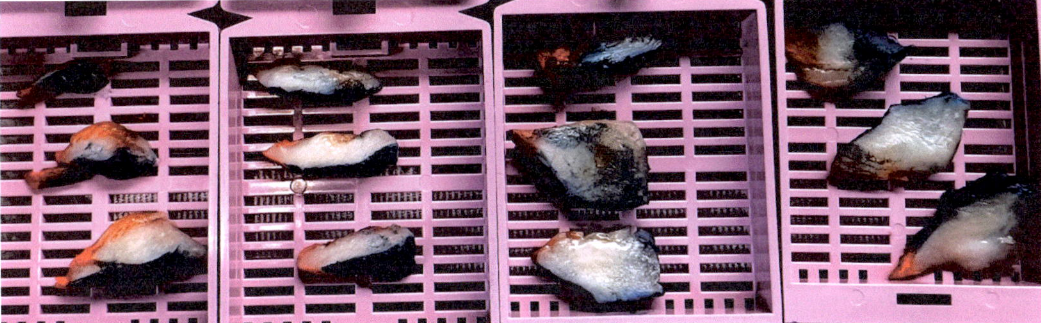

Fig. 8.11   Cervix cassette submission

identified on the 12-3 o'clock quadrant. There is tan-pink ectocervical mucosa on one side. The specimen is radially sectioned to reveal tan-brown cut surfaces.

Ink code
     Orange: endocervical canal margin
     Blue: stroma
Section code
     A1: Cervix 12-3 o'clock
     A2: Cervix 3-6 o'clock
     A3: Cervix 6-9 o'clock
     A4: Cervix 9-12 o'clock

8.5   Endometrial Biopsy: Level IV CPT 88305

The purpose of an endometrial biopsy is to sample and microscopically examine a small amount of the endometrial lining to look for cancer, cellular irregularities, and reasons for abnormal bleeding. These biopsies are an aggregate of tissue and blood.

Step 1: Place the entire specimen in a biopsy bag or divide the specimen into multiple cassettes, if it is a large aggregate of tissue (Fig. 8.12).
Step 2: Describe the tissue and give a three-dimensional measurement.
Step 3: State how the biopsy is submitted in cassettes.

Example Dictation
Specimen A is received in formalin labeled with patient's name, medical record number, "endo-

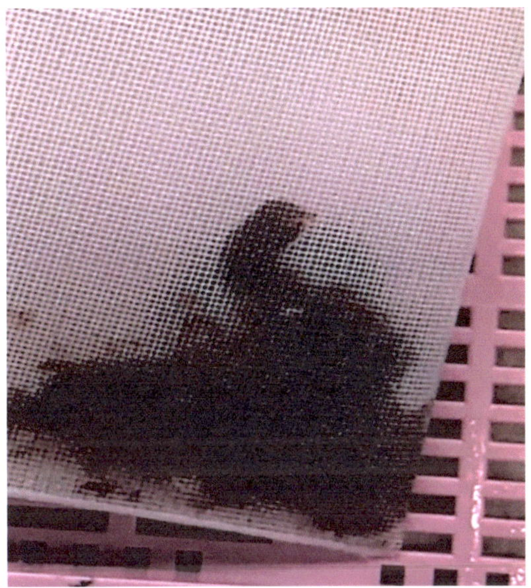

Fig. 8.12   Endometrial biopsy

metrial biopsy" and consists of an aggregate of red-brown, hemorrhagic tissue (1.6 × 1.5 × 0.4 cm) which is submitted in toto in a biopsy bag in A1.

8.6   Uterus, Benign: Prolapse Level IV CPT 88305, Other than Prolapse Level V CPT 88307

The purpose of a benign hysterectomy is to remove the uterus for pain and excessive bleeding or prolapse. One of the primary reasons a hysterectomy is performed is due to fibroids.

Fibroid growth can cause pain and excessive bleeding. Adequate sampling of the fibroids is necessary to assess for necrosis, calcification, or the presence of a leiomyosarcoma.

Patents who have the BRCA1 or BRCA2 gene will often elect to have a hysterectomy prophylactically. The BRCA genes produce proteins that assist in the repair of damaged DNA. People who have inherited the gene have a dramatically increased risk of numerous cancers, especially breast and ovarian cancers. Removing the uterus and ednexa will decrease the risk of those cancers in the future. [3].

A hysterectomy specimen consists of many anatomical structures. Figure 8.13 illustrates the anatomic knowledge essential to properly grossing a hysterectomy.

Step 1: Orient the uterus. There are two ways to orient the uterus. The posterior peritoneal reflection extends more inferiorly toward the cervix than the anterior peritoneal reflection (Fig. 8.14a, b). Also, the fallopian tubes are anterior to the ovaries, and the round ligament is anterior to both the tubes and ovaries (Fig. 8.14c).

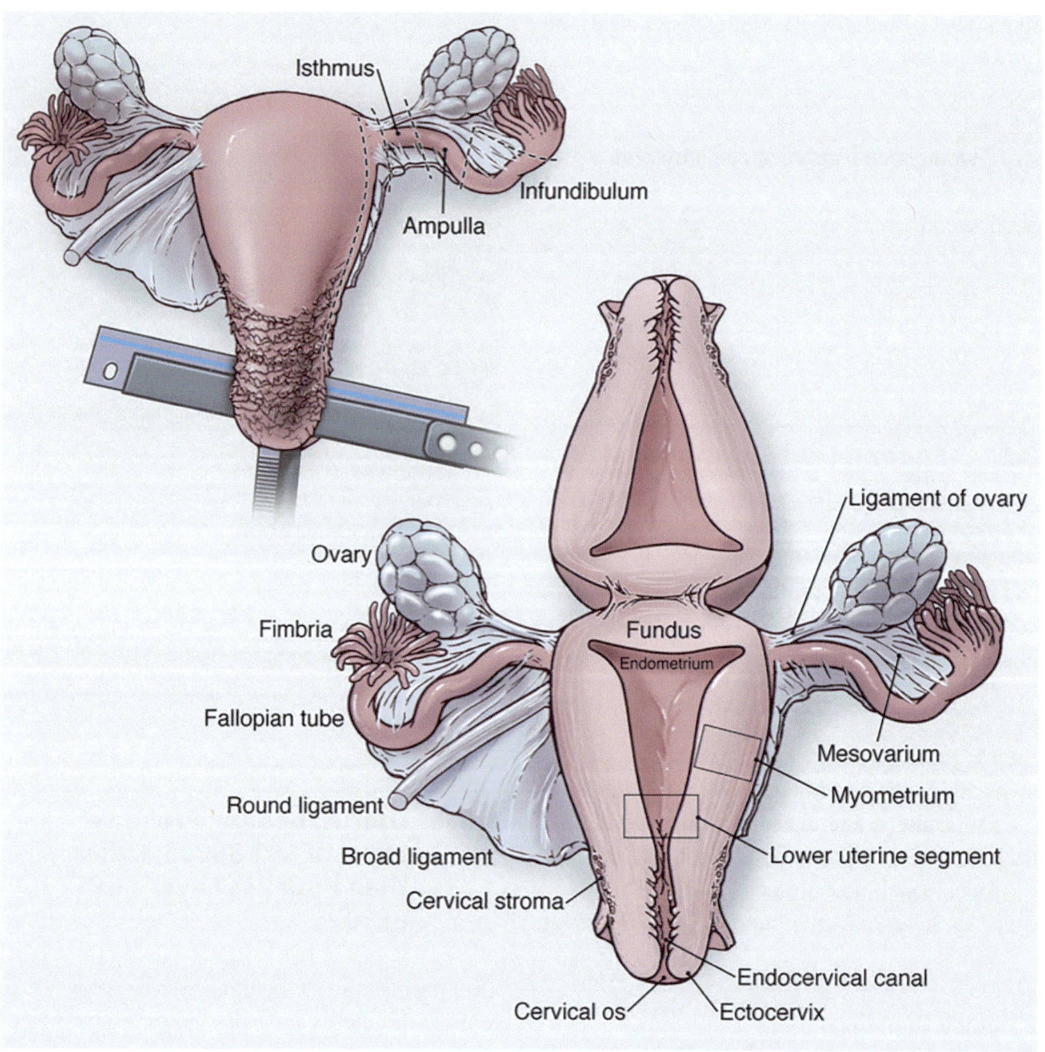

Fig. 8.13 Anatomy for grossing a uterus

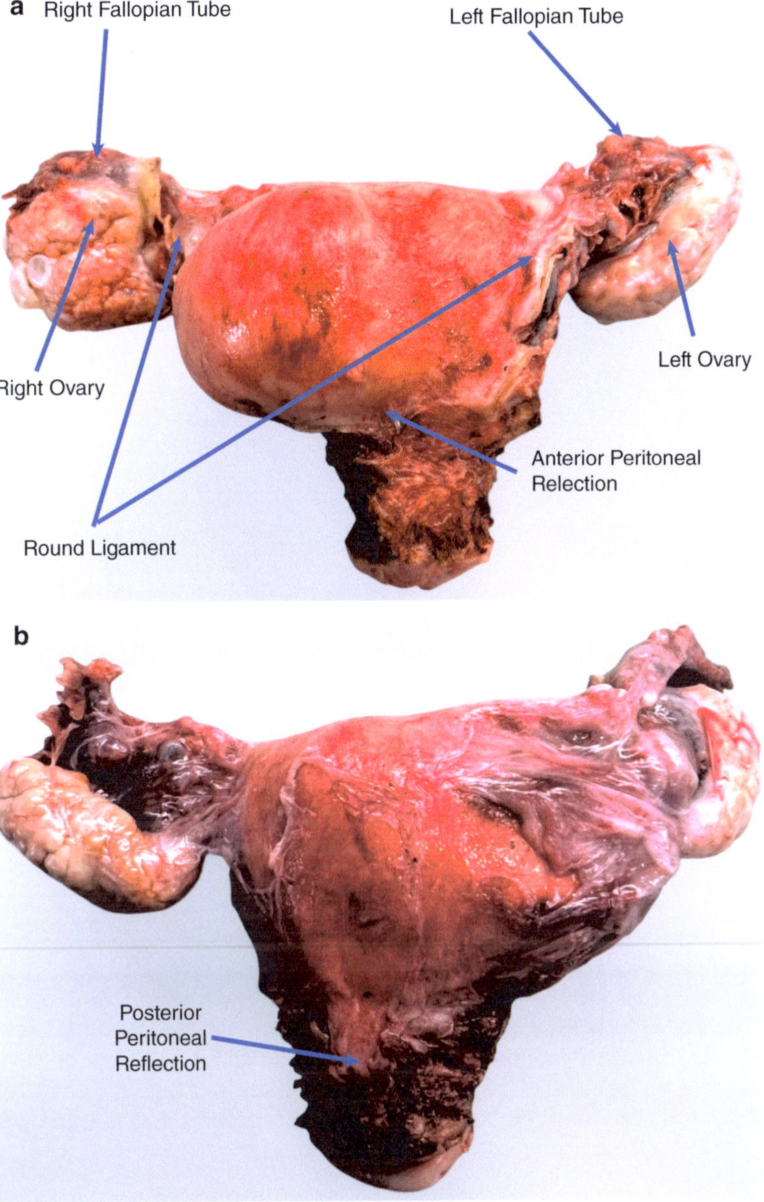

Fig. 8.14 (**a**) Anterior uterus with bilateral adnexa. (**b**) Posterior uterus with bilateral adnexa. (**c**) Adnexa orientation

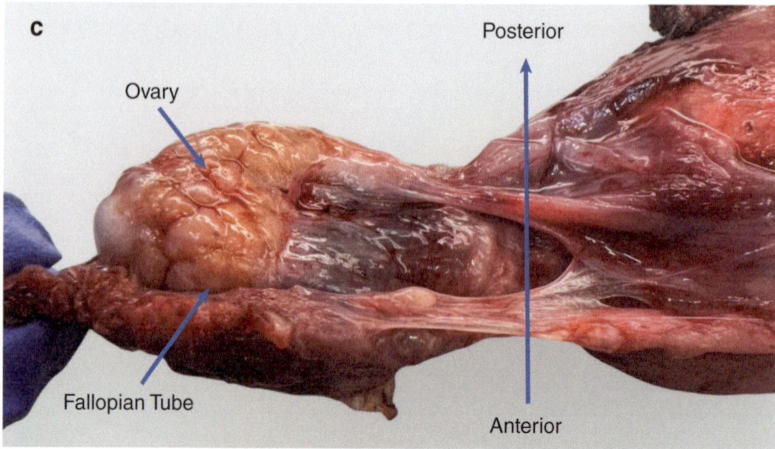

Fig. 8.14 (continued)

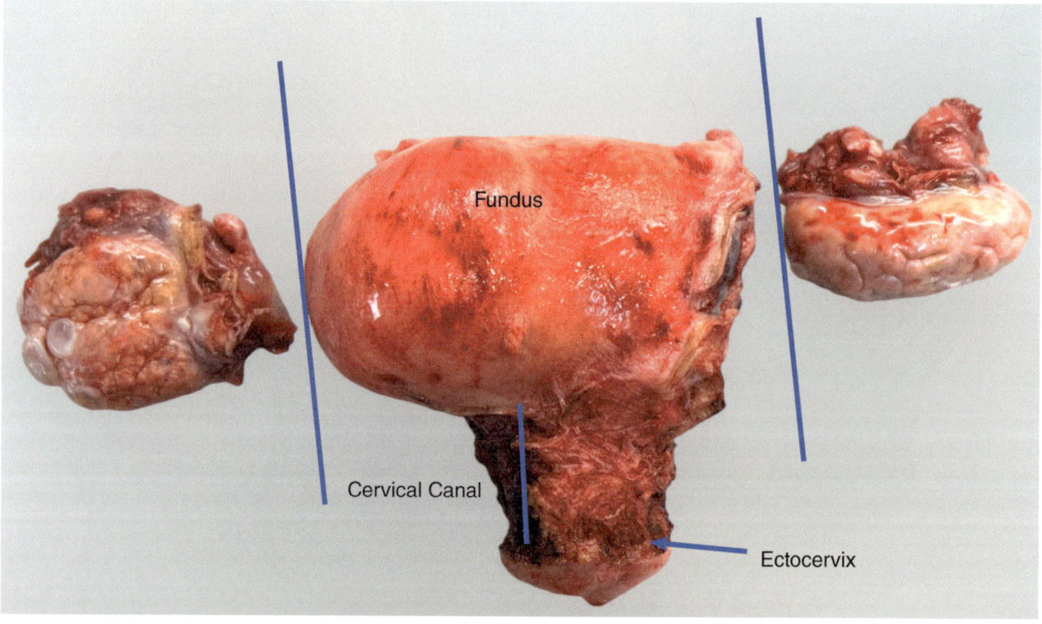

Fig. 8.15 Uterus anatomic locations

Step 2: Dictate the description of the uterus including all anatomic structures that are present.

Step 3: Measure the overall size of the uterus and individually measure the additional structures (cervix, fallopian tubes, ovaries, etc.) (Fig. 8.15).

Step 4: Remove the fallopian tubes and ovaries. Keep the adnexa oriented once removed. Then weigh the uterus (Fig. 8.15).

Step 5: To bivalve the uterus, place large forceps into the cervical os and center the blade between the forceps. Use the forceps as a guide to slice the uterus into anterior and posterior halves. With the forceps in the uterus, it is more likely to slice the cervical canal and endometrial cavity perfectly into anterior and posterior halves (Fig. 8.16).

Step 6: Measure the length of the endocervical canal and the thickness of the myometrium.

The endometrial cavity is then measured in three dimensions with the third dimension being the thickness of the endometrial tissue (Fig. 8.17).

Step 7: Amputate the cervix and then take a longitudinal section of the ectocervix with the

endocervical canal of both the anterior and posterior halves (Fig. 8.18).

Step 8: Serially section the remainder of the uterus looking for leiomyomas or other pathology within the endometrium or myometrium (Fig. 8.19).

Step 9: Two representative sections of anterior and two representative sections of posterior endomyometrium are sufficient. In this case, the endometrium is benign, so the serosal aspect can be removed and two sections of endometrium can be submitted in one cassette (see blue dotted line in Fig. 8.20a). Submit representative sections of the white nodules, if present (Fig. 8.20b).

Step 10: Serially section the fallopian tubes (Fig. 8.21a) and ovaries (Fig. 8.21b). Dictate the gross appearance of each. Representative sections of each can be submitted.

Step 11: Sections submitted are anterior and posterior ectocervix with endocervical canal, 2 sections of each anterior and posterior endomyometrium, and bilateral adnexa (Fig. 8.22).

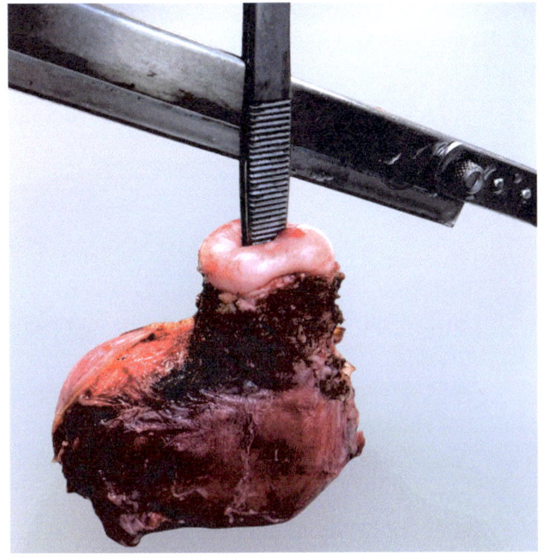

Fig. 8.16 Bivalving the uterus

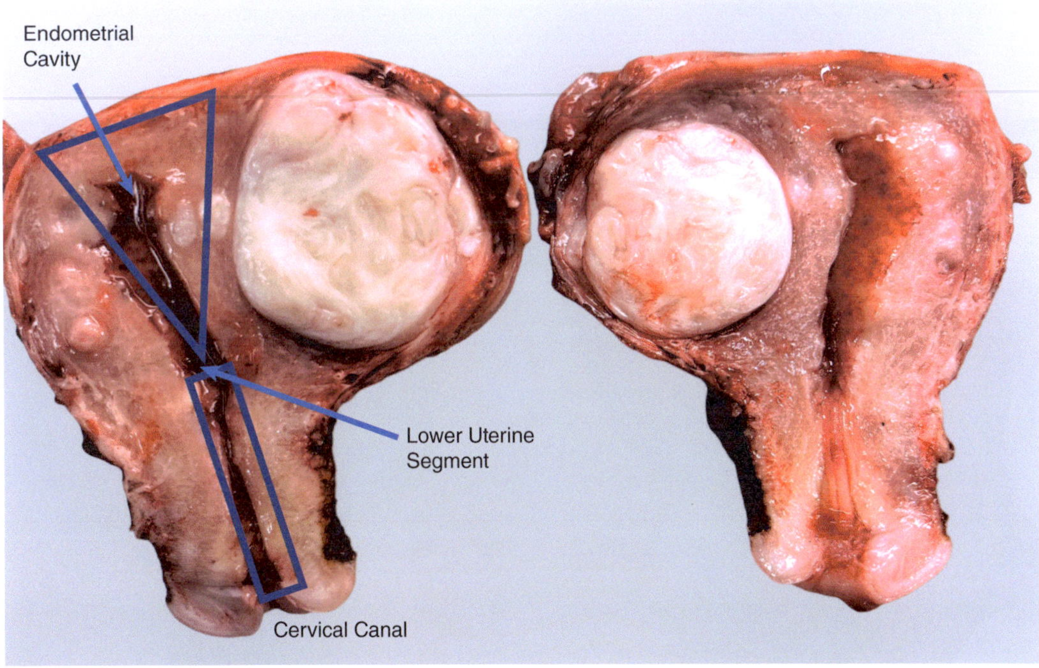

Fig. 8.17 Bivalved uterus

Example Dictation

Specimen A is received in formalin labeled with patient's name, medical record number, "uterus, cervix, bilateral fallopian tubes" and consists of a tan uterus (9.9 × 6.5 × 6.2 cm, 154 g) with attached bilateral fimbriated fallopian tubes (right: 7.4 × 0.6 × 0.5 cm, left: 6.7 × 0.7 × 0.6 cm). The uterine fundus serosal surface is tan-pink and smooth. The ectocervix (3.5 × 3.2 cm) is tan-pink with an eccentrically placed slit-like os (0.9 cm in diameter). The uterus is bivalved to reveal an endocervical canal (4.2 cm in length) which is slightly dilated with herringbone architecture. There are multiple smooth-walled cysts ranging from 0.1 to 0.4 cm present within the cervical stroma, filled with gelatinous material. The endometrial cavity (3.2 × 2.9 × 0.3 cm thick) is scantly hemorrhagic. The myometrium, ranging from 1.1 to 2.4 cm in thickness, is tan-pink and slightly trabeculated on the posterior aspect. The bilateral fallopian tubes are serially sectioned to reveal tan lumens.

Section code

A 1: Anterior ectocervix with endocervical canal.

A 2: Anterior endomyometrium, representative.

A 3: Posterior ectocervix with endocervical canal.

A 4: Posterior endomyometrium, representative.

A 5: Right fallopian tube, representative.

A 6: Left fallopian tube, representative.

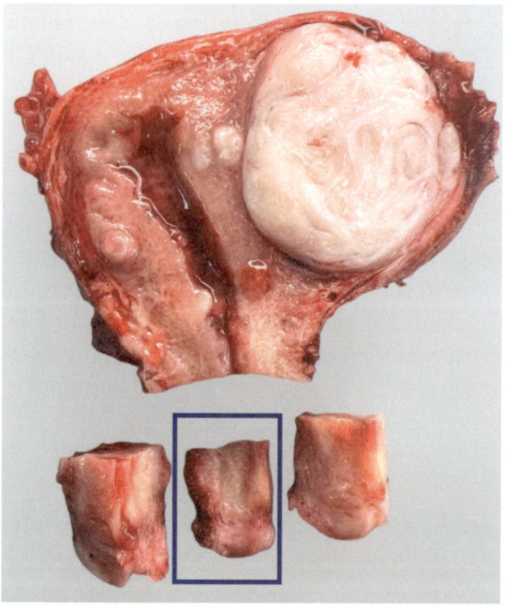

Fig. 8.18 Uterus, cervix sections

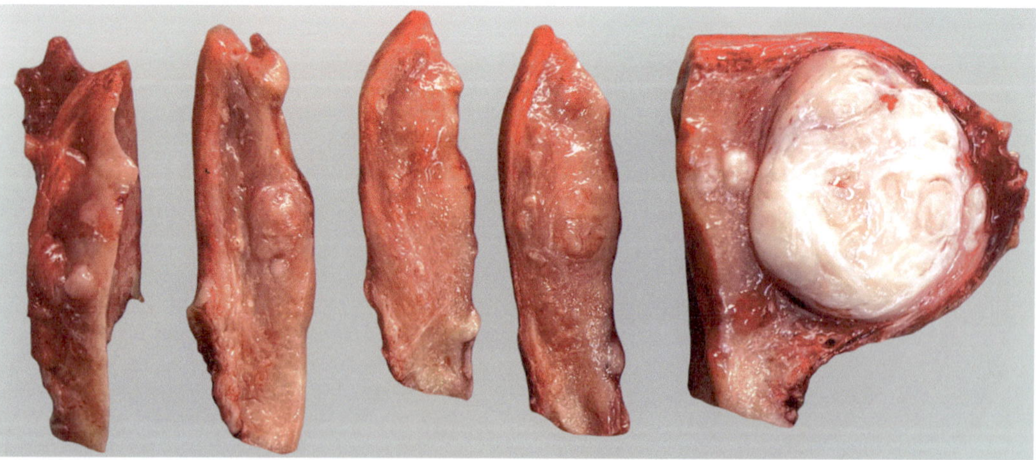

Fig. 8.19 Uterus, serial sections of the uterus

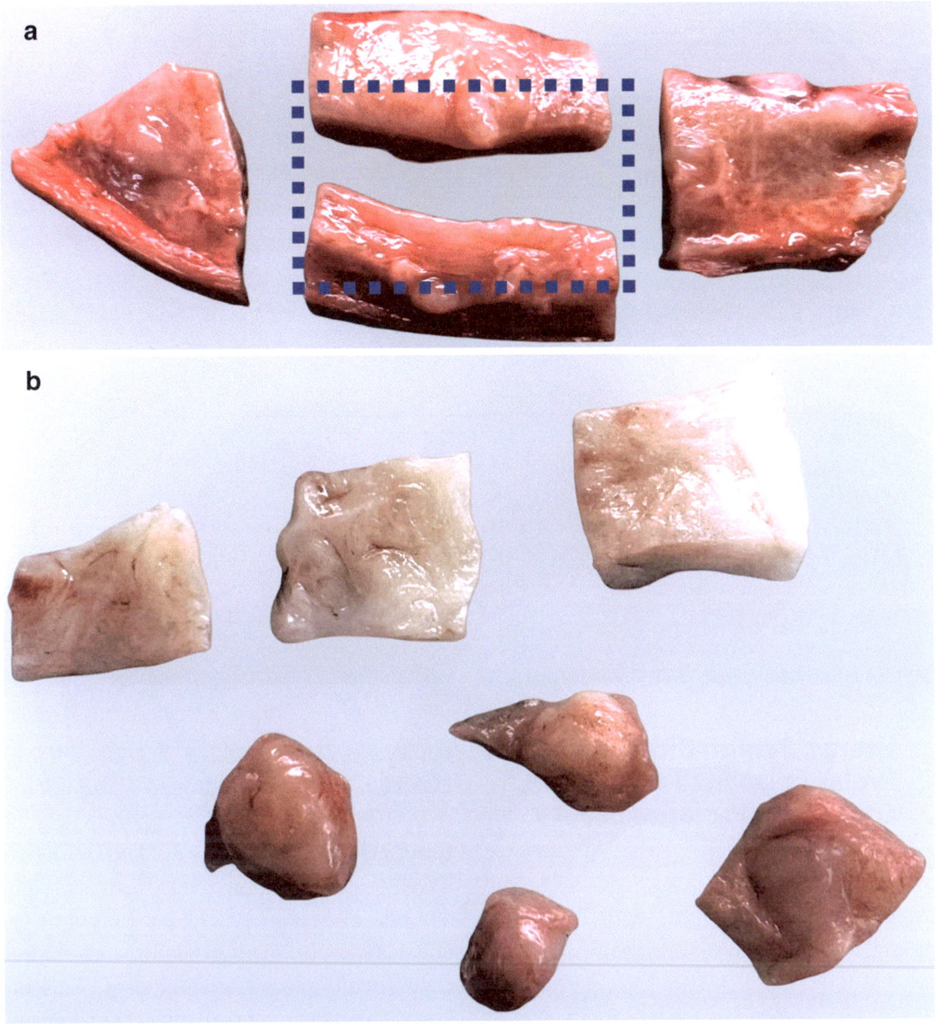

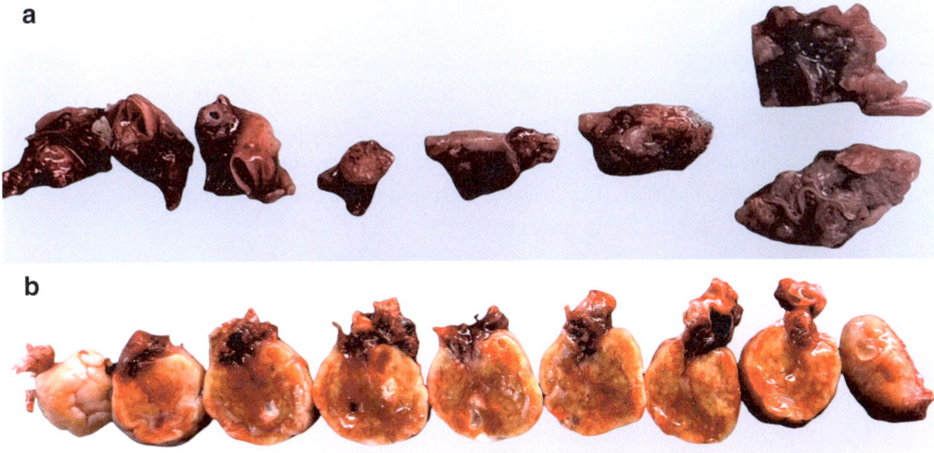

Fig. 8.20 (**a**) Uterus, endometrium sections. (**b**) Uterus, nodule sections

Fig. 8.21 (**a**) Fallopian tube serially sectioned. (**b**) Ovary serially sectioned

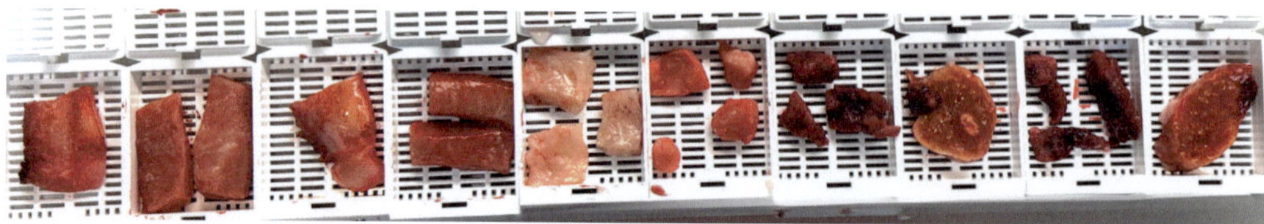

Fig. 8.22 Uterus, cassette submission

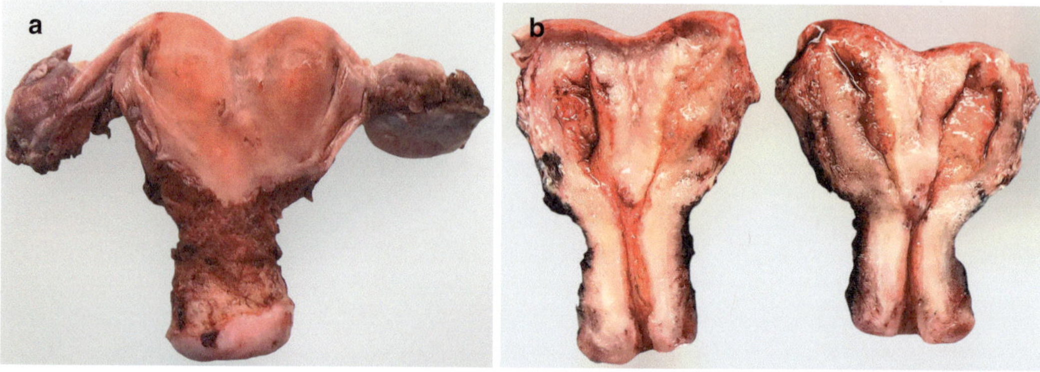

Fig. 8.23 (**a**) Bicornuate uterus. (**b**) Bicornuate uterus, bivalved

8.7 Uterus, Benign Bicornuate: Prolapse Level IV CPT 88305, Other than Prolapse Level V CPT 88307

A bicornuate uterus is a uterus with 2 separate endometrial cavities and/or 2 separate cervical canals.

Step 1: If the uterus is benign, all standard sections of a benign uterus are submitted (Fig. 8.23a). However, sections of the right endometrial cavity and sections of the left endometrial cavity will be submitted separately. The septal division also needs to be identified. In this photo, the septum that divides the right and left endometrial cavities extends down to the lower uterine segment (Fig. 8.23b).

Step 2: See benign uterus for in-depth grossing instructions.

Example Dictation

Specimen A is received in formalin labeled with patient's name, medical record number, "uterus, cervix, bilateral fallopian tubes" and consists of a tan uterus (15.6 × 7.2 × 5.7 cm, 194 g) with attached right fimbriated fallopian tube (6.2 × 0.6 × 0.5 cm) and a separate detached left fimbriated fallopian tube (3.2 × 0.6 × 0.6 cm). The uterine fundus serosal surface is tan-pink and smooth. The ectocervix (3.2 × 3.0 cm) is granular and markedly hemorrhagic surrounding the eccentrically placed, slit-like os (0.9 cm in diameter). The uterus is bivalved to reveal an endocervical canal (3.8 cm in length) with herringbone architecture. The bicornuate endometrial cavities (right cavity: 2.2 × 1.4 × 0.1 cm thick, left cavity: 2.4 × 1.5 × 0.1 cm thick) are scantly hemorrhagic and separated by a 1.6 cm septum. The myometrium, ranging from 0.9 to 1.4 cm, is tan-pink with no identifiable tan-white whorled nodules. The bilateral fallopian tubes are serially sectioned to reveal tan lumens.

Section code

A 1: Anterior ectocervix with endocervical canal.

A 2: Posterior ectocervix with endocervical canal.

A 3: Anterior-right endomyometrium, representative.

A 4: Anterior-left endomyometrium, representative.

A 5: Posterior-right endomyometrium, representative.

A 6: Posterior-left endomyometrium, representative.

A 8: Right fallopian tube, representative.

A 9: Left fallopian tube, representative.

8.8 Uterus, Cervical Dysplasia, and Cervical Cancer: Level VI CPT 88309

The purpose of a total hysterectomy for cervical cancer or cervical dysplasia is to remove the cancerous area of the cervix for staging and treatment. The cervix is typically removed with the uterus to assess invasion of cervical cancer into the cervical stroma and uterus. It is not uncommon for the uterus to be removed for other medical reasons, and cervical dysplasia is identified secondarily. However, the specimen is handled the same way for dysplasia or cancer. The cervix should be radially sectioned and submitted entirely.

Cancer Protocol Breakdown Relative to Grossing Uterus for Cervical Cancer.

Procedure: The resection for cervical cancer can come with additional attached anatomic structures. Typically, the cervix will be attached to the uterus. However bilateral salpingo-oophorectomy, single salpingo-oophorectomy, omentum, and peritoneal tissue can also be included. It is important to note what type of specimen is present and all the anatomical structures.

Tumor site: The cervix is oriented into quadrants (12-3 o'clock, 3-6 o'clock, 6-9 o'clock, and 9-12 o'clock). It is often difficult to grossly identify a lesion on the ectocervix but note any pale or white areas on the mucosa and state which quadrant it is located.

Tumor size: Measure the lesion on the cervical mucosa, if grossly identifiable. Once the cervix is opened, palpate and grossly assess the cervical stroma for invasion, and measure the depth, if applicable, and how close the lesion comes to the surrounding paracervical margin. [2].

Step 1: Dictate the gross appearance of the uterus (Fig. 8.24).

Step 2: Measure the uterus, remove fallopian tubes.

Step 3: Ink the anterior and posterior paracervical margins. Here the anterior half is inked blue, and the posterior half is inked black (Fig. 8.25a, b).

Step 4: Assess the ectocervix for lesions on the mucosa.

Step 5: Remove fallopian tubes and/or ovaries and weigh the uterus and cervix.

Step 6: Place forceps into the cervical os and use forceps as a guide to bivalve the uterus with the blade (Fig. 8.26).

Step 7: Measure and describe the endocervical canal, endometrial cavity, and the thickness of the myometrium (Fig. 8.27).

Step 8: Identify if there is a presence of invasion into the endocervical stroma from the cervical mucosa. No invasion is present in this specimen. However, invasion usually feels firmer than the remaining stroma.

Step 9: Amputate the cervix above the invasion into the cervical stroma (if possible) (Fig. 8.28).

Step 10: Divide the cervix into 4 quadrants in a clock-face fashion as seen in the photo. The cervix is oriented as anterior is 12 o'clock and posterior is 6 o'clock, making the left side 3 o'clock and the right side 9 o'clock (Fig. 8.29).

Step 11: Radially section each quadrant longitudinally around the cervical os, demonstrating

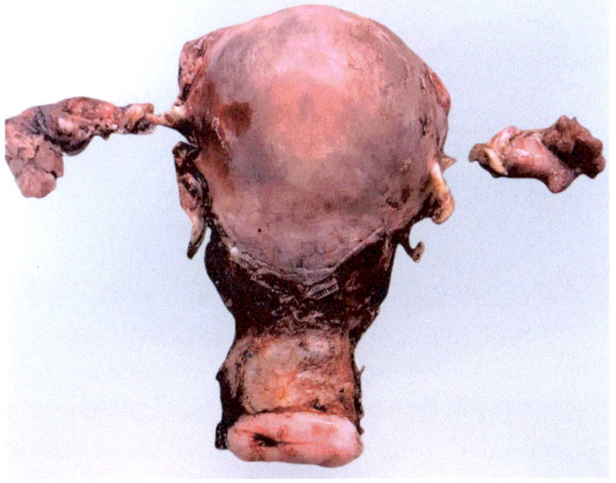

Fig. 8.24 Uterus

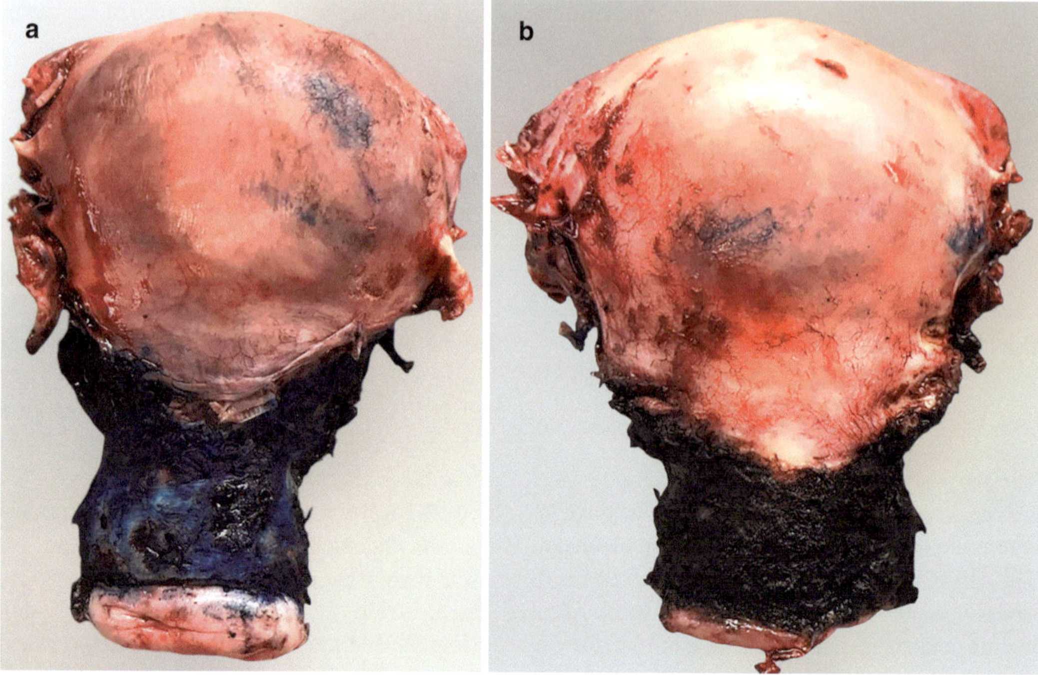

Fig. 8.25 (**a**) Anterior uterus with ink. (**b**) Posterior uterus with ink

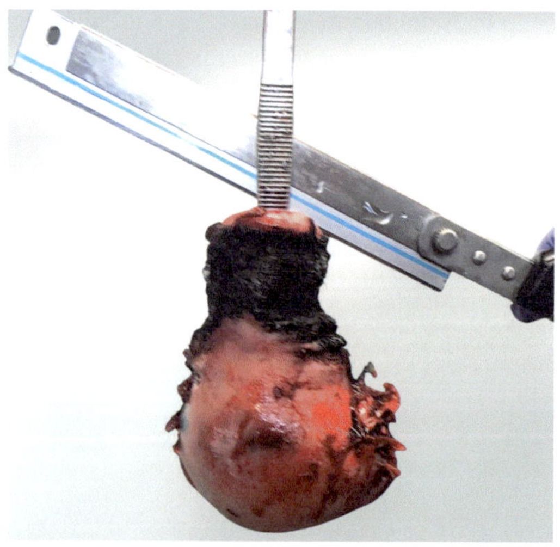

Fig. 8.26 Uterus, bivalve

the ectocervix, paracervical margin, and endocervical canal in each slice (Fig. 8.30).

Step 12: Anterior and posterior lower uterine segments (LUS) are taken perpendicularly and submitted (Fig. 8.31). Note: if the invasion grossly extends to the LUS, the cervix may need to be amputated above the LUS.

Step 13: Serially section the remainder of the endometrial cavity to assess for leiomyomas, polyps, or any lesions (Fig. 8.32).

Step 14: Two representative sections of the anterior and posterior endomyometrium are submitted. In this case, the endometrium is benign so the serosal aspect can be removed and two sections of endometrium can be submitted in one cassette (see blue dotted square) (Fig. 8.33).

Step 15: The fallopian tubes and ovaries (if present) are serially sectioned. Two cross sections of the tube, one half of the bisected fimbria, and one cross section of the ovary are submitted (Fig. 8.34).

Example Dictation

Specimen A is received in formalin labeled with patient's name, medical record number, "uterus, cervix, bilateral fallopian tubes" and consists of a tan uterus (8.6 × 6.8 × 4.7 cm, 124 g) with attached right fimbriated fallopian tube (4.2 × 0.6 × 0.6 cm) and a separate detached left fimbriated fallopian tube (3.6 × 0.8 × 0.7 cm). The uterine fundus serosal surface is tan-pink and

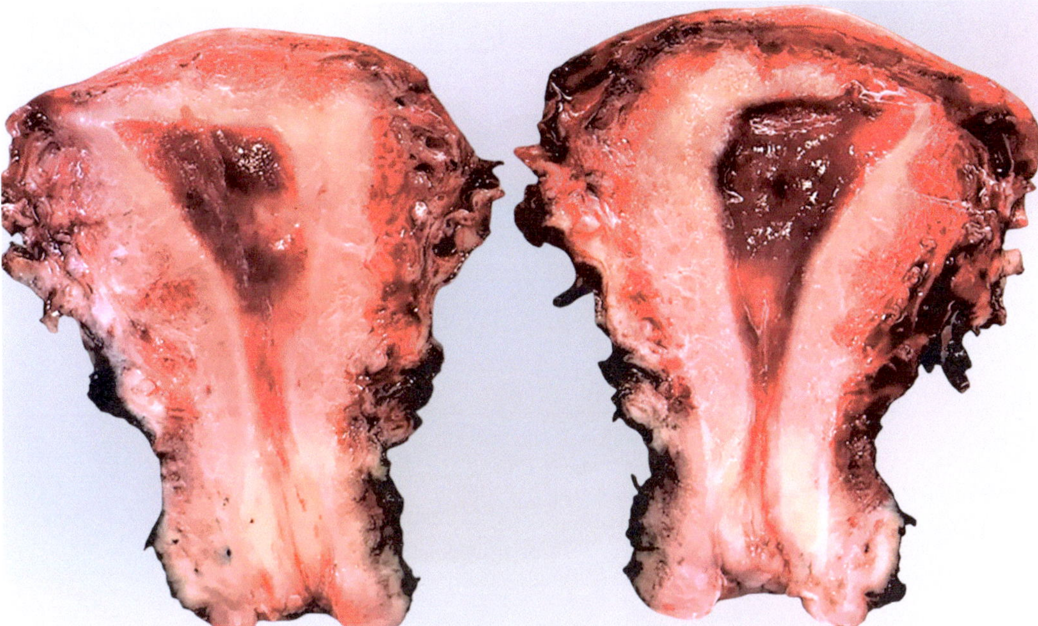

Fig. 8.27 Uterus, bivalved

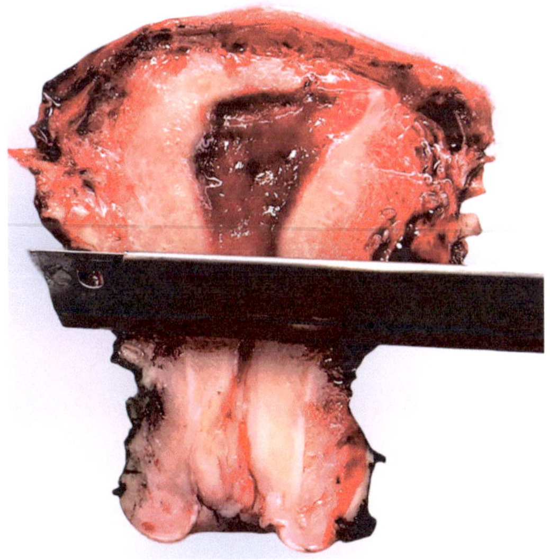

Fig. 8.28 Uterus, amputating the cervix

smooth. The ectocervix (3.1 × 3.0 cm) is granular and markedly hemorrhagic surrounding the eccentrically placed os (0.9 cm in diameter). The uterus is bivalved to reveal an endocervical canal (3.8 cm in length) with herringbone architecture and no grossly identifiable invasion into the cer-

vical stroma. The endometrial cavity (3.2 × 2.6 × 0.1 cm thick) is scantly hemorrhagic. The myometrium, ranging from 0.9 to 1.4 cm, is tan-pink with no identifiable tan-white whorled nodules. The bilateral fallopian tubes are serially sectioned to reveal tan lumens.

Ink code
    Blue: anterior
    Black: posterior
Section code:
    A 1-A 3: Cervix 12-3 o'clock
    A 4-A 6: Cervix 3-6 o'clock
    A 7-A 9: Cervix 6-9 o'clock
    A 10-A 12: Cervix 9-12 o'clock
    A 13: Lower uterine segment, anterior, perpendicular (coinciding with 12 o'clock).
    A 14: Lower uterine segment, posterior, perpendicular (coinciding with 6 o'clock)
    A 15: Anterior endomyometrium, representative
    A 16: Posterior endomyometrium, representative
    A 17: Right fallopian tube, representative
    A 18: Left fallopian tube, representative

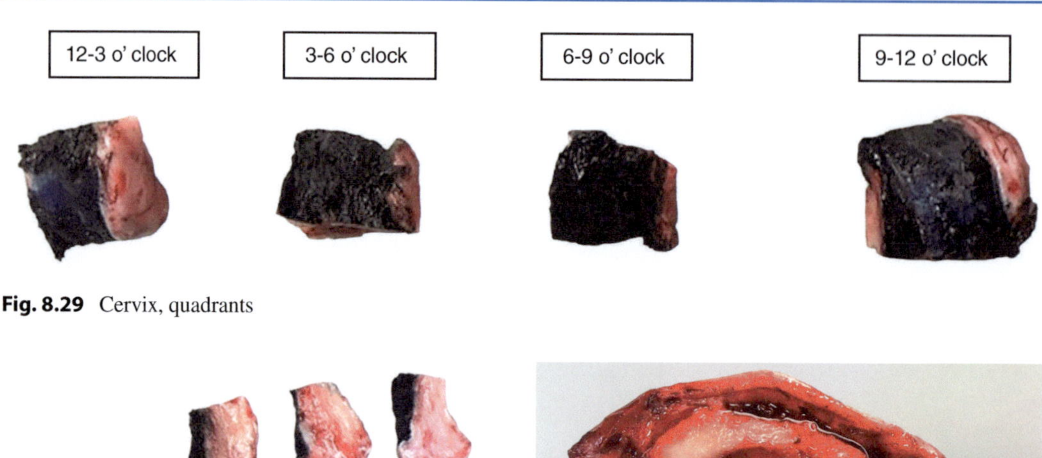

Fig. 8.29 Cervix, quadrants

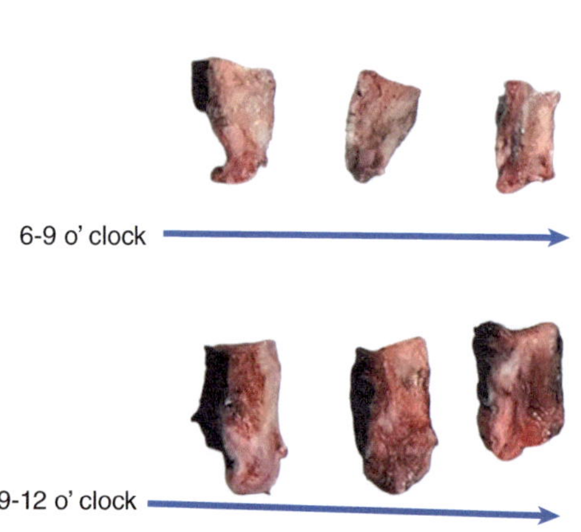

Fig. 8.30 Cervix quadrants, radially sectioned

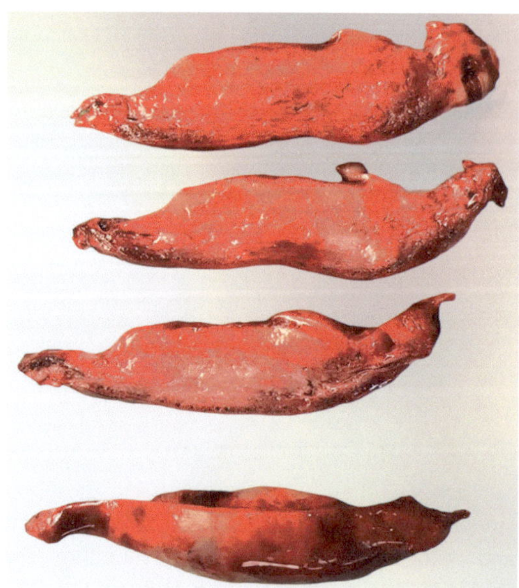

Fig. 8.31 Uterus, lower uterine segment

Fig. 8.32 Uterus, serially sectioned

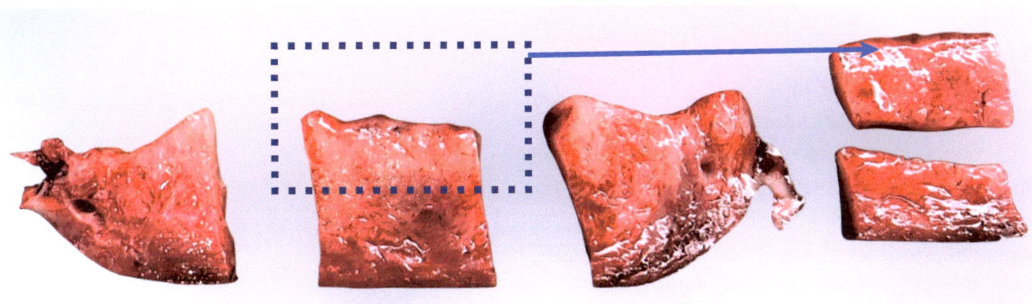

Fig. 8.33 Uterus, endomyometrial sections

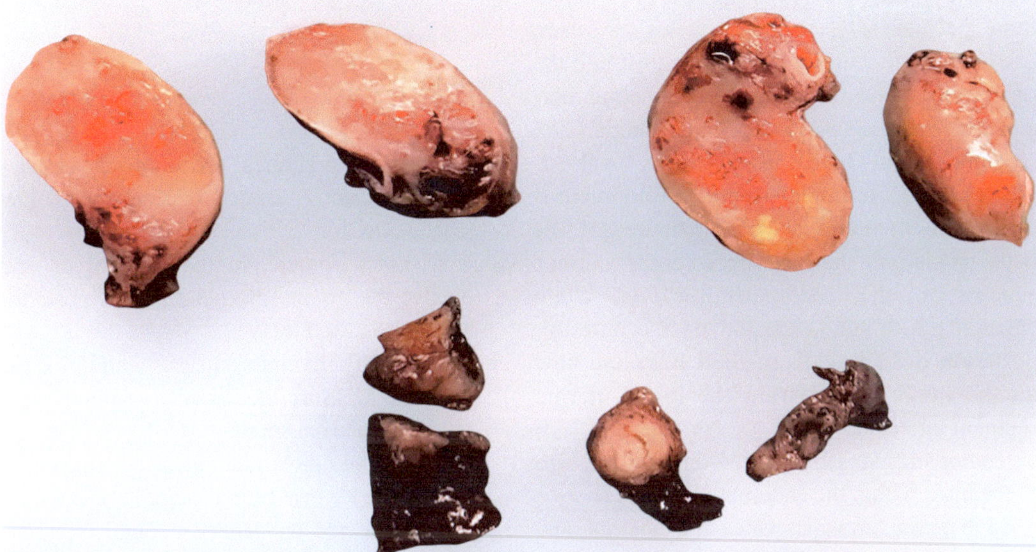

Fig. 8.34 Fallopian tubes and ovaries

8.9 Uterus, Endometrial Hyperplasia, and Endometrial Cancer: Level VI CPT 88309

The purpose of a hysterectomy for endometrial hyperplasia is to assess for evidence of malignancy as described in Table 8.2. In this case, the entire endometrium should be submitted. These sections do not need to be full-thickness to show the serosa but the endometrial cavity should be assessed entirely. The purpose of a hysterectomy for endometrial cancer is for staging and treatment purposes. If endometrial cancer invades greater than 50% of the myometrium, regional

Table 8.2 Tumor gross appearance of uterus

Leiomyoma	Firm, tan-while, fibrous nodules with whorled cut surfaces. Possible areas of necrosis.
Leiomyosarcoma	Large, single, tan-yellow cut surfaces with possible necrosis.
Endometrial carcinoma	Soft, friable, tan-pink, ill-defined mass.
Carcinosarcoma	Large, polypoid, friable, pink-yellow, mostly solid mass that can fill the endometrial cavity.
Adenomatoid tumor	Ill-defined, soft, tan mass within the myometrium, classically near the serosal surface.

lymph nodes are then removed to assess for metastasis.

Cancer Protocol Breakdown Relative to Grossing Uterus for Endometrial Cancer.

Procedure: Hysterectomy specimens for endometrial tumors typically are received with the cervix attached. The bilateral adnexa can also be attached. Additional specimens such as omentum, peritoneal biopsies, and lymph nodes are often received separately. Dictate what anatomical structures are present.

Specimen integrity: Note whether the specimen is received intact, previously opened, or ruptured. If the specimen is received open in any way, there is a potential that tumor cells can embed into the surrounding tissue including the parametrial margins which can cause a false positive margin.

Tumor site: Once the uterus is bivalved, identify the tumor location. Endometrial tumors are often soft and friable making it difficult to identify the location where the tumor adheres to the endometrial cavity. State whether the tumor is present on the anterior, posterior, or both walls of the cavity and how far the tumor comes from the lower uterine segment and cervical os.

Tumor size: Measure a three-dimensional size of the mass within the endometrial cavity.

Myometrial invasion: Once the anterior and posterior aspects of the endometrial cavity are sliced, identify invasion of the tumor into the surrounding myometrium. If invasion is present, measure how deep the invasion is and how close the tumor comes from the closest serosal surface.

Myometrial thickness: Measure the overall thickness of the myometrium.

Percentage of myometrial invasion: Identify if the tumor invasion is greater or less than 50% of the total myometrial thickness. [2].

Step 1: Orient and measure all aspects of the uterus which include uterus, cervix, fallopian tubes, and ovaries. See benign uterus for orientation and anatomy of the uterus (Fig. 8.35).

Step 2: Shave the parametrial margins and submit en face (see blue dotted line) (Fig. 8.36).

Step 3: Remove the fallopian tubes and ovaries and weigh the specimen (see blue solid line) (Fig. 8.36).

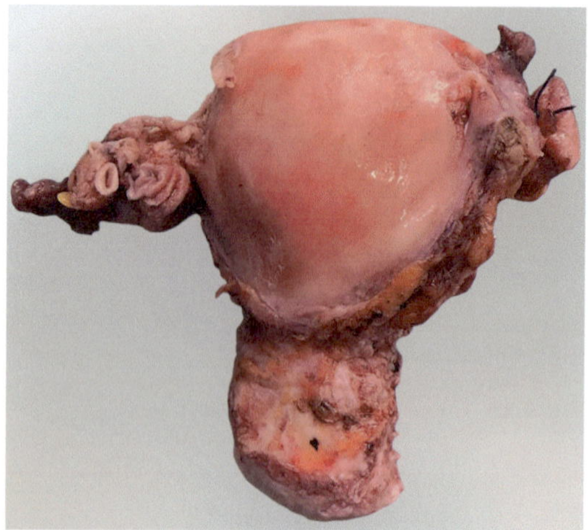

Fig. 8.35 Uterus

Step 4: Ink the peritoneal reflection of the anterior and posterior aspects with separate colors (Fig. 8.37a, b).

Step 5: Place forceps in the cervical os and bivalve the uterus into anterior and posterior halves (Fig. 8.38).

Step 6: Identify the mass, measure, and give the location. Measure the distance of the mass to the lower uterine segment (LUS) and the cervical os. The mass in the figure is in the endometrial cavity (see blue triangle) but does not extend into the endocervical canal (see blue rectangle) (Fig. 8.39).

Step 7: Take anterior and posterior sections of the ectocervix, perpendicular. Take anterior and posterior sections of the mass in relation to the LUS, perpendicular (see blue dotted rectangle). This will allow for microscopic measurement of how close the mass comes to the LUS (Fig. 8.40).

Step 8: Serially section both the anterior and posterior halves of the endometrial cavity. Assess for the greatest depth of invasion on both sides (Fig. 8.41).

Step 9: Measure the depth of invasion and how close the mass comes to the serosal surface. Sections of the greatest depth of invasion are submitted from both anterior and posterior halves. Sections need to be full-thickness (Fig. 8.42) For specimens with endometrial hyperplasia, the entirety of the endometrial cavity is submitted. For endo-

Fig. 8.36 Uterus, parametrial margin

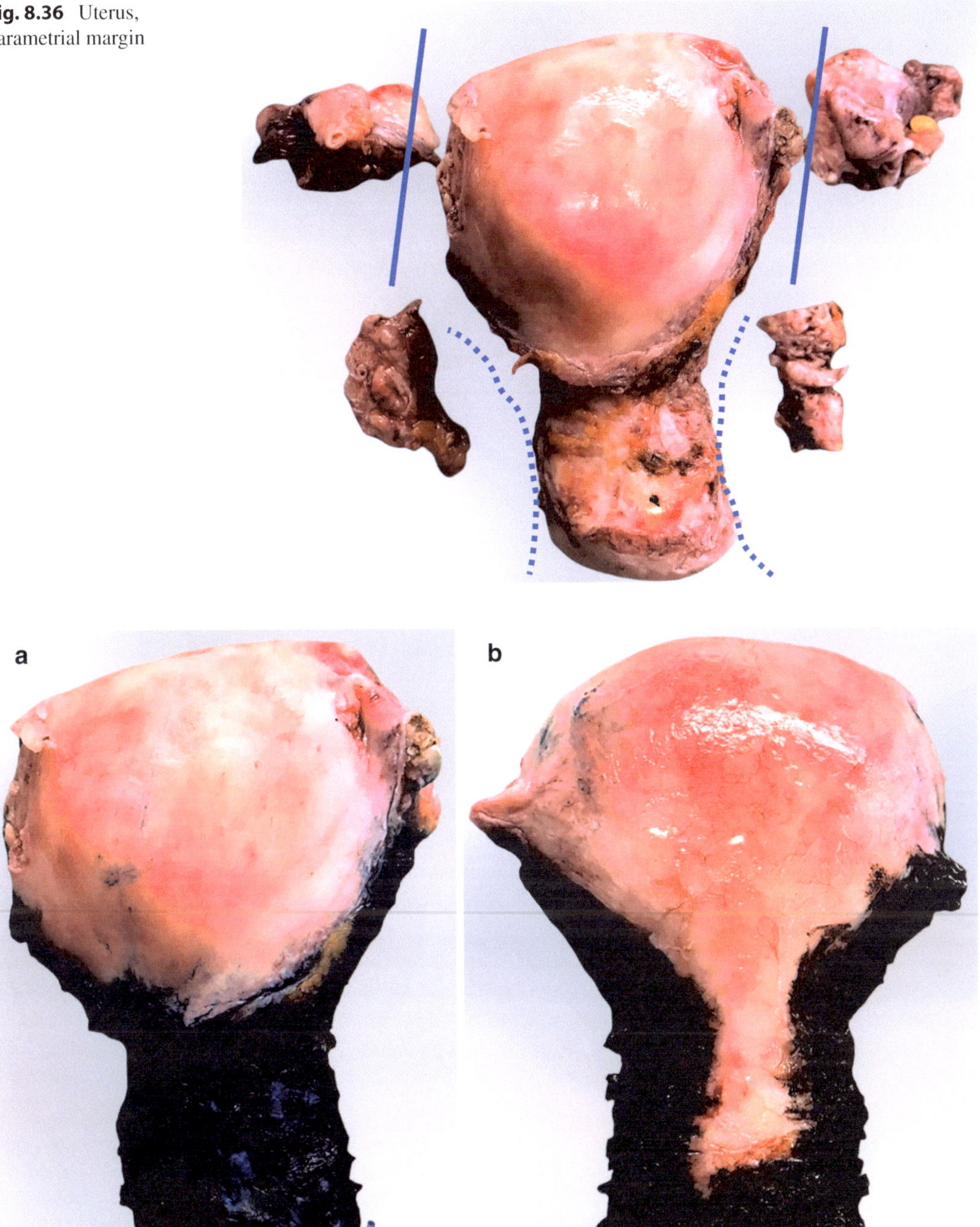

Fig. 8.37 (**a**) Anterior uterus, inked. (**b**) Posterior uterus, inked

metrial cancer, assessing invasion is tricky and takes practice. Invasion is only how far the mass goes into the myometrium. It does not include the exophytic portion of the mass.

Step 10: Serially section the tubes and ovaries as usual. Submit 2 sections of the tube, half of the fimbria, and one full cross section of the ovary as long as the ovary is unremarkable (Fig. 8.43).

Sections submitted are bilateral parametrial shaves, anterior and posterior ectocervix with endocervical canal, anterior and posterior lower uterine segment, anterior and posterior endometrium full-thickness, and bilateral adnexa (Fig. 8.44).

Example Dictation

Specimen A is received in formalin labeled with patient's name, medical record number, "uterus, cervix, bilateral fallopian tubes, and ovaries" and consists of an intact tan-pink uterus

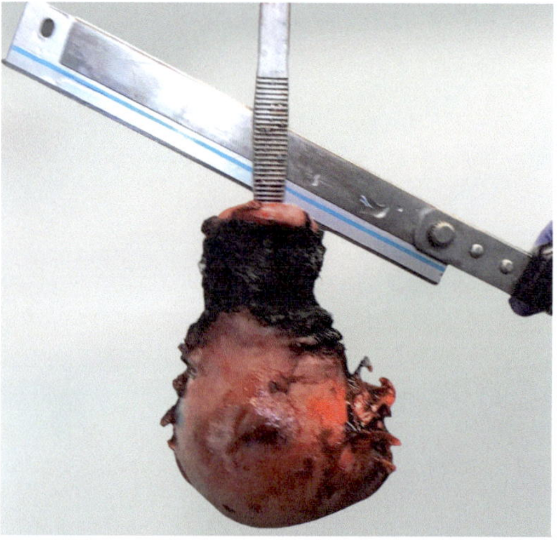

Fig. 8.38 Uterus, bivalve

(9.1 × 6.5 × 3.6 cm, 123 g) with attached bilateral, distal fimbriated fallopian tube segments (right: 1.1 × 0.5 × 0.3 cm, left: 0.9 × 0.5 × 0.4 cm) with previous tubal ligation, and attached bilateral ovaries (right: 2.2 × 1.5 × 1.1 cm, left: 1.4 × 1.0 × 0.8 cm). The uterine fundus serosal surface is tan-pink and smooth. The ectocervix (3.2 × 2.4 cm) is tan-pink with an eccentrically placed slit-like os (1.1 cm in length). The specimen is bivalved to reveal an endocervical canal (3.4 cm in length) with herringbone architecture. There is a single identifiable smooth-walled cyst (0.4 × 0.4 × 0.3 cm) within the cervical stroma, filled with gelatinous material. The endometrial cavity (3.5 × 2.9 × 1.0 cm) contains a tan-yellow, necrotic mass (3.2 × 2.5 × 0.9 cm), adhered to the anterior aspect, coming within 1.2 cm of the lower uterine segment and 4.5 cm from the cervical os. The anterior aspect is serially sectioned to reveal the greatest depth of invasion approximately 0.4 cm, coming within 1.2 cm of the serosal surface and 2.1 cm from the closest anterior parametrial margin. The posterior aspect is serially sectioned to reveal the greatest depth of invasion of less than 0.1 cm, coming within 1.4 cm of the serosal surface and 2.5 cm from the closest posterior parametrial margin with an overall myometrial thickness ranging from 0.9 to 1.4 cm. The bilateral remnants of fimbriated fallopian

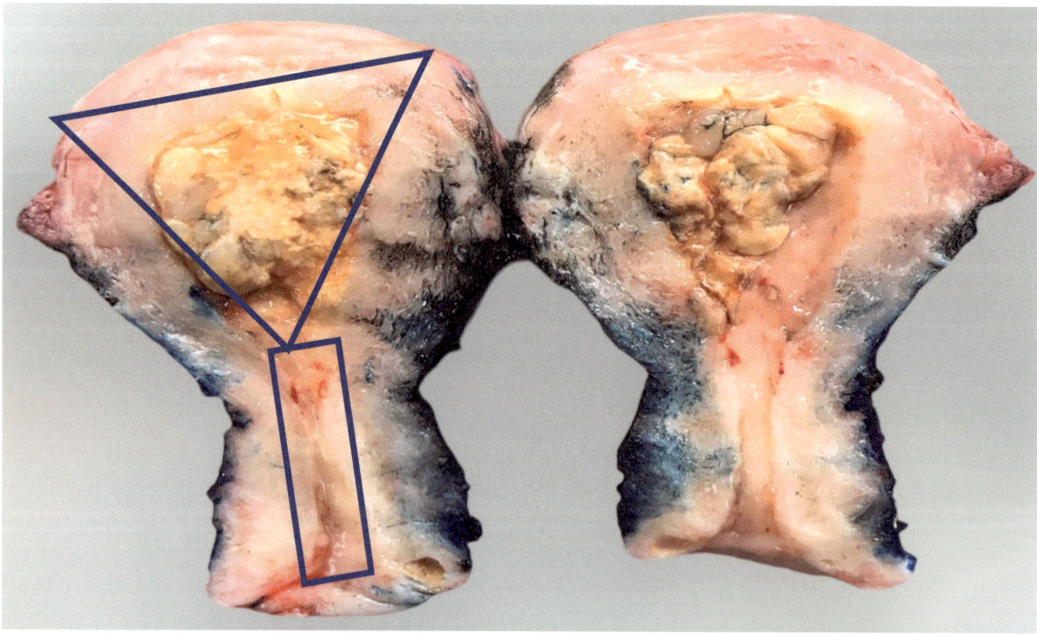

Fig. 8.39 Uterus, bivalved

Fig. 8.40 Uterus, cervical sections

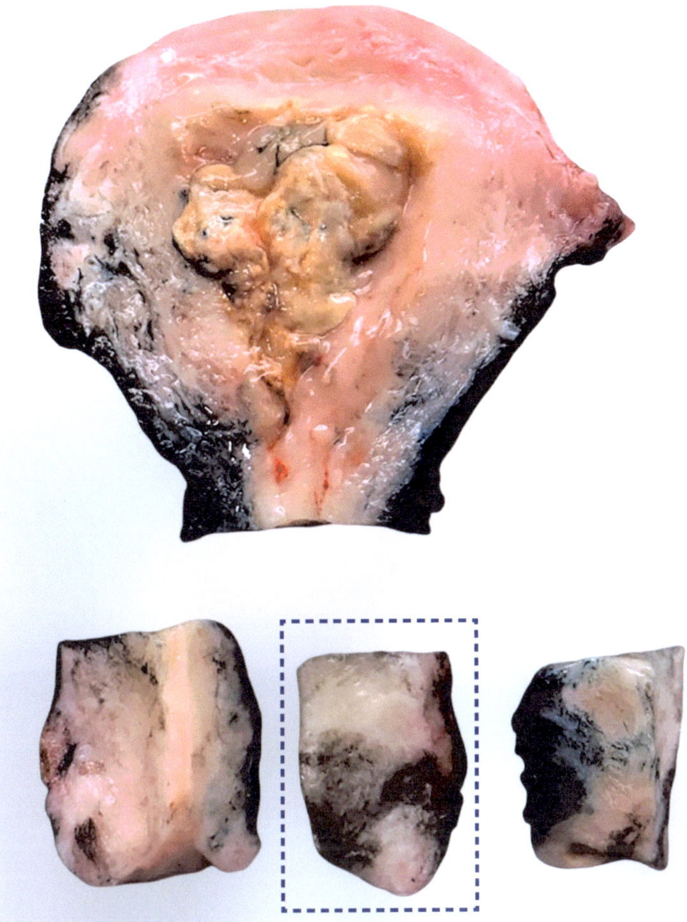

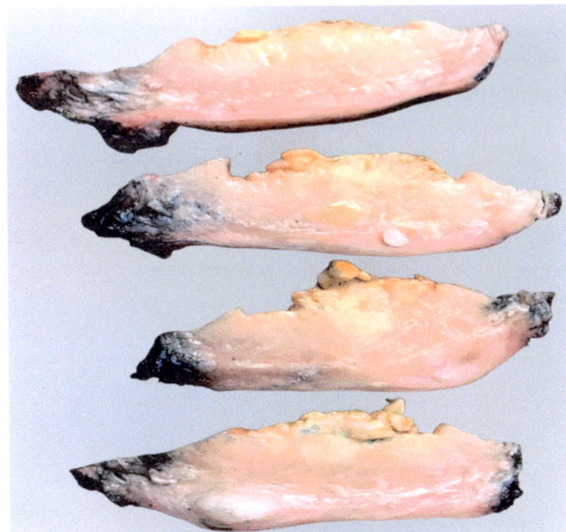

Fig. 8.41 Uterus, serially sectioned

tubes are sectioned to reveal tan lumens. The bilateral ovaries are serially sectioned to reveal tan-white, variegated cut surfaces.

Ink code
>   Blue: anterior
>   Black: posterior

Section code:
>   A 1: Right parametrial shave, en face
>   A 2: Left parametrial shave, en face
>   A 3: Anterior ectocervix with endocervical canal
>   A 4: Anterior lower uterine segment, perpendicular
>   A 5-A 7: Anterior endomyometrium, full-thickness with greatest depth of invasion
>   A 8: Posterior ectocervix with endocervical canal
>   A 9: Posterior lower uterine segment, perpendicular
>   A 10-A 12: Posterior endomyometrium, full-thickness
>   A 13: Right adnexa, representative
>   A 14: Left adnexa, representative

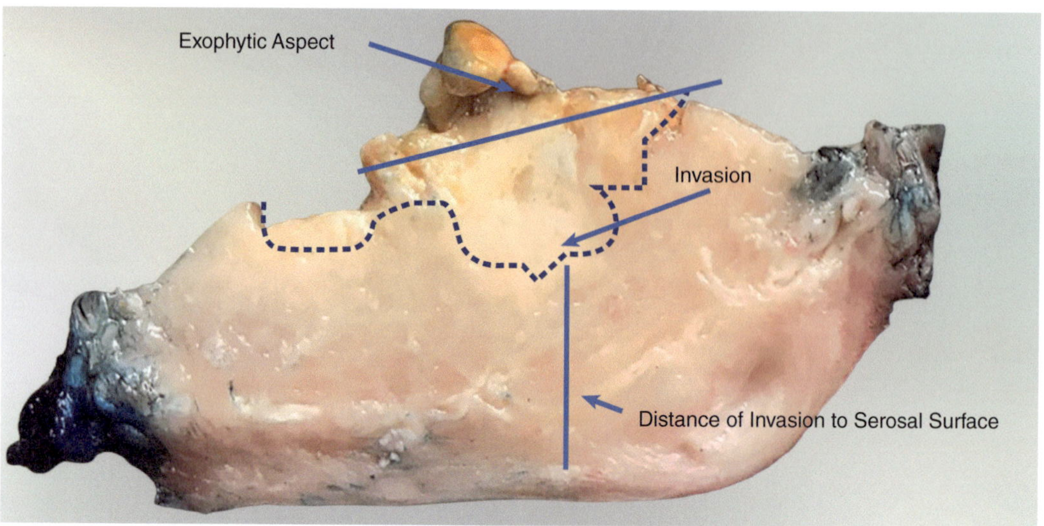

Fig. 8.42   Uterus, depth of invasion

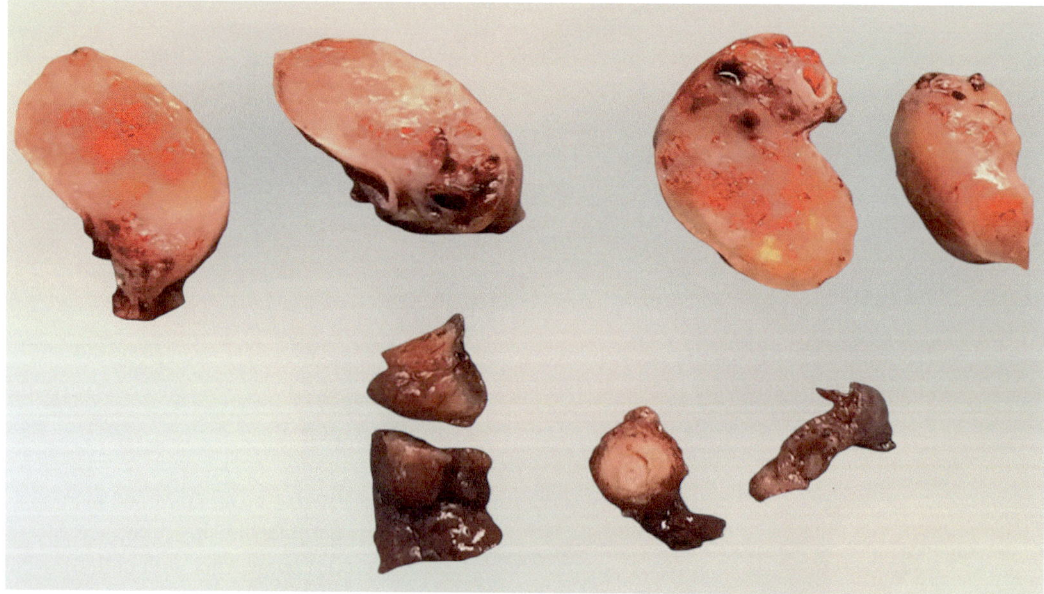

Fig. 8.43   Fallopian tubes and ovaries

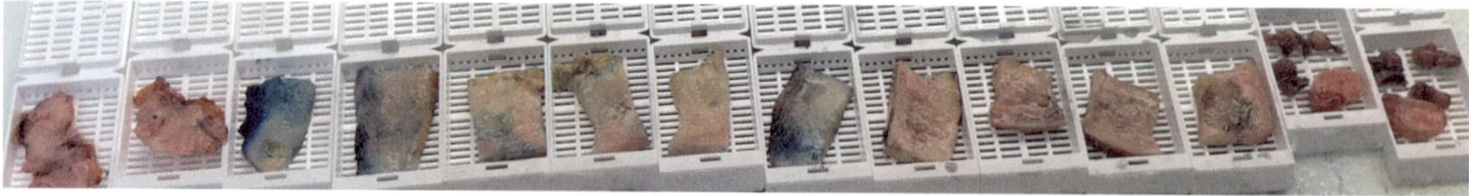

Fig. 8.44   Uterus, sections submitted

8.10   Fallopian Tube with Fimbriae for Sterilization: Level II CPT 88302

Fallopian tubes for sterilization require 1 full cross section of the fallopian tube. If fimbria is present, then one full cross section and one half of the fimbria should be submitted if the pathologist requests the fimbria. If no fimbria is present, then one full cross section of the fallopian tube is necessary. Often two cross sections of the fallopian tube are submitted just in case embedding isn't adequate.

Step 1: Describe the fallopian tube and the presence of fimbria (Fig. 8.45).

Step 2: Measure in three dimensions.

Step 3: Serially section the long axis of the fallopian tube and identify the lumen (see solid blue line) (Fig. 8.46).

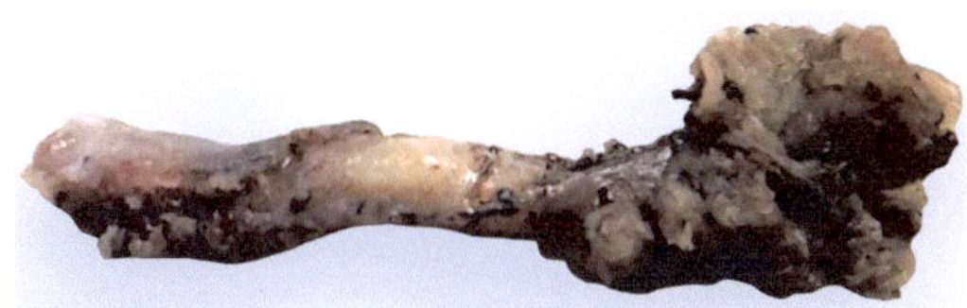

Fig. 8.45 Fallopian tube

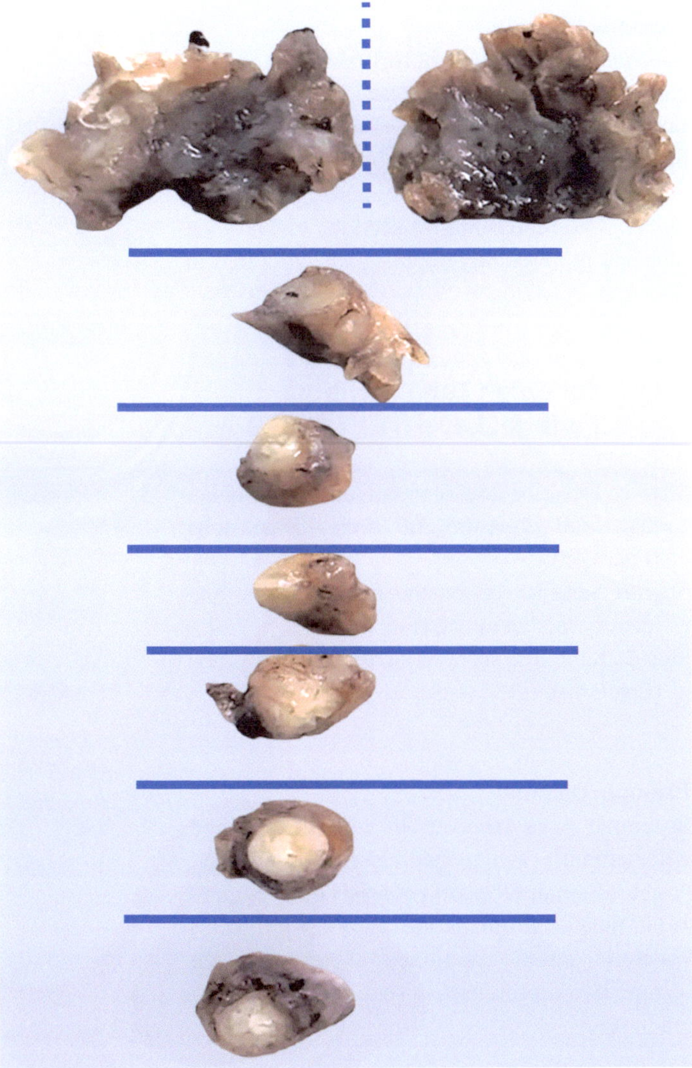

Fig. 8.46 Fallopian tube, serially sectioned

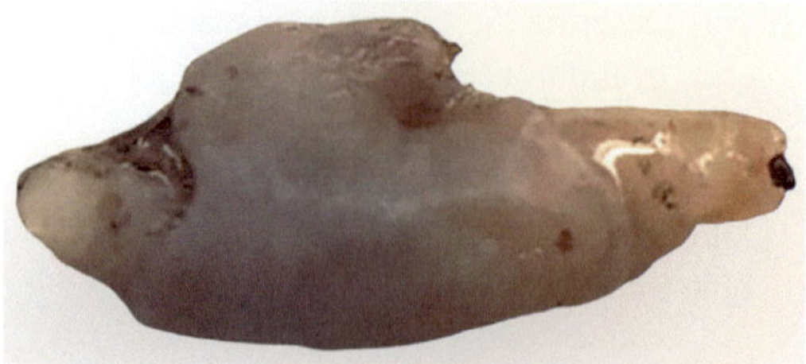

Fig. 8.47 Segment of fallopian tube

Step 4: Bivalve the fimbria (see dotted blue line) (Fig. 8.46).

Step 5: Submit 2 sections of the fallopian tube and 1 half of the fimbria.

Example Dictation

Specimen A is received in formalin labeled with patient's name, medical record number, "right fallopian tube" and consists of a segment of tan-purple fimbriated fallopian tube (5.1 × 0.7 × 0.5 cm) which is serially sectioned to reveal a tan lumen. Two representative sections of fallopian tube and representative fimbria are submitted in A1.

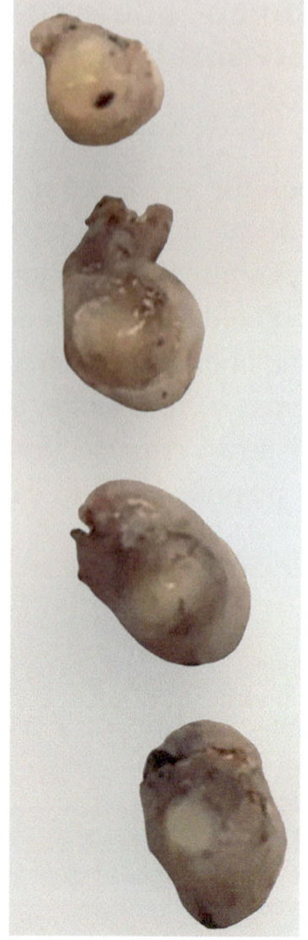

Fig. 8.48 Fallopian tube, serially sectioned

8.11   Fallopian Tube Without Fimbria: Level II CPT 88302

Step 1: Describe the segment of the fallopian tube and measure in three dimensions (Fig. 8.47).

Step 2: Serially section the fallopian tube and identify the tan lumen (Fig. 8.48).

Step 3: Submit 2 sections of the fallopian tube (Fig. 8.49).

Example Dictation

Specimen A is received in formalin labeled with patient's name, medical record number, "right fallopian tube" and consists of a segment of tan-purple fallopian tube (2.1 × 0.7 × 0.5 cm) which is serially sectioned to reveal a tan lumen. Two representative sections are submitted in A1.

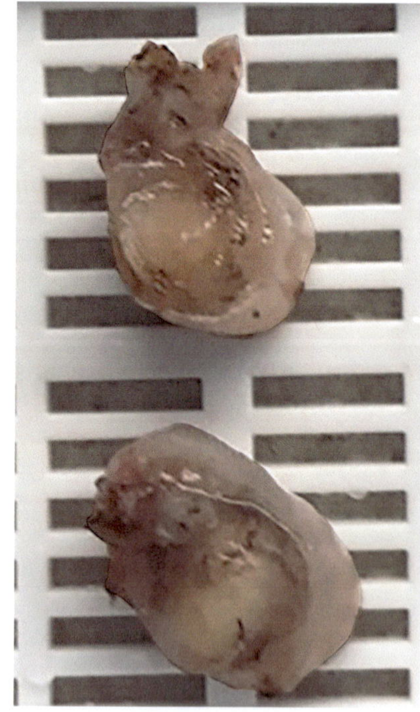

Fig. 8.49 Fallopian tube, cassette submission

8.12   Ovary Cyst/Mass, Non-neoplastic: Level IV CPT 88305, Neoplastic Level V CPT 88307

The purpose of a benign oophorectomy is to remove the entirety of the mass or cyst for the reduction of symptoms. See Table 8.3 for the tumor gross appearance of the ovary. An oophorectomy for malignancy is done to remove the entirety of the cancer for staging and treatment.

Cancer Protocol Breakdown Relative to Grossing Ovary.

Procedure: For ovarian masses, a multitude of specimens and anatomic structures can be sent by the surgeon including total hysterectomy and bilateral salpingo-oophorectomy, single salpingo-oophorectomy, omentum, and peritoneal tissue. It is important to note what type of specimen is present and all the anatomical aspects of the specimen.

Tumor site: The specific site of the tumor should be noted since often many anatomical structures are included.

Specimen integrity: State whether the ovary is received intact or ruptured and if there are any nodules present on the outer surface of the cyst wall.

Tumor Size: When the ovarian mass is grossly identified, a three-dimensional measurement should be included in the description. [2].

Step 1: Describe the ovary and if it is intact or ruptured (Fig. 8.50).
Step 2: Measure the ovary in three dimensions.
Step 3: Describe the fallopian tube and measure in three dimensions.
Step 4: Weigh the ovary if the specimen is intact.
Step 5: Dictate if the outer surface of the ovary is smooth or contains small nodules. Small nodules could be tumor implants on the outer surface.
Step 6: Remove the fallopian tube (Fig. 8.51).
Step 7: Ink the outer surface of the ovary. This step depends on the preference of the pathologists. If the ovary is intact, then it can be inked. If the ovary is ruptured, then inking is not necessary.

Table 8.3 Tumor gross appearance of ovary

Serous tumor	Uniloculated to multiloculated cystic spaces with clear, watery fluid. Can have solid, papillary areas on an otherwise smooth internal cyst wall. Involvement of the outer surface of the cyst may be present consisting of small, flat nodules.
Mucinous tumor	More often multiloculated cystic spaces filled with viscous fluid. Can have solid or papillary areas with necrosis.
Endometrioid tumor	A mix of solid and cystic areas filled with blood and mucinous material.
Brenner tumor	A well-circumscribed, solid, tan-yellow tumor that is usually small in size with possible small cysts on the cut surface.
Teratoma	Typically, uniloculated and contains hair and caseous material. Within the cyst is a solid, fatty protrusion often containing calcified tissue or even teeth.
Dysgerminoma	Typically, solid tumors ranging in size and have tan-yellow to dusky cut surfaces that are soft to the touch.
Endodermal sinus tumor "yolk-sac"	A solid, non-encapsulated tumor that can be tan-pink to yellow with possible necrosis.
Choriocarcinoma	Typically, a smaller tumor with solid hemorrhagic surfaces and necrosis.
Granulosa cell tumor	Can vary in size from microscopic to large, with encapsulated, solid and cystic, tan-yellow surfaces.
Fibroma	A solid, tan-white, fibrous, and well-circumscribed tumor with possible calcification present.
Thecoma	A large, tan-yellow, solid tumor with areas of possible calcification, hemorrhage, cysts, and/or necrosis.
Sertoli-Leydig cell tumor	A solid, pink to golden yellow cut surfaces.

Step 8: Place the ovary near the drain and make a small incision to allow the fluid to drain out. Note the color and consistency of the fluid (Fig. 8.52).
Step 9: Grossly analyze the internal cyst wall. Identify any areas that are solid or papillary.

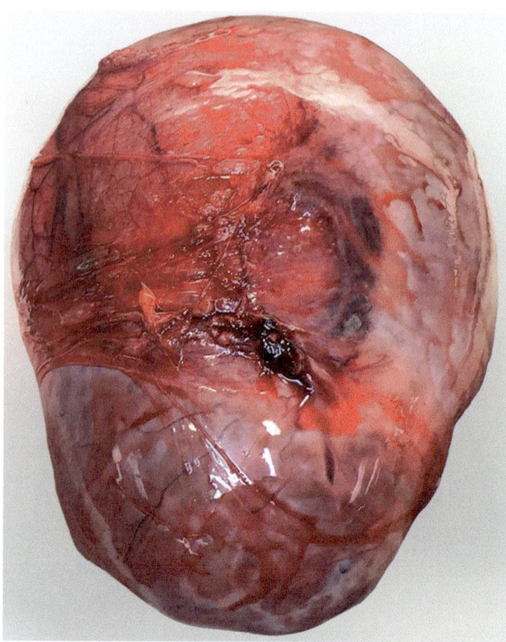

Fig. 8.50 Intact ovarian cyst

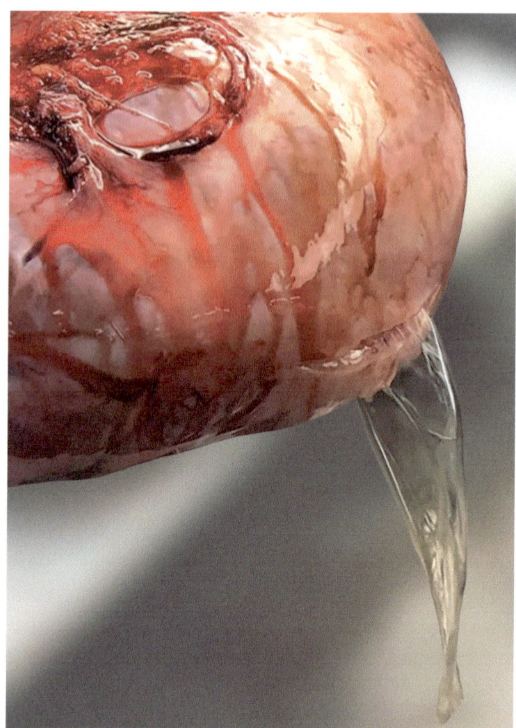

Fig. 8.52 Opening the ovary

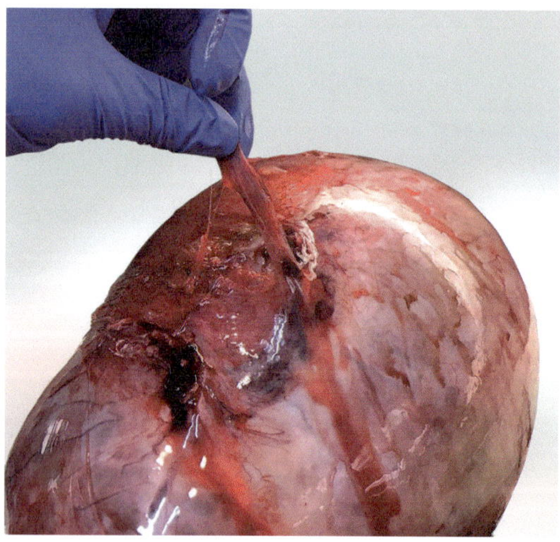

Fig. 8.51 Fallopian tube attached to the ovary

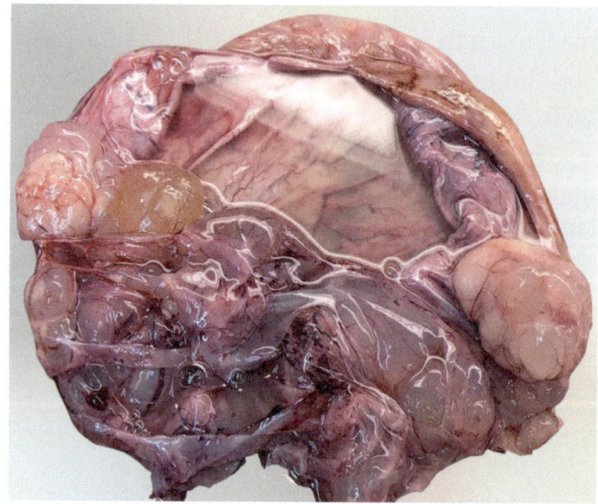

Fig. 8.53 Open ovary

These areas are more concerning than the thin, smooth part of the cyst wall. Dictate the description of the internal ovary using a percentage of how much of the cyst wall is covered in solid or papillary areas (Fig. 8.53).

Step 10: Sections include fallopian tube (2 cross sections of tube and fimbria) and 1 section per 1 cm of overall mass size (Fig. 8.54) focusing more on the solid areas but making sure representative sections of all areas are submitted. If the ovarian mass is 20 cm in the greatest dimension, then 20 sections are to be submitted. However, more than one section can go in 1 cassette, if possible.

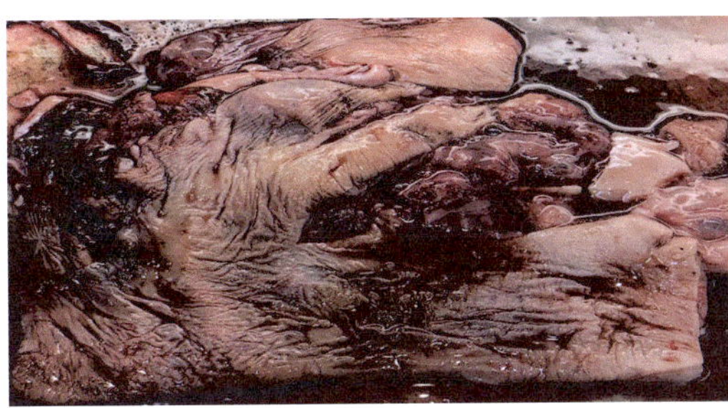

Fig. 8.54 Ovary, internal surface

Example Dictation

Specimen A is received in formalin labeled with patient's name, medical record number, "left fallopian tube and ovary" and consists of an intact, semi-translucent, large cyst (26.1 × 19.5 × 12.2 cm, 3462 g) with a possible overlying fimbriated fallopian tube (4.5 × 0.3 × 0.2 cm) which is markedly stretched along the outer cyst wall. The cyst is opened to reveal a marked amount of semi-translucent fluid. The internal cyst wall is multi-cystic with semi-translucent cysts ranging from 0.5 to 3.9 cm and a focal solid area (3.5 × 3.3 × 1.6 cm) spanning approximately 30% of the cyst wall. No papillary excrescences are identified within the cyst wall. The fallopian tube is serially sectioned to reveal a possible lumen.

Section code
>   A 1-A 5: Representative solid areas
>   A 6-A 15: Representative sections of cyst wall
>   A 16: Possible fallopian tube, entirely

8.13 Products of Conception (POC): Level IV CPT 88305

The purpose of microscopically examining products of conception is to identify the villous tissue. If no villous tissue is identified, it is possible that the procedure was not successful and products are still present in the patient's endometrial cavity.

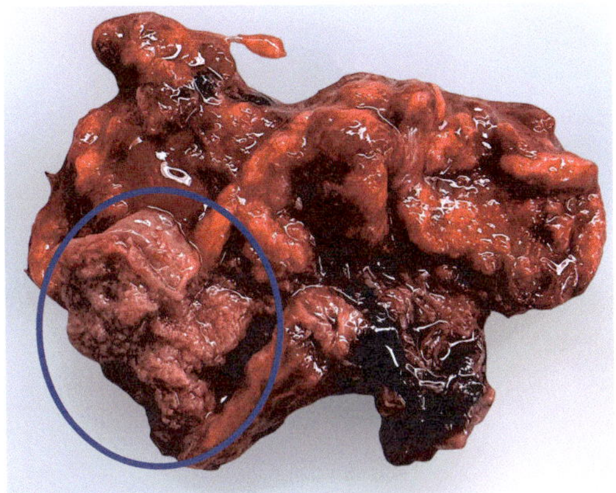

Fig. 8.55 Products of conception, fragmented specimen

Step 1: Describe the aggregate, measure, and weigh the specimen.

Step 2: Representative sections of the tan-pink villous tissue are submitted (see blue circle) (Fig. 8.55).

Specimen A is received fresh labeled with patient's name, medical record number, "POC" and consists of an aggregate of pink-red, hemorrhagic tissue (7.2 × 4.1 × 3.4 cm, 47 g) with identifiable papillary tissue. Representative sections of the papillary tissue are submitted in A1- A2.

Step 1: Missed abortions can also be placentas with or without a fetus. Measure and weigh the placenta. Then measure and weigh the fetus (Fig. 8.56).

Step 2: Submit umbilical cord cross sections. Often, the umbilical cord is too small to grossly assess vessels. Hopefully, vessels will be visible microscopically.

Step 3: If any membranes are present, submit representative sections.

Step 4: Submit representative sections of the placenta. Often, 2-3 full-thickness sections are acceptable.

Step 5: Always address the hospital's policy before submitting fetal structures. If the hospital allows the submission of fetal structures, the fetus can be submitted as well.

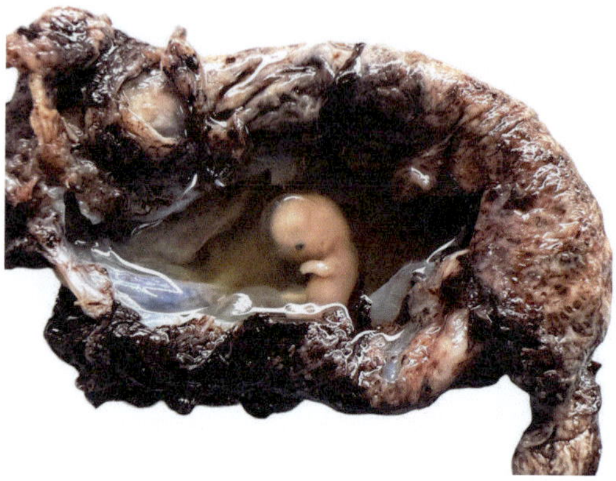

Fig. 8.56 POC, the embryo within the placenta

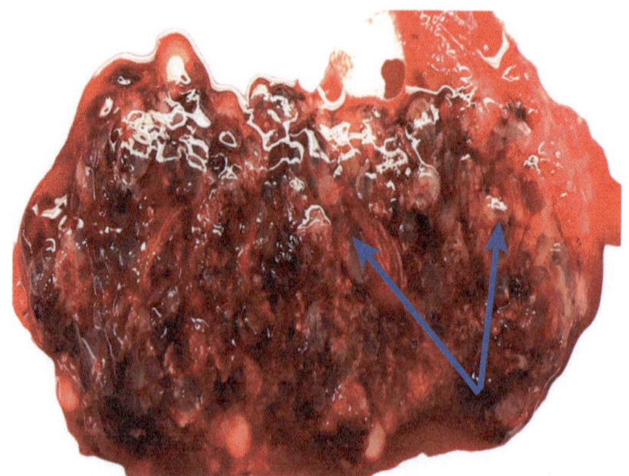

Fig. 8.57 Products of conception, complete mole

Example Dictation

Specimen A is received fresh labeled with patient's name, medical record number, "POC" and consists of a previously ruptured placenta (6.2 × 5.1 × 1.1 cm, 17 grams) with minimal surrounding membranes and complete cotyledons. Attached to the placenta is a small fetal structure (1.9 × 1.0 × 0.9 cm, 1 gram) with a 3.9 cm umbilical cord. The vessels of the umbilical cord are unable to be grossly assessed. The placenta is serially sectioned to reveal red-brown, spongiform cut surfaces. No infarcts are identified.

Section code

    A1: Membranes and umbilical cord, representative

    A2-A3: Placental disc, representative

    A4: Fetus, entirely

8.14 Molar Products of Conception: Level III CPT 88304

A complete molar pregnancy is appreciated with fluid filled, sac-like structures admixed within the specimen. Submit multiple cassettes (4-6 cassettes) of the sac-like structures. In a partial molar pregnancy, fetal structures may be grossly identified such as hands, feet, and organs. In a partial molar pregnancy, submit multiple cassettes (4-6 cassettes) of placental tissue and fetal parts.

Step 1: Describe, measure, and weigh the specimen. This example is a complete molar pregnancy with small, clear sac-like structures present within the aggregate as shown by the blue arrows in Fig. 8.57.

Step 2: Submit representative sections including the sac-like structures.

Example Dictation

Specimen A is received in formalin labeled with the patient's name, medical record number, "POC" and consists of an aggregate of red-brown, hemorrhagic tissue fragments (9.2 × 8.3 × 2.1 cm, 46 grams) with identifiable fluid filled, sac-like structures. Representative sections are submitted in A1-A5.

8.15 Fallopian Tube for Ectopic Pregnancy: Level IV CPT 88305

The main purpose of grossing a fallopian tube with a possible ectopic pregnancy is to identify if there is a rupture of the fallopian tube and villous tissue visible within the fallopian tube or the container.

Step 1: Describe the fallopian tube and measure in three dimensions.

Step 2: Dictate if there is the presence of a rupture site. There is no rupture in Fig. 8.58.

Step 3: Serially section the fallopian tube along the long axis (Fig. 8.59).

Step 4: Identify and dictate the presence/absence of clotted blood and villous tissue (Fig. 8.60).

Step 5: Submit 2-3 sections of the fallopian tube with villous tissue, if present. If villous tissue is not grossly identified, the fallopian tube may be submitted entirely (Fig. 8.61).

Example Dictation

Specimen A is received in formalin labeled with patient's name, medical record number, "fallopian tube, right" and consists of an intact, dusky, enlarged fimbriated fallopian tube (6.4 × 2.1 × 2.0 cm) which is serially sectioned to reveal a dilated lumen (2.0 cm in diameter) filled with clotted blood and a scant amount of villous tissue present within the lumen. Representative sections are submitted in A1-A2.

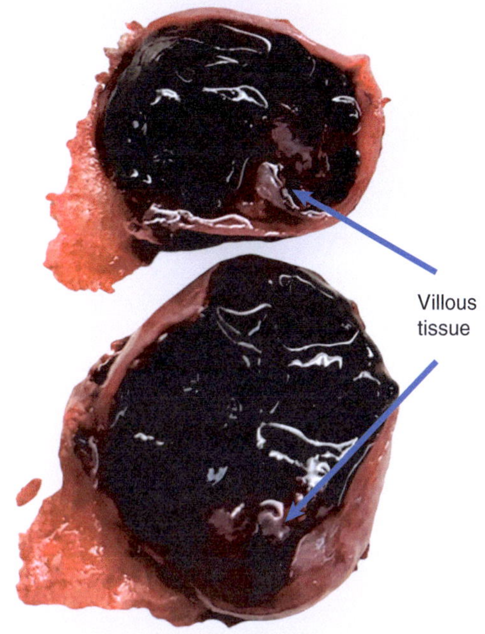

Fig. 8.60   Fallopian tube with ectopic pregnancy, villous tissue

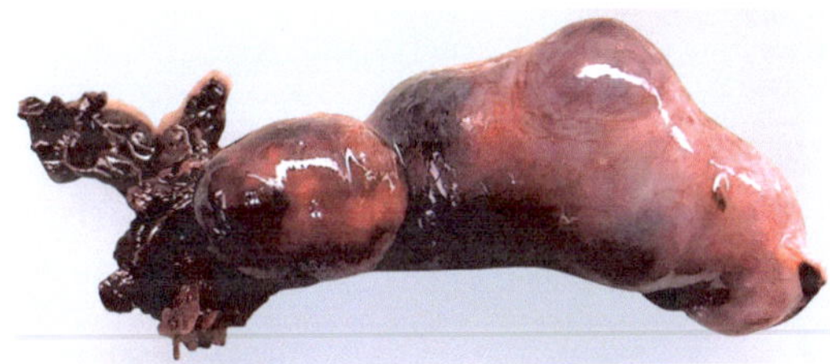

Fig. 8.58   Fallopian tube with ectopic pregnancy

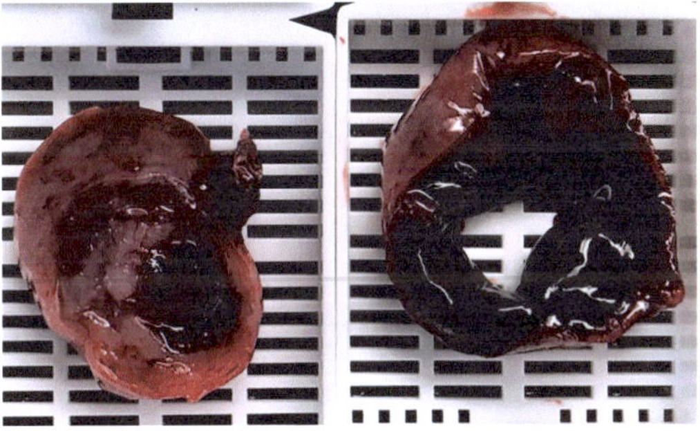

Fig. 8.61   Fallopian tube, cassette submission

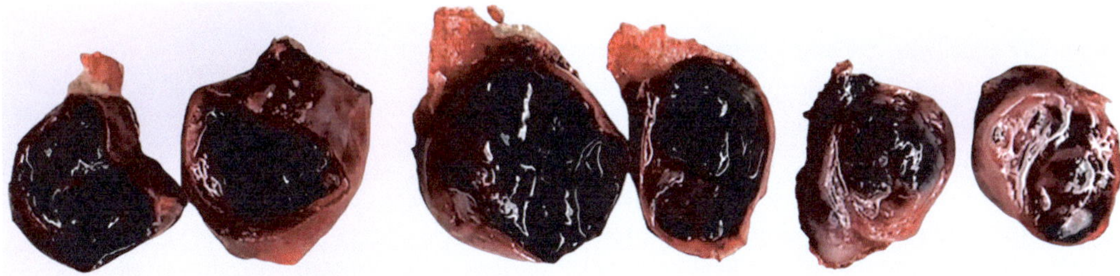

Fig. 8.59   Fallopian tube with ectopic pregnancy, serially sectioned

Fig. 8.62 Singleton placenta

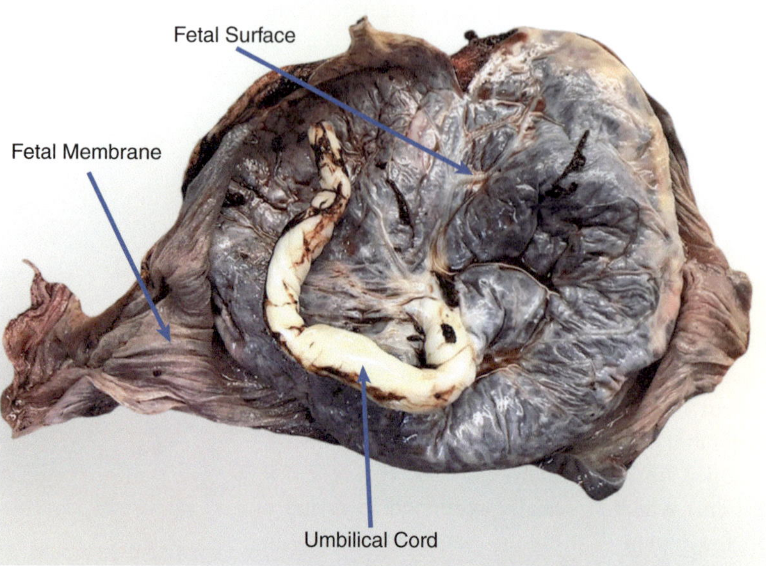

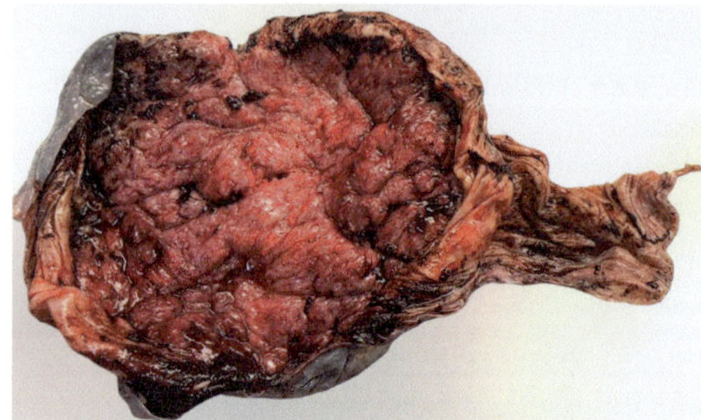

Fig. 8.63 Placenta, maternal surface

8.16 Placenta: 1st and 2nd Trimester Level IV CPT 88305, 3rd Trimester Level V CPT 88307

Examining a placenta can explain the reasons for fetal insufficiencies or fetal death. Complications during pregnancy can extend postpartum and affect both mother and baby.

Step 1: Orient the placenta. In Fig. 8.62, the fetal surface is shown with the umbilical cord and surrounding fetal membranes.

Step 2: Turn the placenta over and note the appearance of the maternal surface (complete or incomplete cotyledons). Fig. 8.63 shows the maternal surface with complete cotyle-

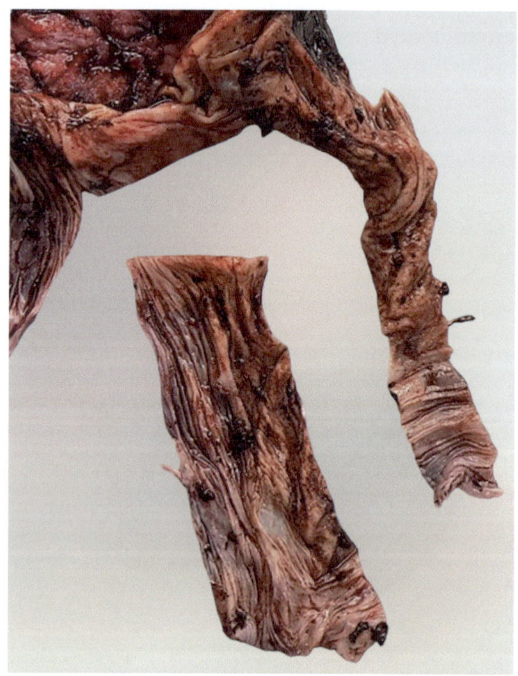

Fig. 8.64 Placental membranes

dons which appear as red, smooth, rounded lobules of placental tissue. If the maternal surface is incomplete, indicate the percentage of incomplete cotyledons.

Step 3: Cut a long, narrow strip of fetal membranes (Fig. 8.64).

Step 4: Clamp one end of the membrane strip tightly with forceps and wrap the membrane around the end of the forceps tightly. Remove the membrane from the forceps (Fig. 8.65).

Step 5: Cut 2 cross sections of the membrane, producing roll-like sections (Fig. 8.66) The remainder of the fetal membranes can now be removed from the placenta.

Step 6: Amputate the umbilical cord where it inserts into the placenta. Section the umbilical cord and note the number of vessels and spirals of the cord. A normal cord has 3 vessels (2 arteries and 1 vein). Two cross sections are to be submitted (Fig. 8.67).

Step 7: Weigh the placental disc, void of fetal membranes and umbilical cord (Fig. 8.68).

Step 8: Serially section the disc and note any areas of hemorrhage or infarcts. If hemor- rhage or infarcts are present, state the area of the cut surface involved in percent (Fig. 8.69).

Step 9: Sections submitted are 2 cross sections of membrane and umbilical cord, and 2 representative full-thickness sections of placenta. If infarcts or hemorrhage are noted, submit representative sections in addition or in place of the original sections (Fig. 8.70).

Example Dictation

Specimen A is received in formalin labeled with patient's name, medical record number, "placenta" and consists of a singleton placenta (16.5 × 16.5 × 2.4 cm) with attached tan-pink, semi-translucent fetal membranes and an eccentrically placed 3-vessel umbilical cord (12.2 × 1.4 × 1.3 cm) inserting 3.5 cm from the disc margin. The fetal surface is tan-blue with vessels spanning the surface. The maternal surface is pink-red with complete cotyledons. The placental disc is serially sectioned to reveal pink-red, spongiform cut surfaces. The placental disc, void of all fetal membranes and umbilical cord is 402 grams.

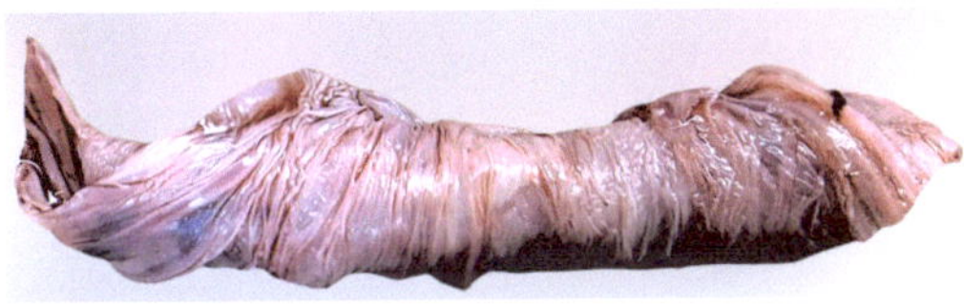

Fig. 8.65   Rolled fetal membranes

Fig. 8.66   Sliced membrane

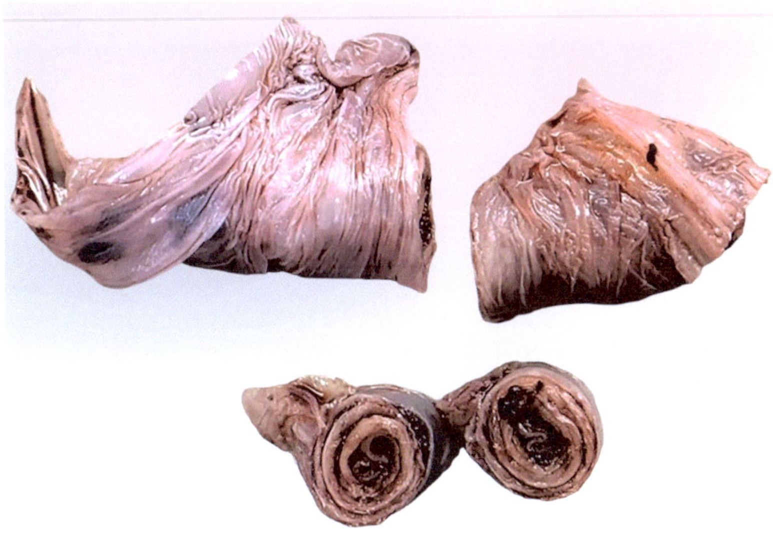

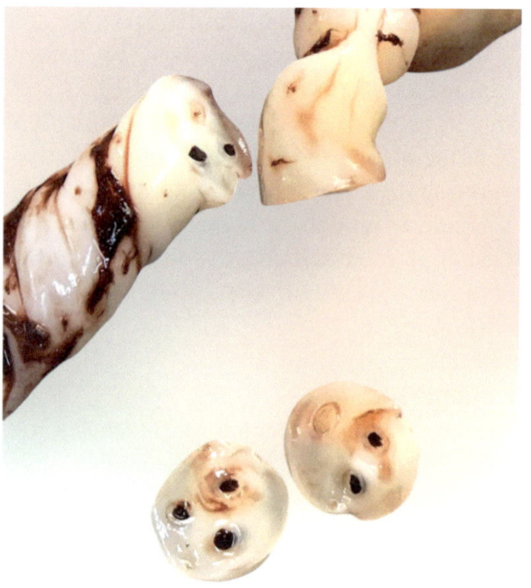

Fig. 8.67 Umbilical cord with three vessels

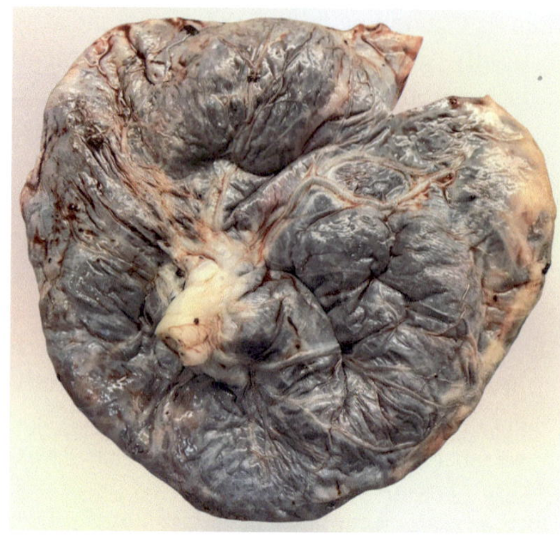

Fig. 8.68 Placenta after removal of umbilical cord and membranes

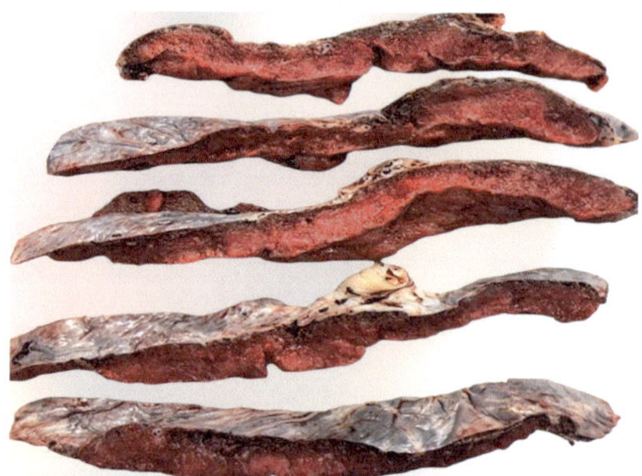

Fig. 8.69 Sliced placental disc

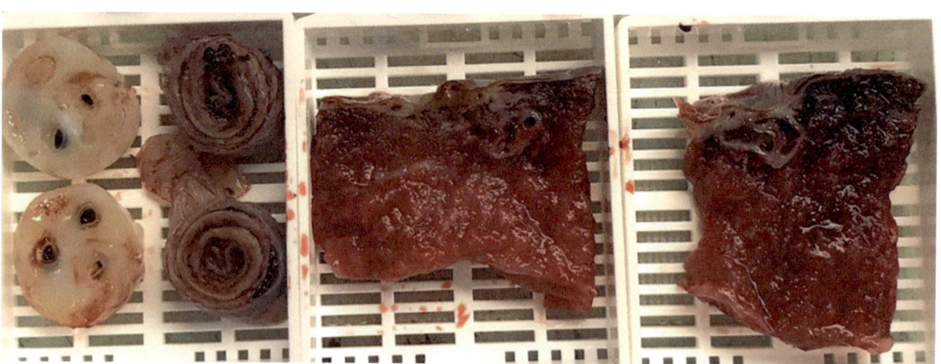

Fig. 8.70 Placenta, sections submission

Section code
  A1: Membrane roll and umbilical cord
  A2-A3: Full-thickness sections

Examples of membrane insertion type (Fig. 8.71).

Examples of cord insertion type (Fig. 8.72).

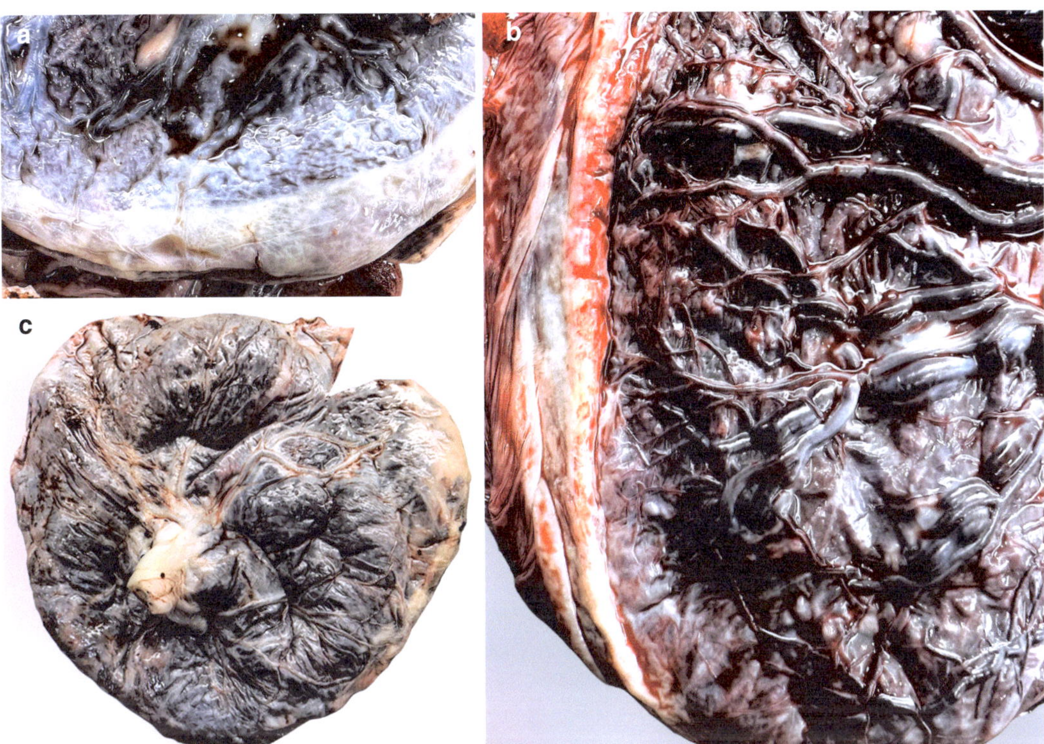

Fig. 8.71 (**a**) Circummarginate insertion: a flattened edge with a ridge of fibrin demarking the edge of the disc. (**b**) Circumvallate insertion: peripheral cup-like insertion of the membranes on the placental surface creating a noticeable ridge. (**c**) Normal insertion: no ridge of any kind is visible

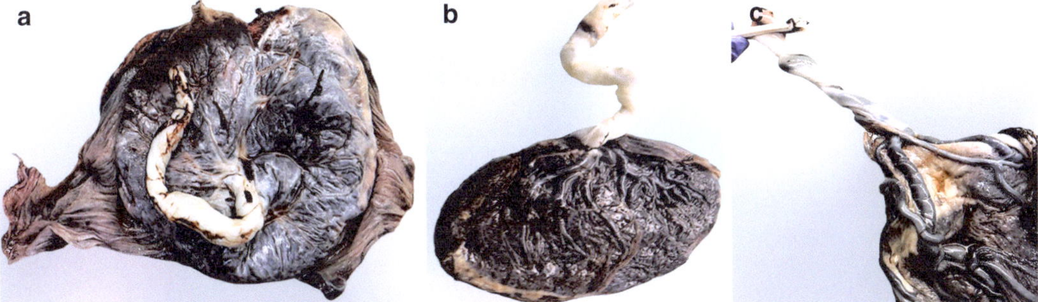

Fig. 8.72 (**a**) Eccentric insertion: cord inserts off center somewhere on the disc. (**b**) Marginal insertion: cord inserts at the absolute edge of the disc. (**c**) Velamentous insertion: cord inserts into the membranes with vessels spanning the membranes and inserting on the disc

8.17 Twin Placenta: 1st and 2nd Trimester Level IV CPT 88305, 3rd Trimester Level V CPT 88307

Fused Disc

Step 1: Orient the specimen. Fused twin placentas are often oriented using the clamps seen on the umbilical cords, typically, as Baby A and Baby B (Fig. 8.73).

Step 2: Take membrane rolls of the dividing membrane. Fused twin placentas will often include a dividing membrane (depending on the type of fused disc) that separates each baby within each placental disc.

Step 3: At this point, you can gross each disc as its own placenta (see singleton placenta).

Step 4: Take representative sections of the transition zone. The area where the 2 discs fuse is called the transition zone.

Specimen A is received in formalin labeled with patient's name, medical record number, "twin placenta" and consists of fused twin placental discs (14.0 × 16.5 × 3.0 cm) with a tan-white dividing membrane. The twin placenta is oriented with 1 clamp on the umbilical cord designating baby A and 2 clamps on the umbilical cord designating baby B.

Placenta twin A (12.0 × 16.0 cm) contains attached tan-brown, semi-translucent fetal membrane, and an eccentrically placed three-vessel umbilical cord (16.0 × 1.0 × 1.0 cm), inserting 3.0 cm from the disc edge. The fetal surface is pink-blue with vessels spanning the surface. The maternal surface is pink-red with complete cotyledons. The placental disc is serially sectioned to reveal pink-red, spongiform cut surfaces.

Placenta twin B (15.0 × 14.0 cm) contains attached tan-brown, semi-translucent fetal membrane and an eccentrically placed three-vessel umbilical cord (16.0 × 0.5 × 0.6 cm), inserting 2.5 cm from the disc edge. The fetal surface is pink-blue with vessels spanning the surface. The maternal surface is pink and ragged with approxi-

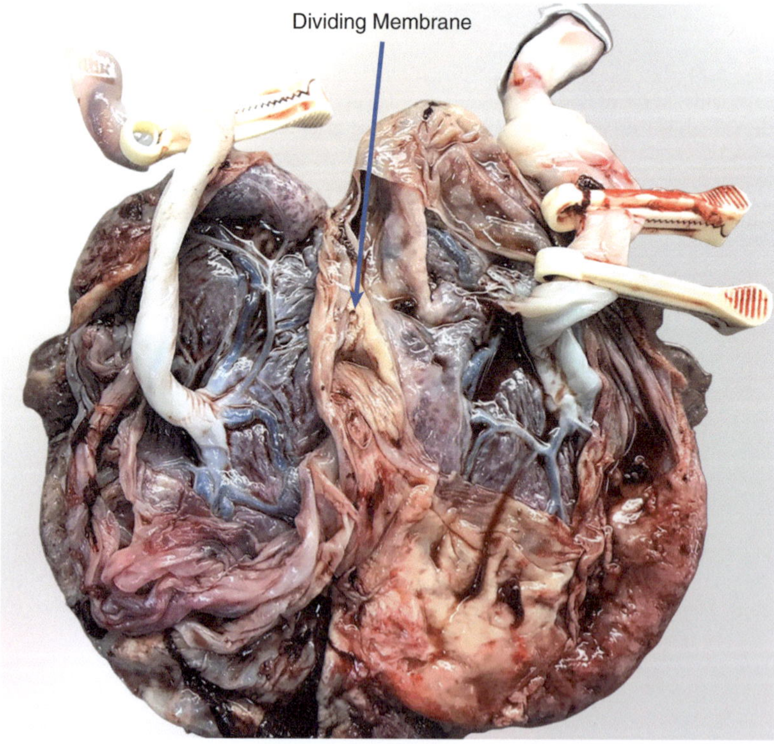

Fig. 8.73 Fused twin placenta

mately 15% incomplete cotyledons. The placental disc is serially sectioned to reveal pink-red, spongiform cut surfaces.

The fused placental disc, void of all fetal membranes and umbilical cord, weighs 505 grams.

Section code
>   A1: Dividing membrane rolls
>   A2: Disc A, membrane rolls and umbilical cord
>   A3-A4: Disc A, full-thickness sections
>   A5: Disc B, membrane rolls and umbilical cord
>   A6-A7: Disc B, full-thickness sections
>   A8: Transition zone

Separate discs Step 1: Orient the specimen. Separate twin placentas are often oriented using the clamps seen on the umbilical cord, typically, as Baby A and Baby B.

Step 2: Take membrane rolls of the dividing membrane as shown by the blue arrow in Fig. 8.74.

Step 3: At this point, you can gross each disc as its own placenta (see singleton placenta).

Separate Discs

Example Dictation

Specimen A is received in formalin labeled with patient's name, medical record number, "twin placenta" and consists of separate twin placental discs with an adhered tan-white dividing membrane. The twin placenta is oriented with 1 clamp on the umbilical cord designating baby A and no clamps on the umbilical cord designating baby B.

Placental disc twin A (16.5 × 16.5 × 2.4 cm) contains attached tan-pink semi-translucent fetal membranes and a velamentously inserted 3-vessel umbilical cord (12.2 × 1.4 × 1.3 cm), inserting 3.5 cm into the membranes from the disc edge. The fetal surface is tan-blue with dilated vessels spanning the surface. The maternal surface is pink-red with complete cotyledons. The placenta disc is serially sectioned to reveal pink-red, spongiform cut surfaces. The placental disc, void of

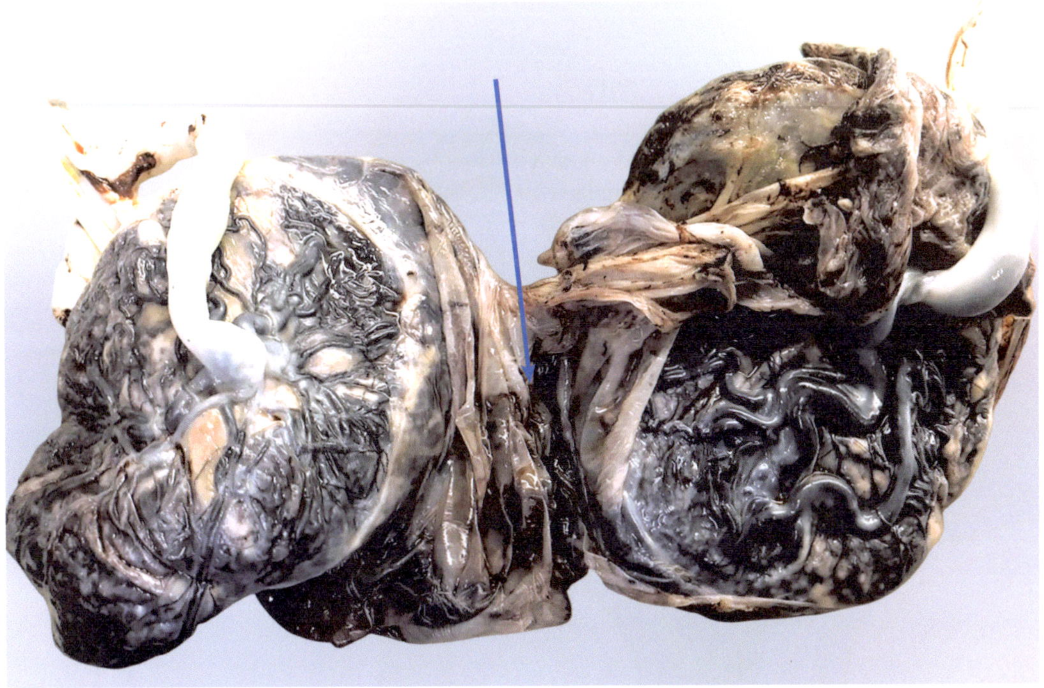

Fig. 8.74 Separate twin placental discs

all fetal membranes and umbilical cord, weighs 402 grams.

Placental disc twin B (17.2 × 16.2 × 2.5 cm) contains attached tan-pink semi-translucent fetal membranes and an eccentrically placed 3-vessel umbilical cord (31.3 × 1.5 × 1.4 cm), inserting 5.3 cm from the disc edge. The fetal surface is tan-blue with vessels spanning the surface. The maternal surface is pink-red with complete cotyledons. The placental disc is serially sectioned to reveal pink-red, spongiform cut surfaces. The placental disc, void of all fetal membranes and umbilical cord, weighs 413 grams.

Section code
  A1: Dividing membrane rolls
  A2: Disc A, membrane rolls, and umbilical cord
  A3-A4: Disc A, full-thickness sections
  A5: Disc B, membrane rolls, and umbilical cord
  A6-A7: Disc B, full-thickness sections

Acknowledgments The author gratefully ackno wledges Veena Shenoy, MD, and Nazar Rahmanov, MD, for their contribution to this chapter.

Quiz Questions

1. A large ovarian mass (15.2 × 14.3 × 13.6 cm) is received for intraoperative consultation. The outer surface is pink and glistening. You take one slice of the mass and a marked amount of clear fluid runs out. Once drained, you finish serially sectioning the mass and see a single smooth tan-pink internal cyst with a small area of papillary excrescences (0.5 × 0.5 × 0.1 cm). Grossly, what is your diagnosis?
   (a) Dysgerminoma
   (b) Mucinous tumor
   (c) Teratoma
   (d) Serous tumor

2. You receive an intact uterus from the operating room with a diagnosis of uncontrolled uterine bleeding. At the gross bench, you follow the steps to bivalve the uterus. The endometrial cavity is slightly thickened and hemorrhagic. Within the myometrium, you note a single tan-yellow, solid, fibrous mass with minimal calcification that you felt when cutting the mass but don't see with the eye. What is your diagnosis?
   (a) Endometrial carcinoma
   (b) Benign uterus with proliferative endometrium
   (c) Leiomyosarcoma
   (d) Bicornuate uterus

3. A uterus is received with no medical history or previous biopsy. You bivalve the uterus into anterior and posterior halves and see Fig. 8.75. What is your gross diagnosis?
   (a) Endometrial polyps
   (b) Endometrial carcinoma
   (c) Benign endometrium
   (d) Third trimester intrauterine pregnancy

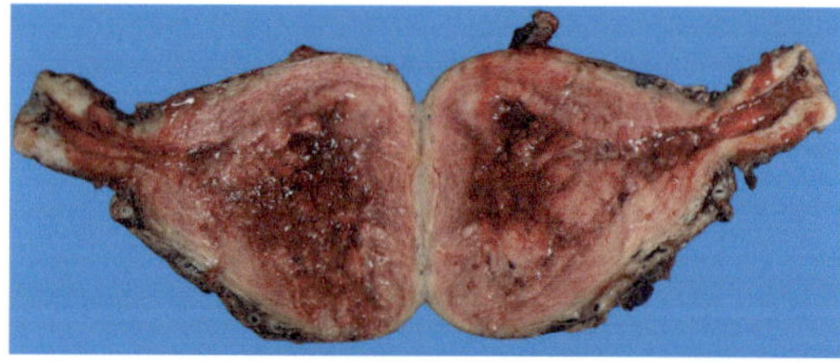

Fig. 8.75 Quiz question

4. During a hysterectomy procedure, the surgeon notices that the right ovary is considerably larger than the left ovary. They bring the specimen to you to gross. You serially section the right ovary and see Fig. 8.76. What is your gross diagnosis?
   (a) Granulosa cell tumor
   (b) Fibroma
   (c) Endodermal sinus tumor "yolk-sac tumor"
   (d) Benign cyst

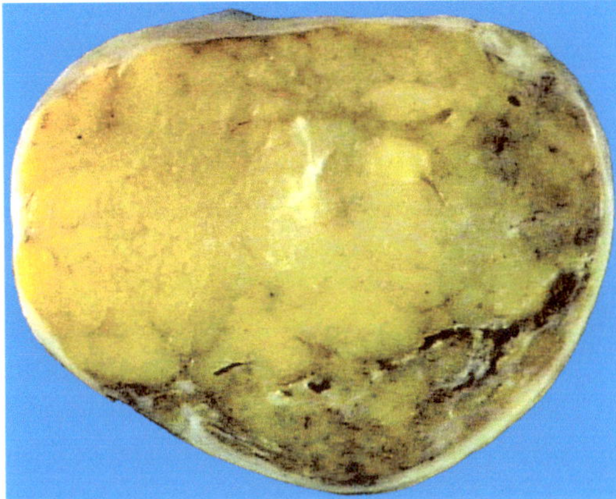

Fig. 8.76 Quiz question

5. A container labeled "products of conception" is received in the lab. You remove the specimen from the container and place it on the gross bench. Friable red-brown, bloody tissue is noted with an innumerable amount of small, clear sac-like structures containing clear fluid. What is your gross diagnosis?
   (a) Benign endometrial tissue
   (b) Complete molar pregnancy
   (c) Partial molar pregnancy
   (d) Clotted blood

6. When grossly assessing products of conception, what type of tissue are you looking for?
   (a) Clotted blood
   (b) Myometrial tissue
   (c) Uterine fibroids
   (d) Villous tissue

7. What needs to be visualized under the microscope to confirm that sterilization of a female patient is successful?
   (a) 1 full cross section of each fallopian tube
   (b) Endometrial tissue
   (c) Unilateral fimbria
   (d) Ectocervical mucosa

8. Which is not a type of placental umbilical cord insertion?
   (a) Eccentric insertion
   (b) Velamentous insertion
   (c) Marginal insertion
   (d) Circumvallate insertion

9. When a physician uses electrocautery to excise a cone-shaped portion of the cervix, this procedure is called what?
   (a) Hysterectomy
   (b) Cervical biopsy
   (c) Loop electrosurgical excision procedure
   (d) Oophorectomy

10. What is the anatomic name for the area where the endocervical canal and the endometrial cavity join?
   (a) Parametrium
   (b) Lower uterine segment
   (c) Cervical os
   (d) Uterine fundus

Answer Key

1. *(d) Serous tumor*
   Explanation: Serous tumors can be uniloculated or multiloculated cysts with clear, watery fluid. Focal papillary excrescences can be noted in an otherwise smooth internal cyst wall. This is why "(d)" is the correct answer. Dysgerminomas are typically solid tumors with a smooth outer capsule. They feel soft to touch and are tan-yellow to gray on cut surface. Focal calcification and focal cystic degeneration can be noted. Mucinous tumors are typically multiloculated cysts filled with thick mucinous fluid with solid areas, papillary excrescences, or focal necrosis. Teratomas are mostly uniloculated containing soft friable caseous material, hair, and calcification with a focal fatty solid area inside the cyst.

2. *(c) Leiomyosarcoma*
   Explanation: Leiomyosarcoma is typically one solid mass within the myometrium

that has a yellow hue. It can often be confused with leiomyomas which are tan-white and often not singular. This is why "(c)" is correct. Endometrial carcinoma is a soft, friable tumor that can be ill-defined spanning the endometrial cavity. Proliferative endometrium is simply increased endometrial tissue. It can occur diffusely or focally within the endometrial cavity and can be confused with endometrial carcinoma. A bicornuate uterus is a uterus with two separate endometrial cavities separated by a myometrial septum. The cavities can converge into a single endocervical canal or have separate endocervical canals and cervical os.

3. *(b) Endometrial Carcinoma*

   Explanation: Endometrial carcinoma is friable and soft to the touch. It can be focal or encompass the entirety of the endometrial cavity even spanning down the cervical canal. This is why "(a)" is correct. Endometrial polyps are typically pink-red polyps arising in the endometrial cavity. They can range in size and number. Benign endometrium is tan-pink, thin, and focally hemorrhagic with a glistening appearance. A third trimester intrauterine pregnancy may contain decidua and/or placental tissue present within the endometrial cavity.

4. *(a) Granulosa cell tumor*

   Explanation: Granulosa cell tumors are variable in size with encapsulated, mostly solid yellow cut surfaces as seen in the photo. This is why "(a)" is correct. Fibromas are tan-white, fibrous, and well circumscribed. Endodermal sinus tumors are solid, non-encapsulated and pink to yellow in color with possible focal necrosis. Benign cysts are smaller in size with a smooth internal cyst wall containing mostly clear fluid.

5. *(b) Complete molar pregnancy*

   Explanation: Complete molar pregnancy grossly looks like clotted blood and pink-red tissue fragments with small clear sacs filled with clear fluid often referred to as "grape-like clusters." Therefore "(b)" is correct. Benign endometrium is tan-pink and hemorrhagic, often with clotted blood. Incomplete molar pregnancy grossly looks like clotted blood and pink-red tissue with identifiable fetal parts such as skin, hands, feet, organs, etc. Clotted blood is dark red-brown and markedly friable when touched.

6. *(d) Villous tissue*

   Explanation: Villous tissue is tan-white finger-like projections that have soft, fluffy appearance. This is indicative of conception; therefore, "(d)" is correct. The remaining answers can all be identified in the uterus, but are not indicative of conception. Clotted blood is friable, dense red-brown material often found in the endometrial cavity. Myometrial tissue is the pink muscular wall of the uterus and uterine fibroids are firm, white, whorled nodules often present within the uterine wall.

7. *(a) 1 full cross section of each fallopian tube*

   Explanation: Microscopically, 1 full cross section of each fallopian tube is acceptable to deem the patient sterile. Therefore, "(a)" is correct. Endometrial tissue is pink-red, friable, hemorrhagic and is present in the endometrial cavity. The fimbria whether unilateral or bilateral is not acceptable for a successful sterilization unless a full cross section of the fallopian tube can be taken from the proximal end first. But this answer only contains one fimbria and not both so the patient cannot be considered sterile. Both the right and left fallopian tubes need to be microscopically visualized for complete sterility. Ectocervical mucosa is present on the cervix only and is tan-pink and shiny.

8. *(d) Circumvallate insertion*

   Explanation: Circumvallate insertion is a type of membrane insertion where the membrane folds over itself at the periphery of the placental disc creating a ridge of tan membrane around the disc. Therefore "(d)" is the correct answer. The remaining options are all forms of umbilical cord insertion. Eccentric insertion is insertion into the placental disc. Velamentous insertion is when the umbilical cord inserts into the membrane before spanning onto the placental disc. Marginal insertion is when the umbilical cord inserts directly into the edge of the placental disc.

9. *(c) Loop electrosurgical excision procedure*

Explanation: LEEP (loop electrosurgical excision procedure) is when a physician removes a cone-shaped portion of the cervix using an electrocautery loop. This makes "(c)" the correct answer. The remaining options are all procedures, but they do not remove a cone-shaped portion of the cervix. A hysterectomy is the removal of the uterus. A cervical biopsy is the excision of a small fragment(s) of ectocervical mucosa. Oophorectomy is the excision of one or both ovaries.

10. *(b) Lower uterine segment*

    Explanation: The junction of the inferior endometrial cavity and the superior endocervical canal is the lower uterine segment. Therefore "(b)" is correct. The remaining options are anatomic structures or locations, but none are present at the junction of the endometrial cavity and the endocervical canal. The parametrium is the large fascia that extends from the outer aspect of the endocervical stroma and attaches to the pelvic wall. The cervical os is the junction of the ectocervical mucosa and the inferior aspect of the endocervical canal. The uterine fundus is the superior aspect of the uterus.

References

1. "FirstPath," 2009–2023. [Online]. Available: https://www.firstpathlab.com/cpt-codes/. Accessed August 2023.
2. "College of Americal Pathologists," December 2022. [Online]. Available: https://www.cap.org/protocols-and-guidelines/cancer-reporting-tools/cancer-protocol-templates. Accessed July 2023.
3. "National Cancer Institute," 19 November 2020. [Online]. Available: https://www.cancer.gov/about-cancer/causes-prevention/genetics/brca-fact-sheet. Accessed 21 August 2023.

Grossing of Ear, Nose, and Throat Specimens

9

Contents

Head and neck specimens can be the most complicated of all surgical pathology. No two cases are alike, and many contain multiple anatomic structures. Keeping orientation from start to finish is necessary as the gross description is the most important supplement to the histologic sections. There are many different CPT codes for ENT so refer to Table 9.1 for the CPT code list.

Table 9.1 CPT codes [1]

Tonsil and/or adenoids	88300 (gross only), 88304 (microscopic)
Nasal mucosa biopsy	88305
Nasopharynx/oropharynx biopsy	88305
Parathyroid	88305
Salivary gland biopsy	88305
Sinus, paranasal biopsy	88305
Thyroglossal duct/brachial cleft cyst	88305
Tongue biopsy	88305
Tonsil biopsy	88305
Trachea biopsy	88305
Salivary gland	88307
Larynx, partial/total resection	88307
Lymph nodes regional resection	88307
Salivary gland	88305 (Biopsy), 88307 (Resection)
Thyroid, total/lobe	88307
Larynx, partial. Total resection with regional lymph nodes	88309
Tongue/tonsil, partial/total resection for tumor	88309
Mandible	88309
Maxilla	88309
Decalcification (list separately in addition to codes for surgical pathology specimen, each count)	88311

9.1 Head and Neck Mucosal Biopsies: Level III CPT 88305

Biopsies of the head and neck include biopsies from the skin, mucosa, bone, and soft tissue from different locations within the head and neck structures. Only mucosal biopsies are discussed here.

Typically, mucosal biopsies are received as multiple unoriented fragments. These specimens are submitted entirely. However, if bone fragments are palpated within the aggregate, separate the bone from the soft tissue and decal the cassette containing the bone only.

Step 1: Describe and measure the specimen. In Fig. 9.1a, there are 3 fragments with a collective measurement.

Step 2: Submit the specimen entirely as shown in Fig. 9.1b. Use a biopsy bag if the specimen is small.

Example Dictation

Specimen A is received in formalin labeled with the patient's name, medical record number, "right true vocal cord" and consists of 3 fragments of irregular, pink-red tissue (1.2 × 0.8 × 0.3 cm) which is submitted in toto in a biopsy bag in A1.

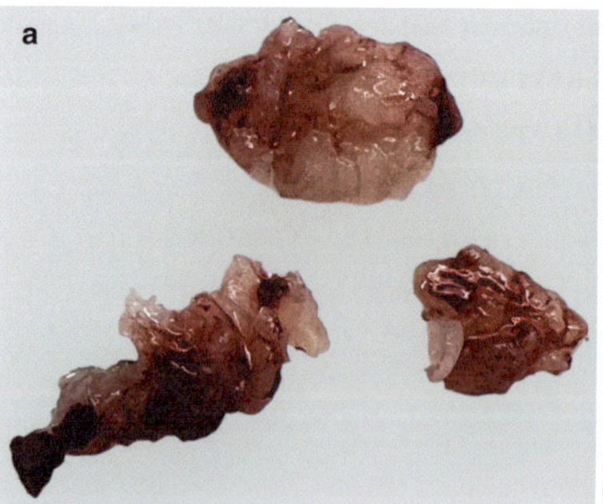
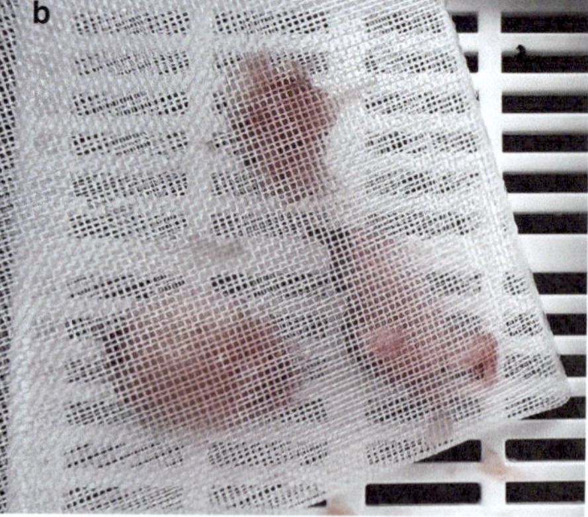

Fig. 9.1 (**a**) Right true vocal cord biopsy; (**b**) right true vocal cord biopsy submission

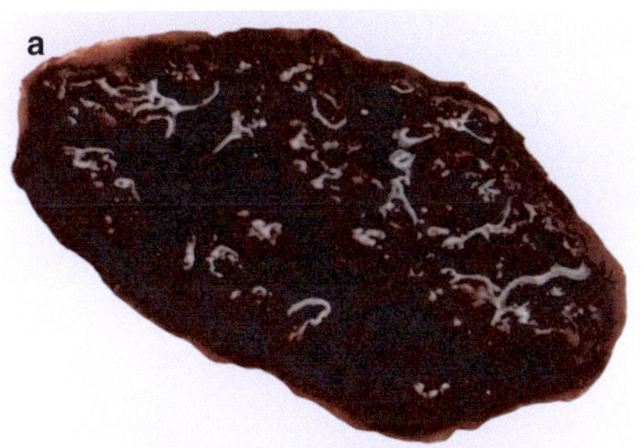

Fig. 9.2 (**a**) Sinus contents; (**b**) sinus contents section submission

9.2 Sinus Contents: Level III CPT 88305

Using an endoscope, sinus contents including mucus, blood, mucosa, and bone are removed to open the passage into the sinuses allowing for better drainage and ventilation for patients with chronic sinusitis.

Step 1: Aggregate the sinus contents. The aggregate can be very minimal to a marked amount.

Step 2: Describe and measure the aggregate as shown in Fig. 9.2a.

Step 3: Submit sections. If the specimen can be submitted entirely in 3-5 cassettes, then submit entirely shown in Fig. 9.2b. Do not ignore or forget the mucoid material – include it in the submission. If the aggregate is larger, then communicate with the pathologist for section submission.

Example Dictation

Specimen A is received in formalin labeled with the patient's name, medical record number, "sinus contents" and consists of an aggregate of markedly hemorrhagic, red-brown tissue fragments (2.2 × 1.9 × 0.3 cm) which is submitted entirely in a biopsy bag in A1.

9.3 Nasopharynx/oropharynx Excision: Level III CPT 88307

A nasopharyngeal/oropharyngeal excision is the removal of a lesion from within the nasopharyngeal/oropharyngeal region. These excisions are typically received oriented and can be handled similarly to a skin excision.

Step 1: Describe and measure the specimen. In this example, the specimen is oriented with a long stitch designating superior and a short stitch designating medial. Fig. 9.3a is the mucosal surface of the excision, and Fig. 9.3b is the deep margin, designated with a blue.

Step 2: Measure the lesion and measure the distance of the lesion to the surrounding peripheral margins.

Step 3: Ink the margins. In Fig. 9.4a, the superior, inferior, medial, and lateral ink is shown and Fig. 9.4b shows the deep margin inked as follows:

Blue: superior
Green: inferior
Orange: lateral
Red: medial
Black: deep

Step 4: Serially section the specimen. In Fig. 9.5, the specimen is serially sectioned from lateral to medial.

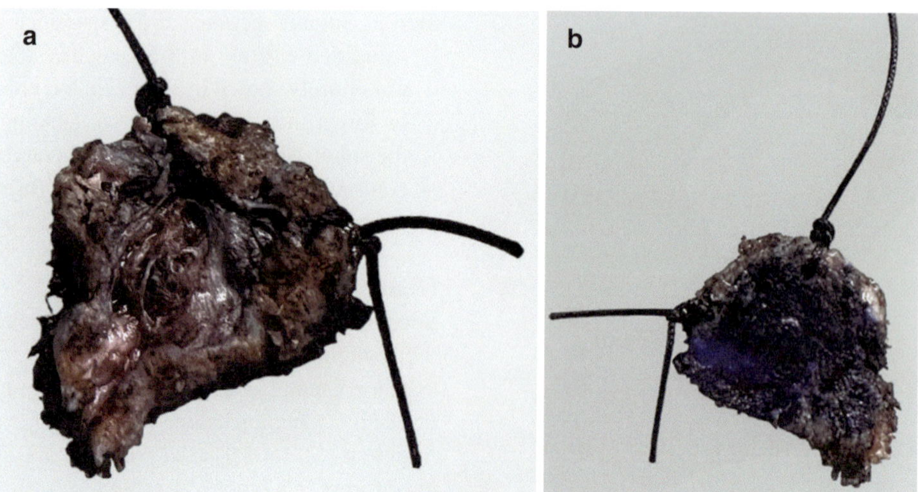

Fig. 9.3 (**a**) Nasopharyngeal excision mucosal surface; (**b**) nasopharyngeal excision deep surface

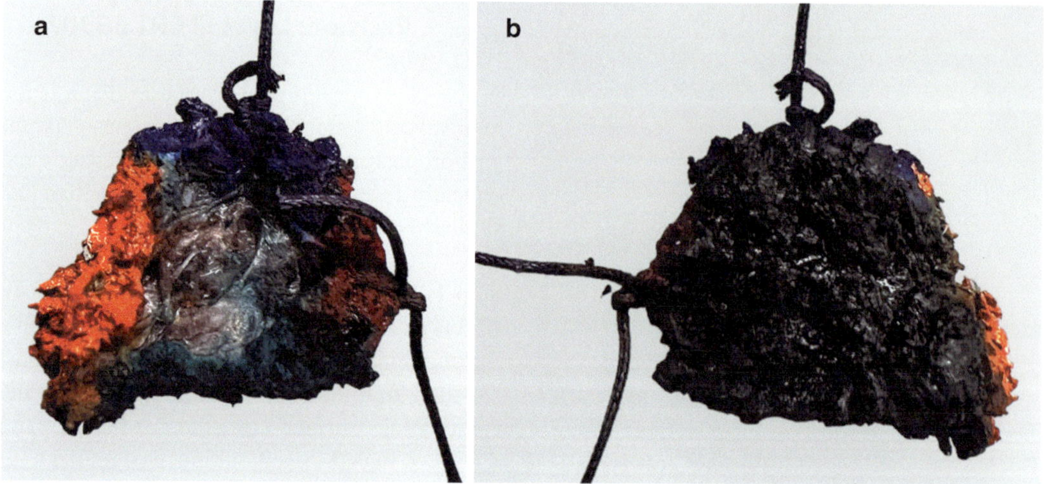

Fig. 9.4 (**a**) Peripheral ink; (**b**) deep ink

Step 5: Measure the greatest depth of invasion and how close the lesion comes from the deep margin. The greatest depth of invasion is designated by a red arrow in Fig. 9.5.

Step 6: Perpendicularly section the end margins as shown in Fig. 9.6. This allows for microscopic measurement of the lesion to the end margins.

Step 7: Submit the specimen entirely as shown in Fig. 9.7. Most nasopharyngeal excisions are small and can be submitted entirely. Communicate with the pathologist, if necessary.

Example Dictation

Specimen A is received in formalin labeled with the patient's name, medical record number, "nasopharyngeal mass" and consists of an excision of tan-brown, irregular, cauterized mucosa (2.1 × 1.8 × 0.6 cm) oriented with a long stitch designating superior, a short stitch designating medial and blue ink designating the deep margin. The mucosal surface contains a markedly ill-defined, ulcerative red-brown lesion (0.7 × 0.4 cm) which comes within 0.4 cm of the superior, medial, and inferior mucosal margins and 0.5 cm from the lateral mucosal margin. The specimen is

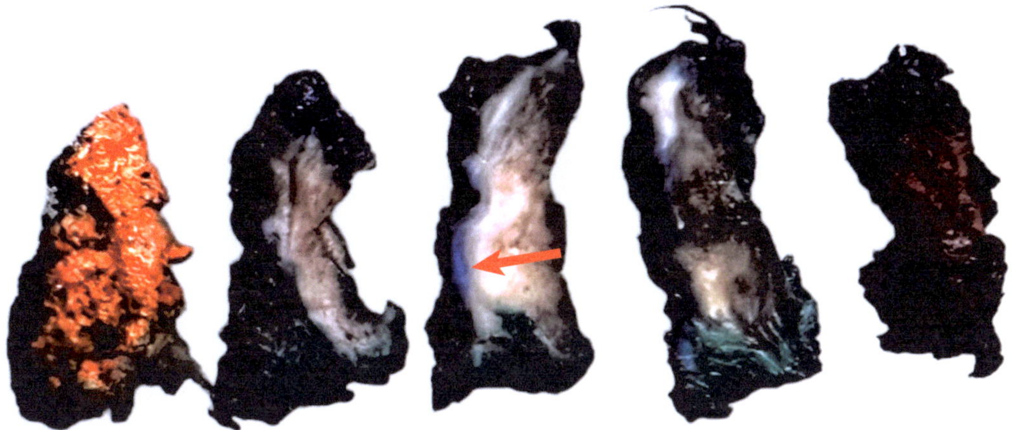

Fig. 9.5 Excision serially sectioned

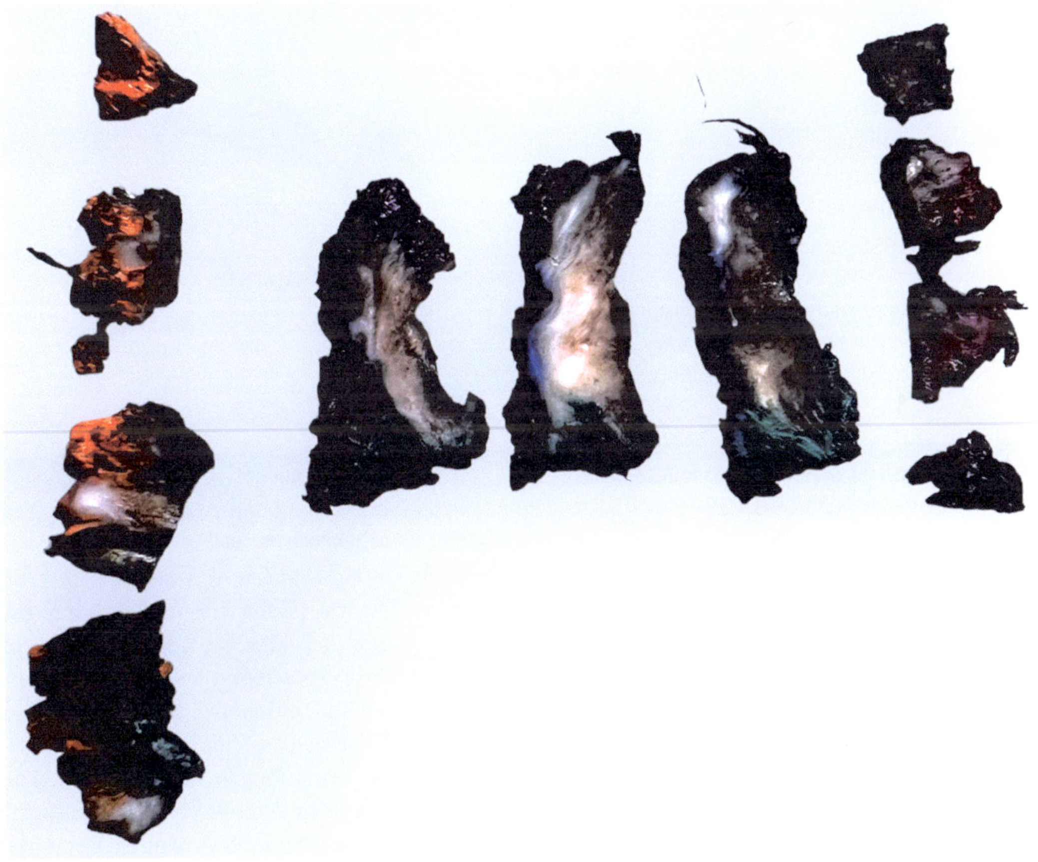

Fig. 9.6 End margins perpendicularly sectioned

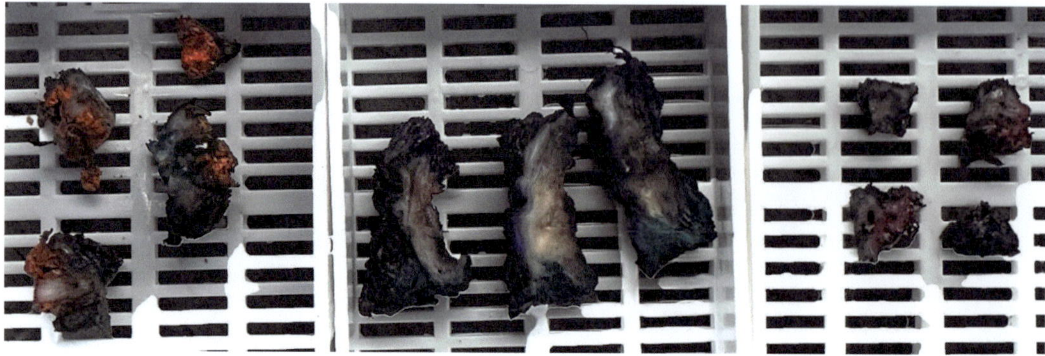

Fig. 9.7 Nasopharyngeal excision section submission

serially sectioned from lateral to medial to reveal the greatest depth of invasion of 0.5 cm, coming within 0.1 cm of the deep margin.

Ink code
> Blue: superior
> Green: inferior
> Orange: lateral
> Red: medial
> Black: deep

Section code
> A1: Lateral margin, perpendicular
> A2: Body of specimen, entirely
> A3: Medial margin, perpendicular

9.4 Floor of the Mouth Excision: Level VI CPT 88309

The floor of the mouth excisions often contains multiple anatomic structures or partial structures depending on the extent of the disease. Keeping strong orientation while grossing these specimens is crucial to obtain appropriate margins and to be able to stage the cancers appropriately.

Step 1: Orient, describe, and measure the specimen. Often these specimens are not obvious in orientation. Communication with the surgeon is key in these cases. A couple of helpful tricks we have used in our practice and commonly in the grossing room include – imagining the resected specimen in one's own mouth to figure out the anatomical landmarks. The sur-

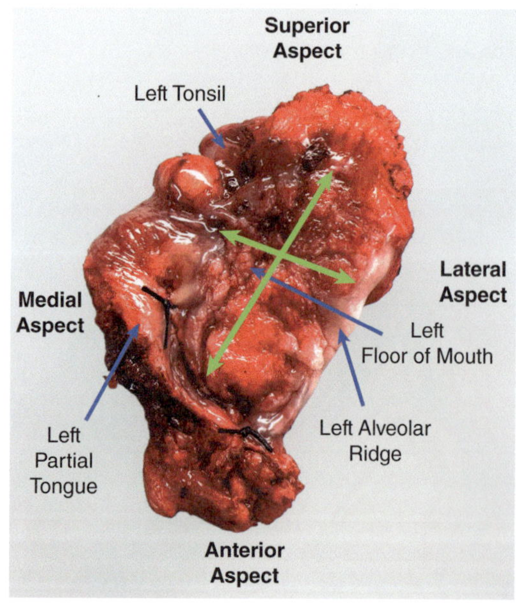

Fig. 9.8 Floor of mouth excision

geons always prefer identification of the margin as a "left alveolar ridge" or "floor of mouth" instead of simply "lateral" or "medial." Figure 9.8 is a floor of mouth excision containing alveolar ridge mucosa, floor of mouth mucosa, left lateral partial tongue, and left tonsil. The slight superior to anterior curve in the specimen represents the in vivo relationship in the mouth.

Step 2: Describe and measure the lesion. In Fig. 9.8, the lesion is identified with green arrows.

Step 3: Measure the lesion to all peripheral mucosal margins.

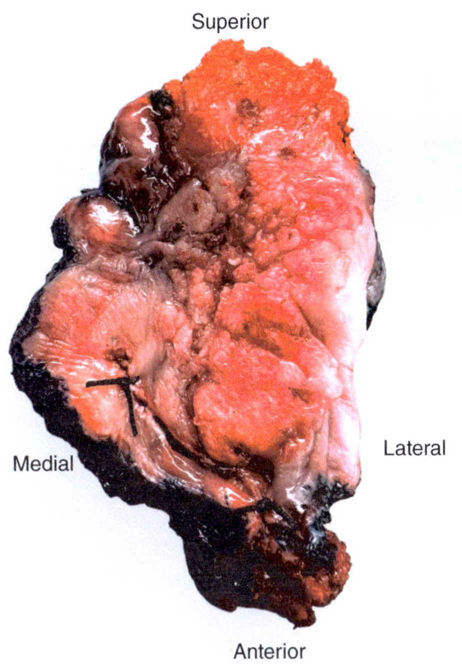

Fig. 9.9 Floor of mouth excision, margins inked

Step 4: Ink the margins. In Fig. 9.9, the ink code is as follows:

    Orange: superior
    Red: anterior
    Blue: medial
    Green: lateral
    Black: deep

Step 5: Serially section the specimen. In Fig. 9.10, the specimen is serially sectioned from superior to anterior.

Step 6: Perpendicularly section the end margins as shown in Fig. 9.11.

Step 7: Identify and measure the greatest depth of invasion of the lesion and measure how close the lesion comes to the deep margin.

Step 8: The end margins are submitted perpendicularly and in this example the slices between are submitted entirely. If the specimen is large, communicate with the pathologist and submit the slices where the lesion is closest to the remaining margins and shows the maximum depth of invasion. Ideally along with the perpendicular margins, at least 2 full face sections are recommended to be able to evaluate the

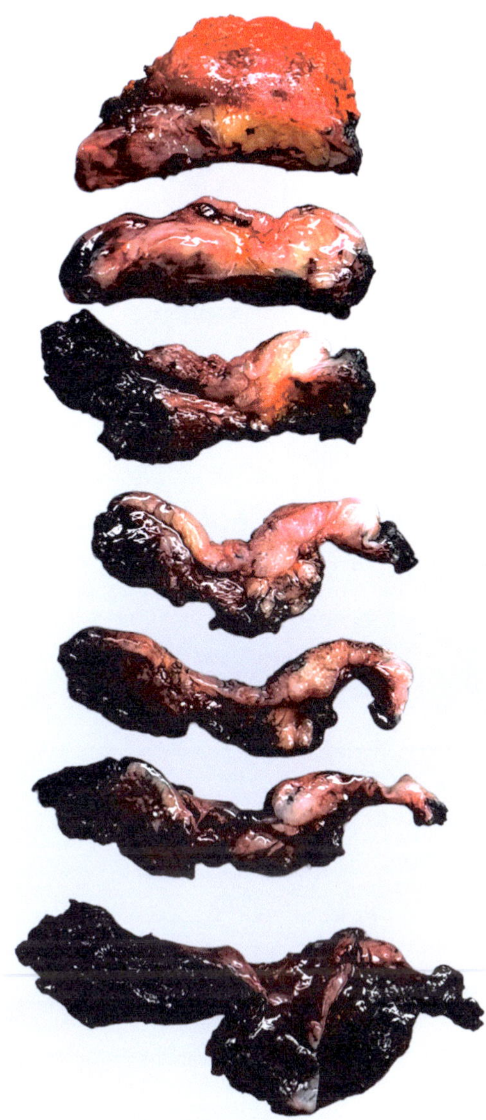

Fig. 9.10 Floor of mouth specimen serially sectioned

depth of invasion in addition to perineural and lymphovascular invasion which are easier to find at the invasive edge of the tumor.

Example Dictation

Specimen A is received in formalin labeled with the patient's name, medical record number, "left floor of mouth excision" and consists of a pink-red, left floor of mouth excision (7.3 × 4.2 × 1.0 cm) containing left tonsil (1.9 × 1.1 × 1.0 cm), left partial tongue (2.9 × 1.9 × 1.5 cm), floor of mouth,

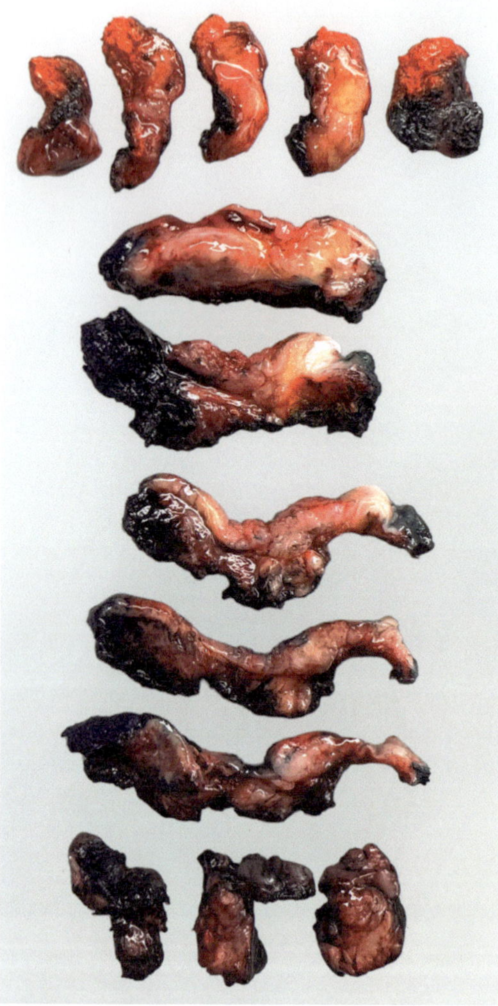

Fig. 9.11 Floor of mouth specimen, perpendicular end margins

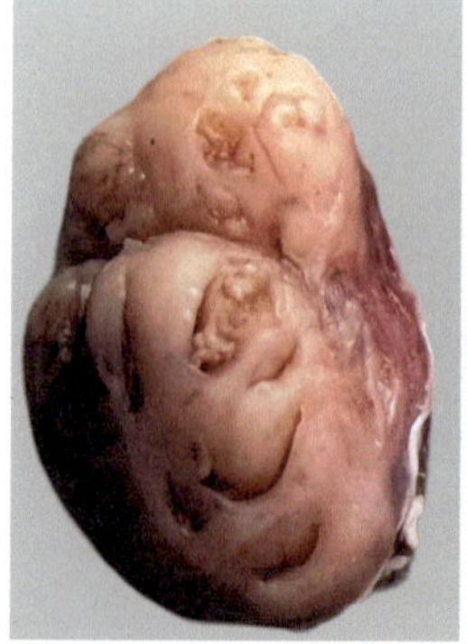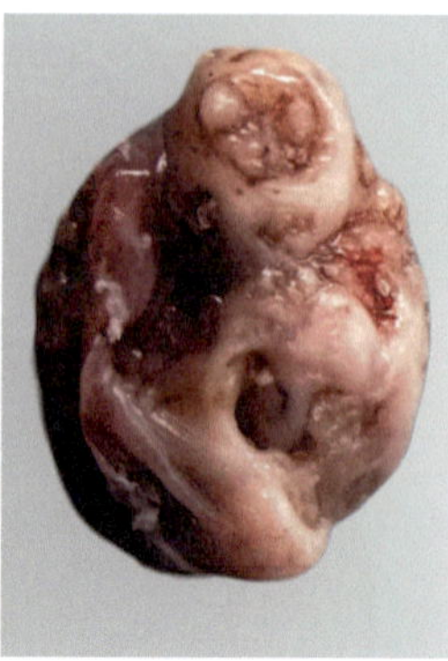

Fig. 9.12 Unoriented tonsils

and left alveolar ridge. The floor of mouth contains a papillary, tan-pink, slightly raised lesion (4.8 × 2.8 cm) which comes within 1.1 cm from the superior mucosal margin, 1.5 from the anterior mucosal margin, 1.9 cm from the medial mucosal margin, and 0.7 cm from the lateral mucosal margin. The specimen is serially sectioned to reveal a greatest depth of invasion of 0.7 cm, coming within 0.1 cm from the deep margin.

Ink code

> Orange: superior
> Red: anterior
> Blue: medial
> Green: lateral

Black: deep

Section code

> A1-A2: Superior margin, perpendicular
> A3-A7: Body of specimen, entirely from superior to anterior
> A8-A9: Anterior margin, perpendicular

9.5 Tonsil, Benign—Level III CPT 88304

Tonsils can be sent to the lab to assess for hyperplasia, cancer, and lymphoma. It is common practice per hospital to treat tonsils under a certain age as gross only specimens. Always be mindful of tonsils that are designated as gross only. If a lesion is identified in such tonsil, sections should be submitted even if it is a gross only specimen. Tonsils that are sent to the lab fresh should first be assessed for possible lymphoma workup before placing the tonsils in formalin.

Step 1: Describe, measure, and weigh each tonsil (Fig. 9.12)

Step 2: Ink the resection margin of each tonsil as shown in Fig. 9.13.

Step 3: Serially section each tonsil as seen in Fig. 9.14.

Step 4: Describe the cut surfaces.

Step 5: Submit a representative section of each unoriented tonsil as shown in Fig. 9.15.

To keep minimal orientation, each tonsil margin can be inked a different color. This is beneficial if a

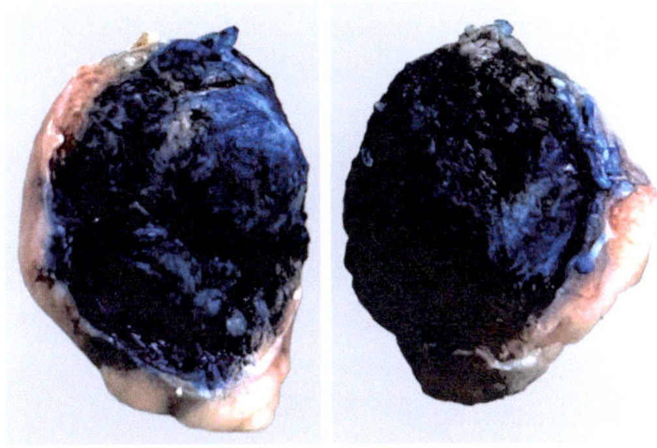

Fig. 9.13 Unoriented tonsils, margins inked

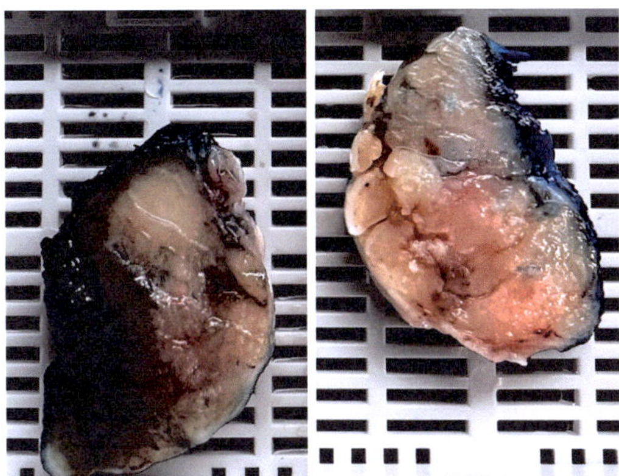

Fig. 9.15 Unoriented tonsil section submission

Example Dictation

Specimen A is received in formalin labeled with the patient's name, medical record number, "bilateral tonsils" and consists of 2 unoriented tan-pink tonsils (2.2 × 1.6 × 1.0 cm, 2 g and 2.3 × 1.7 × 1.1 cm, 2 g). The resection margin of each tonsil is inked blue, and both tonsils are serially sectioned to reveal tan-pink cut surfaces with crypt architecture. A representative section of each tonsil is submitted in A1-A2.

9.6 Radical Tonsillectomy— Level CPT 88309

A radical tonsillectomy is performed for malignancy of the tonsil and includes the tonsil and often additional surrounding mucosa and soft tissue. Radical tonsillectomies can also be performed when a positive lymph node in the head and neck is identified without a known primary lesion. When a lymph node is identified, the tonsils and the floor of the mouth are assessed first for identification of the primary malignancy. These tonsils are often received oriented by the surgeon and margins need to be assessed during grossing and sign out. Pay close attention to the appearance of the tonsil lesion. If the lesion appears fleshy, communicate with the pathologist for possible lymphoma before proceeding.

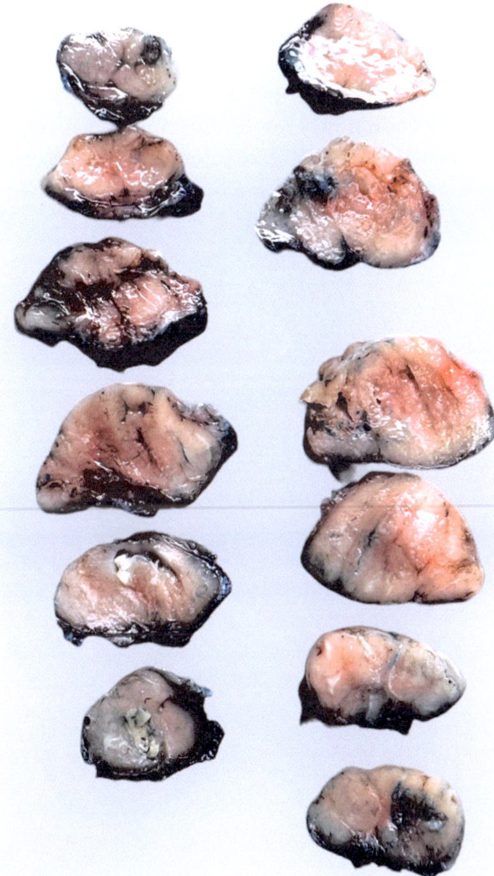

Fig. 9.14 Unoriented tonsils, serially sectioned

lesion is identified on one tonsil. The remainder of the tonsil with the specific ink can then be submitted without needing to submit the other tonsil.

Step 1: Orient the tonsil. In Fig. 9.16, two surgical clips designate the superior margin of the left tonsil.

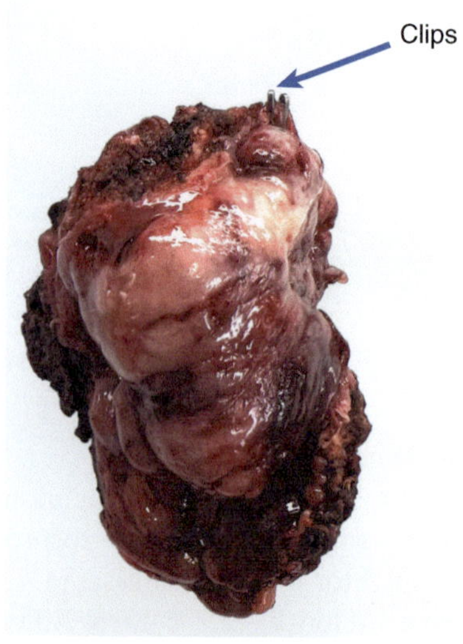

Fig. 9.16 Radical tonsillectomy

Step 2: Describe, measure, and weigh the tonsil.

Step 3: Ink the margins of the tonsil. Figure 9.17a shows the superficial aspect of the inked tonsil, and Fig. 9.17b shows the deep aspect of the inked tonsil. The ink code is as follows:

> Red: superior
> Orange: inferior
> Blue: medial
> Green: lateral
> Black: deep

Step 4: Serially section the tonsil. In Fig. 9.18a, the tonsil is serially sectioned from superior to inferior.

Step 5: Perpendicularly section the ends margins. In Fig. 9.18b, the superior and inferior end margins are perpendicularly sectioned. Perpendicularly sectioning the end margins allows for gross and microscopic measurement of the lesion in relation to the margins.

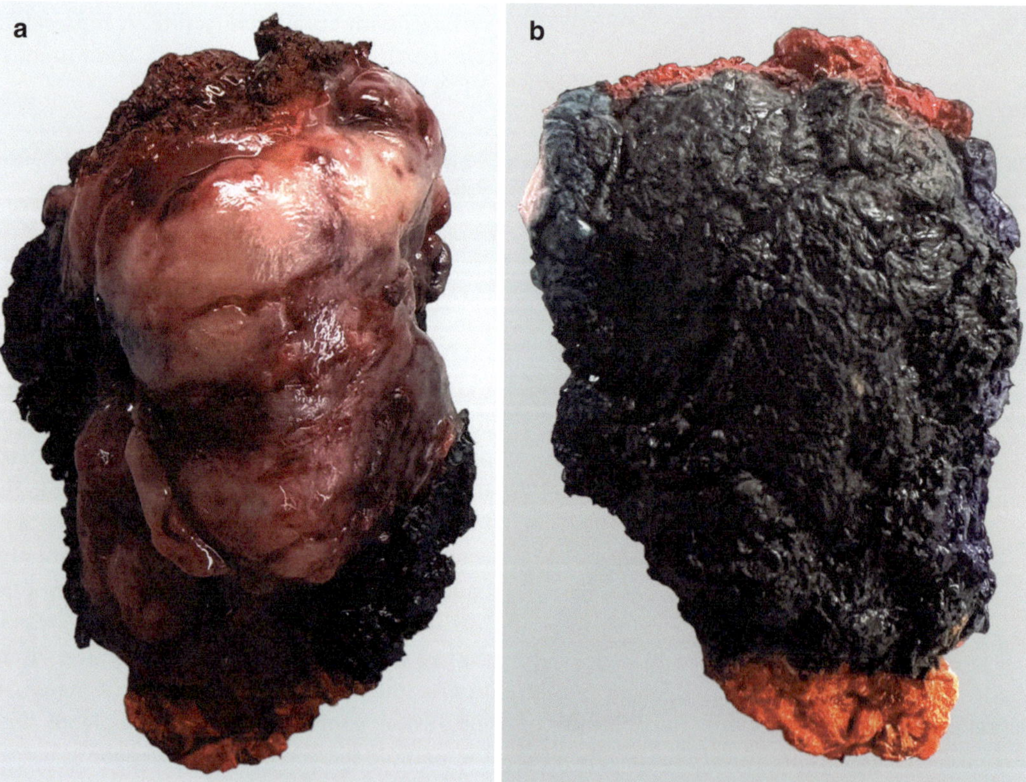

Fig. 9.17 (**a**) Tonsil ink, superficial view; (**b**) Tonsil ink, deep view

Step 6: Describe and measure the lesion. In this example, the lesion is identified by blue arrows in Fig. 9.18a.

Step 7: Measure the lesion to all margins.

Step 8: In tonsils, the identification of the tumor on gross examination may be challenging and therefore if not easily seen, the specimen should be submitted entirely. In Fig. 9.19, the specimen is serially sectioned after submission of the perpendicular margins followed by the remaining slices.

Example Dictation

Specimen A is received in formalin labeled with patient's name, medical record number, "left radical tonsil" and consists of an enlarged, tan-pink tonsil with surrounding soft tissue (5.9 × 3.4 × 2.6 cm) oriented per the surgeon with clips designating superior. The specimen is serially sectioned to reveal a tan-white, solid mass (2.9 × 2.2 × 1.9 cm) which comes within 0.2 cm of the superior mucosal margin, 1.6 cm from the inferior mucosal margin, 0.5 cm from the lateral

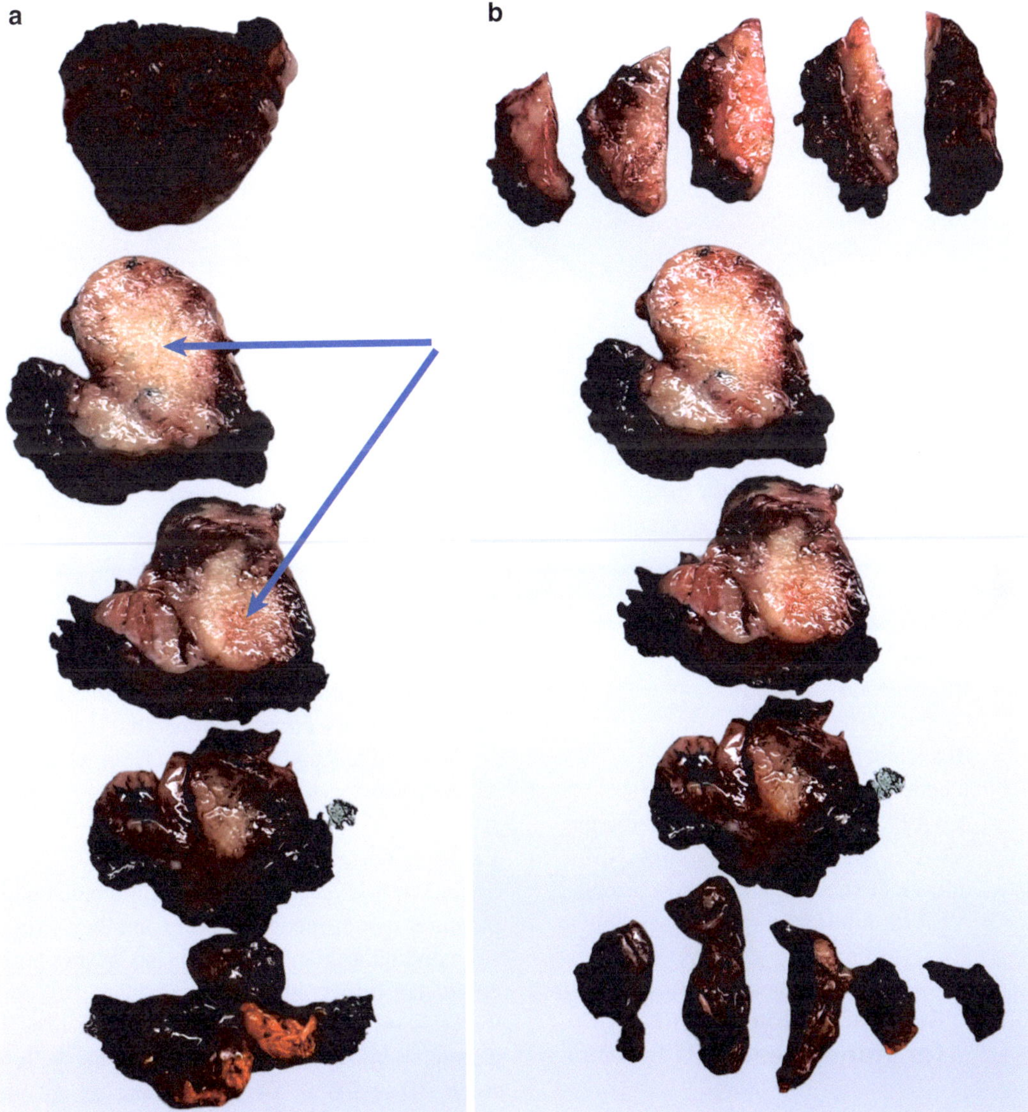

Fig. 9.18 (**a**) Tonsil serially sectioned; (**b**) Tonsil end margins perpendicularly

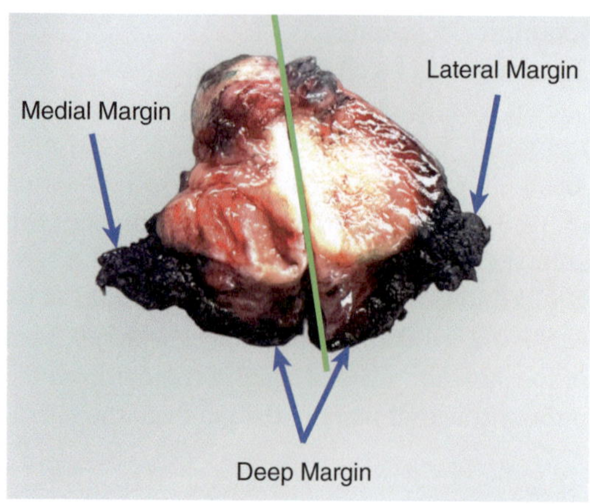

Fig. 9.19 Tonsil section bisected

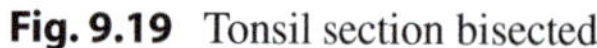

Fig. 9.20 Submandibular gland

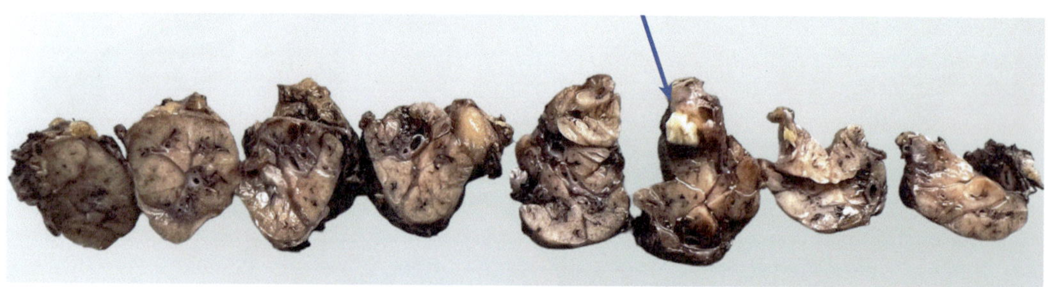

Fig. 9.21 Submandibular gland serially sectioned, containing a stone

mucosal margin, 1.4 cm from the medial mucosal margin, and 0.2 cm from the deep margin.

Ink code
>	Red: superior
>	Orange: inferior
>	Blue: medial
>	Green: lateral
>	Black: deep

Section code
>	A1-A2: Superior margin, perpendicular
>	A3-A8: Tonsil entirely from superior to inferior (1 slice per 2 cassettes, bisected)
>	A9-A10: Inferior margin, perpendicular

9.7   Submandibular Gland for Stones: Level CPT 88300

Submandibular glands are usually removed as part of a neck dissection but can also be separately removed for benign and malignant lesions or stones.

Step 1: Describe and measure the submandibular gland(Fig. 9.20)

Step 2: Serially section the gland as shown in Fig. 9.21.

Step 3: Describe the cut surface of the gland and identify and describe the lesion or stone. The stone is identified by the blue arrow in Fig. 9.21.

Step 4: Submit sections. Remove the stone from the gland and submit sections from where the stone was located.

Example Dictation

Specimen A is received in formalin labeled with patient's name, medical record number, "right submandibular gland" and consists of an unoriented, tan-brown gland (3.9 × 2.2 × 2.1 cm) which is serially sectioned to reveal tan-brown, glandular cut surfaces with a single pale-yellow stone (07 × 0.5 × 0.4 cm) present along one unoriented margin. Representative sections of the gland with the stone capsule are submitted in A1.

9.8 Parotid Gland Unoriented: Level V CPT 88307

The parotid gland is removed for both benign and malignant primary tumors of the salivary gland or possible metastasis to the parotid gland. These specimens can come oriented or unoriented and should be sliced thinly to assess for both tumors and lymph nodes within the parotid gland. The description of the mass in the salivary gland must include details on its circumscription versus infiltrative nature, and involvement of extraglandular soft tissue. If the mass looks like a pleomorphic adenoma (myxoid in appearance), and the patient has a history of rapid growth, look for any area of fibrosis and scarring and submit sections. If the specimen can be submitted entirely within 10 cassettes, do so.

Step 1: Describe, measure, and weigh the specimen. In Fig. 9.22a, the gland is unoriented.
Step 2: Ink the specimen. In Fig. 9.22b, the unoriented gland is entirely inked blue.
Step 3: Serially section the specimen.
Step 4: Describe and measure the mass and how close the mass comes to the closest unoriented margin. In Fig. 9.23, the mass is designated by blue arrows.
Step 5: Assess the gland for lymph node candidates.
Step 6: Submit sections. In this example, the mass is small and is submitted entirely with an extra section of unremarkable parotid gland.

Example Dictation

Specimen A is received in formalin labeled with the patient's name, medical record number, "left parotid gland" and consists of an unoriented, ragged, tan-brown gland (6.8 × 4.3 × 2.0 cm, 12 g) which is entirely inked blue and serially sectioned to reveal a single, encapsulated mass with yellow-tan, friable cut surfaces which comes within 0.1 cm of the nearest unoriented margin. The remainder of the cut surfaces is tan-brown and glandular with no identifiable lymph node candidates.

Section code:
A1-A3: Mass, entirely
A4: Gland, representative

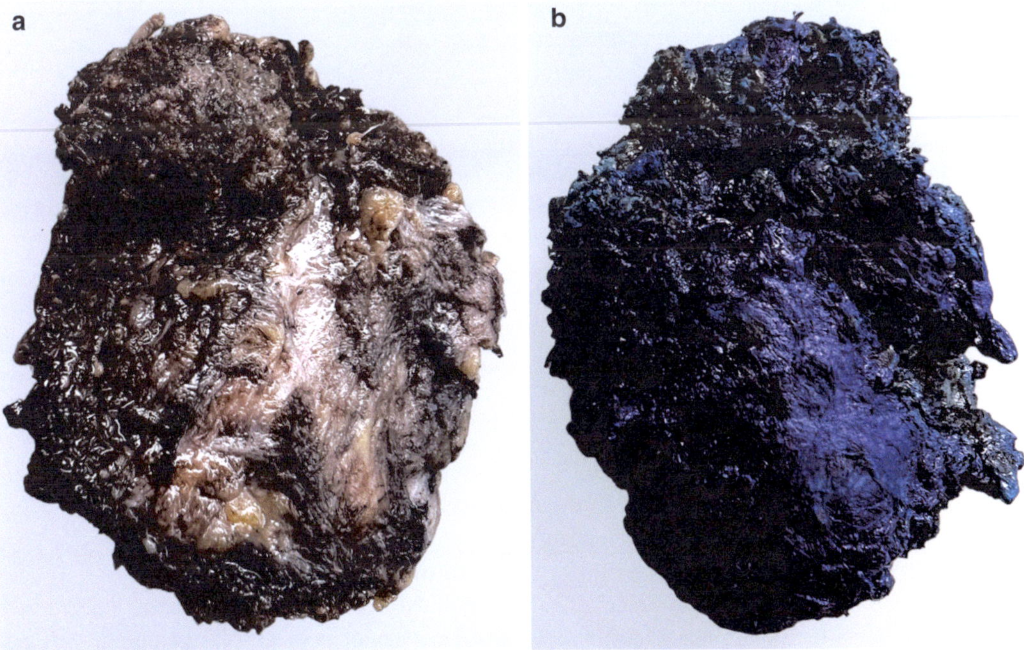

Fig. 9.22 (**a**) Parotid gland unoriented; (**b**) parotid gland inked

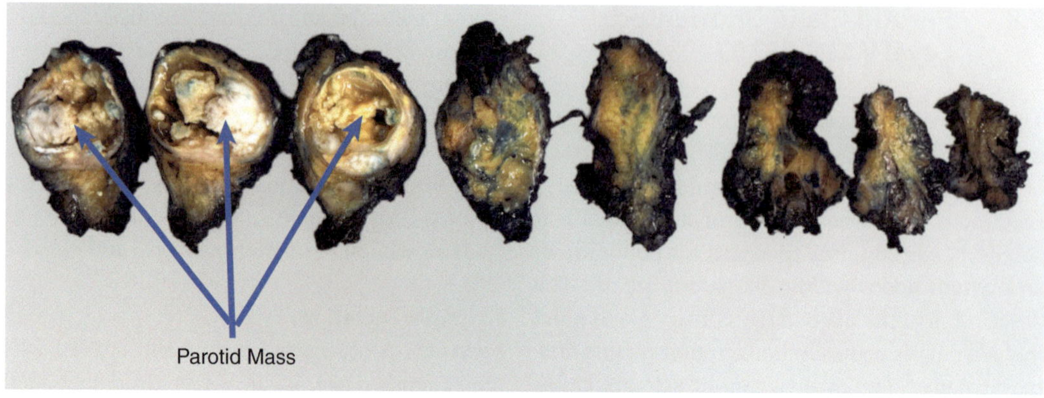

Fig. 9.23   Parotid gland serially sectioned

9.9   Oriented Parotid Gland: Level V CPT 88307

Grossing a parotid gland that is oriented includes a few more steps than an unoriented parotid gland. However, measurements of the mass in relation to the closest margins are the key.

Step 1: Describe, measure, and weigh the specimen.

Step 2: Orient the specimen. In Fig. 9.24, the gland is oriented with a short stitch designating superior and a long stitch designating anterior.

Step 3: Ink the specimen. Figure 9.25a shows the superficial and peripheral inks and Fig. 9.25b shows the deep ink. The ink code is as follows:

> Blue: anterior
> Green: posterior
> Orange: superior
> Red: inferior
> Yellow: superficial
> Black: deep

Step 4: Serially section the specimen perpendicular to the long axis as shown in Fig. 9.26.

Step 5: Describe and measure the lesion in three dimensions. In Fig. 9.27a, the lesion is designated with a blue arrow.

Step 6: Perpendicularly section the superior and inferior margins (end margins). Figure 9.27b shows the superior margin perpendicularly sectioned which will allow the lesion to be measured to the superior margin.

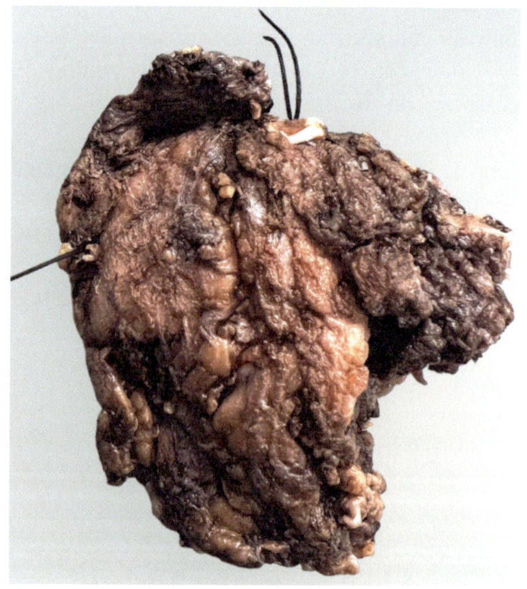

Fig. 9.24   Anterior oriented parotid gland

Step 7: Measure the lesion to all the margins.

Step 8: Describe the remainder of the gland and assess for any lymph nodes that may be present.

Step 9: Section submitted should be the mass in relation to the closest of each margin (Fig. 9.28).

Example Dictation

Specimen A is received in formalin labeled with patient's name, medical record number, "left radical parotidectomy" and consists of a slightly ragged tan-brown gland (6.2 × 5.4 × 2.6 cm, 34 g) oriented with a long stitch designating ante-

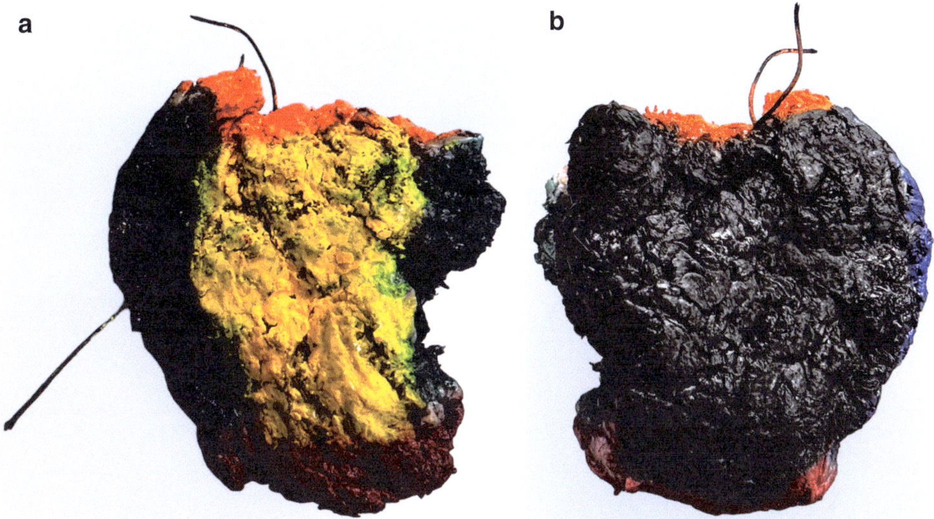

Fig. 9.25 (**a**) Inked parotid anterior view; (**b**) Inked parotid gland posterior view

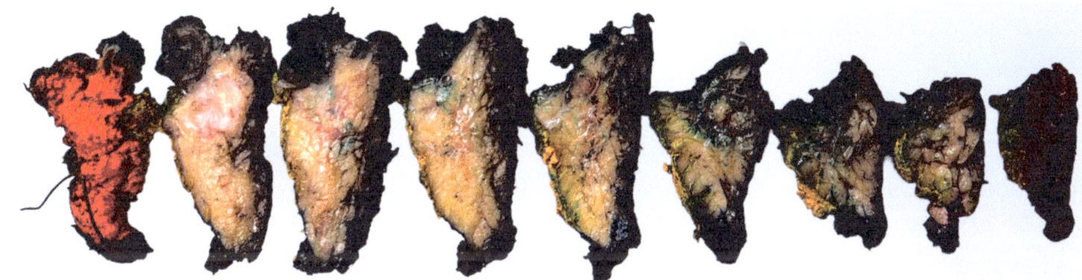

Fig. 9.26 Oriented parotid gland serially sectioned

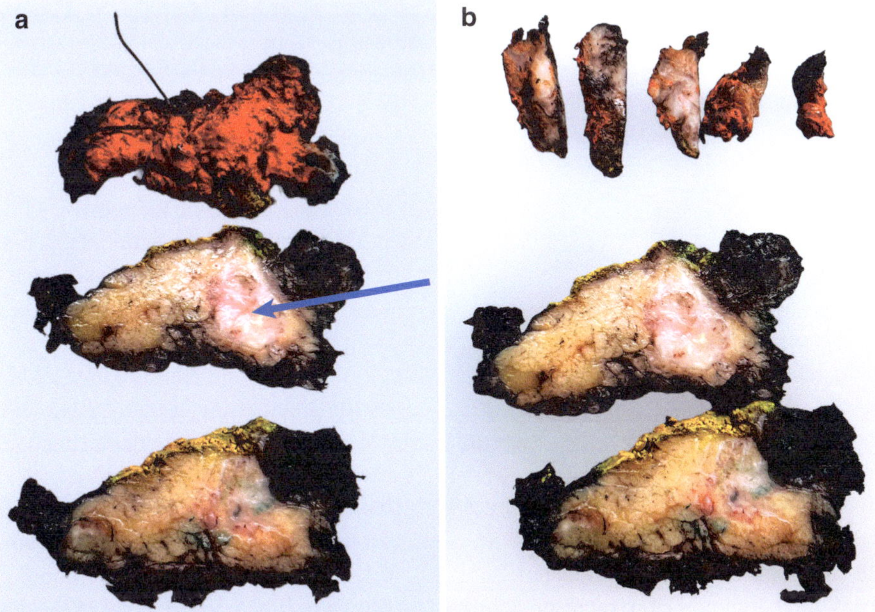

Fig. 9.27 (**a**) Mass in parotid gland; (**b**) superior margin perpendicular

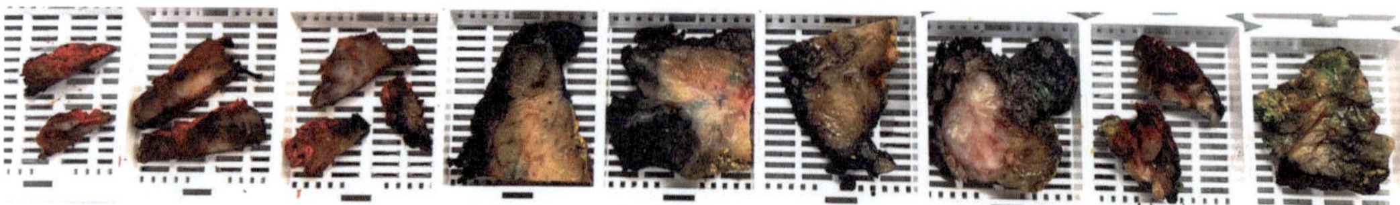

Fig. 9.28 Oriented parotid gland section submission

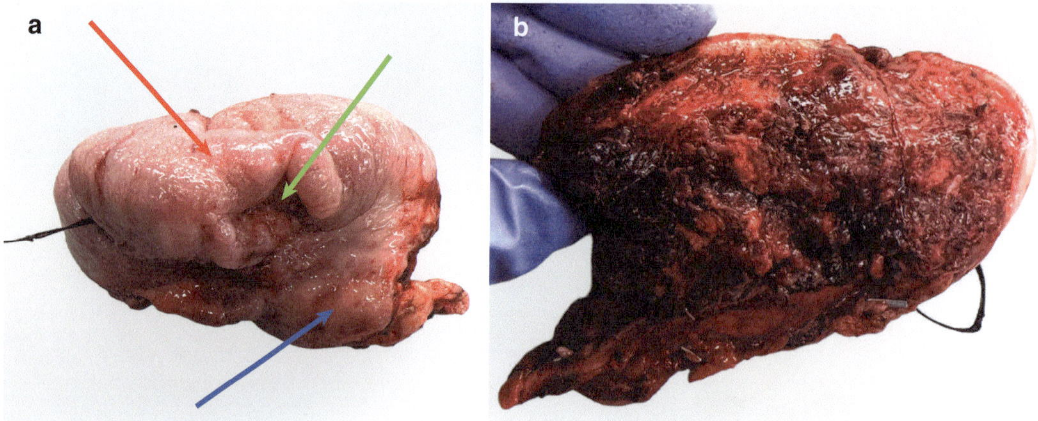

Fig. 9.29 (**a**) Left hemiglossectomy lateral view; (**b**) left hemiglossectomy medial view

rior and a short stitch designating superior. The specimen is serially sectioned to reveal a tan-white, ill-defined lesion (1.5 × 1.4 × 1.0 cm) which comes within 0.3 cm of the superficial margin, 0.2 cm from the deep margin, 2.6 cm from the anterior margin, 0.5 cm from the posterior margin, 0.2 cm from the superior margin, and 4.6 cm from the inferior margin. The remaining cut surfaces are tan-brown and glandular with no additional lesions identified.

Ink code
    Blue: anterior
    Green: posterior
    Orange superior
    Red: inferior
    Yellow: superficial
    Black: deep
Section code
    C1-C4: Mass in relation to superior margin
    C5-C 8: Mass entirely (1 slice per 2 cassettes, bisected)
    C 9: Inferior margin, perpendicular
    C10: Unremarkable gland, representative

9.10 Hemiglossectomy: Level VI CPT 88309

A hemiglossectomy is the excision of approximately half of the tongue and can include surrounding mucosal structures such as floor of mouth mucosa or alveolar ridge mucosa.

Step 1: Orient the specimen. In Fig. 9.29a, the stitch designates anterior tongue of the left hemiglossectomy. Figure 9.29b shows the medial margin of the tongue.

Step 2: Describe and measure the specimen. The red arrow in Fig. 9.29a designated the left tongue, and the blue arrow designates the left floor of mouth.

Step 3: Describe and measure the lesion as noted by the green arrow in Fig. 9.29a.

Step 4: Measure how close the lesion comes to all the mucosal margins. Mucosal margins include anterior tongue, posterior tongue, dorsal tongue, anterior floor of mouth, lateral floor of mouth, and posterior floor of mouth as shown in Fig. 9.30. Margins of head and neck

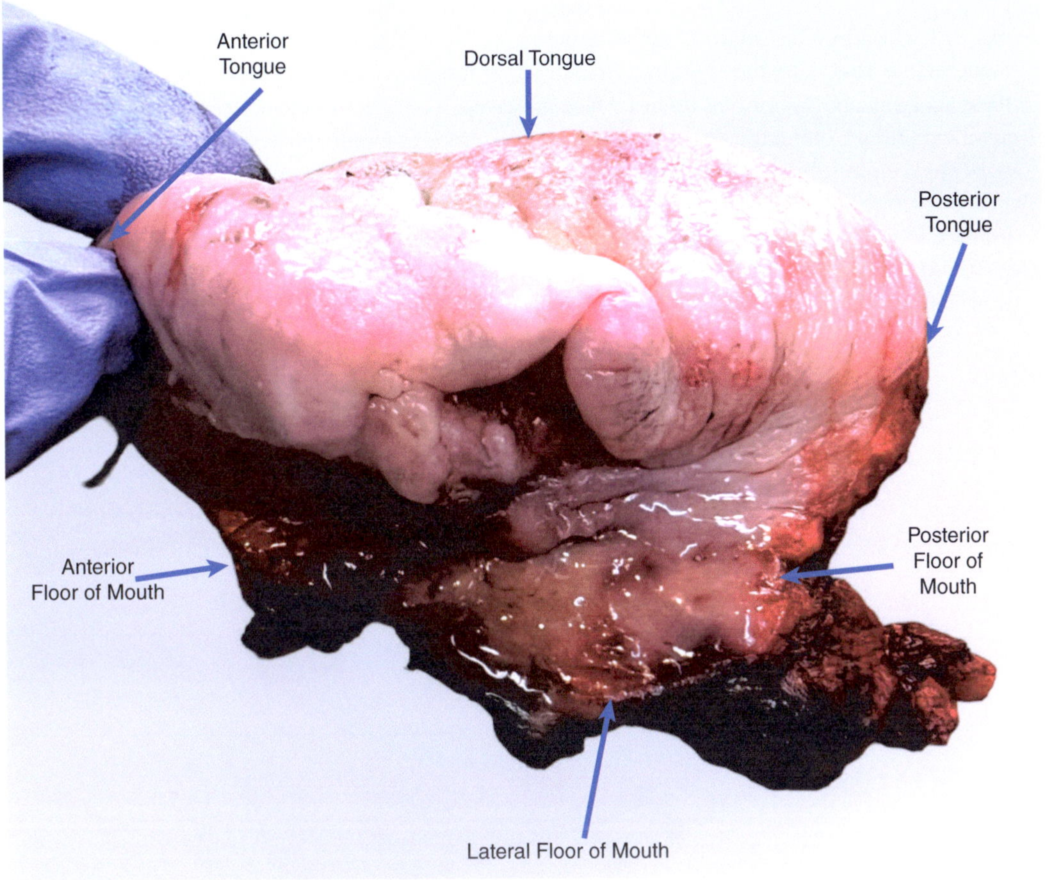

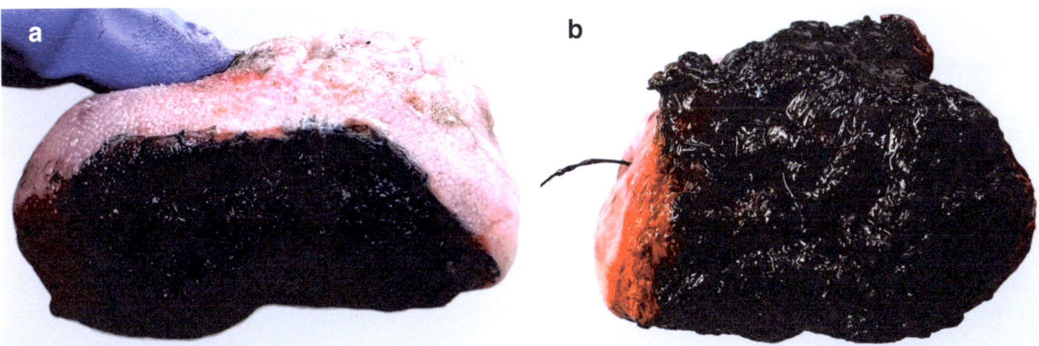

Fig. 9.30 Left hemiglossectomy lateral view with ink

Fig. 9.31 (**a**) Left hemiglossectomy medial view with ink; (**b**) left hemiglossectomy inferior

specimens are numerous, and keeping orientation is absolute key to grossing the specimen.

Step 5: Ink the anterior, lateral, and posterior margins as shown in Fig. 9.30.

Step 6: Ink the medial (Fig. 9.31a) and inferior (Fig. 9.31b) margins.

Step 7: Serially section the specimen from anterior to posterior. Lay each slice flat and keep orientation.

Step 8: Perpendicularly section the anterior tongue, anterior floor of mouth, posterior tongue, and posterior floor of mouth as shown in Fig. 9.32. Perpendicularly sectioning these margins will allow for microscopic measurement of the lesion to the margins. Shaving these margins and submitting them en face is another option. Communicate with the pathologist for section submission.

Step 9: Describe and measure the lesion in 3 dimensions.

Step 10: Measure how close the lesion comes from the soft tissue margins. In this example, the soft tissue margins are anterior tongue and floor of mouth, posterior tongue and floor of mouth, medial tongue, and inferior tongue.

Step 11: Submit the anterior tongue, anterior floor of mouth, posterior tongue, and posterior floor of mouth perpendicular margins.

Step 12: Submit 1 or 2 full cross sections of the tongue with the closest margins. In Fig. 9.33, the margins included are lateral floor of mouth mucosa and soft tissue (blue arrow), inferior

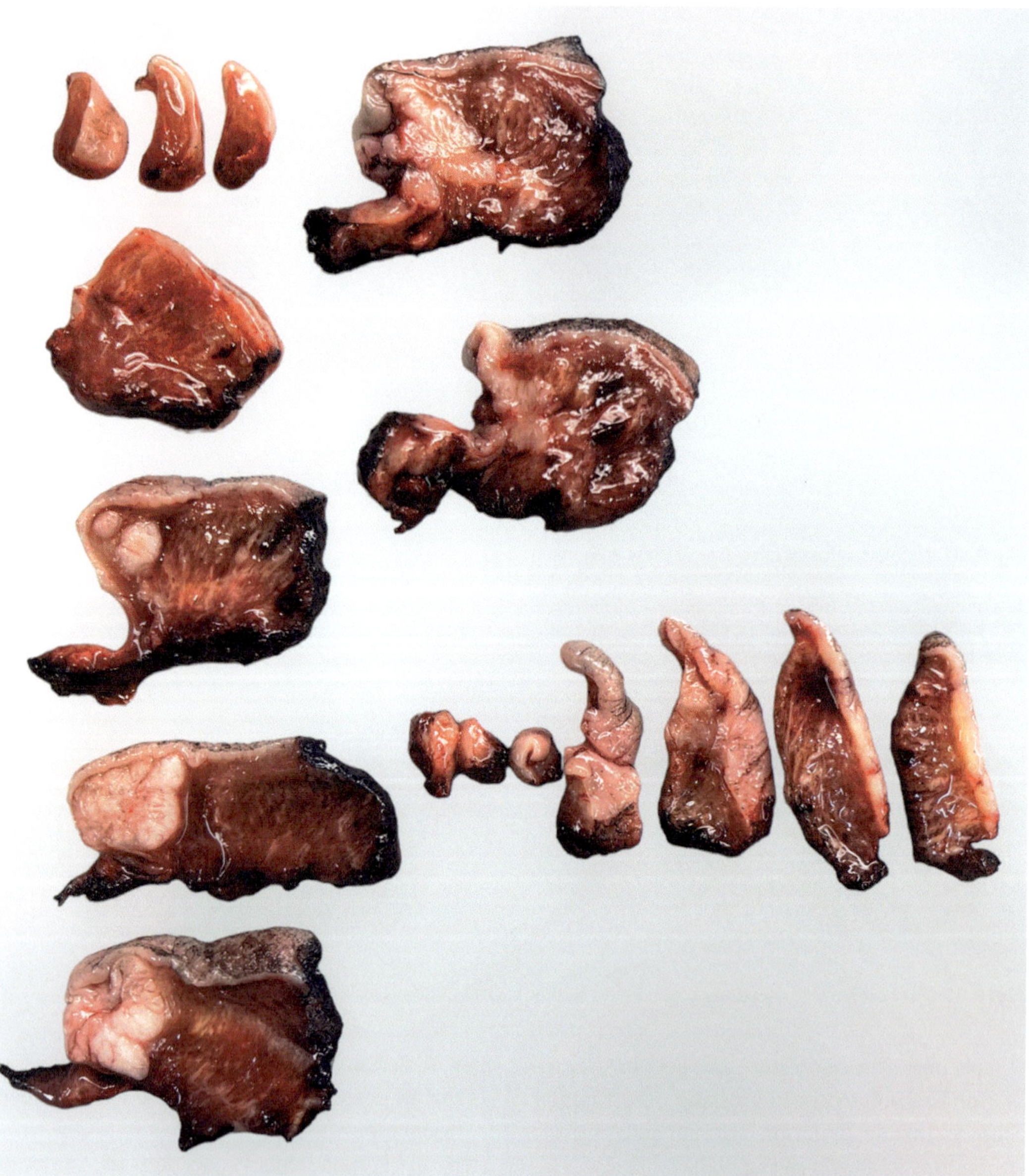

Fig. 9.32 Left hemiglossectomy serially sectioned

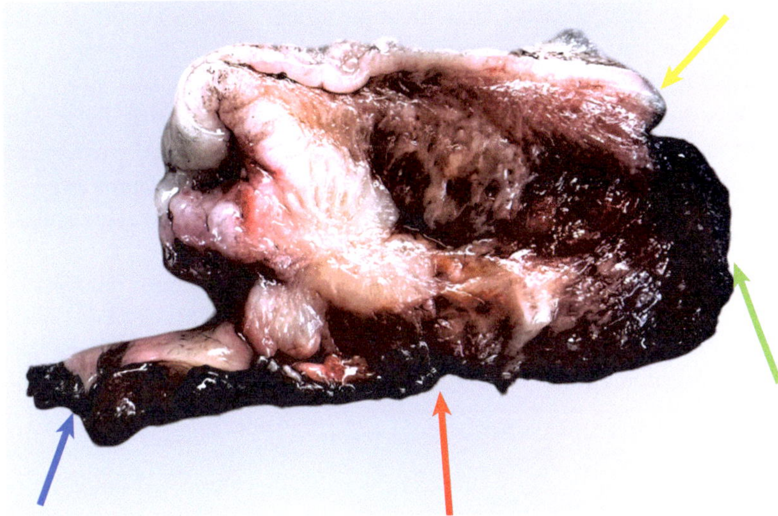

Fig. 9.33 Left hemiglossectomy slice with mass

soft tissue (red arrow), dorsal tongue mucosa (orange arrow), and medial tongue soft tissue (green arrow). Often these slices will need bisected or trisected to fit in the cassettes.

Example Dictation

Specimen A is received fresh for intraoperative consultation labeled with patient's name, medical record number, "left hemiglossectomy" and consists of a left hemiglossectomy ($7.1 \times 4.4 \times 3.2$ cm) with left lateral attached floor of mouth (4.2×1.6 cm) and a stitch designating anterior. At the lateral tongue is an ulcerative tan-pink lesion (2.6×2.0 cm) which is centrally ulcerated with raised borders. The lesion comes within 2.1 cm from the dorsal tongue mucosal margin, 0.4 cm from the lateral floor of mouth mucosal margin, 0.5 cm from the anterior floor of mouth mucosal margin, 1.9 cm from the posterior floor of mouth mucosal margin, 2.9 cm from the anterior tongue, and 2.5 cm from the posterior tongue mucosal margin. The specimen is serially sectioned to reveal a greatest depth of invasion approximately 1.6 cm, coming within 2.2 cm of the medial margin and 0.3 cm from the inferior/deep margin

Ink code
  Blue: medial tongue
  Red: posterior tongue and posterior floor of mouth
  Green: lateral

Orange: anterior tongue and anterior floor of mouth
Black: inferior

Section code
  A1: Anterior floor of mouth, perpendicular
  A 2: Posterior floor of mouth, perpendicular
  A3: Posterior tongue margin, perpendicular
  A4-A6: Frozen section remnant fullface section of lesion with greatest depth of invasion and closest lateral, inferior/deep and medial margins, trisected from lateral to medial.
  A7-A9: Fullface section of tongue from lateral to medial
  A10-A12: Fullface section of tongue from lateral to medial
  A13: Anterior tongue, perpendicular (no tumor present)

9.11   Neck Mass: Level CPT 88307

A neck mass excision is an ambiguous term for the excision of many benign or malignant tumors or other lesions like enlarged/infected lymph nodes, metastatic lesions, and developmental anomalies within the neck. No matter the pathology, excision with clear margins is the goal.

Step 1: Describe, measure, and orient the specimen. In Fig. 9.34, the specimen is oriented with a short stitch designating superior and a long stitch designating medial.

Step 2: Ink the specimen. In this example, the specimen is inked in 6 colors. Figure 9.35a shows the superficial and peripheral view, and Fig. 9.35b shows the deep view of the specimen. The ink code is as follows:

    Yellow: superficial

    Blue: superior

    Green: inferior

    Orange: medial

    Red: lateral

    Black: deep

Step 3: Serially section the specimen. In Fig. 9.36, the specimen is serially sectioned from superior to inferior.

Step 4: Perpendicularly section the end margins. In this example, the superior (Fig. 9.37) and inferior margins are sectioned perpendicularly.

Step 5: Describe and measure the lesion. In Fig. 9.38, the lesion is the pale, yellow, slightly ill-defined area.

Step 6: Measure the lesion to all the margins.

Step 7: Submit representative sections of the lesion to the closest of each margin. This includes superficial, deep, superior, inferior, medial, and lateral margins.

Example Dictation

Specimen A is received in formalin labeled with the patient's name, medical record number, "left posterior neck mass" and consists of an excision of tan-yellow soft tissue and skeletal muscle (9.2 × 7.8 × 3.1 cm) oriented with a short stitch designating superior and a long stitch designating medial. The specimen is serially section from superior to inferior to reveal a single, pale-yellow,

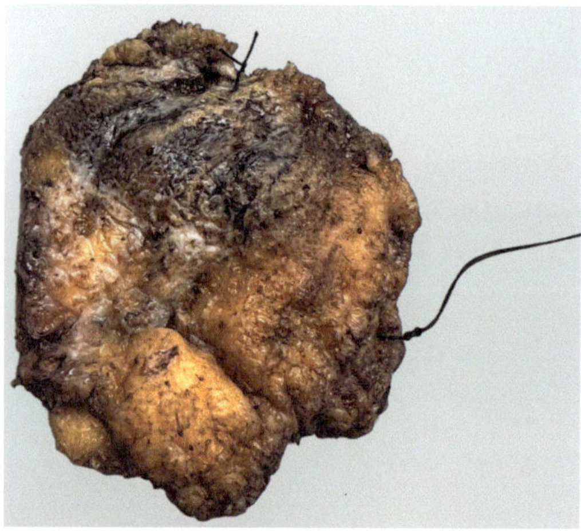

Fig. 9.34 Oriented neck mass excision

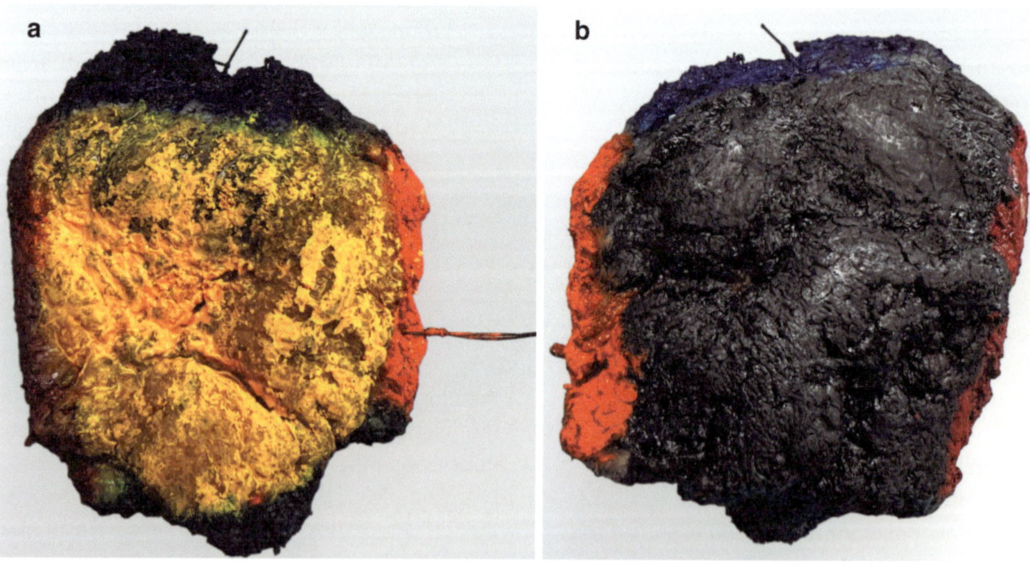

Fig. 9.35 (**a**) Neck mass inked, superficial view; (**b**) neck mass inked, deep view

Fig. 9.36 Neck mass serially sectioned

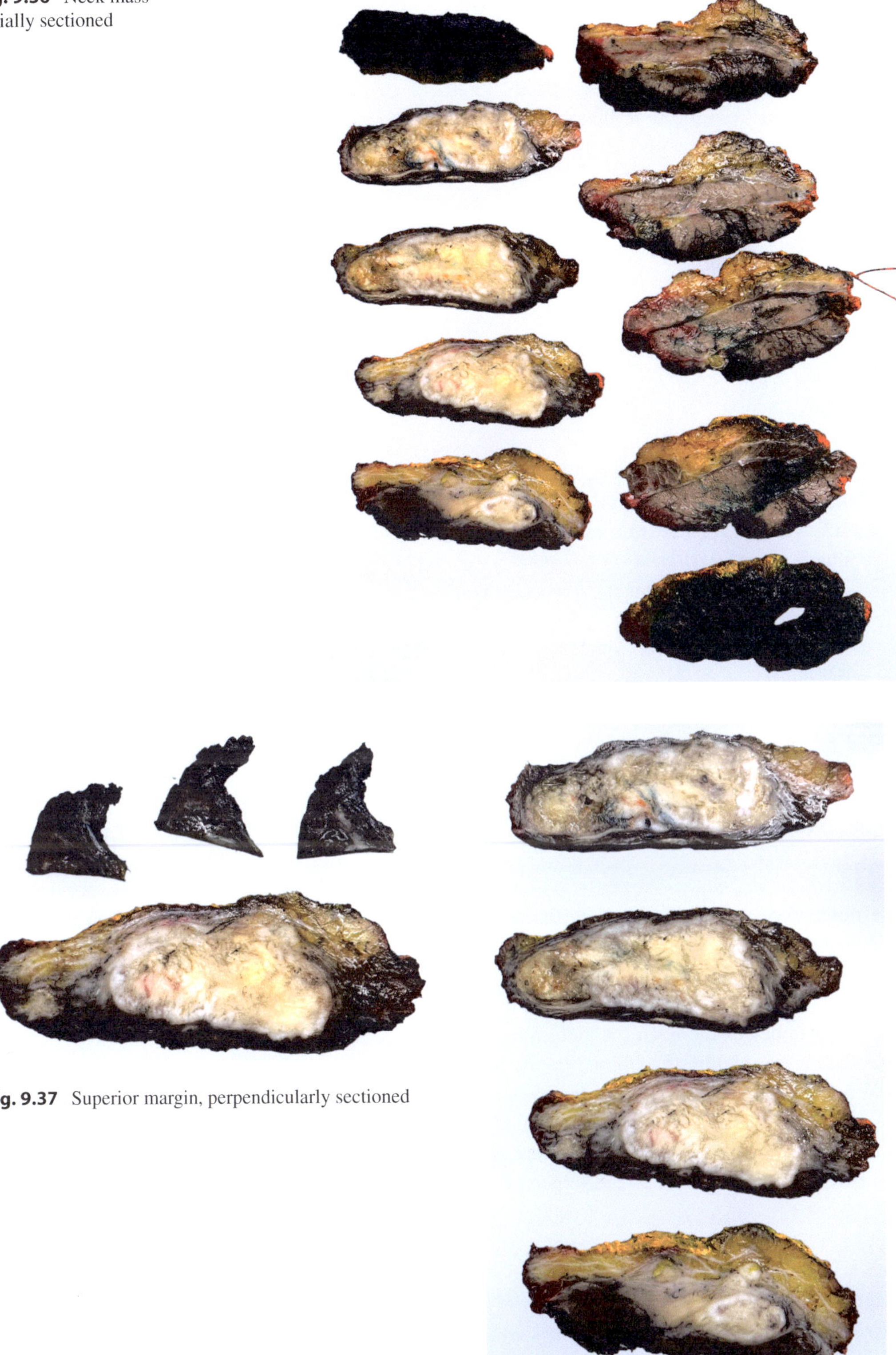

Fig. 9.37 Superior margin, perpendicularly sectioned

Fig. 9.38 Neck mass cut surface of lesion

soft and slightly irregular mass (6.3 × 5.2 × 2.1 cm) which comes within 1.6 cm from the superior margin, 4.1 cm from the inferior margin, 1.1 cm from the medial margin, 1.9 cm from the lateral margin, 0.1 cm from the superficial margin, and 0.2 cm from the deep margin, surrounded by adipose tissue and skeletal muscle.

Ink code

    Yellow: superficial

    Blue: superior

    Green: inferior

    Orange: medial

    Red: lateral

    Black: deep

Section code

    A1: Superior margin, perpendicular

    A2: Inferior margin, perpendicular

    A3: Mass in relation to closest superficial margin

    A4: Mass in relation to closest deep margin

    A5: Mass in relation to closest medial margin

    A6: Mass in relation to closest lateral margin

9.12 Neck Dissection: Level V CPT 88307

The removal of the lymph nodes in the neck is called a neck dissection, and it is a common surgery performed along with many head and neck oncologic resections. The purpose is to assess the lymph nodes of the neck for metastatic disease. If cancer is identified in these lymph nodes, additional treatment such as radiation may be necessary. The neck dissection is oriented by levels, and each level should be oriented or divided into separate levels by the surgeon in the OR (Fig. 9.39).

Step 1: Describe and measure the overall size of the neck dissection.

Step 2: Identify and orient the neck dissection. In Fig. 9.40a, lines are drawn on the specimen and labels are placed to identify each level.

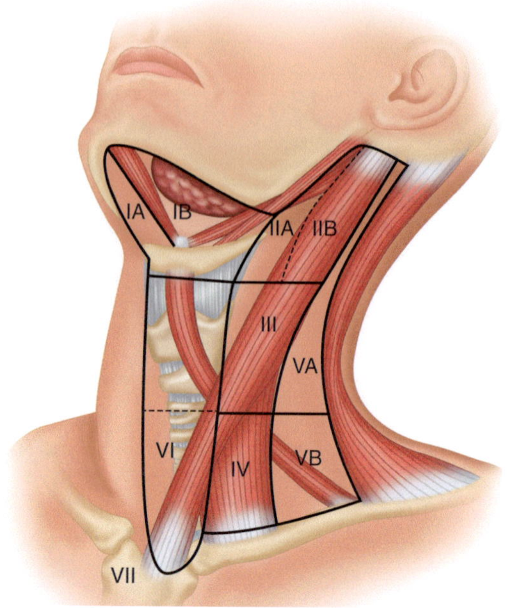

Fig. 9.39 Illustration of neck dissection levels orientation

Step 3: Divide the neck dissection into the designated levels. In Fig. 9.40b, the neck is divided into levels II-V.

Step 4: Palpate and separate each lymph node per level as shown in Fig. 9.41.

Step 5: Section larger lymph nodes. In Fig. 9.42, the large lymph node in level II is sectioned to reveal cystic, soft cut surfaces.

Step 6: Submit all lymph nodes per level as shown in Fig. 9.43. Large lymph nodes that are grossly positive for metastasis can be representatively.

Step 7: Submit the remainder of the adipose tissue after palpating. This step is dependent on the pathologist and presence of the number, size, and laterality of grossly positive lymph nodes. Communicate for instruction. Additionally, level 1 almost always has submandibular salivary gland which if uninvolved and unremarkable (as is in most cases) should be only representatively submitted.

Example Dictation

Specimen A is received in formalin labeled with the patient's name, medical record number, "right neck" and consists of a single fragment of adi-

Fig. 9.40 (**a**) Neck dissection; (**b**) neck dissection divided

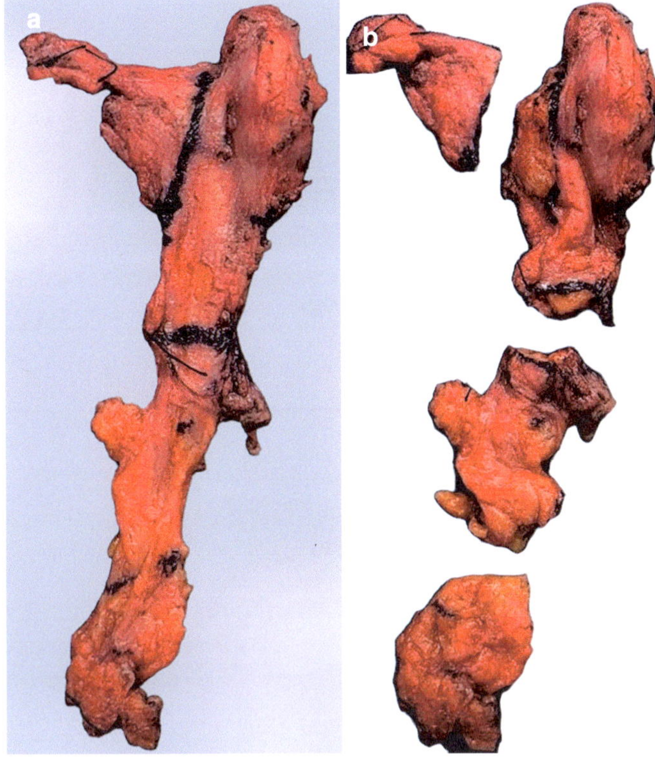

Fig. 9.41 Lymph nodes palpated per level

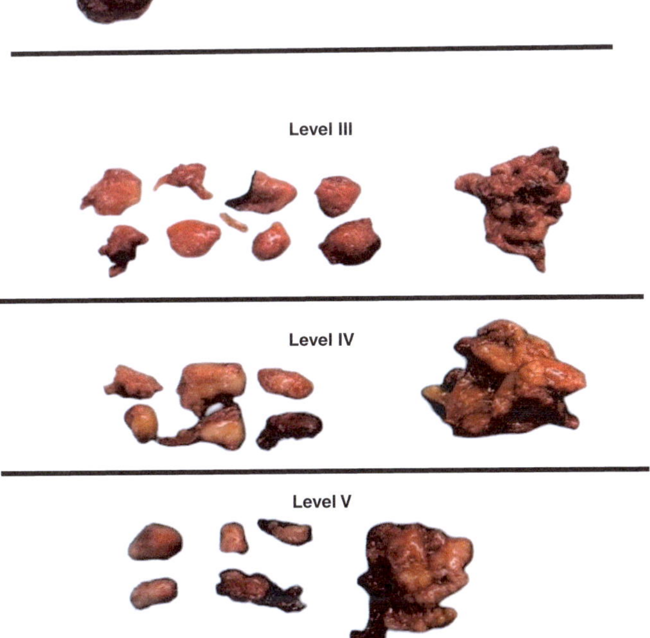

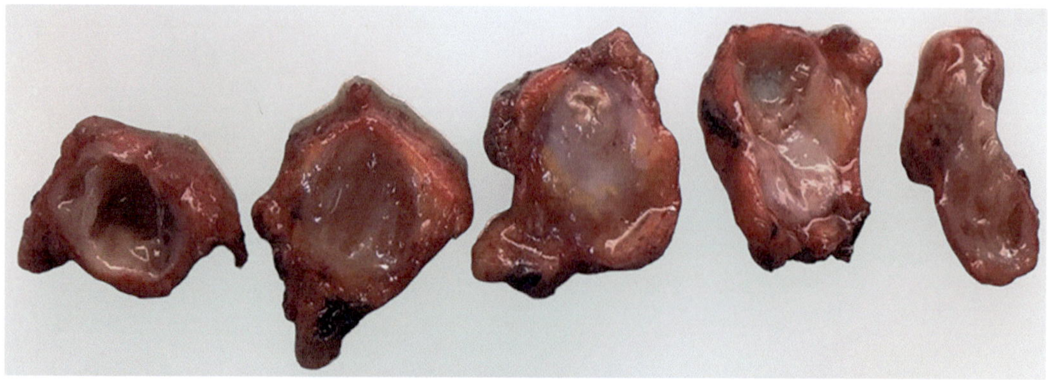

Fig. 9.42 Large lymph node serially sectioned

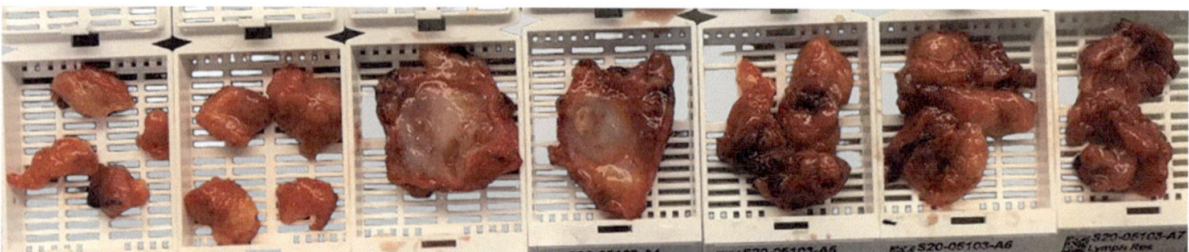

Fig. 9.43 Neck dissection section submission

pose tissue (10.9 × 4.2 × 1.7 cm) oriented per the surgeon into levels II-V. Level II is palpable for 9 lymph node candidates ranging from 0.2 to 2.1 cm. The largest level II lymph node candidate is sectioned to reveal soft, tan-white, cystic cut surfaces. Level III is palpable for 8 lymph node candidates ranging from 0.1 to 2.1 cm. The largest level III lymph node candidate is sectioned to reveal soft, tan-white, cystic cut surfaces. Level IV is palpable for 11 lymph node candidates ranging from 0.2 to 0.7 cm. Level V is palpable for 5 lymph node candidates ranging from 0.3 to 0.6 cm.

Section code

A1-A2: Level II, 3 lymph node candidates per cassette, whole

A3: Level II, 2 lymph node candidates, whole

A4-A5: Level II, 1 large lymph node candidate, representative

A6: Level II, remainder of soft tissue

A7-A8: Level III, 4 lymph node candidates per cassette, whole

A9: Level III, remainder of soft tissue

A10-A11: Level IV, 3 lymph node candidate per cassette, whole

A12: Level IV, remainder of soft tissue

A13: Level V, 3 lymph node candidates, whole

A14: Level V, 2 lymph node candidates, whole

A15: Level V, remainder of soft tissue

9.13 Parathyroid: Level III CPT 88305

Parathyroid is removed due to overactivity called hyperparathyroidism. One or more parathyroid glands can be removed during surgery depending upon the etiology of the hyperparathyroidism. Rarely parathyroid glands can be removed for malignancy,

Step 1: Describe and measure the specimen. Figure 9.44a shows an intact slightly enlarged parathyroid gland.

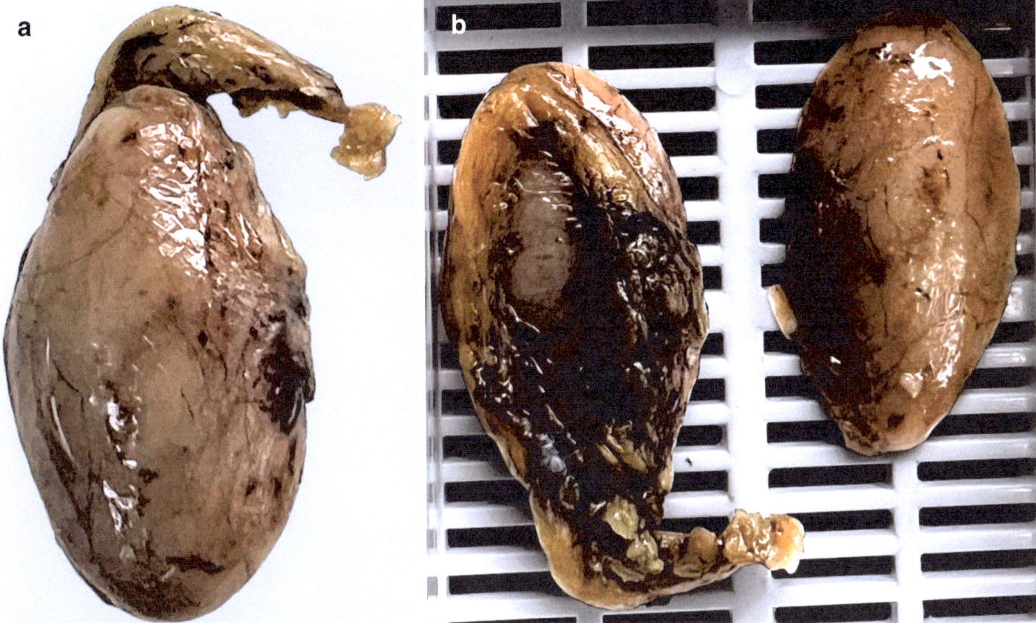

Fig. 9.44 (a) Parathyroid gland; (b) parathyroid gland section submission

Step 2: Weigh the specimen. This requires a scale that is calibrated in milligrams.

Step 3: Submit the parathyroid. If the specimen is large, bivalve the parathyroid gland and submit as shown in Fig. 9.44b.

Example Dictation

Specimen A is received in formalin labeled with the patient's name, medical record number, "right superior parathyroid gland" and consists of an intact, tan-brown parathyroid gland candidate (1.9 × 1.1 × 0.9 cm, 866 mg) which is bivalved to reveal homogenous cut surfaces. The specimen is submitted entirely in A1.

9.14 Thyroglossal Duct Cyst: Level III CPT 88305

A thyroglossal duct cyst is an embryologic remnant that leads to the formation of a cyst in the anterior neck near the hyoid bone due to the failure of the closure of the thyroglossal duct.

Step 1: Describe and measure the specimen. A typical thyroglossal duct cyst contains a small fragment or portion of hyoid bone which is designated by the blue arrow in Fig. 9.45a and attached soft tissue containing the cyst.

Step 2: Ink the specimen entirely. In Fig. 9.45b, the specimen is entirely inked blue.

Step 3: Serially section the specimen perpendicular to the hyoid bone as shown in Fig. 9.46. This will result in hyoid bone and cyst in each section.

Step 4: Describe the cut surface. In Fig. 9.46, there is a multiloculated, intact cyst containing hemorrhagic material.

Step 5: Submit 1 or 2 fullface representative sections as shown in Fig. 9.47. The sections containing hyoid bone will need to be decalcified before submitting.

Example Dictation

Specimen A is received in formalin labeled with patients name, medical record number, "thyroglossal duct cyst" and consists of an unoriented fragment of soft tissue (3.1 x 2.0 x 1.8 cm) with attached segment of hyoid bone (1.1 x 0.8 x 0.5 cm). The specimen is entirely inked blue and serially sectioned to reveal a multiloculated cystic space (2.1 x 1.5 cm) filled with red-brown material. Representative sections are submitted in A 1- A 2, post decalcification.

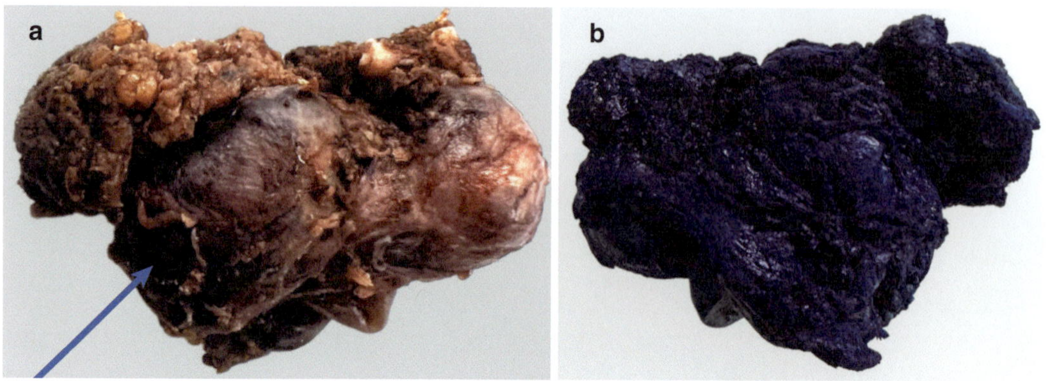

Fig. 9.45 (a) Thyroglossal duct cyst; (b) thyroglossal duct cyst inked

Fig. 9.46 Thyroglossal duct cyst serially sectioned

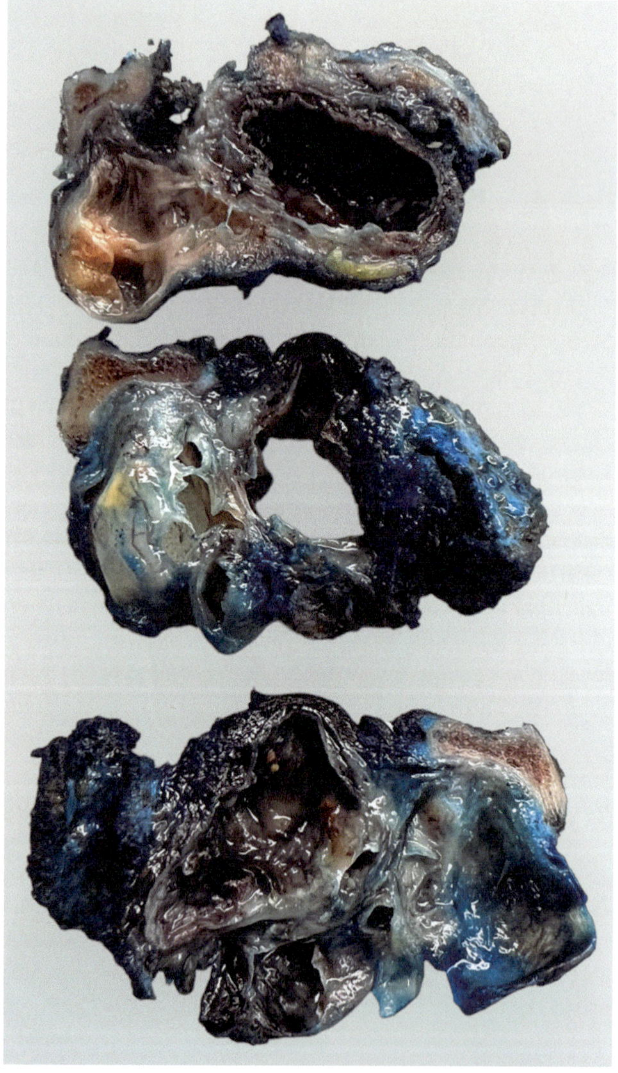

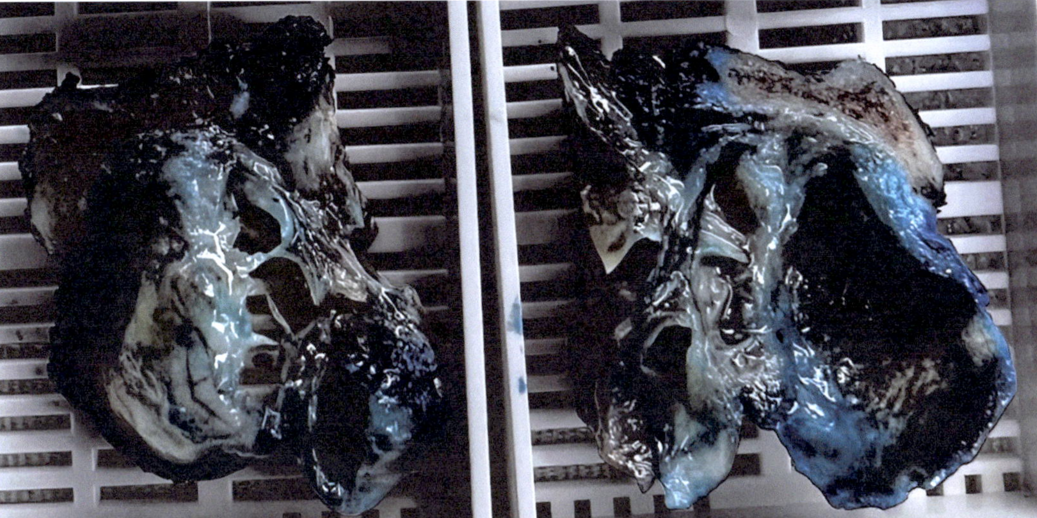

Fig. 9.47 Thyroglossal duct cyst section submission. Specimen A is received in formalin labeled with patients name, medical record number, "thyroglossal duct cyst" and consists of an unoriented fragment of soft tissue (3.1 x 2.0 x 1.8 cm) with attached segment of hyoid bone (1.1 x 0.8 x 0.5 cm). The specimen is entirely inked blue and serially sectioned to reveal a multiloculated cystic space (2.1 x 1.5 cm) filled with red-brown material. Representative sections are submitted in A 1- A 2, post decalcification

9.15   Thyroid for Follicular Nodular Disease/Goiter: Level V CPT 88307

Thyroid follicular nodular disease is the most common disease of the thyroid gland which can lead to diffuse or nodular enlargement of the thyroid gland. Refer to Table 9.2 for gross descriptions of all thyroid lesions.

Cancer Protocol Relative to Grossing Thyroid Procedure:

Partial excision—the removal of a portion of a thyroid lobe.

Lobectomy—the removal of either the left or the right thyroid lobe.

Lobectomy with isthmusectomy the removal of either the left or the right thyroid lobe including the isthmus.

Subtotal or near total thyroidectomy—the removal of one thyroid lobe, the isthmus, and a portion of the opposing thyroid lobe.

Total thyroidectomy—the removal of the entire thyroid including right lobe, isthmus, and left lobe.

Completion thyroidectomy—the removal of the remainder of the thyroid lobe after the previ-

Table 9.2 Tumor gross appearance of thyroid lesions

Goiter	Pink to amber, gelatinous nodules varying in size with possible calcification
Papillary thyroid carcinoma	Solid, tan-white with possible cystic or calcified areas
Follicular thyroid carcinoma	Encapsulated tan-brown, mostly solid mass
Medullary thyroid carcinoma	Solid, non-encapsulated, well-circumscribed, tan-white mass
Anaplastic thyroid carcinoma	Ill-defined, firm, tan mass with areas of possible necrosis

ous surgery which removed the thyroid lobe with the lesion.

Tumor focality: Dictate the number of separate lesions present and measure the size of each lesion.

Tumor site: Dictate where the lesion is present. This can include the right lobe, left lobe, isthmus, or pyramidal lobe.

Tumor size: Overall lesion size should be dictated in centimeters.

Extrathyroidal extension: Dictate if any soft tissue is present surrounding the thyroid and if the lesion grossly extends outside the thyroid and into the surrounding soft tissue.

Margin status: Dictate how close the lesion comes from the superior pole, inferior pole, and anterior and posterior thyroid and from the isthmus resection margin in hemithyroidectomy cases.

pT Category

For follicular tumors

pT1: Tumor size less than or equal to 2 cm in greatest dimension, limited to thyroid.

pT2: Tumor greater than 2 cm but less than or equal to 4 cm in greatest dimension, limited to thyroid pT3a: Tumor greater than 4 cm limited to the thyroid.

pT3b: Gross extrathyroidal extension invading only strap muscles (sternohyoid, sternothyroid, thyrohyoid, or omohyoid muscles) from a tumor of any size.

pT4a: Gross extrathyroidal extension invading subcutaneous soft tissues, larynx, trachea, esophagus, or recurrent laryngeal nerve from a tumor of any size.

pT4b: Gross extrathyroidal extension invading prevertebral fascia or encasing the carotid artery or mediastinal vessels from a tumor of any size.

For medullary tumors

pT1: Tumor size less than or equal to 2 cm in greatest dimension, limited to thyroid.

pT2: Tumor greater than 2 cm but less than or equal to 4 cm in greatest dimension.

pT3a: Tumor greater than 4 cm in greatest dimension limited to the thyroid.

pT3b: Tumor of any size with gross extrathyroidal extension invading only strap muscles (sternohyoid, sternothyroid, thyrohyoid, or omohyoid muscles).

pT4a: Moderately advanced disease; tumor of any size with gross extrathyroidal extension into the nearby tissues of the neck, including subcutaneous soft tissue, larynx, trachea, esophagus, or recurrent laryngeal nerve.

pT4b: Very advanced disease; tumor of any size with extension toward the spine or into nearby large blood vessels, gross extrathyroidal extension invading the prevertebral fascia, or encasing the carotid artery or mediastinal vessels.

Step 1: Orient the thyroid specimen. Figure 9.48a shows the anterior aspect of the thyroid and Fig. 9.48b shows the posterior aspect of the thyroid.

Step 2: Describe and measure each lobe and isthmus, and weigh the specimen.

Step 3: Ink the thyroid specimen. In this example, Fig. 9.49a is the anterior thyroid which is inked blue and Fig. 9.49b is the posterior thyroid which is inked black.

Step 4: Separate the right lobe, isthmus and left lobe as shown in Fig. 9.50. Keep each lobe oriented.

Step 5: Serially section each lobe as shown in Fig. 9.51. The right and left lobes are serially sectioned from superior to inferior, and the isthmus is serially sectioned from right to left.

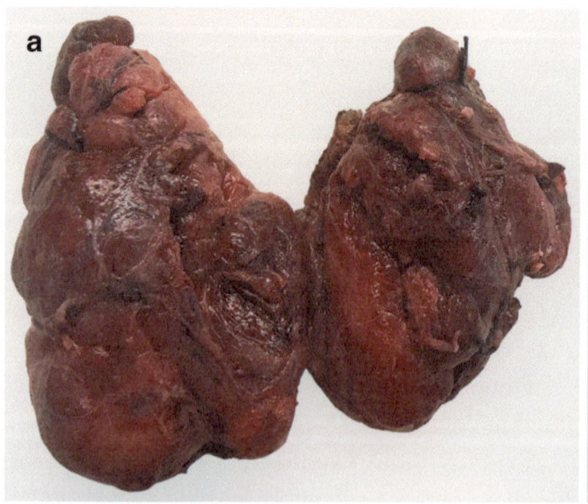
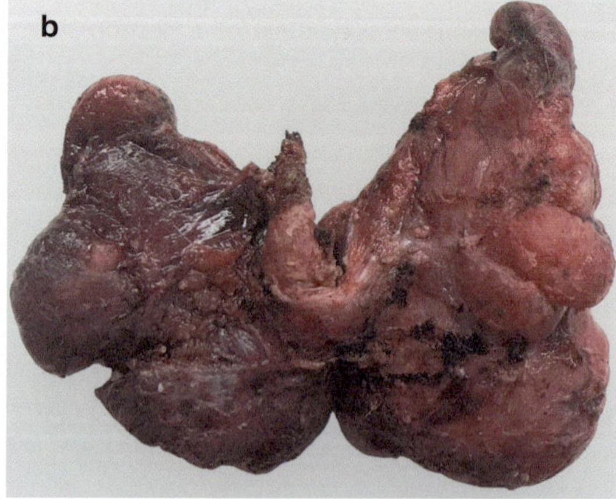

Fig. 9.48 (**a**) Total thyroid anterior view; (**b**) total thyroid posterior view

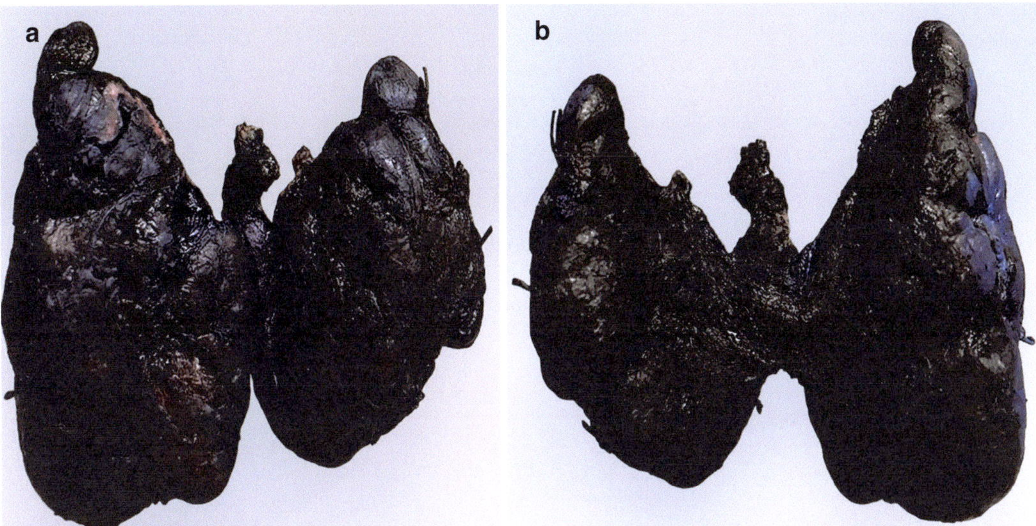

Fig. 9.49 (**a**) Anterior ink; (**b**) posterior ink

Fig. 9.50 Separating
right, isthmus and left
thyroid lobes

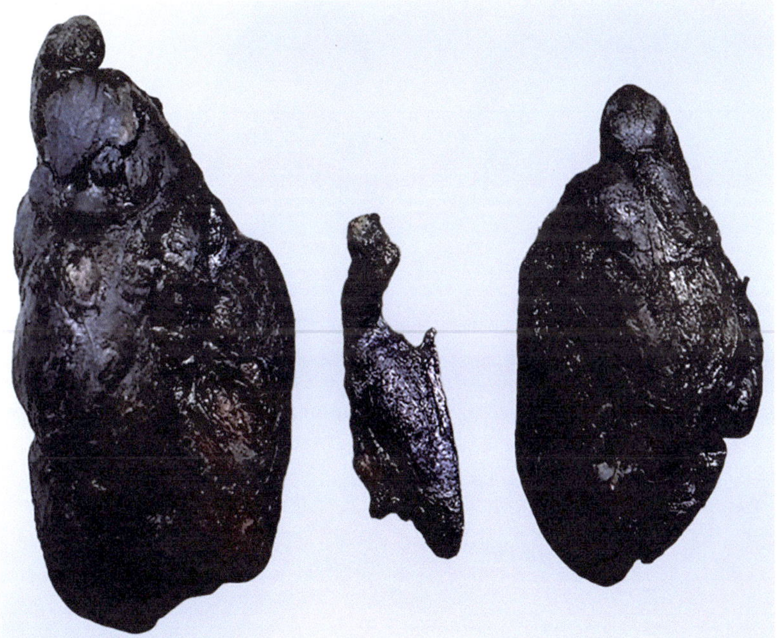

Step 6: Perpendicularly section the superior and inferior poles of each thyroid lobe as indicated by the blue arrows in Fig. 9.51.

Step 7: Describe the cut surfaces. In Fig. 9.51, the right lobe contains a single large goiter nodule that becomes hemorrhagic and slightly cavitary toward the inferior aspect of the nodule.

Step 8: Measure the nodules and measure how close the closest nodule comes from the ante-rior and posterior thyroid and the superior and inferior thyroid poles.

Step 9: Describe the remaining thyroid parenchyma.

Step 10: Submit sections. Submit the bilateral superior and inferior thyroid poles and representative sections of each lobe and isthmus which include the goiter (Fig. 9.52).

Fig. 9.51 Total thyroid serially sectioned

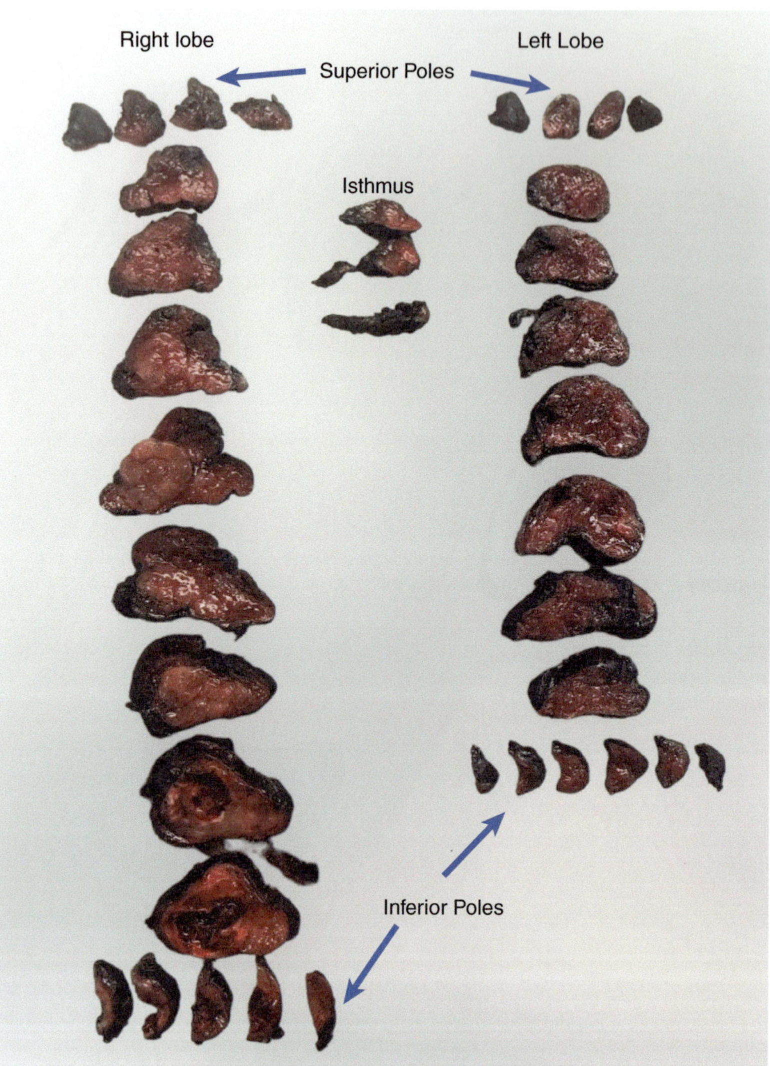

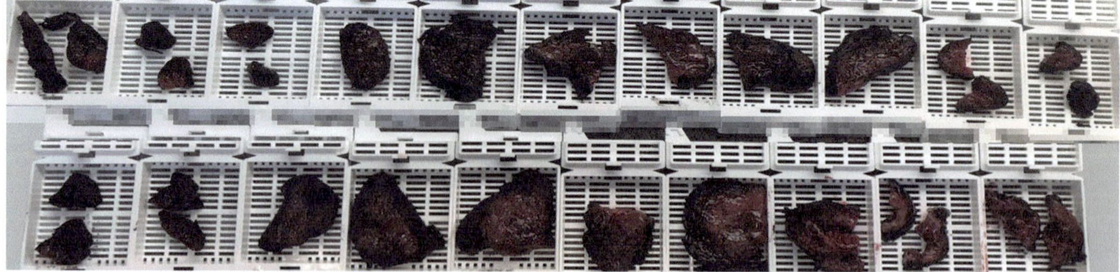

Fig. 9.52 Total thyroid section submission

9.16   Total Thyroid for Papillary Thyroid Carcinoma: Level V CPT 88307

Papillary thyroid cancer (PTC) is a relatively common thyroid neoplasm with a good general outcome. PTC lesions are solid, tan-white, usually single lesions within the thyroid gland. The significant feature of PTC is the ability to invade into the lymphatics with metastatic spread into the lymph nodes of the neck [2]

Step 1: Orient the thyroid specimen. Figure 9.53a shows the anterior aspect of the thyroid and Fig. 9.53b shows the posterior aspect of the thyroid. In this example, there is also a stitch designating the left superior pole.

Step 2: Describe, measure each lobe and isthmus, and weigh the specimen.

Step 3: Ink the thyroid specimen. In this example, Fig. 9.54a is the anterior thyroid which is inked blue and Fig. 9.54b is the posterior thyroid which is inked black.

Step 4: Separate the right lobe, isthmus and left lobe as shown in Fig. 9.55. Keep each lobe oriented. In this example, the separation sites, which are false margins, are inked red to identify these areas as false margins microscopically.

Step 5: Serially section each lobe as shown in Fig. 9.56. The right and left lobes are serially

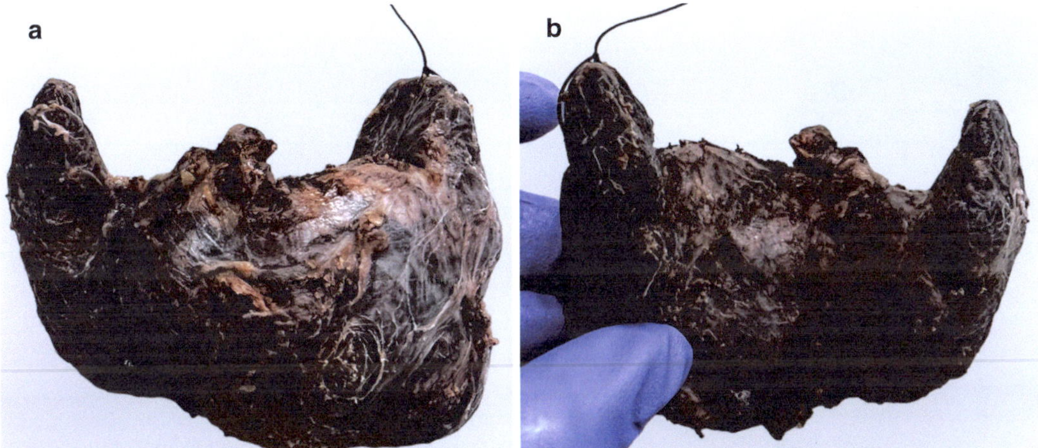

Fig. 9.53   (a) Thyroid anterior view; (b) thyroid posterior view

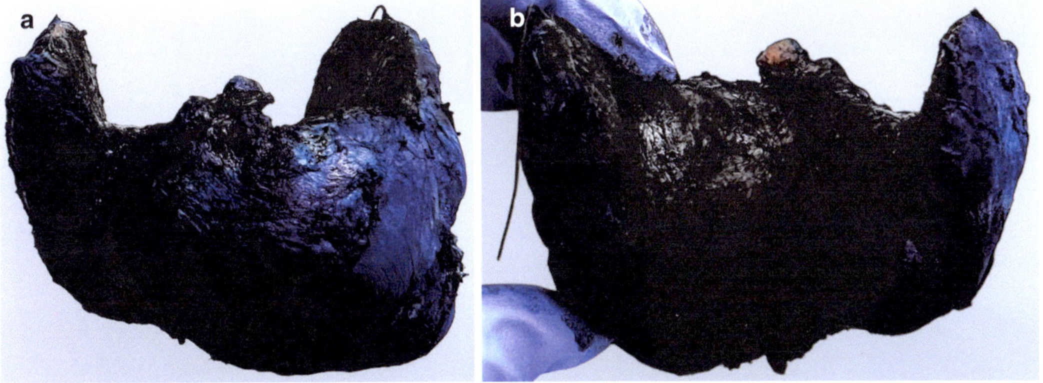

Fig. 9.54   (a) Thyroid anterior ink; (b) thyroid posterior ink

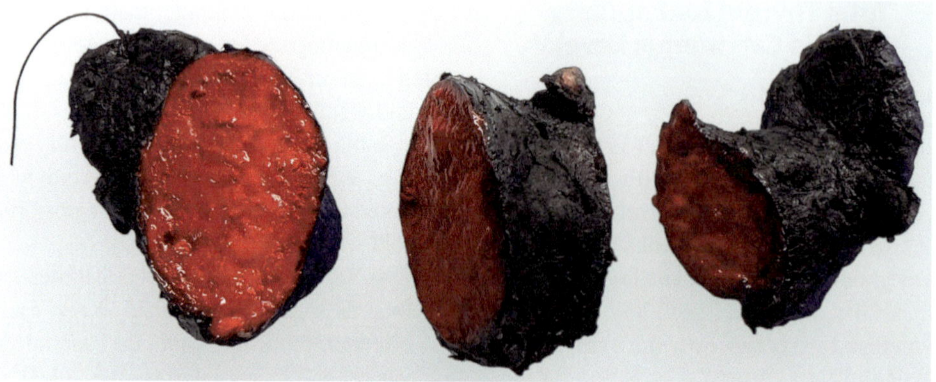

Fig. 9.55 Separation of right, isthmus and left thyroid lobes with false margin ink

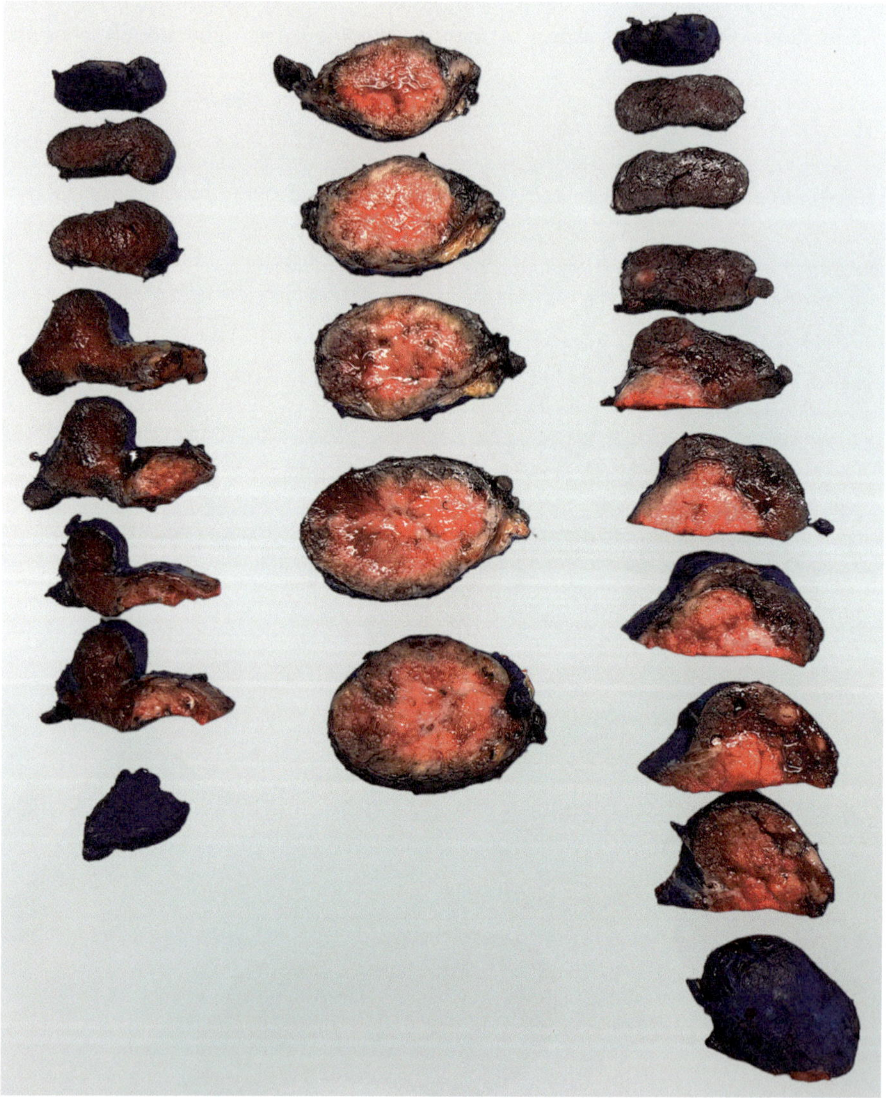

Fig. 9.56 Thyroid serially sectioned

sectioned from superior to inferior and the isthmus is serially sectioned from right to left.

Step 6: Perpendicularly section the superior and inferior poles of each thyroid lobe as indicated by the blue arrows in Fig. 9.57.

Step 7: Describe the cut surfaces. In Fig. 9.57, there is a large mass in the isthmus which extends into the right and left thyroid lobes.

Step 8: Measure the mass, state the location and measure how close the nodule comes from the anterior and posterior thyroid and the superior and inferior thyroid poles.

Step 9: Describe the remaining thyroid parenchyma.

Example Dictation

Specimen A is received in formalin labeled with patient's name, medical record number, "total thyroidectomy" and consists of a ragged total thyroid (right lobe: 5.4 × 3.0 × 1.7 cm, left lobe:

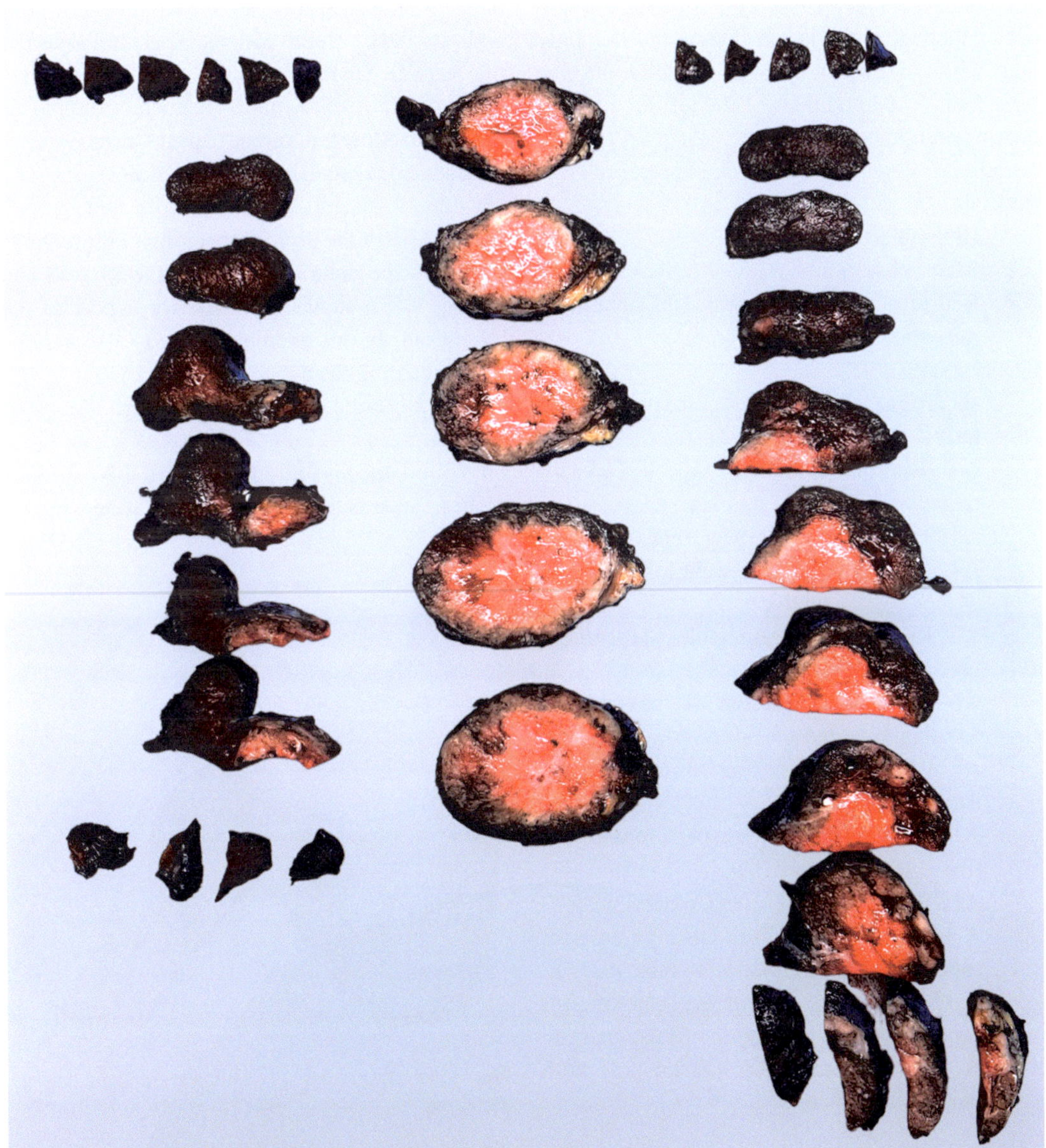

Fig. 9.57 Thyroid poles perpendicularly sectioned

5.6 × 3.5 × 3.0 cm, isthmus: 5.2 × 4.1 × 2.7 cm, 74 g) with a stitch designating the left superior pole. The thyroid lobe is serially sectioned to reveal a large, slightly ill-defined tan-white mass (5.3 × 4.5 × 3.1 cm) with scant calcification present, encompassing the entirety of the isthmus, and extending into the medial aspect of the right lobe. The mass comes within 2.2 cm of the superior pole of the left lobe and abuts the inferior pole of the left lobe. Additionally, the isthmus portion of the mass comes within 0.1 cm of the anterior aspect and posterior margin. The remainder of the right lobe is red-brown and homogenous with 0.5 cm extension of the mass into the right lobe. The remainder of the left lobe is red-brown and homogeneous.

Ink code

    Blue-anterior

    Black-posterior

    Red-false margin (separation of right, isthmus and left lobes)

Section code

    A1: Right lobe, superior pole, perpendicular

    A 2: Right lobe, superior aspect, representative

    A3: Right lobe, mid aspect, representative

    A4: Mass in relation to right lobe, inferior aspect, representative

    A5: Right lobe, inferior pole, perpendicular

    A6-A7: Fullface section of mass within isthmus, bisected

    A8-A9: Fullface section of mass within isthmus, bisected

    A10: Left lobe, superior aspect, representative

    A12: Left lobe, mid aspect, representative

    A 13-A 14: Mass within left lobe, inferior aspect, bisected in relation to false margin

    A 15-A 16: Mass within left lobe, inferior aspect, bisected in relation of false margin

    A 17-A 20: Left lobe, inferior pole with mass, perpendicular

9.17 Hemithyroidectomy for Follicular Nodules: Level V CPT 88307

Follicular nodules of the thyroid need to be handled slightly different from the other thyroid nodules. The capsule of the nodule is imperative to proper diagnosis. Nodules that are encapsulated or have a previous fine needle aspiration (FNA) diagnosis of follicular neoplasm need to have the capsule of the nodule submitted entirely. In cases where the nodule is large, the capsule can be sectioned into strips and submitted entirely without the central aspect of the lesion. Smaller nodules can be submitted entirely. The following specimen example is grossed to allow for optimal capsule surface area to be assessed microscopically (Fig. 9.58).

Step 1: Orient the thyroid specimen. Figure 9.59a shows the anterior aspect of the thyroid and Fig. 9.59b shows the posterior aspect of the thyroid. In this example, there is also a stitch designating the superior pole.

Step 2: Describe, measure, and weigh the specimen.

Step 3: Ink the thyroid specimen. In this example, Fig. 9.60a is the anterior thyroid lobe which is

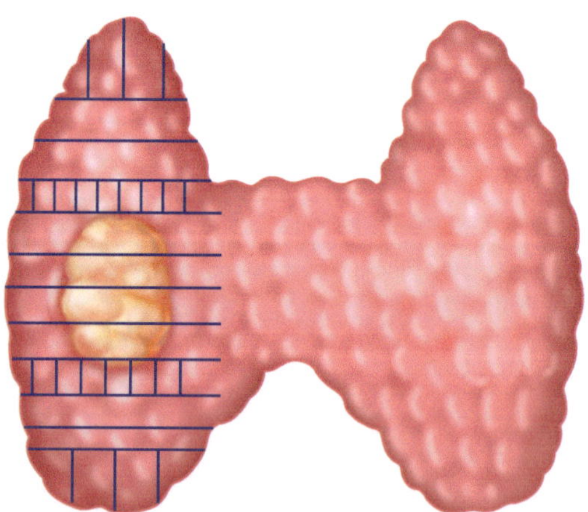

Fig. 9.58 Illustration of follicular nodule capsule sectioning

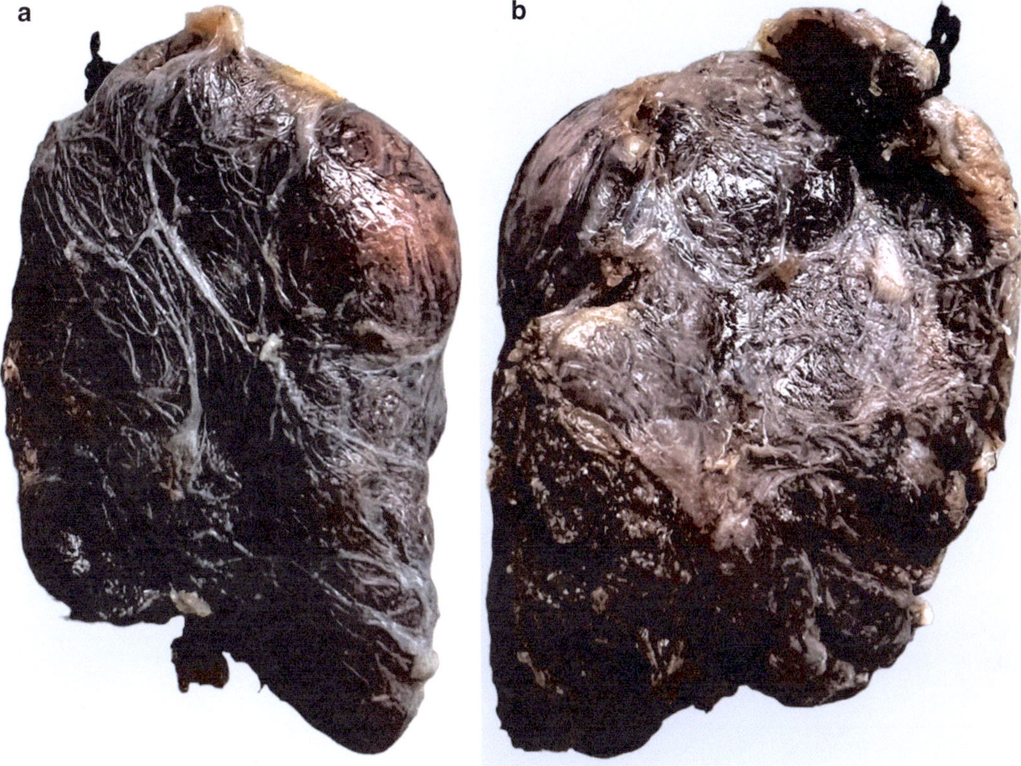

Fig. 9.59 (**a**) Right thyroid lobe, anterior view; (**b**) right thyroid lobe, posterior view

inked blue, and Fig. 9.60b is the posterior thyroid lobe which is inked black. The orange ink is present on the partial isthmus which is a true margin for hemithyroidectomy specimens.

Step 4: Serially section the thyroid lobe from superior to inferior as shown in Fig. 9.61.

Step 5: Perpendicularly section the superior and inferior poles of the thyroid lobe which is indicated by the blue arrows in Fig. 9.62.

Step 6: Perpendicularly section the slices that contain the superior and inferior aspects of the encapsulated nodule as shown in Fig. 9.62 by the red arrow. Notice in Fig. 9.62, the superior aspect of the encapsulated nodule is present at the superior pole (which is already perpendicularly sections) so now only the inferior aspect of the encapsulated nodule needs to be perpendicularly sectioned.

Step 7: Describe and measure the lesions. In Fig. 9.62, there is a follicular appearing lesion in the superior to mid right thyroid lobe and a separate papillary appearing lesion present in the inferior aspect of the right thyroid lobe. Describe where each lesion is and how far apart the lesions are from each other.

Step 8: Describe the remaining thyroid parenchyma.

Step 9: Submit the thyroid poles perpendicular and submit the follicular lesion capsule entirely. In this example, the thyroid lobe is small, so the specimen is submitted entirely (Fig. 9.63).

Example Dictation

Specimen A is received in formalin labeled with patient's name, medical record number, "right hemi thyroid" and consists of a slightly ragged tan-brown thyroid lobe (4.0 × 2.9 × 2.3 cm, 11 g) with attached portion of isthmus (1.9 × 0.7 × 0.6 cm) and a stitch designating the superior pole. The specimen is serially sectioned to reveal an encapsulated tan-pink nodule (1.9 × 1.2 × 1.2 cm) on the

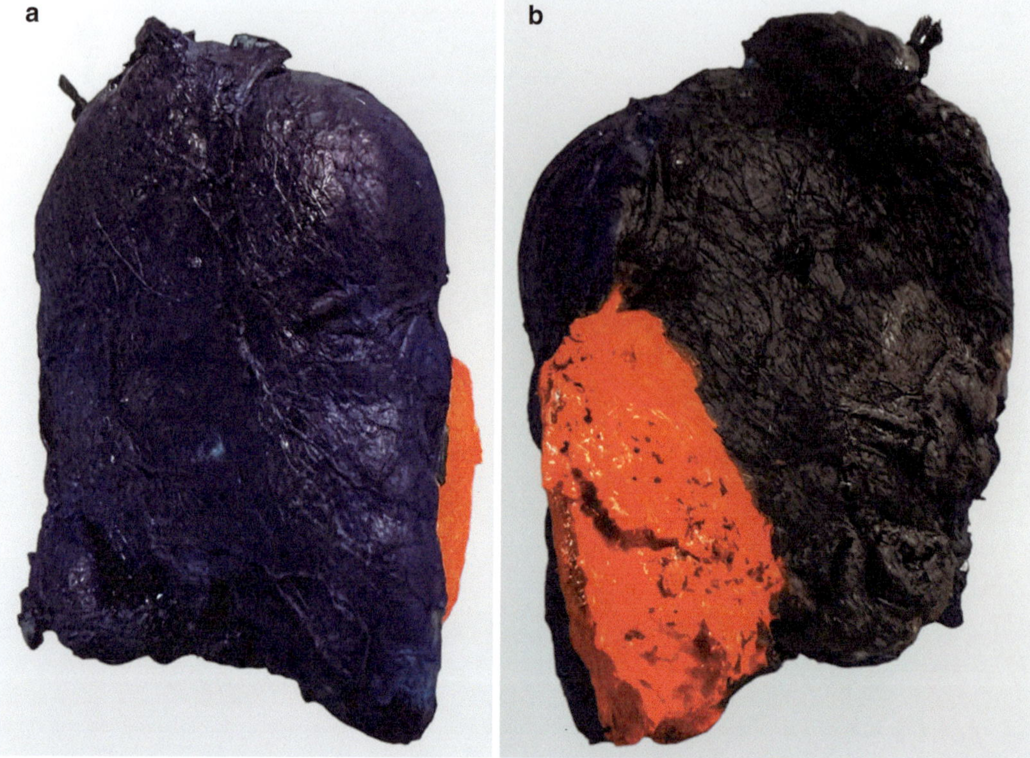

Fig. 9.60 (**a**) Right thyroid lobe, anterior ink; (**b**) right thyroid lobe, posterior ink with isthmus

medial aspect of the thyroid lobe, coming within 0.1 cm of the superior pole. There is a separate ill-defined tan-white lesion (0.7 × 0.5 × 0.5 cm) present in the inferior aspect coming within 1.3 cm of the inferior pole and a proximally 0.6 cm from the well-circumscribed superior nodule. The remaining cut surfaces are red-brown and homogenous.

Ink code
  Blue: anterior
  Black: posterior
  Orange: isthmus
Section code
  A1-A 2: Superior pole, perpendicular
  A3-A8: Thyroid lobe entirely from superior to inferior, perpendicular inferior aspect nodule in A5-A6
  A9-A10: Inferior pole, perpendicular

Cancer Protocol Relative to Grossing Oral Cavity Lesions
  Procedure:

Excision—the removal of the lesion with surrounding unremarkable tissues.

Glossectomy—the removal of part or most of the tongue.

Buccal mucosa resection—the removal of the lesion with surrounding unremarkable tissues of the cheek mucosa.

Mandibulectomy—the removal of a portion of the mandibular bone typically with the overlying mucosa.

Maxillectomy—the removal of a portion of the maxillary bone typically with underlying mucosa.

Palatectomy—the removal of a portion of the hard and/or soft palate with the attached mucosa.

It is not common to receive a composite resection which includes several of the above types in one resected specimen. In all oral cavity cancer resection specimens, it is important to remember that the final pathologic stage depends upon the

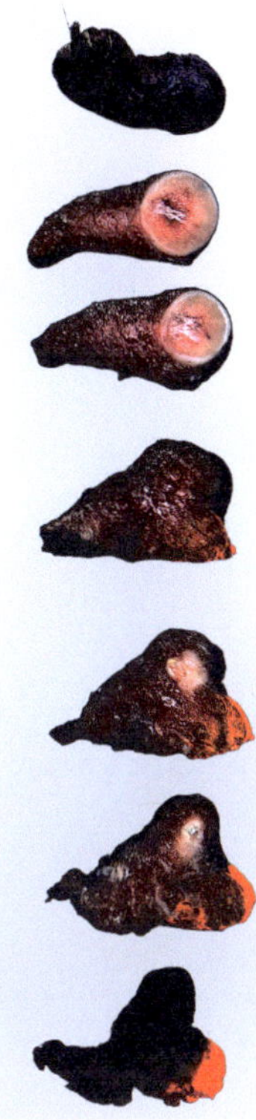

Fig. 9.61 Right thyroid lobe serially sectioned from superior to inferior

size of the tumor and the depth/extent of tumor invasion. Keeping this in mind is important when grossing these specimens.

Tumor focality: Dictate the number of separate lesions present and measure the size of each lesion.

Multiple primary sites: Dictate if there is one lesion or if there are multiple lesions which are completely separate from one another.

Tumor site: Dictate all anatomical structures the lesion involved. This can include mucosa of lip, tongue, gingiva, floor of mouth, hard palate, buccal mucosa, vestibule of mouth, alveolar ridge, and retromolar area.

Tumor laterality: Dictate what side the lesion is present which can include left side, right side, midline, or more than one.

Tumor size: Overall lesion size should be dictated in centimeters.

Margin status: Dictate the distance of the lesion to all margins.

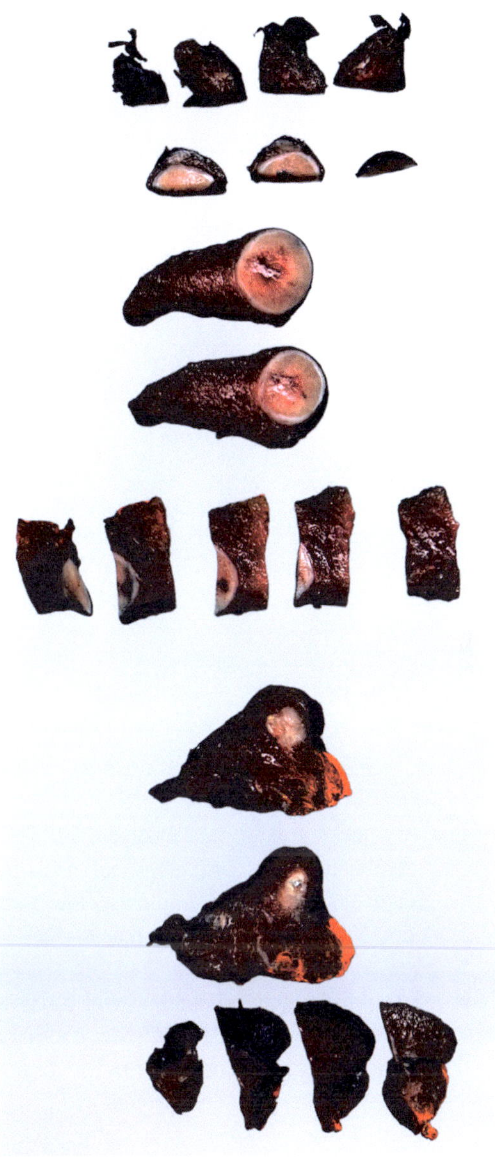

Fig. 9.62 Right thyroid lobe, perpendicular sections of superior and inferior poles and slice with capsule edge

pT Category

pTis: Carcinoma in situ

pT1: Tumor less than or equal to 2 cm with depth of invasion less than or equal to 5 mm

pT2: Tumor less than or equal to 2 cm with depth of invasion greater than 5 mm or tumor greater than 2 cm and less than or equal to 4 cm with depth of invasion less than or equal to 10 mm

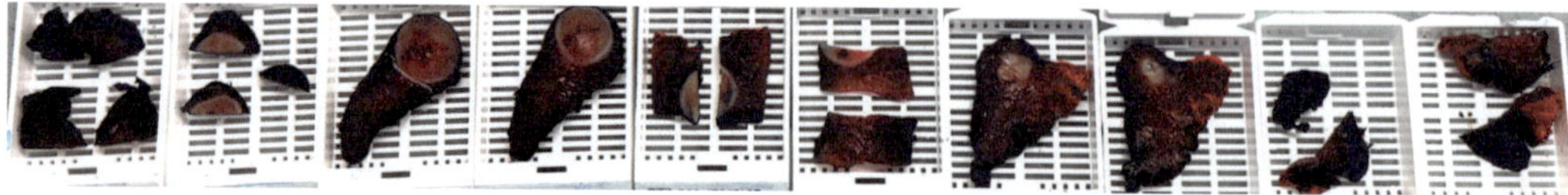

Fig. 9.63 Right thyroid lobe section submission

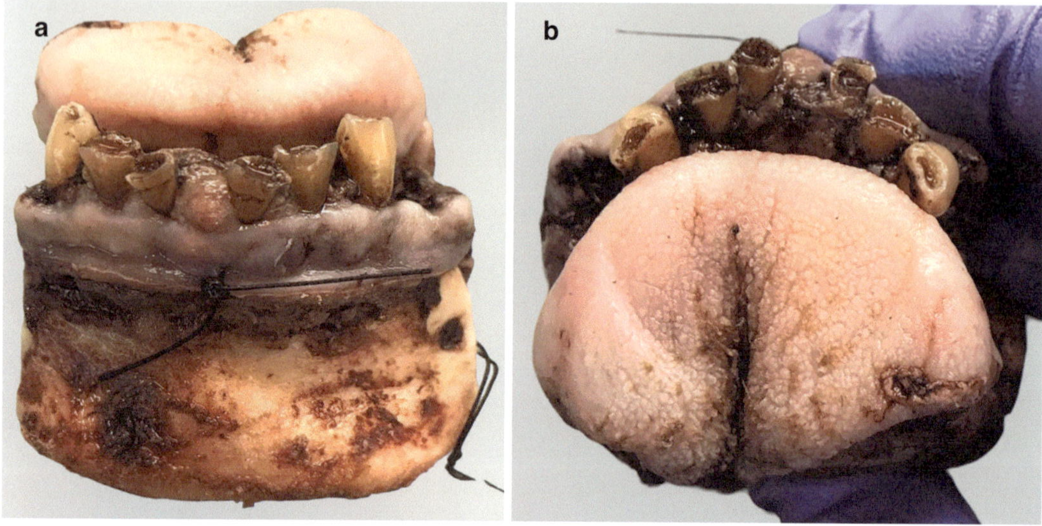

Fig. 9.64 (**a**) Mandible anterior view; (**b**) mandible posterior view

pT3: Tumor greater than 2 cm and less than or equal to 4 cm with depth of invasion greater than 10 mm or tumor greater than 4 cm with depth of invasion less than or equal to 10 mm

pT4a: Moderately advanced local disease. Tumor greater than 4 cm with depth of invasion greater than 10 mm or tumor invades adjacent structures only.

pT4b: Tumor invades masticator space, pterygoid plates, or skull base, and/or encases internal carotid artery.

9.18 Anterior Mandible: Level VI CPT 88309

Grossing of all mandible specimens follow the same necessary rules but can be grossed differently. Each mandible specimen has mucosal margins, soft tissue margins, and bone margins. Whether these margins are shaved and submitted en face or perpendicularly sectioned and submit-

ted on edge is to the discretion of the pathologist. The example is grossed showing mucosal margins shaved and submitted en face.

Step 1: Orient the specimen. Figure 9.64a shows a single stitch designating anterior mandible and a double stitch designating left lateral.

Step 2: Describe and measure the specimen, dictating all the anatomic structures present. Figure 9.64b shows partial anterior tongue and 6 anterior teeth in addition to the mandible.

Step 3: Describe and measure the lesion. Figure 9.65 shows a large anterior floor of mouth lesions extending onto the posterior mandible and ventral tongue.

Step 4: Measure the lesion to all mucosal margins. In this case, the mucosal margins are anterior mandible mucosa, right and left floor of mouth mucosa, right and left tongue mucosa, and dorsal tongue mucosa.

Step 5: Ink the specimen. Figure 9.66a shows the anterior mandible ink, and Fig. 9.66b shows the posterior mandible ink. The ink code is as follows:

Yellow: anterior mandible
Blue: posterior tongue margin
Red: right lateral margin
Orange: left lateral margin
Black: Inferior margin

Step 6: Shave the anterior mandible and posterior tongue mucosal margins. In this example, all mucosal margins are shaved and submitted en face. Figure 9.67a, b show the anterior mandible and posterior tongue mucosal margins shaved, respectively.

Step 7: Shave the right and left floor of mouth mucosal margins, Fig. 9.68a, b show the right and left floor of mouth mucosal margins shaved, respectively.

Step 7: Shave the right and left tongue mucosal margins, Fig. 9.69a, b show the right and left tongue mucosal margins shaved, respectively.

Step 8: Shave the right and left osseous margins and submit en face as shown in Fig. 9.70.

Step 9: Serially section the specimen from right to left and perpendicularly section the right and left ends as shown in Fig. 9.71.

Step 10: Measure the greatest depth of invasion and measure the lesion to all the soft tissue margins.

Step 11: Dictate if the lesion extends into the mandible. In Fig. 9.72, the lesion does extend into the superior aspect of the mandibular bone as indicated by the blue arrow.

Step 12: Submit sections. Submit a fullface section of the lesion in relation to the closest margins and including the maximum depth of invasion (at least two fullface sections are recommended). Sections of tumor in relation to the bone are very important especially if on

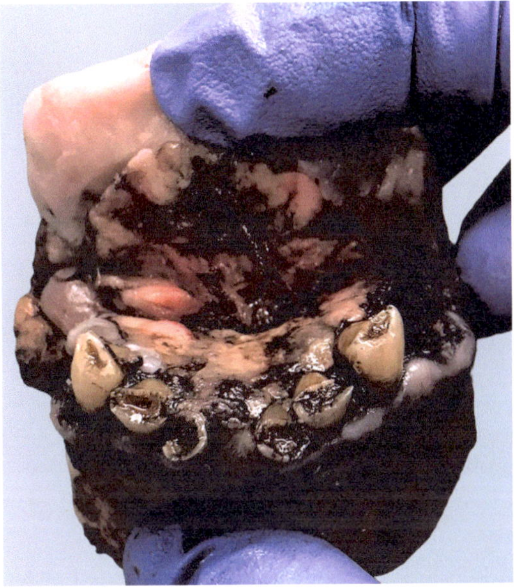

Fig. 9.65 Anterior floor of mouth lesion

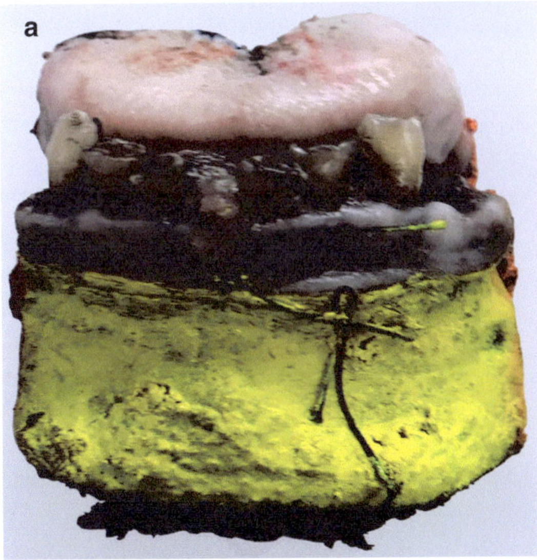

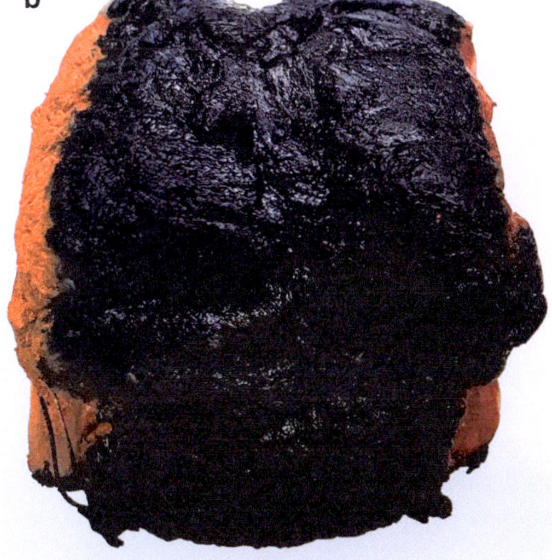

Fig. 9.66 (**a**) Anterior ink; (**b**) posterior ink

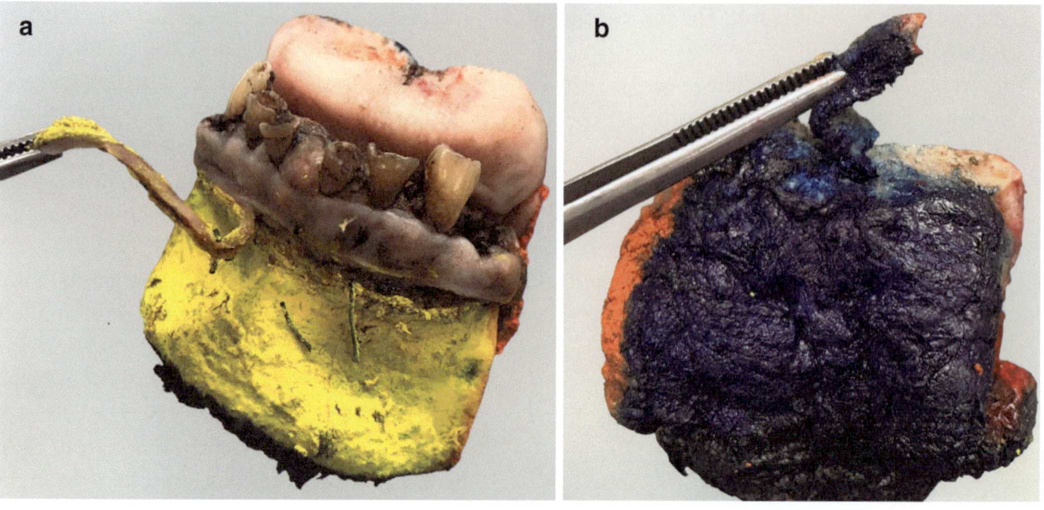

Fig. 9.67 (a) Anterior shave margin; (b) posterior shave margin

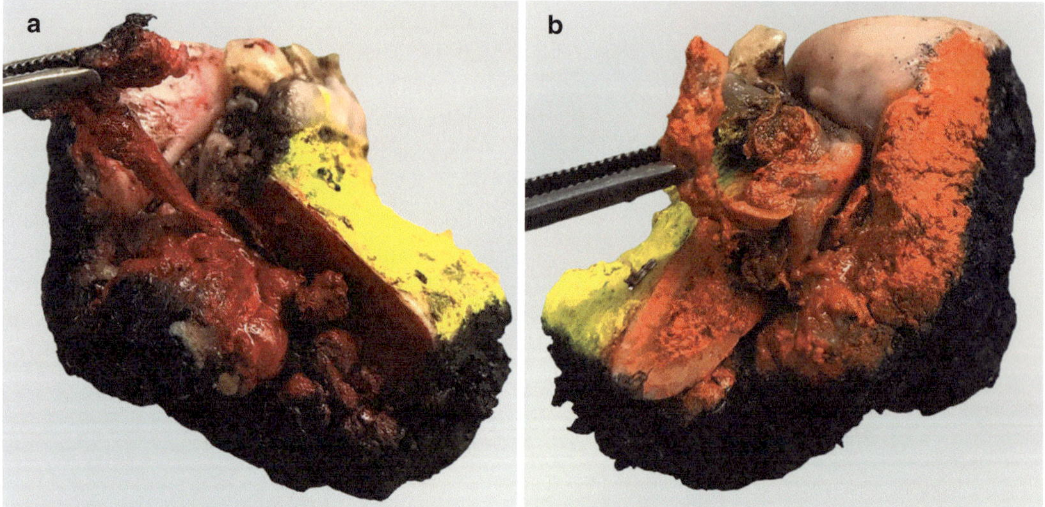

Fig. 9.68 (a) Right floor of mouth shave margin; (b) posterior floor of mouth shave margin

imaging bone invasion is suspected and the tumor is close or approaches the bone on gross evaluation. Figure 9.73 shows these slices quadrisected to fit into the cassettes. In addition, the shaved mucosal margins are submitted en face, and the osseous margins are submitted en face.

Step 13: All cassettes containing bone need to be decalcified before submitting.

Example Dictation

Specimen A is received in formalin labeled with the patient's name, medical record number, "anterior mandible with tongue" and consists of an anterior floor of mouth resection (6.3 × 5.9 × 5.4 cm) including anterior tongue and 6 anterior teeth. The anterior floor of mouth contains a flat, pink-white, soft lesion (4.3 × 3.8 × 0.2 cm) which extends onto the posterior mandibular mucosa 0.9 cm from the right and onto

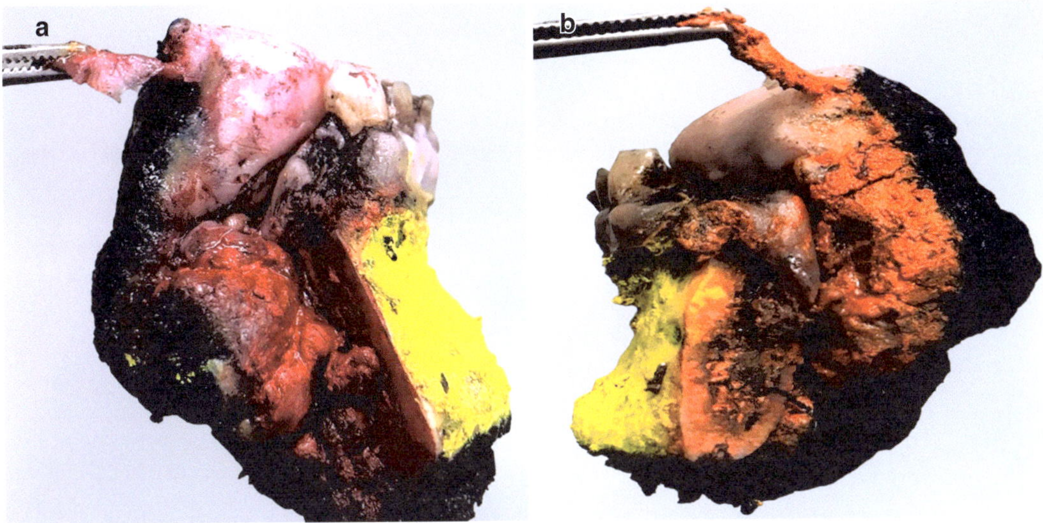

Fig. 9.69 (**a**) Right tongue shave margin; (**b**) left tongue shave margin

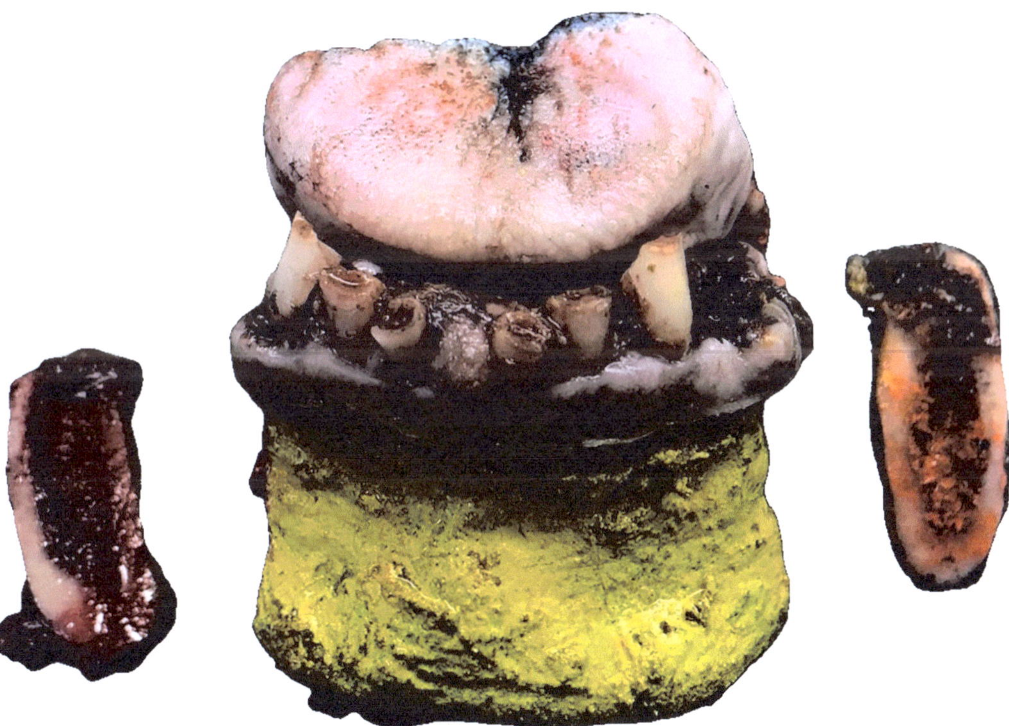

Fig. 9.70 Right and left osseous shave margins

the ventral tongue 1.6 cm. The lesion comes within 0.9 cm from the right lateral floor of mouth mucosal margin, 0.8 cm from the left lateral floor of mouth mucosal margin, 1.1 cm from the anterior mandibu-lar mucosal margin, and 3.1 cm from the dorsal tongue mucosal margin. The specimen is serially section from right to left to reveal the greatest depth of invasion of 0.6 cm, coming within 0.4 cm of the

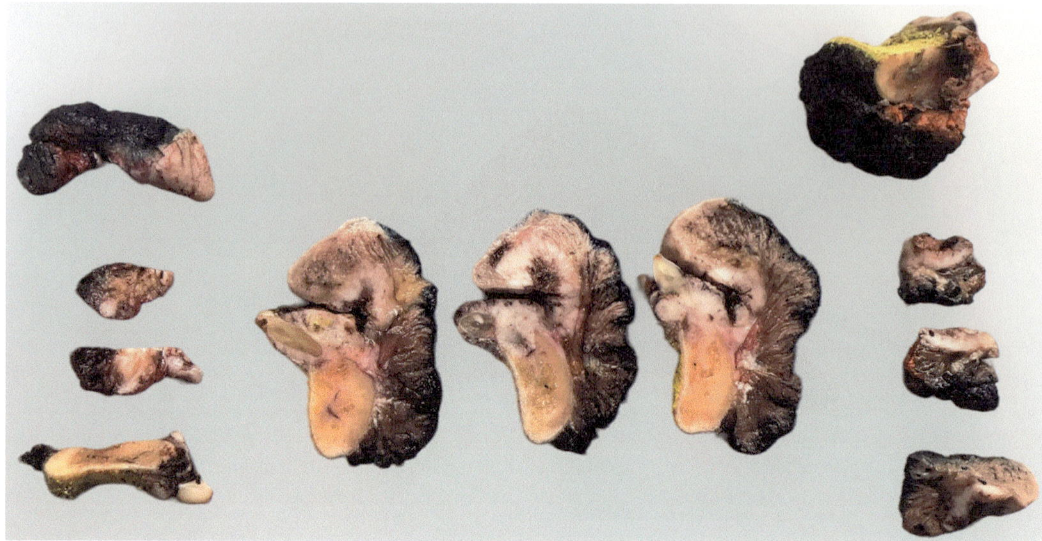

Fig. 9.71 Mandible serially sectioned

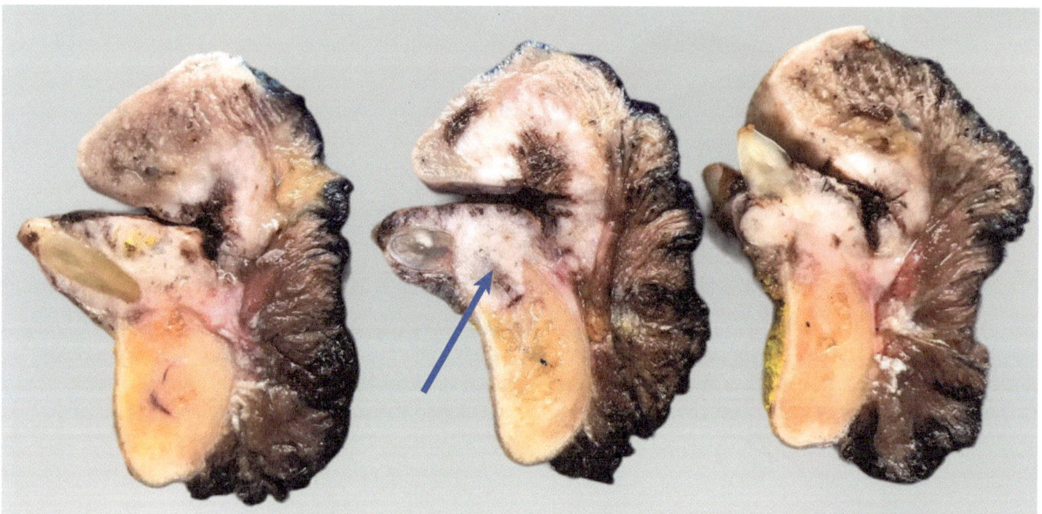

Fig. 9.72 Floor of mouth lesion.

anterior soft tissue margin, 1.1 cm from the posterior tongue soft tissue margin, 1.0 cm from the right floor of mouth soft tissue margin, 0.7 cm from the left floor of mouth soft tissue margin. The lesion invades into the superior aspect of the mandible coming within 2.1 cm of the inferior aspect of the mandible, 0.9 cm from the right osseous margin, and 0.6 cm from the left osseous margin.

Ink code

 Yellow: anterior mandible
 Blue: posterior tongue margin
 Red: right lateral margin
 Orange: left lateral margin
 Black: inferior margin

Section code

 A1: Anterior mandible mucosal margin, en face
 A2: Dorsal tongue mucosal margin, en face
 A3: Right floor of mouth mucosal margin, en face
 A4: Left floor of mouth mucosal margin, en face
 A5: Right tongue mucosal margin, en face

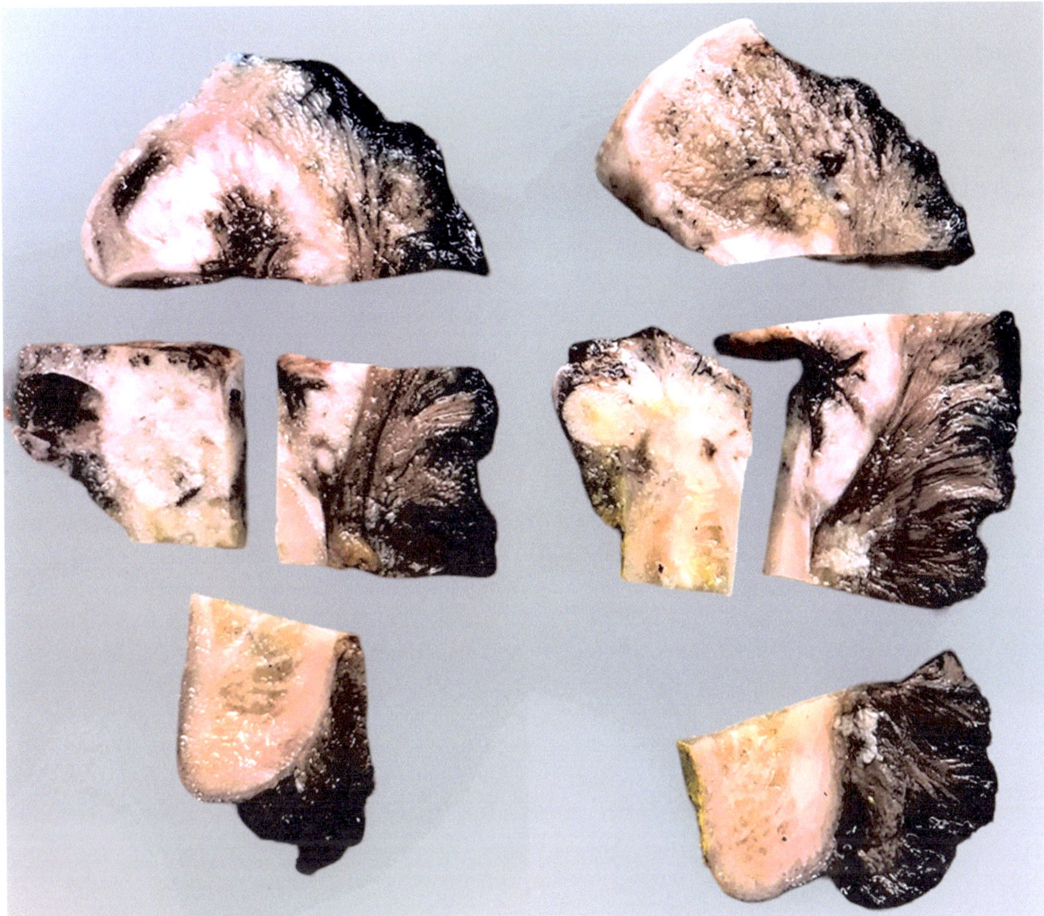

Fig. 9.73 Floor of mouth section submission

A6: Left tongue mucosal margin, en face
A7: Right osseous margin, en face
A8: Left osseous margin, en face
A9-A12: Fullface section, quadrisected
A13-A16: Fullface section, quadrisected

Cassettes containing bone are decalcified prior to submission.

9.19 Right Mandible: Level VI CPT 88309

In the example of the right mandible, the margins are all submitted in a perpendicular manner. This allows the pathologists to microscopically measure the distance from the tumor to each margin.

Always communicate with the pathologist before grossing the specimen and discuss how margins should be submitted.

Step 1: Orient the specimen. Figure 9.74 does contain orientation with a long stitch designating lateral and a short stitch designating anterior. However, one end of the specimen is disarticulated and is therefore posterior at the temporomandibular joint. The disarticulated posterior end is not an osseous margin.

Step 2: Describe and measure the specimen, dictating all the anatomic structures present. Figure 9.75 is the superior view and shows lateral buccal mucosa, alveolar ridge, 1 tooth, retromolar trigone and medial floor of mouth.

Step 3: Describe and measure the lesion. The lesion is present on the alveolar ridge, posterior to the 1 tooth as designated by the blue circle in Fig. 9.75.

Step 4: Measure the lesion to all mucosal margins. In this example, the mucosal margins are anterior mucosal, floor of mouth mucosal, buccal mucosal, and retromolar trigone mucosal margins.

Step 5: Ink the specimen. Figure 9.76a shows the lateral mandible ink, and Fig. 9.76b shows the inferior and medial mandible inks. The ink code is as follows:

Orange: anterior
Blue: lateral
Green: medial
Red: posterior
Black: Inferior

Step 6: Serially section the specimen from anterior to posterior as shown in Fig. 9.77.

Step 7: Measure the greatest depth of invasion designated by the blue arrow in Fig. 9.78 and measure the lesion to all the soft tissue margins. In this example, the soft tissue margins are anterior, posterior, medial, lateral, and inferior.

Step 8: Dictate if the lesion extends into the mandible. The arrow in Fig. 9.78 also shows the mass extending into the mandible bone.

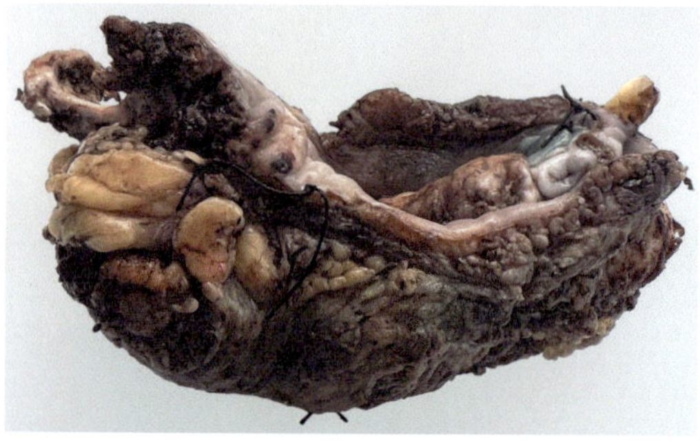

Fig. 9.74 Right mandible lateral view

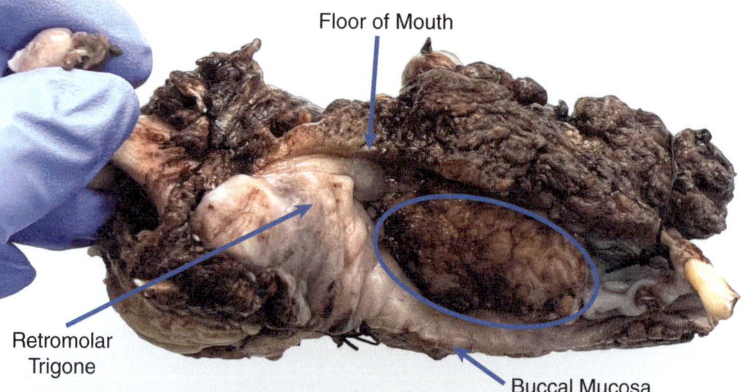

Fig. 9.75 Right mandible superior view

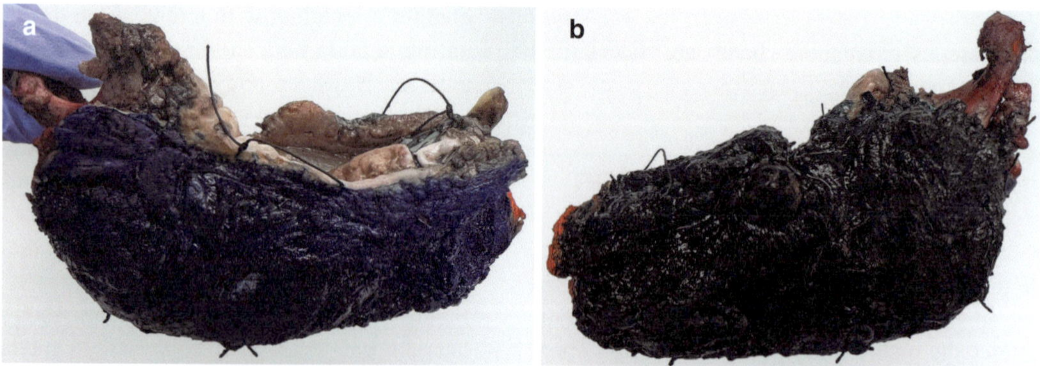

Fig. 9.76 (**a**) Right mandible lateral ink; (**b**) right mandible inferior and medial ink

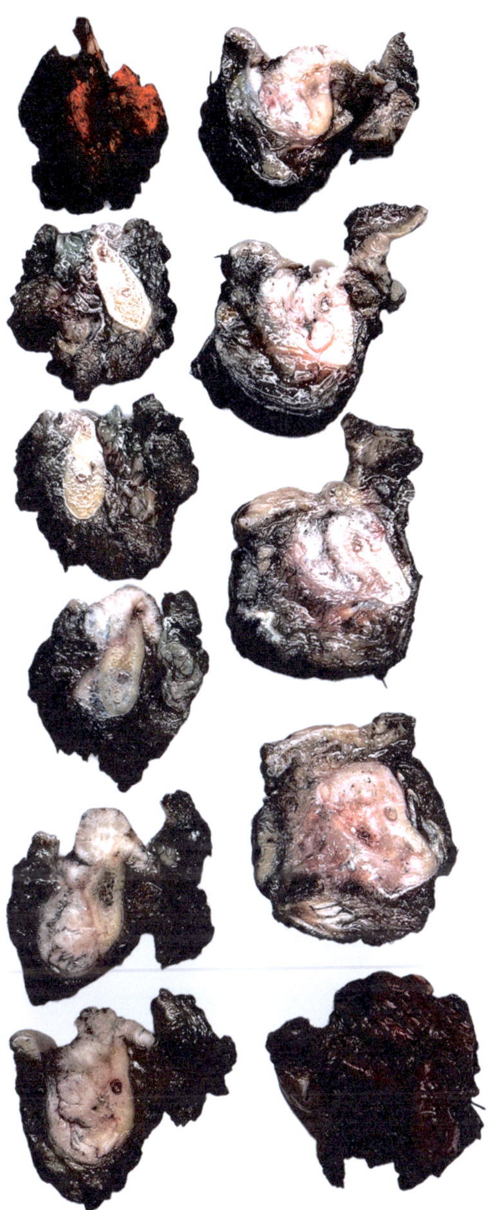

Fig. 9.77   Right mandible serially sectioned

Step 9: Shave the anterior bone margin and submit en face. Perpendicularly section the anterior mucosal and soft tissue margin and submit on edge as shown in Fig. 9.79.

Step 10: Perpendicularly section the posterior mucosal and soft tissue margin and submit on edge. Remember, in this example, there is no posterior osseous margin.

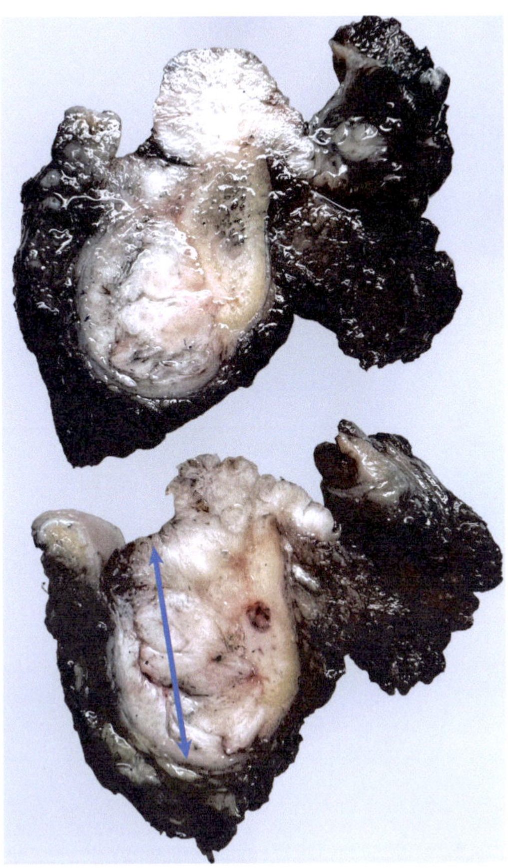

Fig. 9.78   Right mandible with greatest extent of mass

Step 11: Submit sections. Submit a fullface section of the lesion in relation to the closest margins and include the maximum depth of invasion (at least two fullface sections are recommended). Sections of tumor in relation to the bone are very important especially if on imaging bone invasion is suspected and the tumor is close or approaches the bone on gross evaluation. Figure 9.80 shows these slices quadrisected to fit into the cassettes. In this example, medial, lateral, and inferior margins are included in the slices. Anterior and posterior sections are submitted separately. No margin is shaved and submitted en face in this example.

Step 12: All cassettes containing bone need to be decalcified before submitting.

Example Dictation

Specimen A is received in formalin labeled with patient's name, medical record number, "right

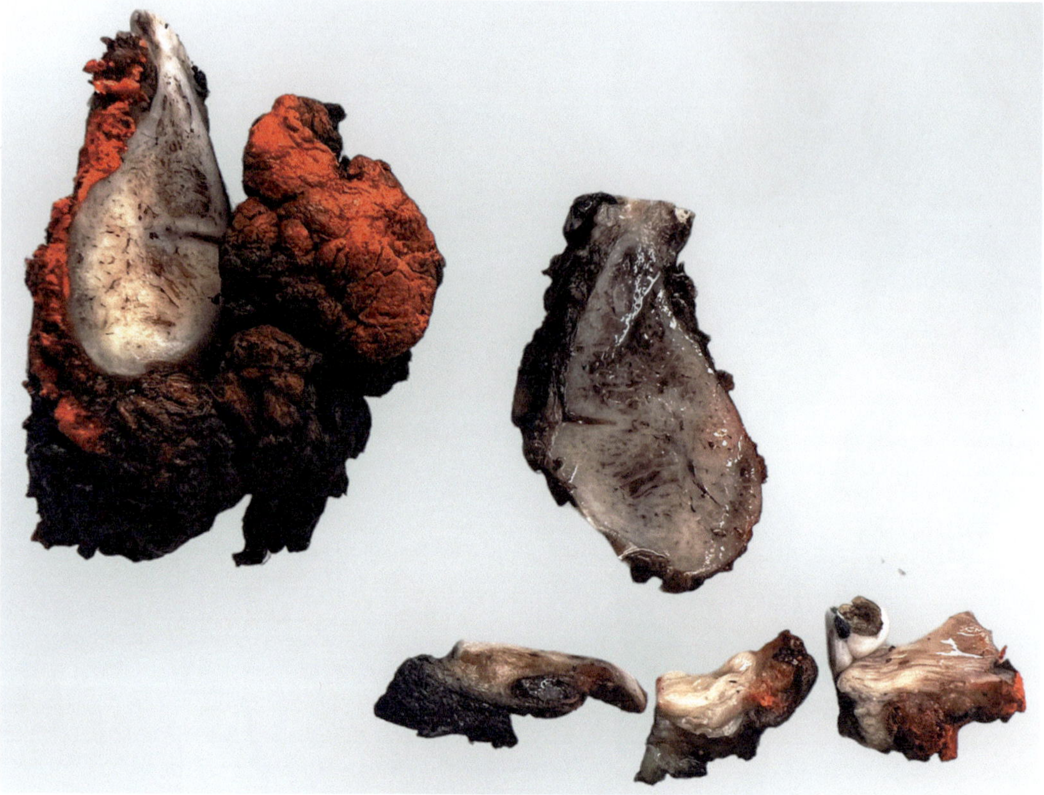

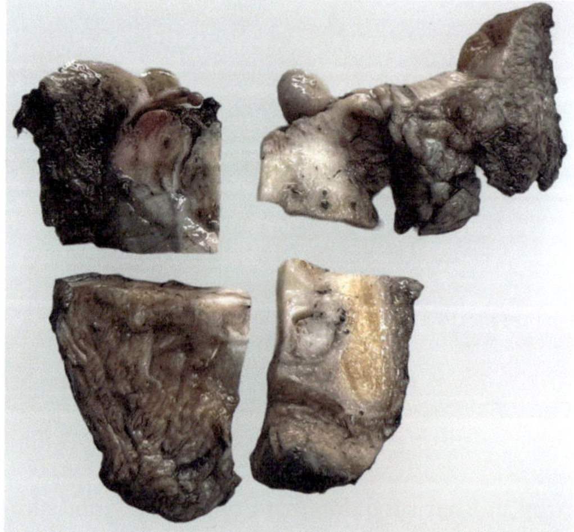

Fig. 9.79 Right mandible anterior margins

mandible" and consists of a segment of right mandible (12.5 × 6.5 × 5.5 cm) with 1 stitch designating anterior and 2 stitches designating lateral and is cleanly transected at the anterior margin and disarticulated posteriorly. There is 1 intact anterior tooth present at the anterior osseous margin. The superior aspect is covered in overlying tan-pink mucosa (9.2 × 5.5 cm) containing floor of mouth, alveolar ridge, buccal and retromolar trigone mucosa. Within the mucosa is a raised tan-brown, firm lesion (4.3 × 2.5 × 0.9 cm) which comes within 2.5 cm of the anterior mucosal margin, 2.2 cm from the medial floor of mouth mucosal margin, 5.1 cm from the posterior-superior retromolar trigone mucosal margin, and 1.2 cm from the lateral-superior buccal mucosal margin. The mandible is serially sectioned to reveal lesion extension of an ill-defined tan-white, soft mass (8.2 × 3.5 × 2.6 cm) which comes within 3.0 cm from the anterior soft tissue margin, 1.6 cm from the posterior soft tissue mar-

Fig. 9.80 Right mandible section quadrisected

gin, 0.7 cm from the lateral soft tissue margin, 0.5 cm from the medial soft tissue, and 0.1 cm from the inferior soft tissue margin.

Ink code
   Blue: lateral
   Green: medial
   Black: inferior
   Orange: anterior
   Red: posterior

A1: Anterior osseous margin, en face
A2: Anterior mucosal margin, perpendicular
A3: Anterior soft tissue margin, perpendicular
A4: Posterior mucosal margin, perpendicular
A5: Posterior soft tissue margin, perpendicular
A6-A9: Fullface section in relation to medial, lateral, and inferior, quadrisected
A10-A13: Fullface section in relation to medial, lateral, and inferior, quadrisected
A14-A17: Fullface sections in relation to medial, lateral, and inferior, quadrisected, post decalcification

9.20 Maxillomandibular Resection: Level CPT 88309

Large resections involving multiple anatomic sites are common for head and neck. Remember that in all head and neck specimen, there are a set of mucosal, soft tissue and possible bone margins. Keeping the orientation and using the margins present in the resection as a check list for how to perform the gross is key to completing the specimen (Fig. 9.81).

Step 1: Orient the specimen. Figure 9.82a is the medial view of the specimen which includes maxilla, buccal mucosa, and partial mandible. Figure 9.82b is the superior view showing the inferior aspect of the maxillary sinus and nasal septum.

Step 2: Describe and measure the specimen. Include the overall three-dimensional measurement and identify all the anatomic structures present.

Step 3: Describe and measure the lesion. Figure 9.83 is an internal view of the specimen with a large lesion present in the hard palate extending through the upper teeth into the anterior gingiva and extending onto the soft palate and buccal mucosa within the blue circle.

Step 4: Measure the lesion to all mucosal margins of the maxilla, buccal mucosa, and mandible. Margins include:

   Maxilla: Anterior mucosal margin, medial hard palate mucosal margin, posterior soft palate mucosal margin.
   Buccal: Anterior mucosal margin.
   Mandible: Anterior mandible mucosal margin, anterior floor of mouth mucosal margin,

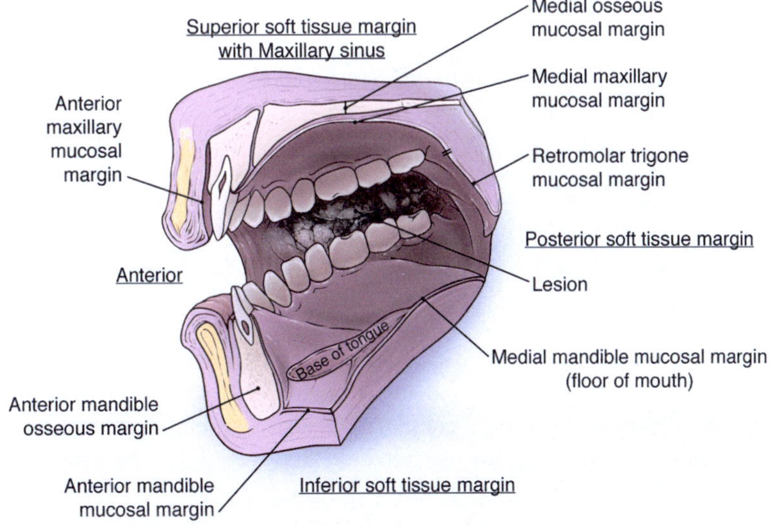

Fig. 9.81 Illustration of maxillomandibular resection

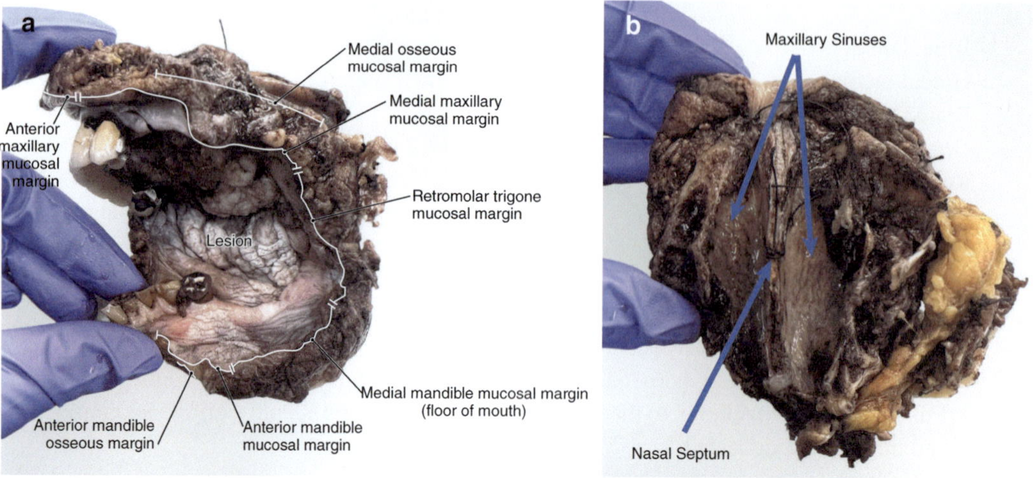

Fig. 9.82 (**a**) Right maxillomandibulectomy, medial view; (**b**) right maxillomandibulectomy, superior view

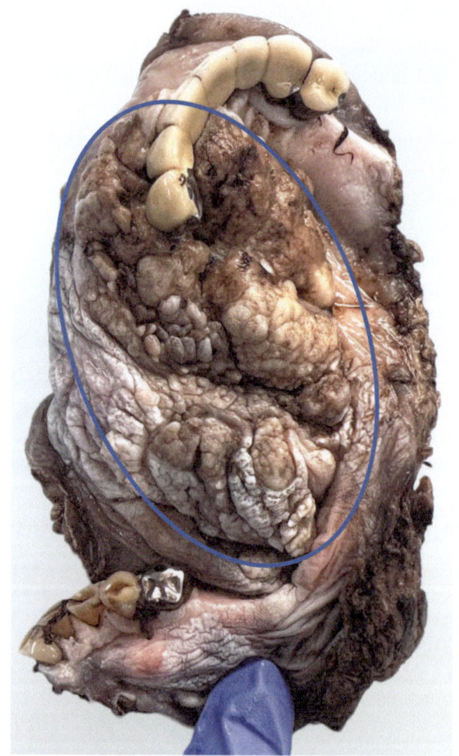

Fig. 9.83 Right maxillomandibulectomy, internal mucosal view

medial floor of mouth mucosal margin, posterior retromolar trigone mucosal margin.

Step 5: Ink the anterior, posterior, and lateral margins. Figure 9.84a shows the anterior aspect inked, and Fig. 9.84b shows the posterior and lateral aspects inked. Ink code is as follows:

Red-anterior maxilla buccal mucosa and mandible

Blue-medial hard palate, soft palate and mandible

Black-posterior maxilla and posterior soft tissue

Green-lateral mandible and lateral buccal soft tissue

Step 6: Ink the superior and inferior margins. Figure 9.85a shows the superior aspect inked which does not include the internal sinus mucosa, and Fig. 9.85b shows the inferior aspect inked. Ink code is as follows:

Yellow-superior maxilla

Orange-inferior mandible

Step 7: Shave the superior maxillary sinus margins as shown in Fig. 9.86 and submit en face. This includes the nasal septum and the right and left lateral maxillary bone.

Step 8: Serially section the specimen from anterior to posterior as shown in Fig. 9.87. Sectioning in this direction will allow for complete slices that include maxilla, buccal mucosa, and mandible.

Step 9: Perpendicularly section the anterior aspect. The anterior aspect is shown in Fig. 9.88a, and the perpendicular sections are

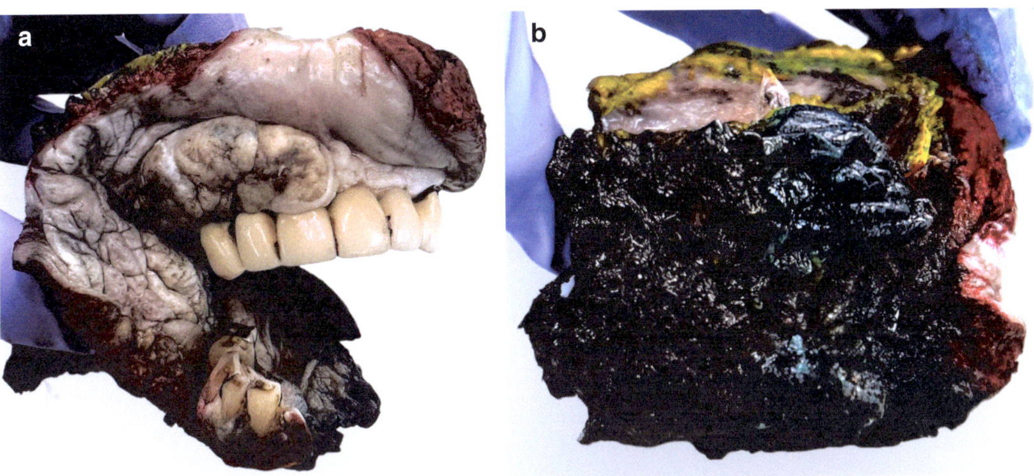

Fig. 9.84 (**a**) Right maxillomandibulectomy, anterior ink; (**b**) right maxillomandibulectomy, posterior ink

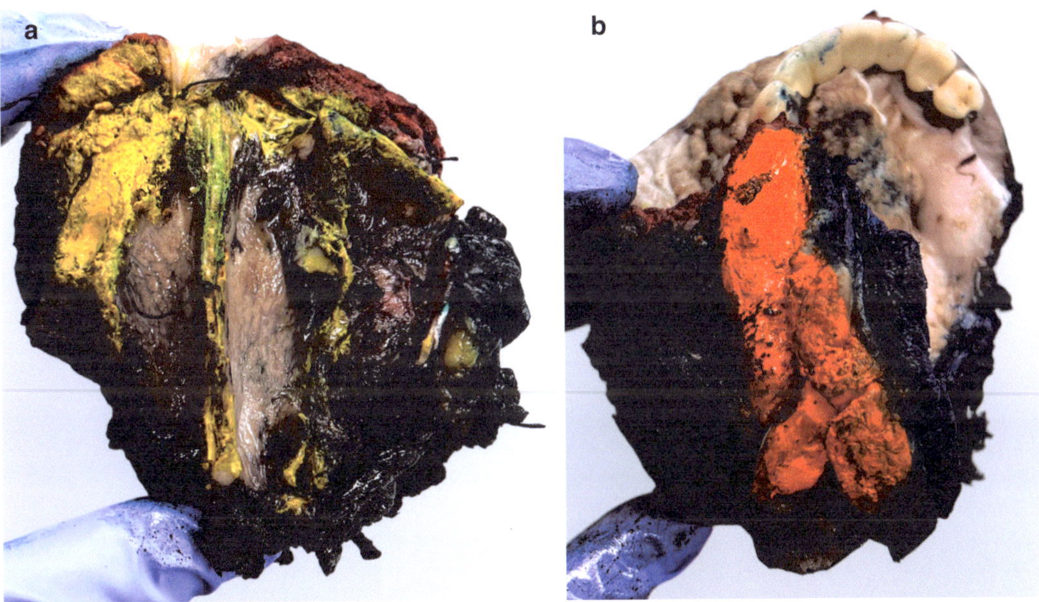

Fig. 9.85 (**a**) Right maxillomandibulectomy, superior ink; (**b**) right maxillomandibulectomy

shown in Fig. 9.88b. Always keep orientation and order when taking perpendicular sections as designated in Fig. 9.88b.

Step 10: Perpendicularly section the posterior aspect. The posterior aspect is shown in Fig. 9.89a, and the perpendicular sections are shown in Fig. 9.89b. Always keep orientation and order when taking perpendicular sections as designated in Fig. 9.89b.

Step 11: Measure the greatest depth of invasion and include invasion into the maxilla and mandible bones.

Step 12: Measure the distance of the lesion to the bone margins. In Fig. 9.90, the lesion extends into the right side of the maxilla, coming close to the right sinus cavity (not a margin) and close to the right lateral sinus bone margin. The lesion does not extend into the mandible bone.

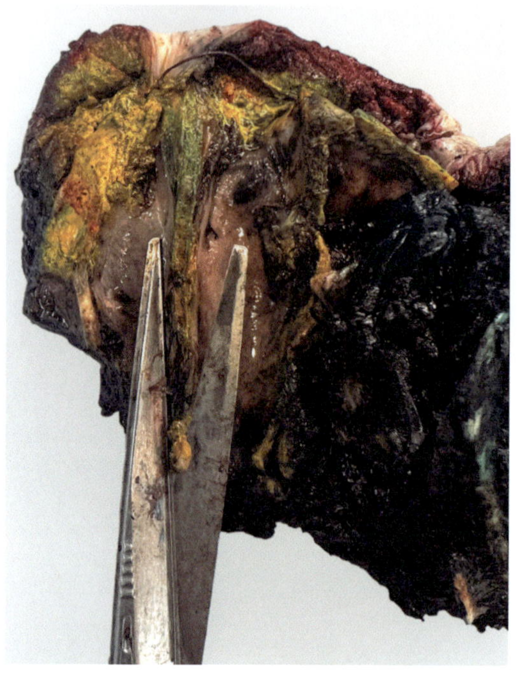

Fig. 9.86 Right maxillomandibulectomy, superior maxilla margins

Fig. 9.87 Right maxillomandibulectomy serially sectioned

Step 13: Submit sections. All margins are submitted either en face or perpendicular. Communicate with attending for instruction. Figure 9.91 is an example of a full cross section of the specimen which has been mapped for visual confirmation. Mapping specimen does take extra time but is incredibly helpful for complicated specimens.

Example Dictation

Specimen A is received in formalin labeled with patient's name, medical record number, "right maxilla and right mandible" and consists of a wide excision of right partial mandible, buccal mucosa, and bilateral maxilla (11.2 × 7.5 × 5.5 cm) with 5 teeth on the mandibular segment with partial underlying mandible and 7 teeth on the maxilla. The specimen is oriented with 1 stitch designating anterior and 2 stitches designating superior. The superior aspect contains bilateral inferior aspects of the nasal maxilla with identifiable septum. Within

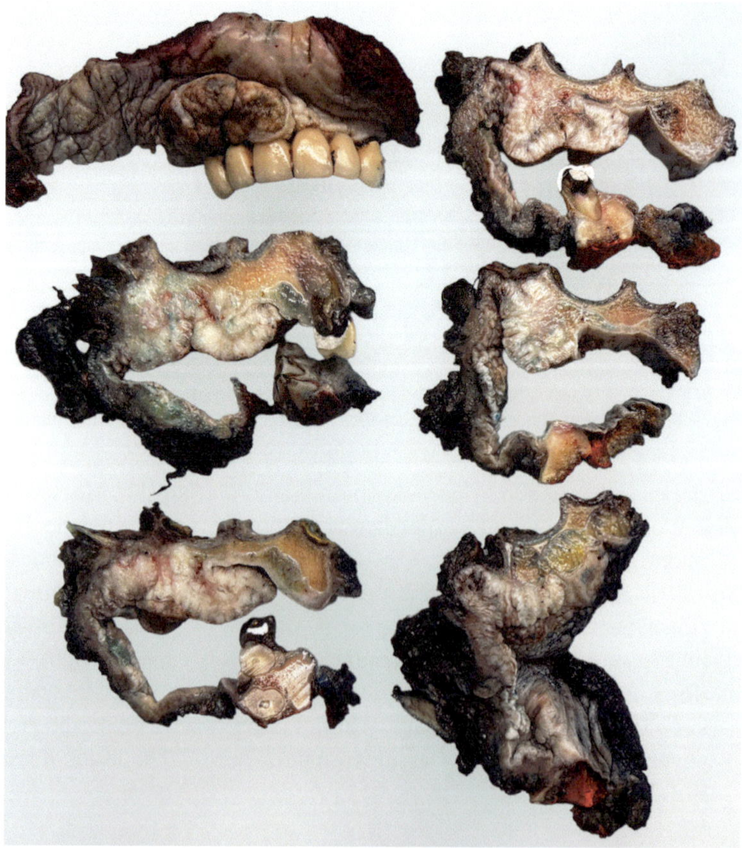

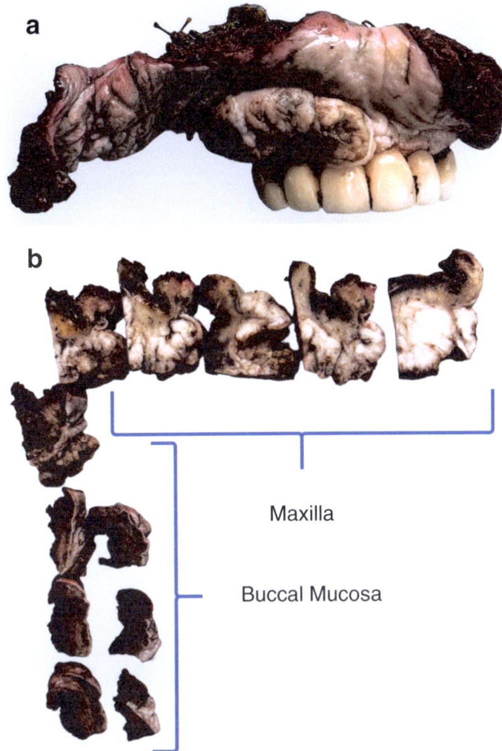

Fig. 9.88 (**a**) Right maxillomandibulectomy anterior, whole; (**b**), right maxillomandibulectomy, anterior perpendicularly sectioned

the hard palate is a large, fungating tan-brown mass (7.2 × 5.1 × 1.1 cm) extending the entirety of the right aspect of the maxilla, crossing the maxillary midline and extending into the right side of proximally 1.5 cm. The mass extends through the maxillary alveolar ridge and teeth, extending onto the right lateral gingival mucosa approximately 1.6 cm. Additionally, the mass extends through the entirety of the left and mid aspect of the soft palate and into the right lateral buccal mucosa, with scant extension onto the retromolar trigone. The mass comes within 1.9 cm of the anterior maxillary mucosal margin, 1.5 cm from the medial maxillary mucosal margin, 1.0 cm from the lateral maxillary mucosal margin, 1.6 cm from the posterior retromolar trigone mucosal margin, 0.6 cm from the anterior buccal mucosal margin, 2.6 cm from the medial floor of mouth mucosal margin, and 3.8 cm from the anterior mandible

mucosal margin. The specimen is serially sectioned to reveal maxillary bone invasion superiorly greatest depth of invasion approximately 0.6 cm, coming within 0.6 cm of the right superior maxillary sinus osseous margin, 0.9 cm from the nasal septum margin, and 1.5 cm from the left superior maxillary sinus osseous margin. The mass invades laterally approximately 0.3 cm, coming within 0.5 cm of the lateral buccal soft tissue margin. The mass invades inferiorly, proximally 0.2 cm, coming within 0.4 cm of the mandibular bone, without mandibular bone involvement.

Ink code
    Yellow: superior maxilla
    Red: anterior maxilla buccal mucosa and mandible
    Blue: medial hard palate, soft palate and mandible
    Black: posterior maxilla and posterior soft tissue
    Orange: inferior mandible
    Green: lateral mandible and lateral buccal soft tissue

A1: Right superior maxillary sinus margin, en face
A2: Left superior maxillary sinus margin, en face
A3: Nasal septum margin, en face
A4-A5: Mass in relation to anterior maxillary mucosal margin
A6: Anterior buccal mucosal margin, perpendicular (no mass present)
A7: Anterior floor of mouth, shave, en face
A8: Anterior mandible, perpendicular
A9: Mass in relation to posterior and medial hard palate, perpendicular
A10: Mass in relation to posterior and medial soft palate, perpendicular
A11: Mass in relation to posterior and medial floor of mouth
A12-A17: Full face section of mass from maxilla to mandible

Sections containing bone are decalcified prior to submission.

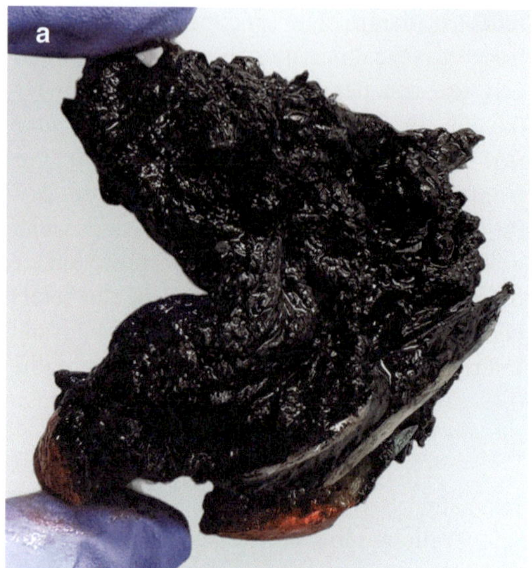

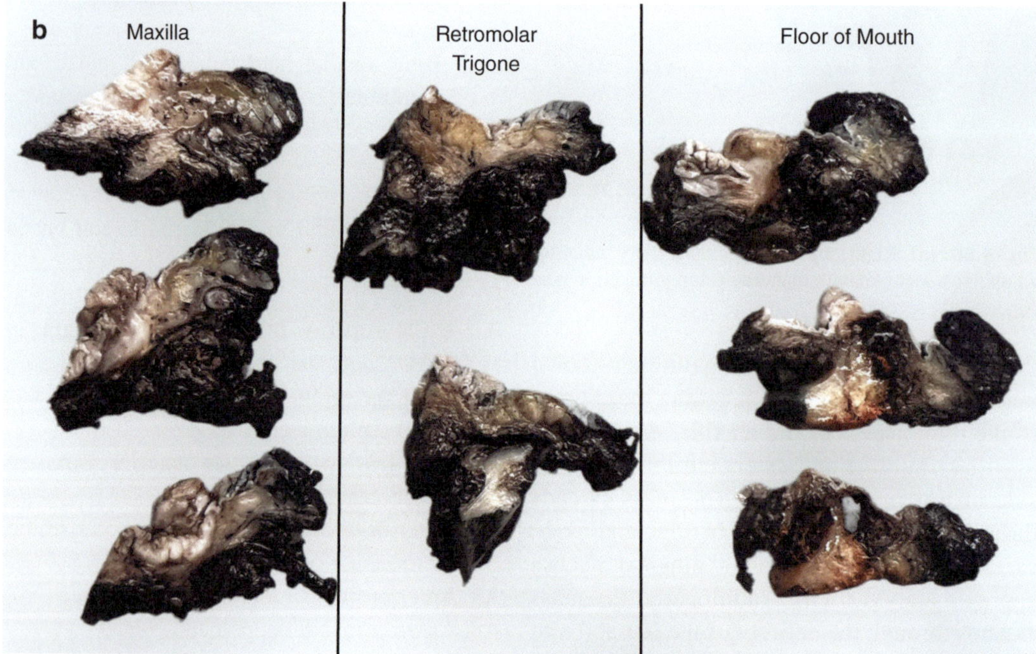

Fig. 9.89 (**a**) Right maxillomandibulectomy posterior, whole; (**b**) right maxillomandibulectomy, posterior perpendicularly sectioned

Cancer Protocol Relative to grossing the Larynx.

Procedure:

Endolaryngeal excision—the removal of the lesion transorally with preservation of the vocal cords.

Transoral laser excision—the piecemeal removal of a lesion using a carbon dioxide laser transorally.

Supraglottic laryngectomy—the removal of the supraglottic aspect of the larynx which includes from the epiglottis to the false cords.

Supracricoid laryngectomy—the removal of the thyroid cartilage with the attached vocal cords.

Vertical hemilaryngectomy—the removal of either the right or the left vocal cords with the attached thyroid cartilage.

Partial laryngectomy—the removal of only a portion of the larynx containing the lesion.

Total laryngectomy—the removal of the entire laryngeal structures with some trachea.

Tumor focality: Dictate the number of separate lesions present, if applicable and measure the size of each lesion.

Tumor Site: Primary site of origin

Extent of invasion: Dictate all anatomical structures the lesion involves. This includes the supraglottis, epiglottis, aryepiglottic folds, arytenoids, bilateral true and false vocal cords, ventricle, and anterior and posterior commissure. For accurate staging of laryngeal tumor, the extent of invasion is important and therefore must be included in the gross description. Besides the involvement for separate subsites, extra laryngeal extension, invasion of the hypopharynx, thyroid, and cricoid cartilage should be included.

Transglottic extension: Tumor involving supraglottis, glottis, and/or subglottis.

When subglottic extension is identified, extend of invasion from true vocal cord should be measured and included in the gross description.

Tumor laterality: Dictate which side the lesion is present including left side, right side, midline, or more than one.

Tumor size: Overall lesion size should be dictated in centimeters.

Margin status: Dictate the distance of the lesion to all margins.

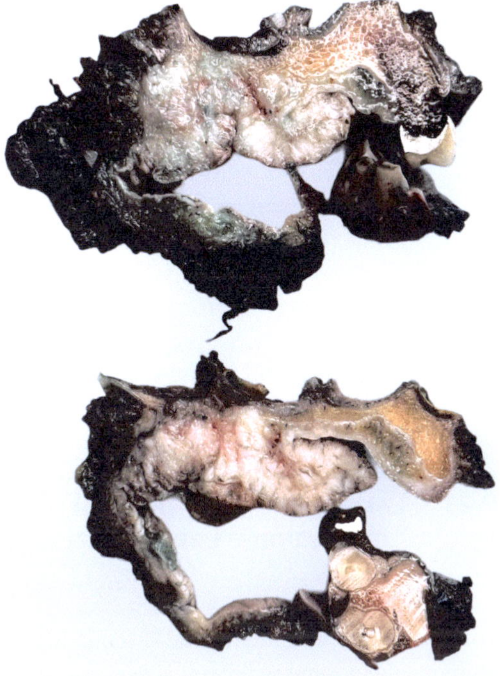

Fig. 9.90 Right maxillomandibulectomy serially sectioned

Fig. 9.91 Right maxillomandibulectomy section map

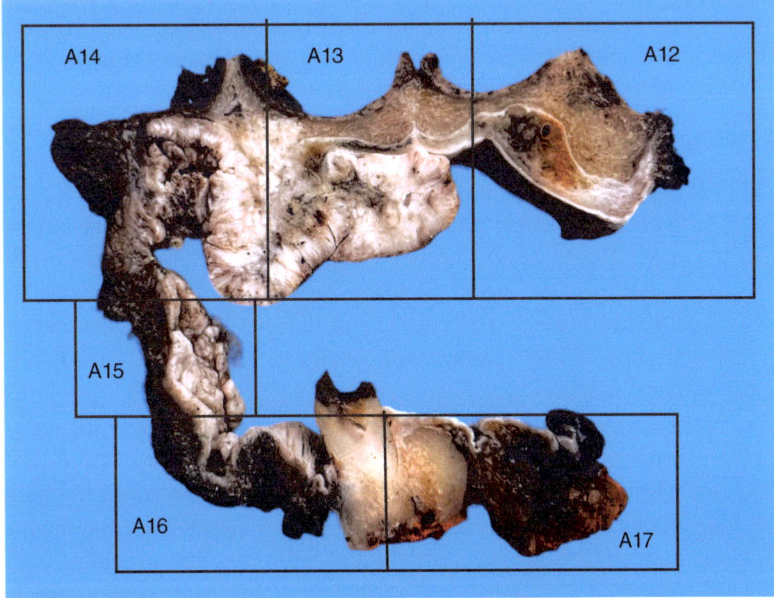

pT Category

Supraglottic lesions

pT1: Tumor limited to one subsite of supraglottis with normal vocal cord mobility.

pT2: Tumor invades mucosa of more than one adjacent subsite of supraglottis or glottis or region outside the supraglottis without fixation of the larynx.

pT3: Tumor limited to larynx with vocal cord fixation and/or invades any of the following: postcricoid area, preepiglottic space, paraglottic space, and/or inner cortex of thyroid cartilage.

pT4a: Moderately advanced local disease. Tumor invades through the thyroid cartilage and/or invades tissues beyond the larynx (e.g., trachea, soft tissues of neck including deep extrinsic muscle of tongue, strap muscles, thyroid, or esophagus)

pT4b: Very advanced local disease. Tumor invades prevertebral space, encases carotid artery, or invades mediastinal structures.

Glottic Lesions

pT1: Tumor limited to the vocal cords with normal mobility.

pT1a: Tumor limited to one vocal cord.

pT1b: Tumor involves both vocal cords.

pT2: Tumor extends to supraglottis and/or subglottis and/or with impaired vocal cord mobility.

pT3: Tumor limited to the larynx with vocal cord fixation and/or invasion of paraglottic space and/or inner cortex of the thyroid cartilage.

pT4a: Moderately advanced local disease. Tumor invades through the outer cortex of the thyroid cartilage and/or invades tissues beyond the larynx (e.g., trachea, cricoid cartilage, soft tissues of neck including deep extrinsic muscle of the tongue, strap muscles, thyroid, or esophagus).

pT4b: Very advanced local disease. Tumor invades prevertebral space, encases carotid artery, or invades mediastinal.

Subglottic lesions

pT1: Tumor limited to subglottis.

pT2: Tumor extends to vocal cord with normal or impaired mobility.

pT3: Tumor limited to larynx with vocal cord fixation and/or invasion of paraglottic space and/or inner cortex of the thyroid cartilage.

pT4a: Moderately advanced local disease. Tumor invades cricoid or thyroid cartilage and/or invades tissues beyond the larynx (e.g., trachea, soft tissues of neck including deep extrinsic muscles of the tongue, strap muscles, thyroid, or esophagus)

pT4b: Very advanced local disease. Tumor invades prevertebral space, encases carotid artery, or invades mediastinal structures.

9.21 Laryngectomy with Vocal Cord Lesion—Level VI CPT 88309

The anatomy of the larynx is complicated. Studying the normal structures is key to grossing a laryngectomy appropriately. Section submission changes based on location of the lesion and lesion involvement of structures of the larynx. See Fig. 9.92a, b for a review of anatomical structures of the larynx.

Step 1: Describe and measure the specimen. Figure 9.92a shows the anterior aspect of the larynx, and Fig. 9.92b shows the posterior aspect of the larynx.

Step 2: Note the presence or absence of the thyroid gland and/or a tracheostomy site. There is no tracheostomy site noted in Fig. 9.92a.

Step 3: Describe and measure the lesion. In Fig. 9.93, the lesion is slightly hemorrhagic, present in the right false cord designated with a blue arrow.

Step 4: Dictate where the lesion is located including all anatomic structures, present in the supraglottic, glottic, or subglottic space and whether the lesion crosses the anterior

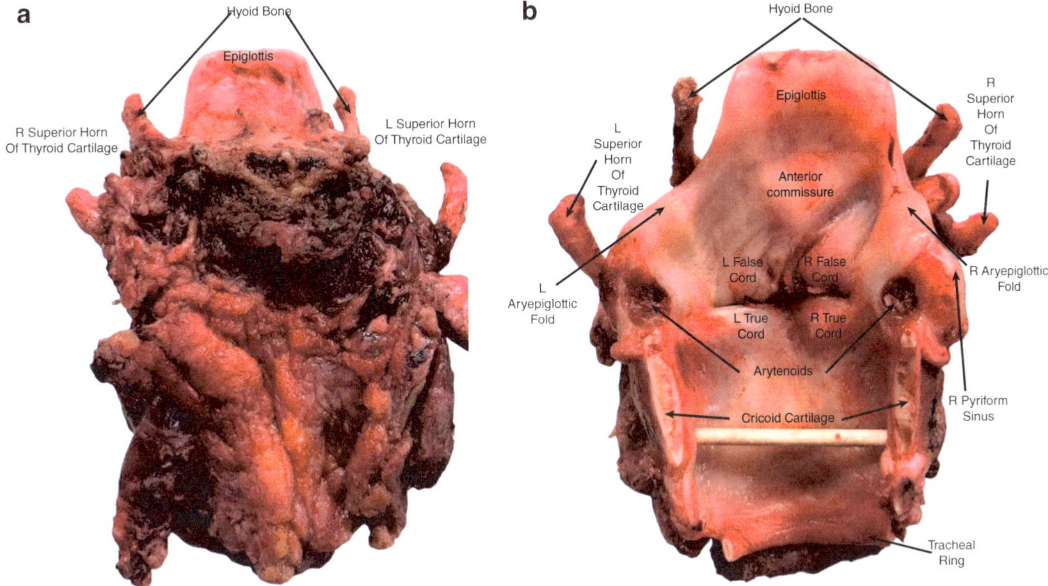

Fig. 9.92 (**a**) Larynx anterior view; (**b**) larynx posterior view

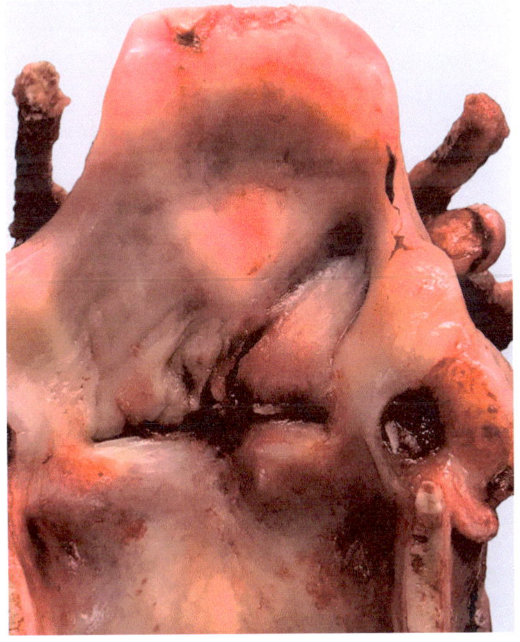

Fig. 9.93 Right false vocal cord lesion

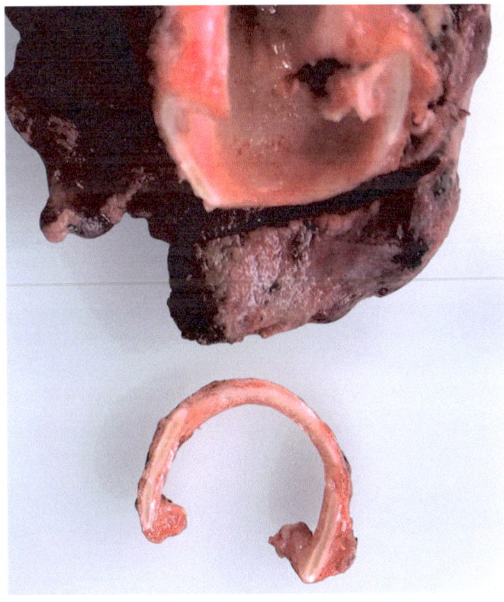

Fig. 9.94 Tracheal margin

or posteriorly. In Fig. 9.93, the lesion is present grossly in the right true and false vocal cords, spanning the supraglottic and glottic space and crossing the anterior commissure.

Step 5: Measure the lesion to all mucosal margins which includes the base of tongue, right and left lateral mucosa, posterior-inferior mucosa, and inferior tracheal margins.

Step 6: Shave the tracheal margin and submit en face as shown in Fig. 9.94.

Step 7: Shave the base of tongue (Fig. 9.95a) mucosal margin and the posterior-inferior (Fig. 9.95b) mucosal margin and submit en face.

Step 8: Shave the left (Fig. 9.96a) and right (Fig. 9.96b) lateral mucosal margins and submit en face.

Step 9: Ink the resection margin. In this example, the entire resection margin is inked blue. Figure 9.97a is the anterior view, and Fig. 9.97b is the posterior view.

Step 10: Remove the hyoid bone. Using a scalpel blade, resect the hyoid bone from the larynx. This step is optional depending on pathologist's preference.

Step 11: Ink the false margin on the larynx and hyoid bone as seen in Fig. 9.98.

Step 12: Take representative sections of the left (Fig. 9.99a) and right (Fig. 9.99b) aryepiglottic fold with pyriform sinus. This section will show the presence or absence of tumor in the areas.

Step 13: Take a section of the posterior commissure longitudinally as shown in Fig. 9.100. This will show the presence or absence of tumor crossing the posterior commissure midline.

Step 14: Take the anterior commissure full length slice as shown in Fig. 9.101. Cut through both sides of the anterior commissure to remove the central anterior slice. This shows the presence or absence of tumor crossing the anterior commissure (midline).

Step 15: Longitudinally section the remaining left side of the larynx as shown in Fig. 9.102.

Step 16: Longitudinally section the remaining right side of the larynx as shown in Fig. 9.103.

Step 17: Measure the greatest depth of invasion of the lesion which is designated with a blue arrow in Fig. 9.104 and measure how close the lesion comes to the surrounding inked margin and the hyoid false margin.

Step 18: Take representative sections of the hyoid bone in the area there the tumor would come closest as shown in Fig. 9.105.

Step 19: Submit sections. In addition to the mucosal margins, full length sections of the mass in relation to the closest margins, bilateral vocal cords, anterior/posterior commissure, tracheostomy, and thyroid closest to lesion should be submitted. These sections can be photographed and mapped, if necessary.

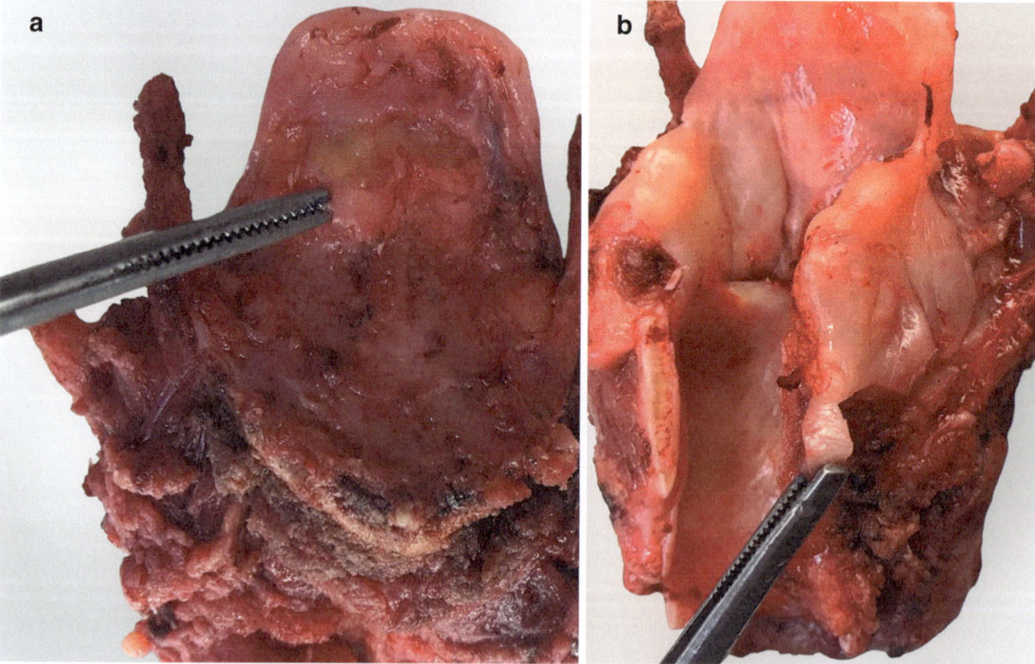

Fig. 9.95 (**a**) Base of tongue mucosal margin; (**b**) posterior-inferior mucosal margin

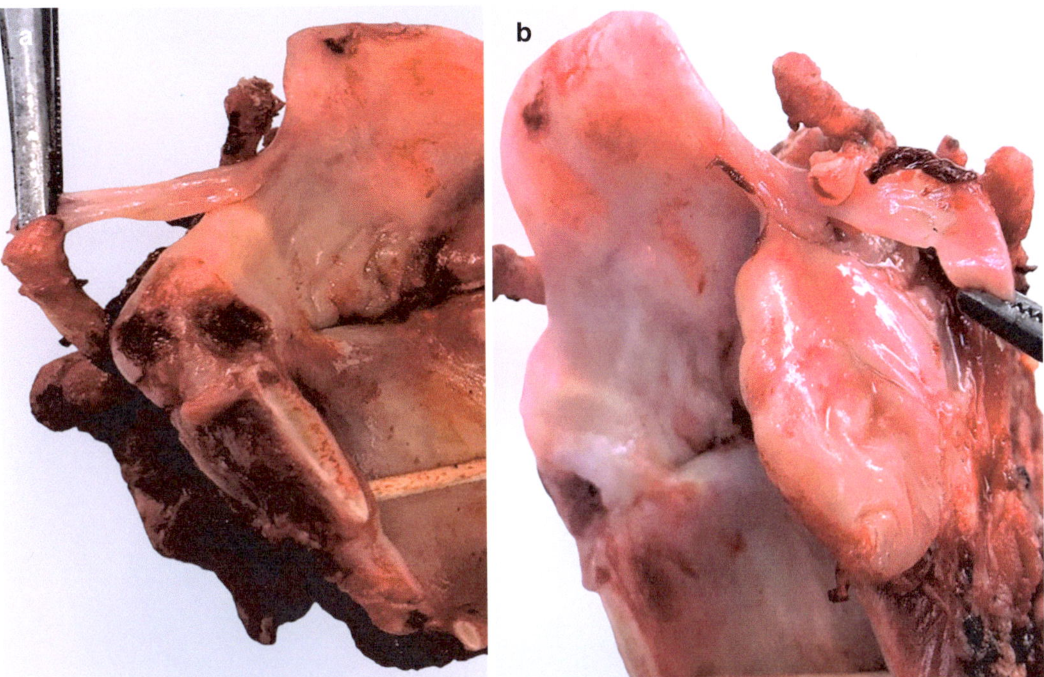

Fig. 9.96 (**a**) Left lateral mucosal margin; (**b**) right lateral mucosal margin

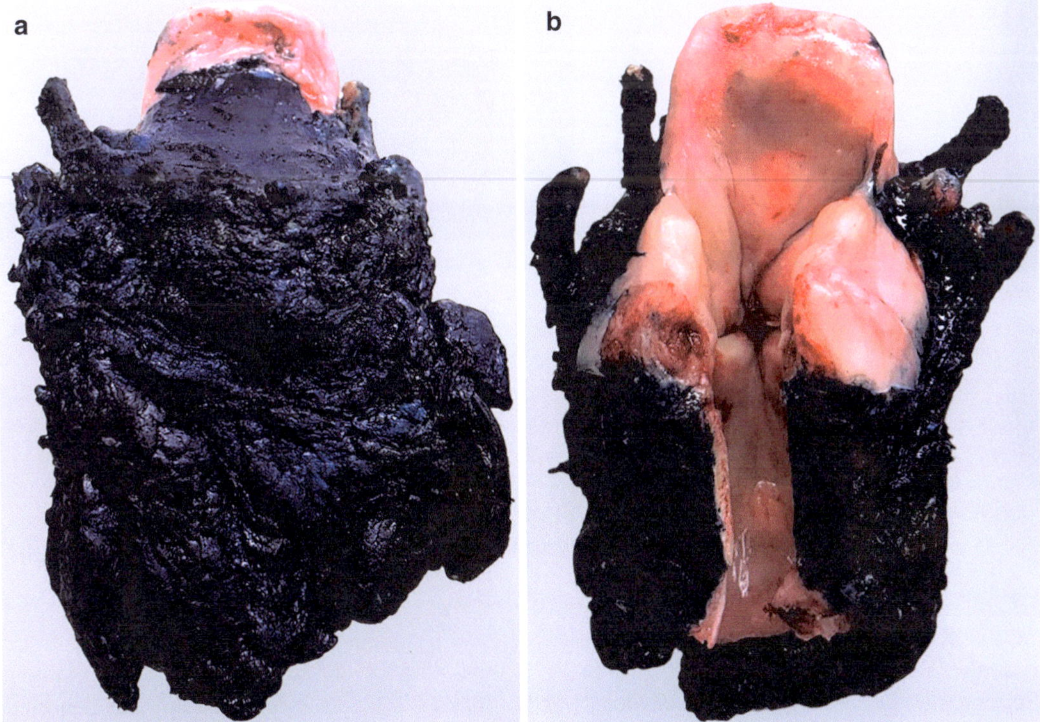

Fig. 9.97 (**a**) Anterior ink; (**b**) posterior ink

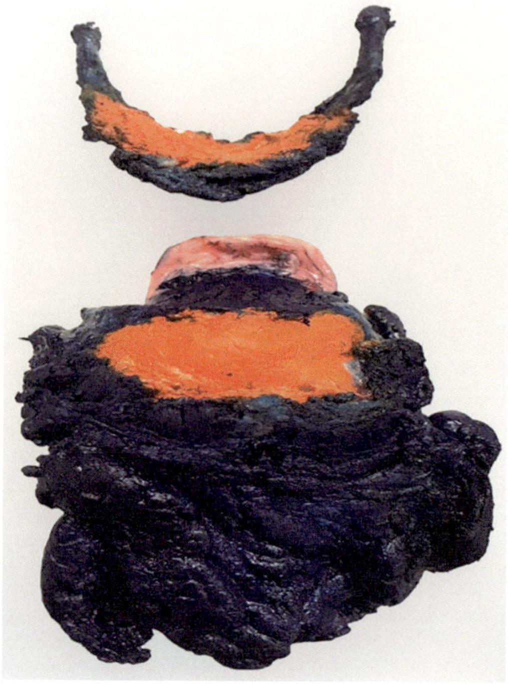

Fig. 9.98 Removal and ink of hyoid bone

Fig. 9.100 Posterior commissure

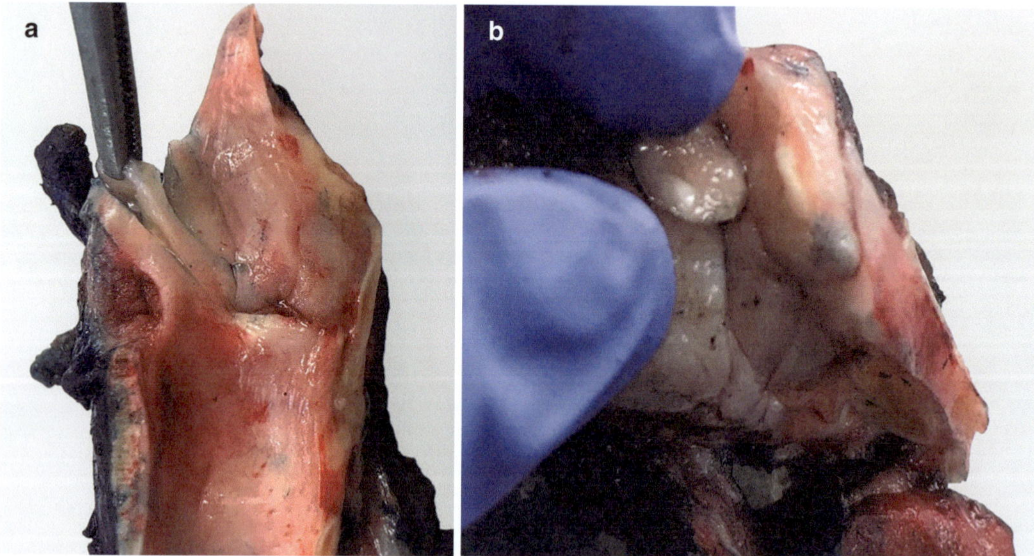

Fig. 9.99 (**a**) Left aryepiglottic fold; (**b**) right aryepiglottic fold

Example Dictation

Specimen A is received fresh labeled with patient's name, medical record number, "total laryngectomy" and consists of a total laryngectomy (7.5 × 2.9 cm in diameter) including anterior soft tissue (1.1–1.9 cm thick), right thyroid lobe (3.5 × 1.4 × 1.1 cm), and isthmus (2.0 × 1.5 × 1.1 cm) with no ostomy site identified. The specimen is previously opened posteriorly to reveal a hemorrhagic, slightly ulcerative pink-red lesion (0.9 × 0.7 cm) present in the supraglottic right false cord, abutting the anterior commissure

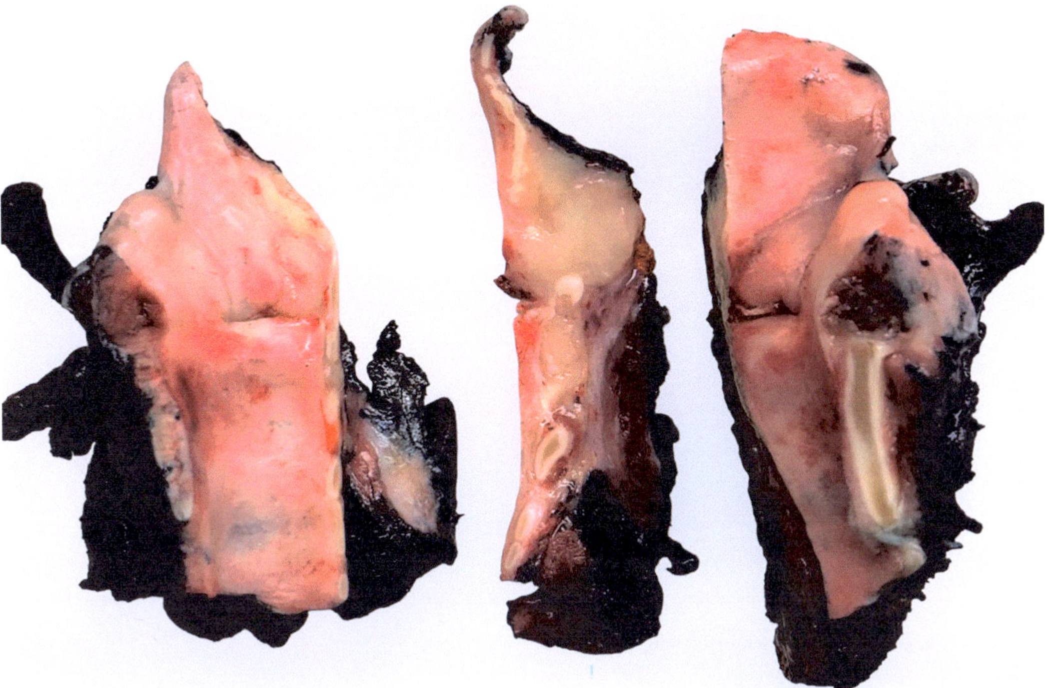

Fig. 9.101   Anterior commissure

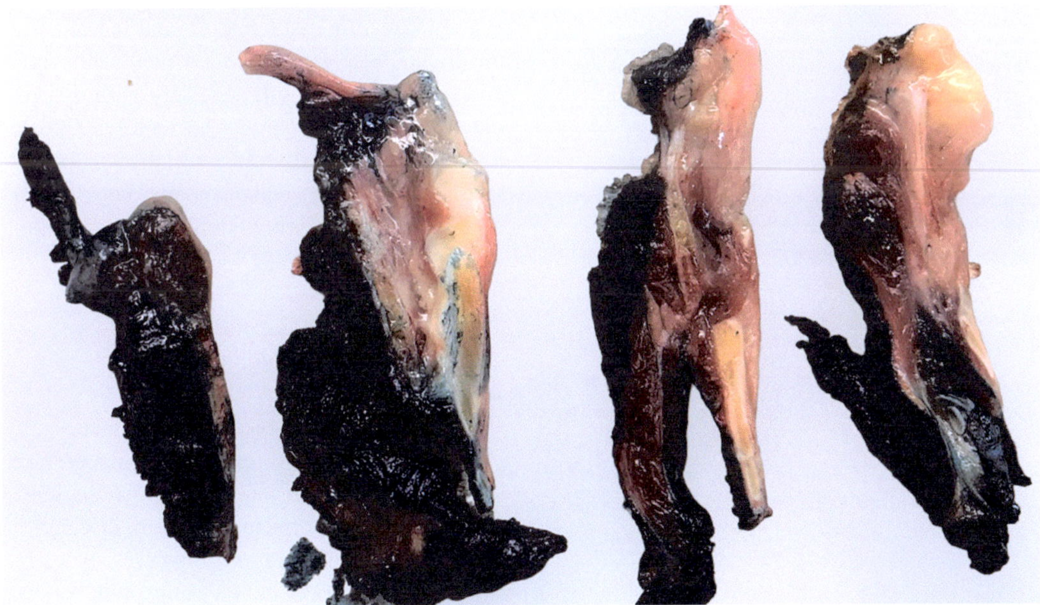

Fig. 9.102   Left side serially sectioned longitudinally

with slight invasion into the right true cord. The lesion comes within 2.4 cm from the tip of the epiglottis, 3.6 cm from the tracheal resection margin, 1.2 cm from the right aryepiglottic fold, and 4.2 cm from the right lateral mucosal margin. The larynx is serially sectioned to reveal a greatest depth of invasion approximately 1.6 cm, creating an overall mass size 3.2 × 2.1 × 1.6 cm,

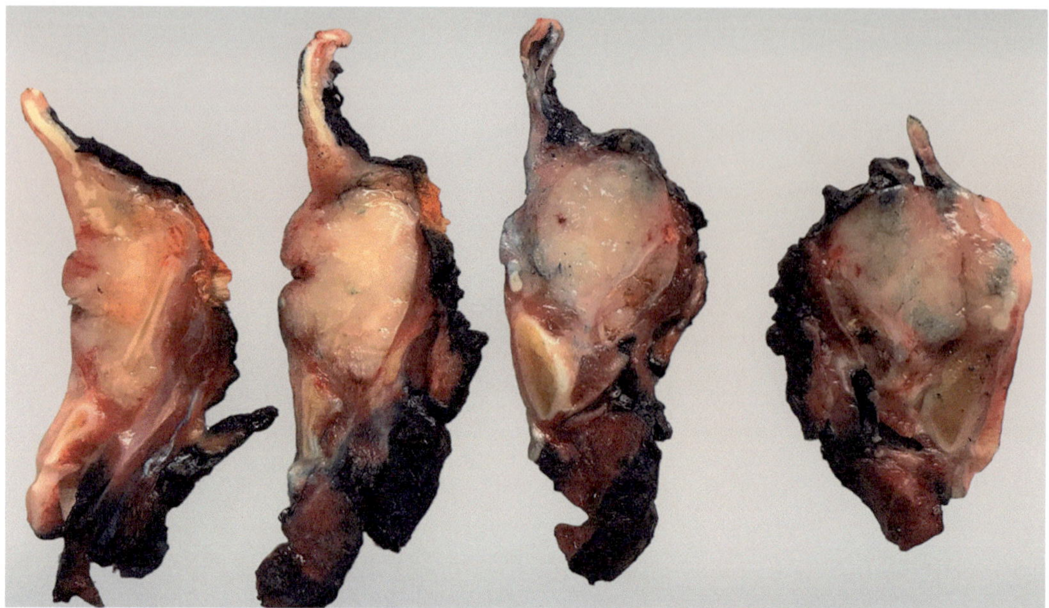

Fig. 9.103 Right side serially sectioned longitudinally

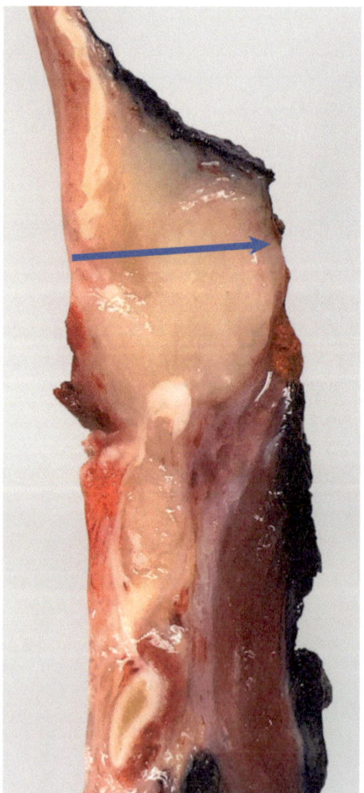

Fig. 9.104 Mass to closest margin

submucosally invading under the right true cord and abutting the thyroid cartilage with possible cortical invasion and comes within 0.2 cm of the supraglottic soft tissue margin and 0.3 cm from the hyoid false margin. Additionally, the mass crosses the midline submucosally with approximately 0.1 cm of submucosal invasion into the left false cord. The thyroid is serially sectioned to reveal red-brown, homogeneous cut surfaces with no masses present within the thyroid lobe.

Ink code

    Blue: surrounding margin

    Orange: hyoid false margin

Section code

    A1: Base of tongue margin, en face

    A2: Right lateral mucosal margin, en face

    A3: Left lateral mucosal margin, en face

    A4: Posterior mucosal margin, bisected,

    A5: Tracheal margin, en face

    A6: Posterior commissure with cricoid cartilage

    A7: Left aryepiglottic fold, inferior pyriform sinus

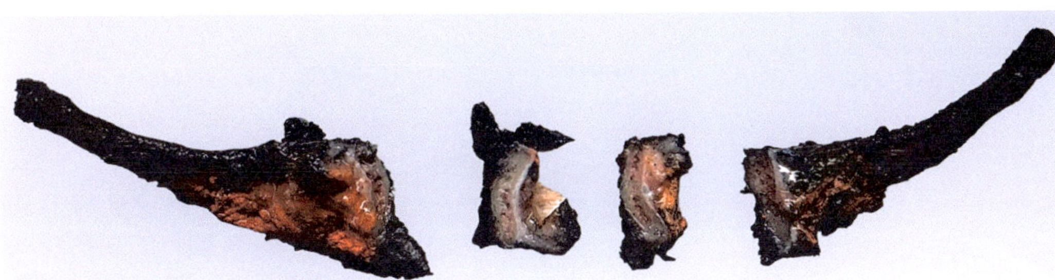

Fig. 9.105 Hyoid bone sections

A8: Left true and false vocal cords

A9-A10: Mass within anterior commissure, including epiglottis, anterior commissure, ventricles and anterior soft tissue margin, bisected

A11-A14: Full length section of right side (11: Epiglottis and hyoid false margin, 12: True and false right vocal cord, 13: Mass invading thyroid cartilage and unremarkable cricoid cartilage, 14: Unremarkable cricoid cartilage)

A15: Mass in relation to right aryepiglottic fold

A16: Hyoid bone, post decalcification

A17: Thyroid, representative

9.22 Laryngectomy and Partial Pharyngectomy—Level VI CPT 88309

The pharynx and larynx are closely associated so pharyngeal lesions are frequently resected with the larynx. These specimens contain the same laryngeal margins and sections but have additional pharyngeal margins and sections. In this example, the specimen is fixed in formalin and then decalcified intact, leaving the hyoid bone attached to the larynx for sectioning.

Step 1: Describe and measure the specimen. This includes the larynx and the right partial pharynx as shown in Fig. 9.106. The partial pharynx is designated with a blue circle in Fig. 9.106.

Step 2: Note the presence or absences of the thyroid gland and/or a tracheostomy site.

Step 3: Ink the surrounding soft tissue resection margin as shown in Fig. 9.107.

Step 4: Describe and measure the lesion shown in Fig. 9.108.

Step 5: Measure the lesion to all the surrounding mucosal margins. In this example, the lesion is present in the right partial pharynx, extending onto the right aryepiglottic fold and into the right side of the epiglottis. The margins of the pharynx are anterior-superior, lateral, and posterior-inferior mucosa.

Step 6: Shave the margins that are greater than 2 cm from the lesion and submit en face. In this example, the posterior-inferior larynx mucosal margin (Fig. 9.109a), the left lateral larynx mucosal margin (Fig. 9.109b), and the tracheal margin (Fig. 9.109c) are greater than 2 cm from the lesion. These margins are shaved and submitted en face.

Step 7: Remove the anterior-superior and lateral mucosal margins of the pharynx and submit perpendicularly. Notice in Fig. 9.110a, these margins are cut from the main specimen approximately 1 cm thick and then perpendicularly sectioned as shown in Fig. 9.110b.

Step 8: Remove the posterior-inferior right partial pharynx margin and submit perpendicularly as shown in Fig. 9.111.

Step 9: Take a longitudinal section of the posterior commissure as shown in Fig. 9.112a. This section shows if the lesion has extended into the posterior aspect of the larynx and has or has not crossed the midline (posterior commissure).

Step 10: Take a longitudinal section of the anterior commissure as shown in Fig. 9.112b. This section shows if the lesion has extended into

Fig. 9.106 Larynx with right partial pharyngectomy

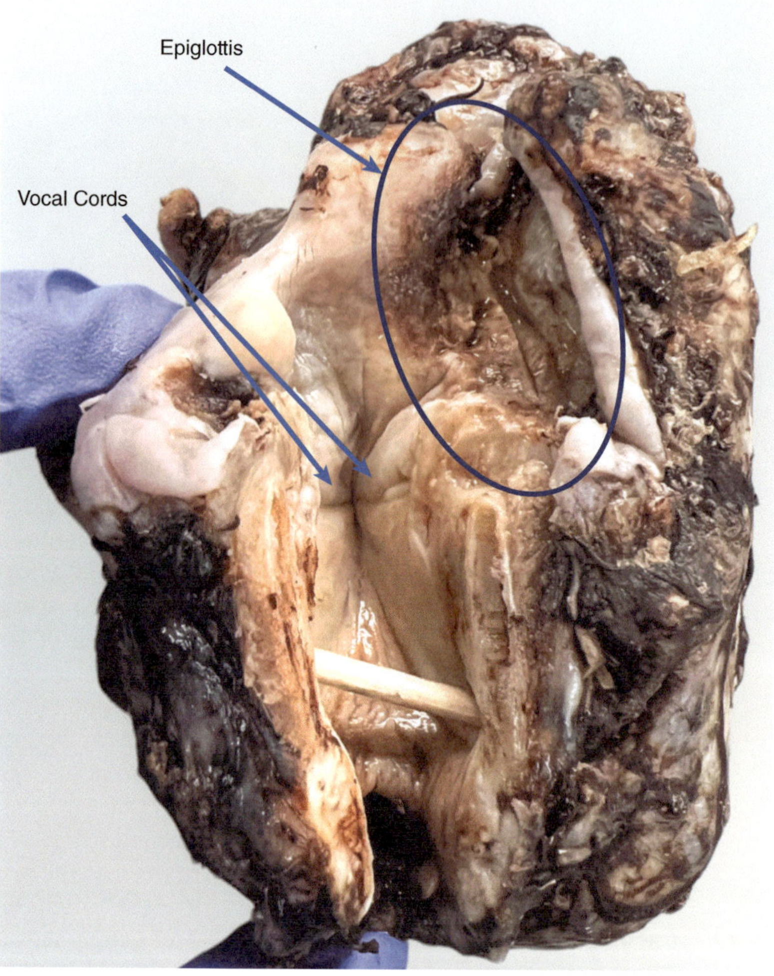

the anterior aspect of the larynx and has or has not crossed the midline (anterior commissure). This section is the anterior central slice of the larynx.

Step 11: Longitudinally serially section the right and left larynx as shown in Fig. 9.113. The pharynx on the far-right side will remain intact.

Step 12: Assess extension of the lesion from the partial pharynx into the larynx. In Fig. 9.114, the blue arrow shows lesion extension from the partial pharynx into the right epiglottis and right base of tongue.

Step 13: Serially section the remainder of the right larynx and partial right pharynx from superior to inferior as shown in Fig. 9.115a.

Step 14: Measure the greatest depth of invasion of the pharynx lesion and how close the lesion comes from the deep pharynx soft tissue margin. In Fig. 9.115b, the greatest depth of invasion is designated by the blue arrow.

Step 15: Submit representative sections of the pharynx with the greatest depth of invasion.

Step 16: Serially section the thyroid, if present. In Fig. 9.116, the thyroid is sectioned and contains a separate nodule designated with a blue arrow.

Step 17: Describe and measure the nodule.

Step 18: Submit representative sections of the thyroid nodule.

Example Dictation

Specimen A is received freshly labeled with patient's name, medical record number, "total laryngectomy and right partial pharyngectomy" and consists of a total laryngectomy (7.2 × 5.5 × 4.4 cm)

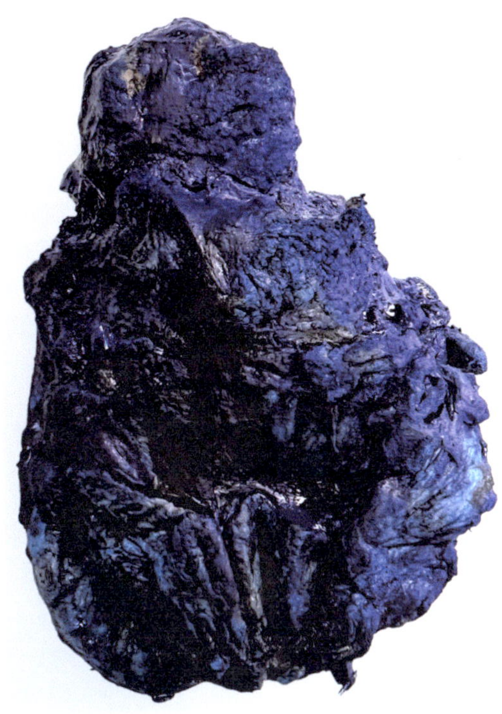

Fig. 9.107 Larynx specimen inked, anterior view

with attached portion of right pharynx (5.2 × 3.1 × 1.5 cm), anterior ostomy site (1.4 cm in diameter) surrounded by tan-brown skin and attached right thyroid lobe (4.2 × 1.9 × 1.8 cm). The right pharynx contains an ulcerative tan-brown lesion (3.0 × 2.4 cm) which comes within 1.8 cm of the anterior-superior pharyngeal wall, 0.6 cm from the right lateral pharyngeal wall, and 0.9 cm from the posterior-inferior pharyngeal wall, extending medially through the aryepiglottic fold and into the right aspect of the epiglottis, without extension into the right bilateral vocal cords and coming within 5.0 cm of the tracheal margin. The specimen is serially sectioned to reveal the greatest depth of invasion within the pharynx approximately 0.3 cm, coming within 0.8 cm of the deep pharyngeal soft tissue margin, abutting the right thyroid cartilage with no extension into the cricoid cartilage. Additionally, the mass extends to within 0.9 cm of the right base of tongue soft tissue margin. The attached right thyroid lobe is serially sectioned to reveal a tan-white, well-circumscribed nodule (1.2 × 1.1 × 0.9 cm)

Fig. 9.108 Larynx specimen inked, posterior view

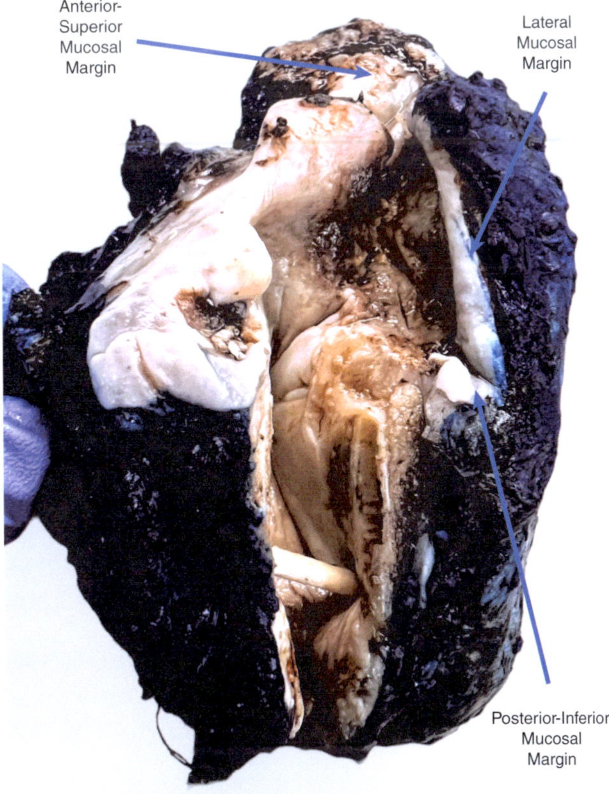

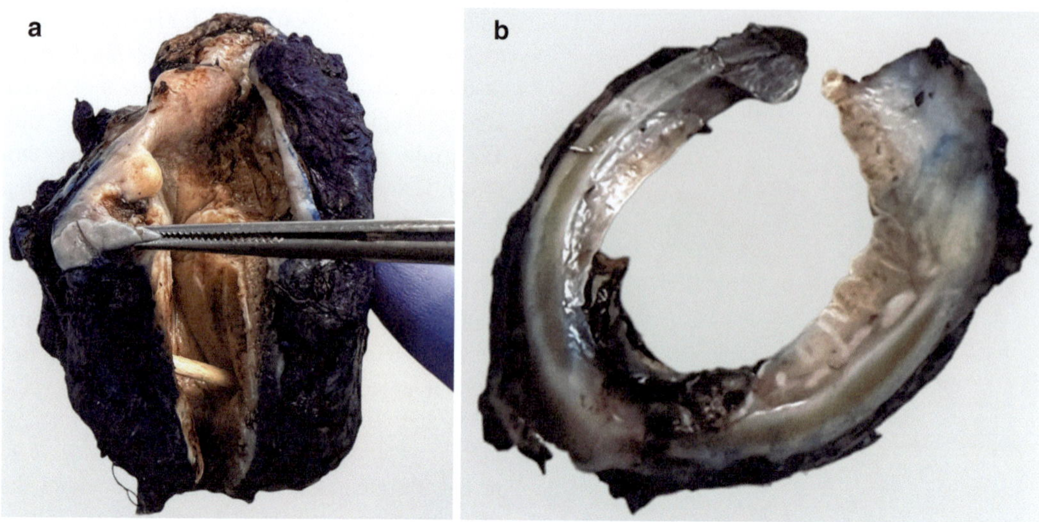

Fig. 9.109 (**a**) Posterior-inferior mucosal margin; (**b**) left lateral mucosal margin; (**c**) tracheal margin

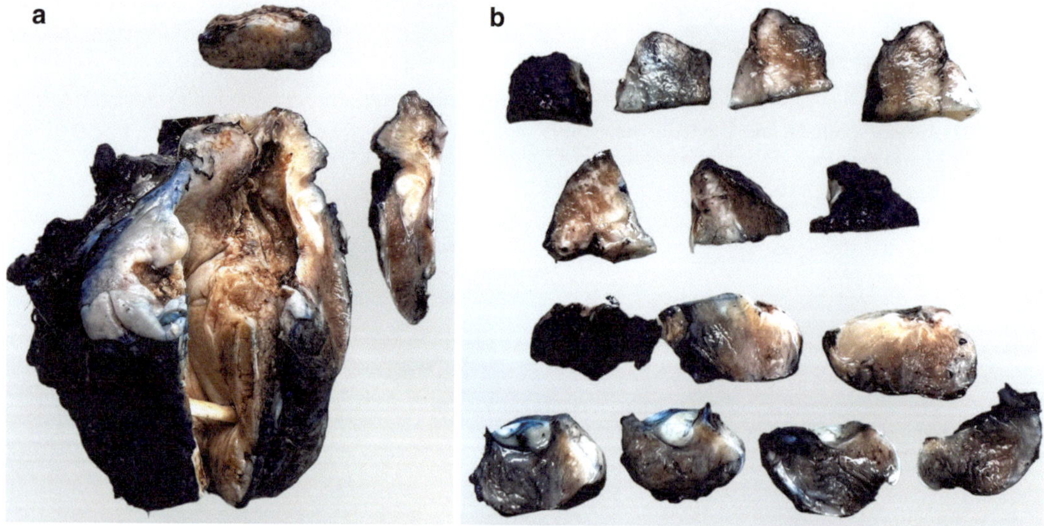

Fig. 9.110 (**a**) Anterior-superior and lateral right partial pharynx mucosal margin, shaved; (**b**) anterior-superior and lateral right partial pharynx mucosal margin, perpendicularly sectioned

present mid lobe, coming within 1.1 cm of the superior pole and 1.0 cm of the inferior pole surrounded by red-brown thyroid parenchyma.

Section code

A 1: Tracheal margin, en face

A2-A3: Anterior-superior pharyngeal margin, perpendicular

A4-A6: Right lateral pharyngeal margin, perpendicular

A7: Posterior-inferior pharyngeal margin, perpendicular

A8: Posterior commissure, representative

A9: Unremarkable left true and false vocal cords, representative

A10-A11: Central slice superior aspect including epiglottis and anterior commissure

A12-A14: Right side, full length from superior to inferior, post decalcification

Fig. 9.111 Posterior-inferior partial pharynx margin, perpendicular

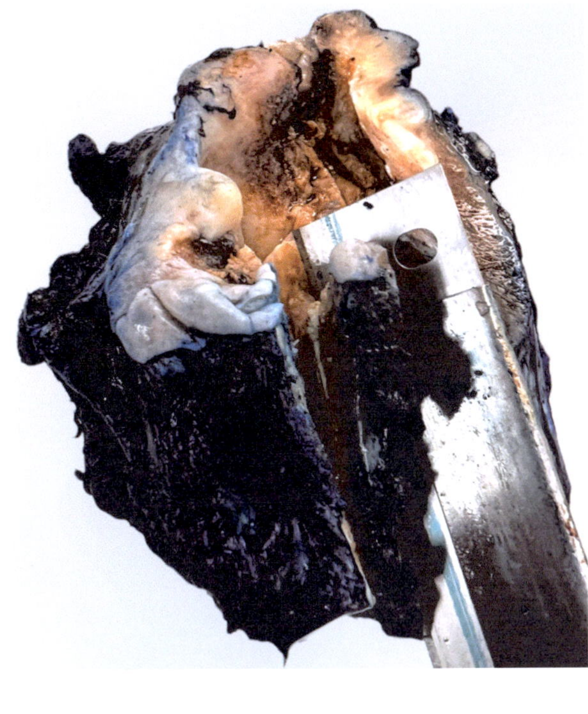

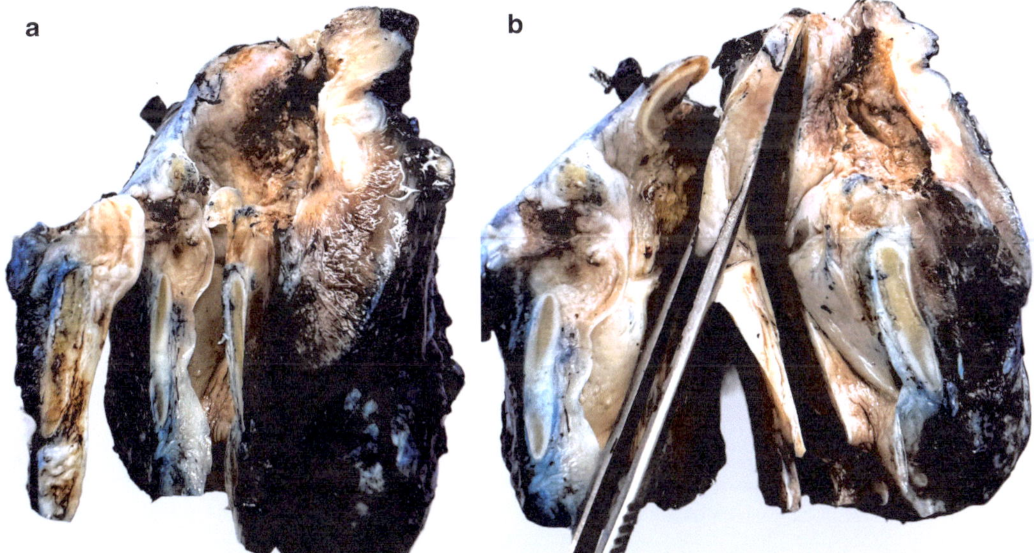

Fig. 9.112 (**a**) Posterior commissure section; (**b**) anterior commissure section

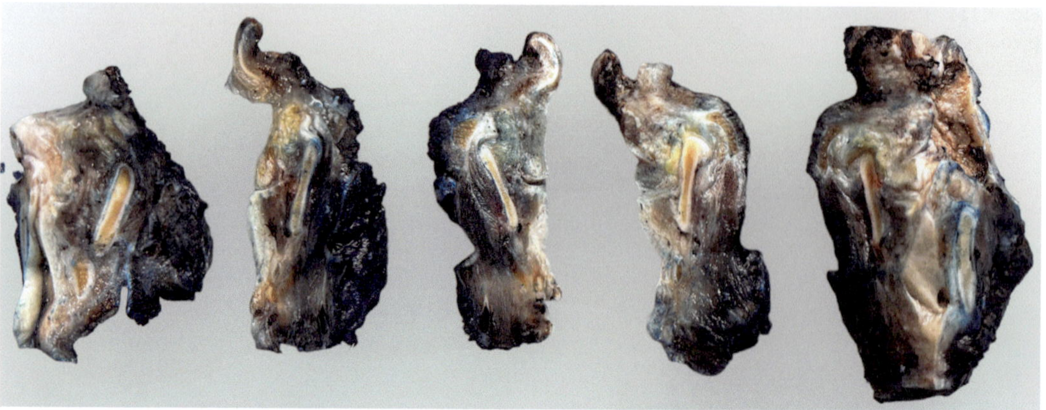

Fig. 9.113 Larynx serially sectioned

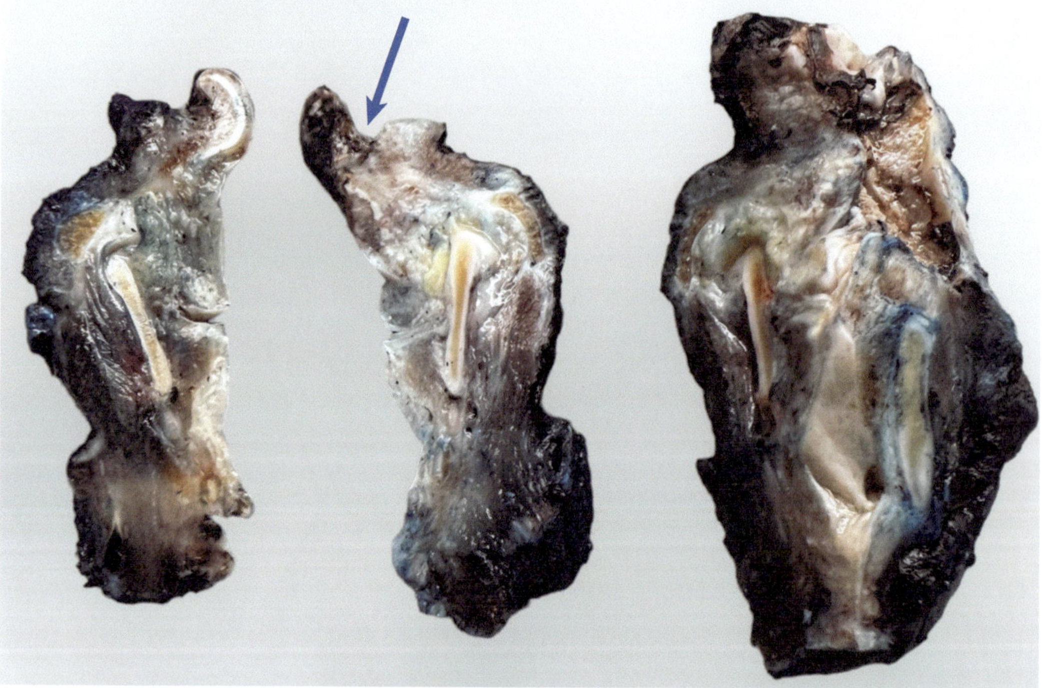

Fig. 9.114 Right side of larynx with lesion

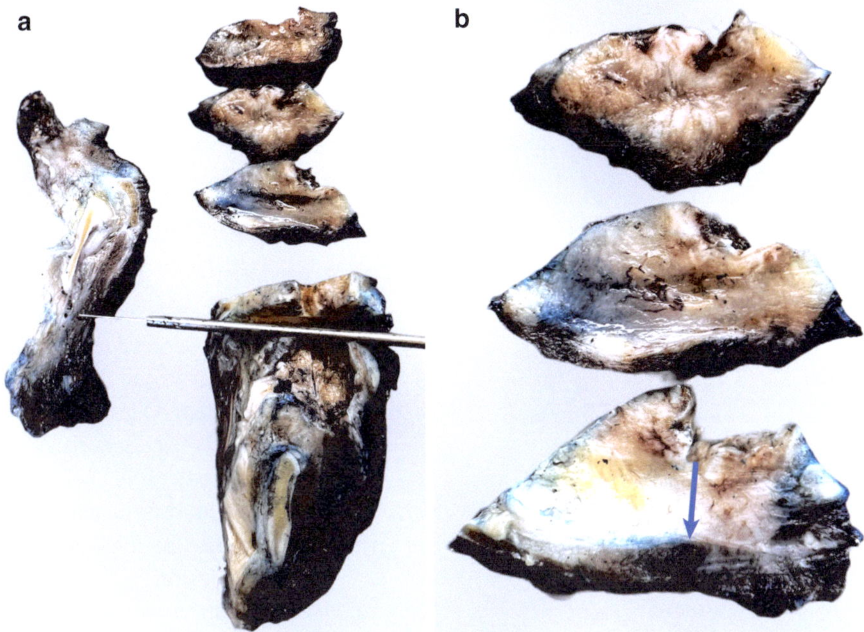

Fig. 9.115 (**a**) Right partial pharynx, serially sectioned; (**b**) right partial pharynx sections with lesion.

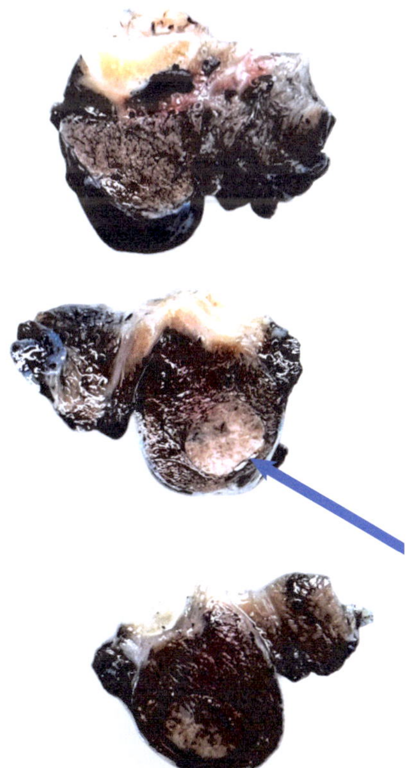

Fig. 9.116 Thyroid serially sectioned

A15-A19: Pharyngeal mass in relation to pharyngeal deep margin from superior to inferior

A20-A22: Right thyroid lobe nodule, entirely

Acknowledgment The author gratefully acknowledges Varsha Manucha, MD, and A. Wajdan Baqir, MD, for their contribution to this chapter.

Quiz Questions

1. Based on the gross characteristics of the thyroid nodule in Fig. 9.117, what is the most likely diagnosis?
   (a) Follicular thyroid carcinoma
   (b) Papillary thyroid carcinoma
   (c) Goiter
   (d) Anaplastic thyroid carcinoma

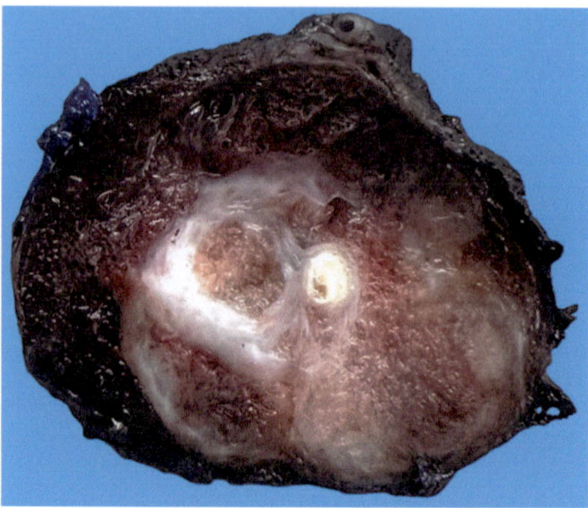

Fig. 9.117 Quiz question 1

2. What structure is designated by the red arrow in Fig. 9.118?
   (a) Anterior commissure
   (b) Left pyriform sinus
   (c) Cricoid cartilage
   (d) Left false vocal cord

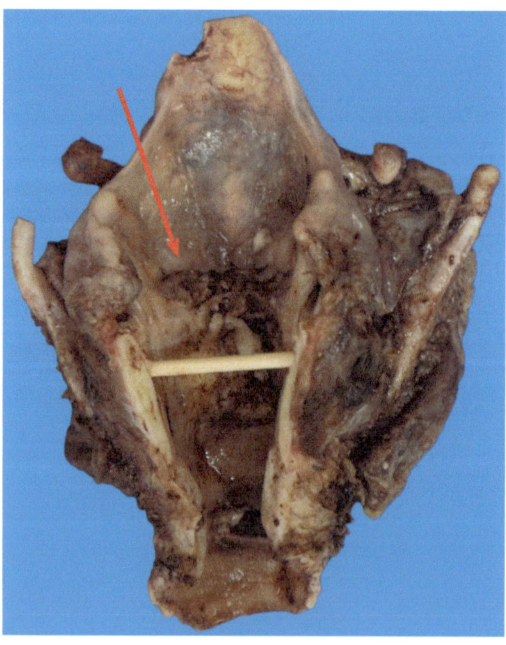

Fig. 9.118 Quiz question 4

3. A right neck dissection is received in the lab unoriented. While palpating lymph nodes, the grossing person encounters a 3.0 cm gland within the soft tissue. What neck level contains this gland?
   (a) Bilateral level IA
   (b) Level IB
   (c) Level II
   (d) Level III

4. A total thyroid is received in the lab. An FNA was done before surgery resulting in a diagnosis of follicular lesion. Upon sectioning a 4.0 cm encapsulated lesion is identified in the right lobe. What sections of the lesion must be submitted?
   (a) One representative section
   (b) One full slice of the thyroid lobe containing the lesion
   (c) 4 Representative sections of the center aspect of the lesion
   (d) The lesion capsule entirely

5. A 2.0 cm segment of anterior mandible contains what two osseous margins?
   (a) Floor of mouth and anterior osseous margins
   (b) Anterior and medial osseous margins
   (c) Floor of mouth and right osseous margins
   (d) Left and right osseous margins

6. Which type of margin allows for histologic measurement of the lesion to the margin?
   (a) En face margin
   (b) Perpendicular margin
   (c) Osseous margin
   (d) Shave margin

7. What is the osseous margin of the mandibulectomy specimen in Fig. 9.119?

   (a) Posterior
   (b) Gingival
   (c) Anterior
   (d) Hard palate

8. The anterior central slice of a larynx with tumor is present in Fig. 9.120. How would you grossly stage this patient based on the image?

   (a) pT2
   (b) pT3
   (c) pT4a
   (d) pT4b

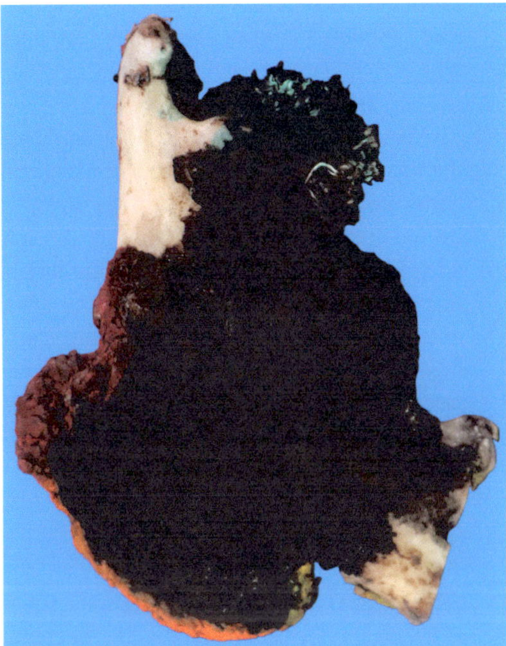

Fig. 9.119 Quiz question 7

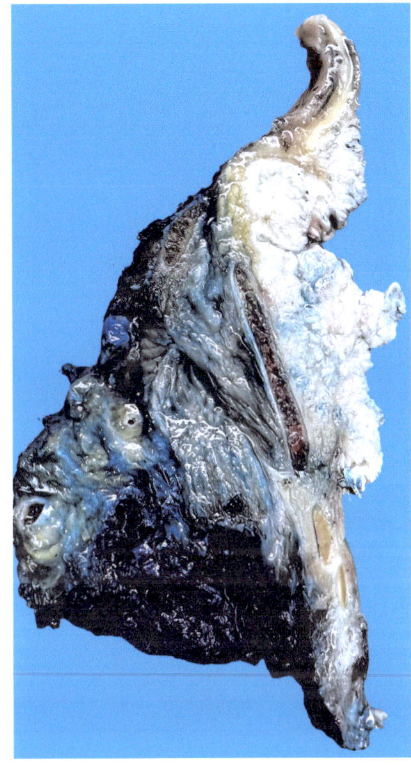

Fig. 9.120 Quiz question 8

9. A right radical tonsillectomy is received with surgical clips designating superior. What is the margin designated by the red arrow in Fig. 9.121 below?
   (a) Medial
   (b) Inferior
   (c) Lateral
   (d) Anterior

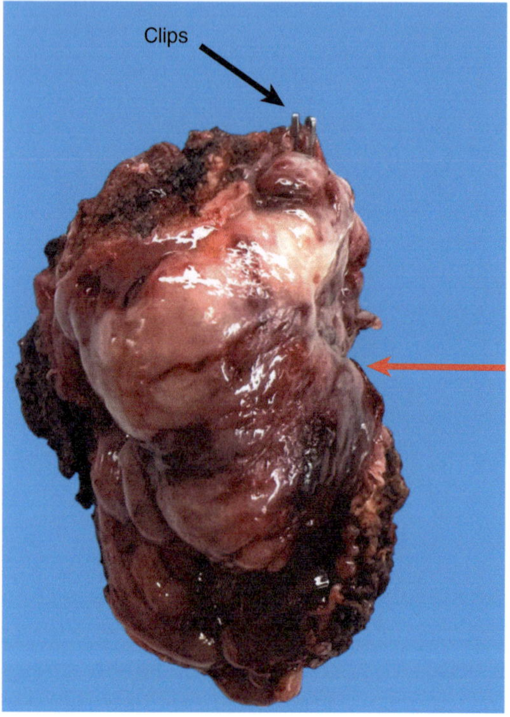

Fig. 9.121 Quiz question 9

10. Bilateral tonsils on a 22-year-old female are received in the laboratory concerning for tonsillitis. Both tonsils are received in one container and are unoriented. The pathologists ask to have sections of each tonsil submitted for histology. What is the CPT code for this specimen?
    (a) 88300
    (b) 88301
    (c) 88304
    (d) 88305

Answer Key

1. *(b) Papillary lesion.*

   Explanation: The solid, tan-white, focally calcified nodule is grossly consistent with a papillary thyroid carcinoma. Follicular thyroid carcinoma is also encapsulated but is tan-brown and solid. Goiter nodules are pink to amber and gelatinous while anaplastic thyroid carcinoma is ill-defined at the periphery with possible necrosis.

2. *(d) Left false vocal cord.*

   Explanation: The superior vocal cards are the false vocal cords, and the interior vocal cords are the true vocal cords. The arrow is on the left superior cord which is the left false vocal cord. The anterior commissure is just medial to the arrow in the central anterior aspect of the larynx. The cricoid cartilage is located posterior-lateral within the larynx, and the left pyriform sinus is located left lateral to the left false cord on the external aspect of the larynx between the larynx and the thyroid cartilage.

3. *(b) Level IB.*

   Explanation: Anatomically, the submandibular gland is present in level IB, so answer B is correct. Occasionally, the identification of the gland can help guide further orientation of an unoriented neck dissection.

4. *(d) The lesion capsule entirely.*

   Explanation: The diagnosis between a benign follicular lesion and a malignant follicular lesion is the microscopic identification of invasion through the lesions capsule. Invasion through the capsule is diagnostic of a malignant follicular lesion but invasion can be minimal so the entirety of the capsule needs to be submitted for histologic examination to be certain of present or absence of invasion; therefore, answer D is correct. The remaining answers do not include the capsule being submitted entirely and are therefore incorrect.

5. *(d) Right and left osseous margins*

    Explanation: A short 2.0 segment of anterior mandible is anatomically located at the central mandible; therefore, right and left are the best designation of osseous margins, answer D. Retromolar trigone is a mucosal anatomic location and anterior and posterior osseous margins are present when one side (right or left side) of the mandible is removed.

6. *(b) Perpendicular margin*

    Explanation: A perpendicular section is a section of the lesion to the margin. This allows microscopic visualization of the edge of the lesion to the margin and therefore can be measured. En face is the orientation of a shave margin which means the true margin is placed down in the cassette and allows for broad visualization of the margin only. If the en face margin contains lesional cells, then the margin is positive but no measurement can be taken. Osseous margins are bone margins and are typically submitted en face.

7. *(c) Anterior*

    Explanation: Notice that one end of the mandible is disarticulated. The mandible contains two disarticulation sites, right posterior and left posterior. No matter if the mandible segment is right or left, the disarticulated aspect is posterior. The surgically transected osseous margin that is opposite will be the anterior osseous margin, so C is correct.

8. *(a) pT3*

    Explanation: The lesion is present in the glottis invading superior into the supraglottis and inferior into the subglottis. Additionally, the lesion invades the preglottic space and paraglottic space with "vocal cord fixation." Additionally, the tumor abuts the thyroid cartilage without extension into the thyroid cortex which can be grossly stages as pT3.

    Glottic Lesions

    pT1: Tumor limited to the vocal cords with normal mobility.

    pT1a: Tumor limited to one vocal cord.

    pT1b: Tumor involves both vocal cords.

    pT2: Tumor extends to supraglottis and/or subglottis and/or with impaired vocal cord mobility.

    pT3: Tumor limited to the larynx with vocal cord fixation and/or invasion of paraglottic space and/or inner cortex of the thyroid cartilage.

    pT4a: Moderately advanced local disease. Tumor invades through the outer cortex of the thyroid cartilage and/or invades tissues beyond the larynx (e.g., trachea, cricoid cartilage, soft tissues of neck including deep extrinsic muscle of the tongue, strap muscles, thyroid, or esophagus)

    pT4b: Very advanced local disease. Tumor invades prevertebral space, encases carotid artery, or invades mediastinal.

9. *(a) Medial*

    Explanation: Note the tonsil is designated as right tonsil. Tonsils are present on the right and left side of the posterior-lateral aspect of the oropharynx. Tonsillar mucosa covers the anterior aspect of the specimen. In the image, with clips designating superior and mucosa on the anterior surface of the right tonsil, the red arrow designated medial. The margin opposite of the arrow is lateral, and the margin opposite of the clips is inferior. The margin (not pictured) that is on the opposite side of the mucosal surface is the deep (posterior).

10. *(c) 88304*

    Explanation: Tonsils with sections submitted is CPT code 88304, so C is correct. Tonsils received as gross only is CPT 88300 and a radical tonsillectomy for cancer is CPT 88309.

References

1. "FirstPath," 2009–2023. [Online]. Available: https://www.firstpathlab.com/cpt-codes/. Accessed August 2023.

2. Limaiem F, Rehman A, Anastasopoulou C, Mazzoni T. Papillary Thyroid Carcinoma, StatPearls, 1 January 2023.

Contents

The meticulous handling of hepatopancreatobiliary (HPB) gross specimens is paramount in delivering optimal patient care following major procedures. These specimens serve as crucial components in the diagnostic process, necessitating precise description and submission for histologic evaluation to obtain an accurate microscopic diagnosis. While managing HPB specimens, particularly the intricate Whipple specimen, can pose challenges for trainees, a grasp of fundamental principles can lay the groundwork for effective handling. Presented below is a systematic, stepwise approach to managing HPB gross specimens:

1. Recognition of importance: Acknowledge the critical role of HPB specimens in patient care, emphasizing the need for careful handling and accurate reporting.

2. Understanding specimen variability: Appreciate the diverse nature of HPB specimens, recognizing the variations encountered in different clinical scenarios.

3. Attention to detail: Exercise meticulousness in specimen description, ensuring thorough documentation of relevant features to aid in precise diagnosis.

4. Adherence to protocols: Follow established protocols for specimen handling and processing, adhering to standardized procedures to minimize errors.

5. Whipple specimen considerations: Recognize the complexity of Whipple specimens and the specific requirements for handling these intricate specimens with meticulous care.

By adhering to these fundamental principles and adopting a systematic approach, the trainee

Table 10.1 CPT codes [1]

Liver biopsy	88307
Liver partial resection	88307
Liver explant	88307
Liver total	88309
Gallbladder	88304
Pancreas biopsy	88307
Pancreas, total/subtotal resection	88309

can navigate the complexities of handling HPB gross specimens effectively, ultimately contributing to improved patient outcomes and diagnostic accuracy. Also see Table 10.1 for CPT codes.

10.1 Liver Biopsy: Level V CPT 88307

A liver biopsy procedure is performed for many reasons such as possible cysts, liver diseases, or malignancy. A long biopsy needle is inserted through the abdominal skin and into the liver. A liver core is produced from the biopsy. If there is a history of lymphoma, make sure to put a portion in RPMI for additional studies, if necessary.

Step 1: Describe, count, and measure the number of cores (Fig. 10.1).

Step 2: Submit core entirely as shown in Fig. 10.2. If more than one core is present, it is best to divide the cores among 2–3 cassettes (Fig. 10.2). Communicate with the pathologist for instructions.

Example Dictation

Specimen A is received in formalin labeled with patients' name, medical record number, "liver biopsy" and consists of a single tan-brown core (2.1 × 0.1 × 0.1 cm) which is submitted in toto in a biopsy bag in A 1.

10.2 Gallbladder: Level III CPT 88304

A cholecystectomy is the procedure of removing the gallbladder. This can be performed laparoscopically or as an open abdomen procedure. Symptomatic cholelithiasis and cholecystitis are

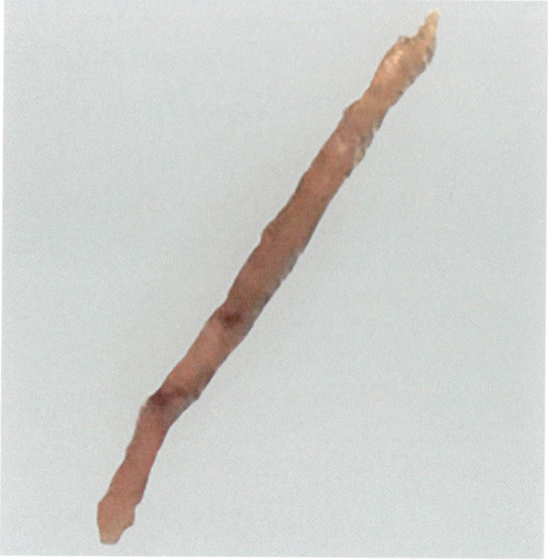

Fig. 10.1 Liver core biopsy

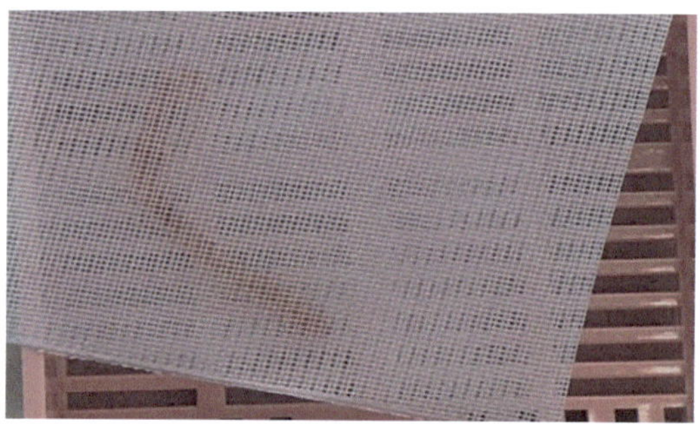

Fig. 10.2 Liver core biopsy cassette submission

the most common reasons for gallbladder removal but malignancy can also occur in the gallbladder. Pay special attention to the thickness of the wall, anything >0.4 cm, additional sections should be submitted to rule out dysplasia.

Step 1: Describe and measure the gallbladder.

Step 2: Dictate if the gallbladder is received intact or ruptured.

Step 3: Orient the gallbladder. The serosal surface is the side of the gallbladder visible on the liver (Fig. 10.3a) while the adventitial surface is the side that adheres the liver (Fig. 10.3b).

Step 4: For gallbladder resections concerning for cancer, ink the adventitial margin as seen in Fig. 10.4.

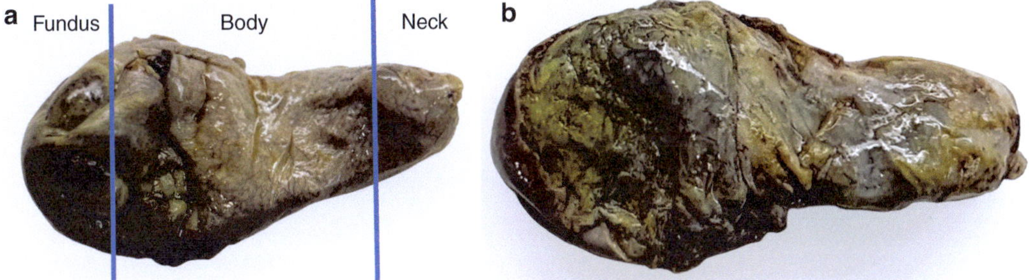

Fig. 10.3 (**a**) Gallbladder serosal surface; (**b**) gallbladder adventitial margin

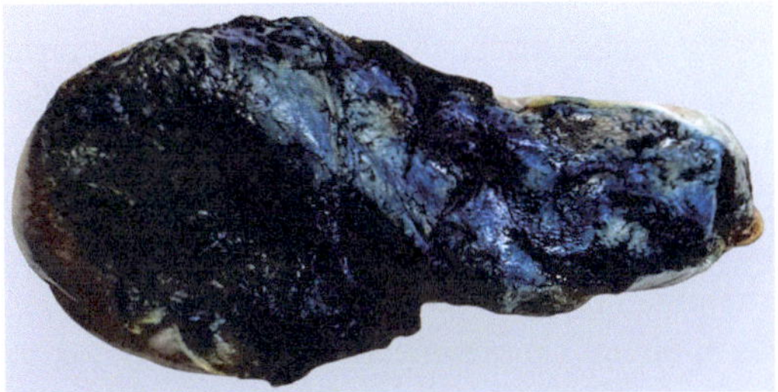

Fig. 10.4 Gallbladder adventitial surface inked

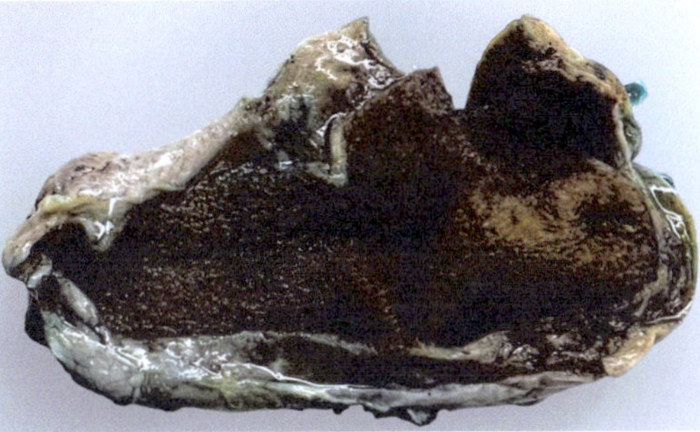

Fig. 10.6 Gallbladder open

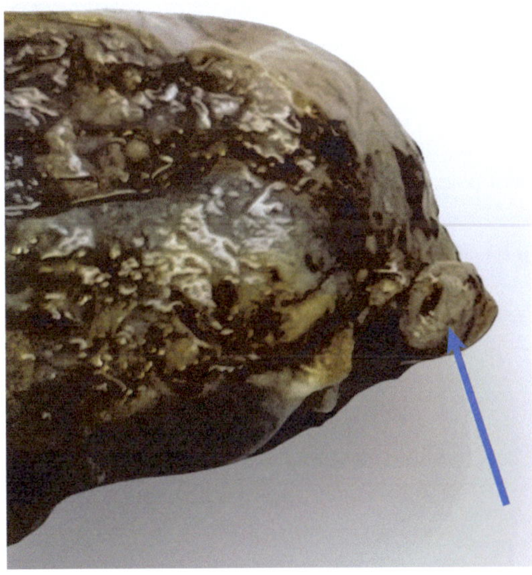

Fig. 10.5 Gallbladder cystic duct margin

Step 5: Identify and shave the cystic duct margin (Fig. 10.5). Submit the cystic duct margin en face.

Step 6: Open the gallbladder as seen in Fig. 10.6. Start at the gallbladder fundus and cut along the edge of the serosal surface toward the cystic duct.

Step 7: Describe the mucosal surface, evidence of stones, presence or absence of bile and measure the wall thickness. If a mass is present, describe and measure the size and measure how close it comes from the cystic duct margin. After sectioning the mass, measure the depth of invasion into the gallbladder wall.

Step 8: Submit two representative sections of the gallbladder wall in the same cassette as the cystic duct margin as seen in Fig. 10.7. Submit the mass entirely, if applicable.

Step 9: Palpate the gallbladder neck for a periductal lymph node. If identified, submit entirely.

Example Dictation

Specimen A is received in formalin labeled with patients' name, medical record number, "gallbladder" and consists of an intact, tan-green gallbladder (6.2 × 2.5 × 2.4 cm) which is opened to reveal a wall thickness ranging from 0.2 to 0.4 cm, tan-green velvety mucosa and scant bile. No periductal lymph node is identified. Representative sections are submitted in A 1.

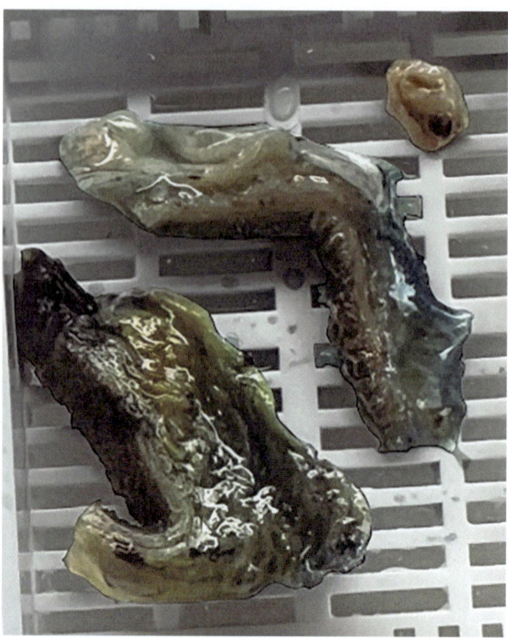

Fig. 10.7 Gallbladder section submission

Table 10.2 Tumor gross appearance of liver lesions

Adenoma	Single or multiple, tan brown, circumscribed, unencapsulated
FNH and fibrolamellar carcinoma	Tan-brown lesion with central scar
Hepatocellular carcinoma	Single or multiple, tan yellow to green, circumscribed, may be encapsulated or infiltrative, sometimes occur in the background of cirrhotic liver
Cholangiocarcinoma	Tan white firm nodules

10.3 Liver Wedge: Level V CPT 88307

A liver wedge resection can be performed on peripheral primary or metastatic lesions that do not involve the greater vessels of the liver. These resections include the lesion with the over lying liver capsule and resection margin.

Cancer Protocol Breakdown Relative to Grossing Liver

The cancer protocol for liver specimens is only used for carcinomas of the liver.

Procedure: Liver lesions can be removed by wedge resection, major partial hepatectomy (3+ segments excised), minor partial hepatectomy (less than 3 segments excised), or total hepatectomy. See Table 10.2 for tumor descriptions.

Tumor site: The site of the mass is identified by lobes which are the right lobe, left lobe, caudate lobe, or quadrate lobe. The site can also be identified by the 8 liver anatomical surgical segments.

Tumor size: Dictate the three-dimensional size of the mass. The cancer protocol requires the largest dimension be identified.

Treatment effect: Analyze the patient's chart to see if the patient received any presurgery treatments such as chemotherapy. If treatment is received, the mass should be submitted entirely or 1 section per 1 centimeter of mass should be submitted if the mass is large to assess for treatment effect. Communicate with the pathologists for instruction.

Tumor extent: Dictate what anatomical areas are involved by the mass. The mass can be confined to the liver or extend into adjacent structures such as the hepatic and portal vein, peritoneum, gallbladder, diaphragm, or another adjacent organ.

Margins: Measure the mass to the parenchymal resection margin. [2].

pT Category

pT Not assigned

pT0: No evidence of primary tumor

pT1: Solitary tumor less than or equal to 2 cm

pT1b: Solitary tumor greater than 2 cm without vascular invasion

pT2: Solitary tumor greater than 2 cm with vascular invasion, or multiple tumors, none greater than 5 cm

pT3: Multiple tumors, at least one of which is greater than 5 cm

pT4: Single tumor or multiple tumors of any size involving adjacent structures [2]

Step 1: Describe, measure, and weigh the specimen (Fig. 10.8).

Step 2: Identify the liver capsule and the resection margin.

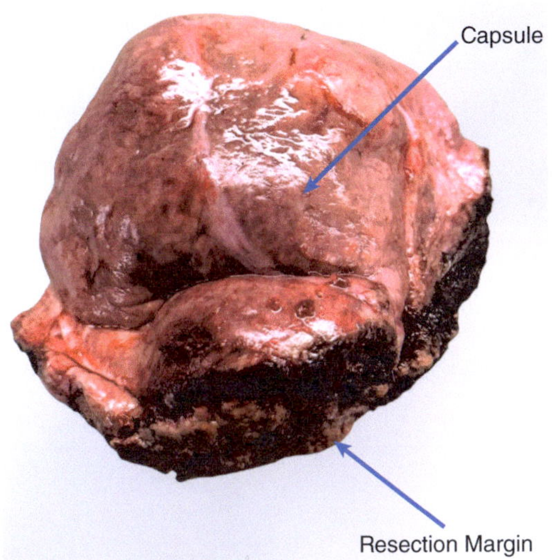

Fig. 10.8 Liver wedge

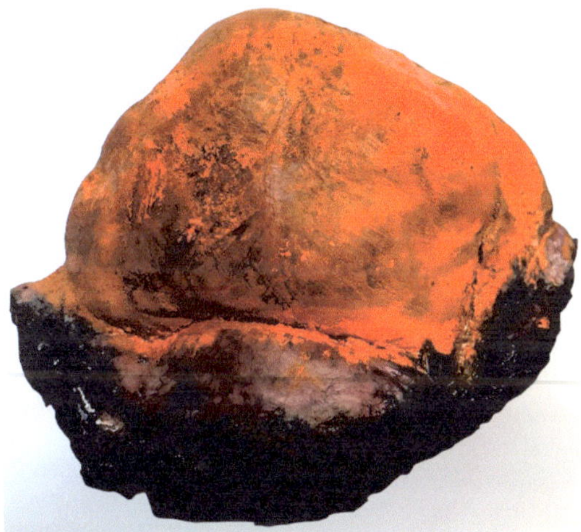

Fig. 10.9 Inked liver wedge

Step 3: Ink the resection margin and any bulging or puckered area on the capsule surface. In Fig. 10.9, the resection margin is inked blue, and the bulging area of the liver capsule is inked orange.

Step 4: Serially section the specimen perpendicular to the resection margin. The slices in Fig. 10.10 show both the liver capsule (orange) and the resection margin (blue) in each slice.

Step 5: Measure the mass in three dimensions and measure how close the mass comes to the liver capsule and the resection margin is identified by the blue arrow in Fig. 10.11.

Step 6: Assess the remaining liver and describe the parenchyma.

Step 7: Submit representative sections of the mass in relation to the resection margin and liver capsule. Additional sections of mass in relation to liver parenchyma and of just mass can be submitted (Fig. 10.12).

Example Dictation

Specimen A is received in formalin labeled with patients' name, medical record number, "liver wedge" and consists of an unoriented liver wedge (9.6 × 8.5 × 7.7 cm, 32 g) with a bulging area on the liver capsule (4.4 × 3.9 cm). The specimen is serially sectioned to reveal an irregular, tan-white, solid mass (4.4 × 3.9 × 2.9 cm) which bulges the overlying liver capsule without invasion through and comes within 1.8 cm from the resection margin. The remaining cut surfaces are red-brown and slightly variegated.

Ink code
  Blue: resection margin
  Orange: liver capsule
Section code
  A1-A3: Mass in relation to closest resection margin, representative.
  A4-A6: Mass in relation to liver capsule
  A7: Mass in relation to liver parenchyma, representative
  A8: Mass, representative

Fig. 10.10 Liver wedge serially sectioned

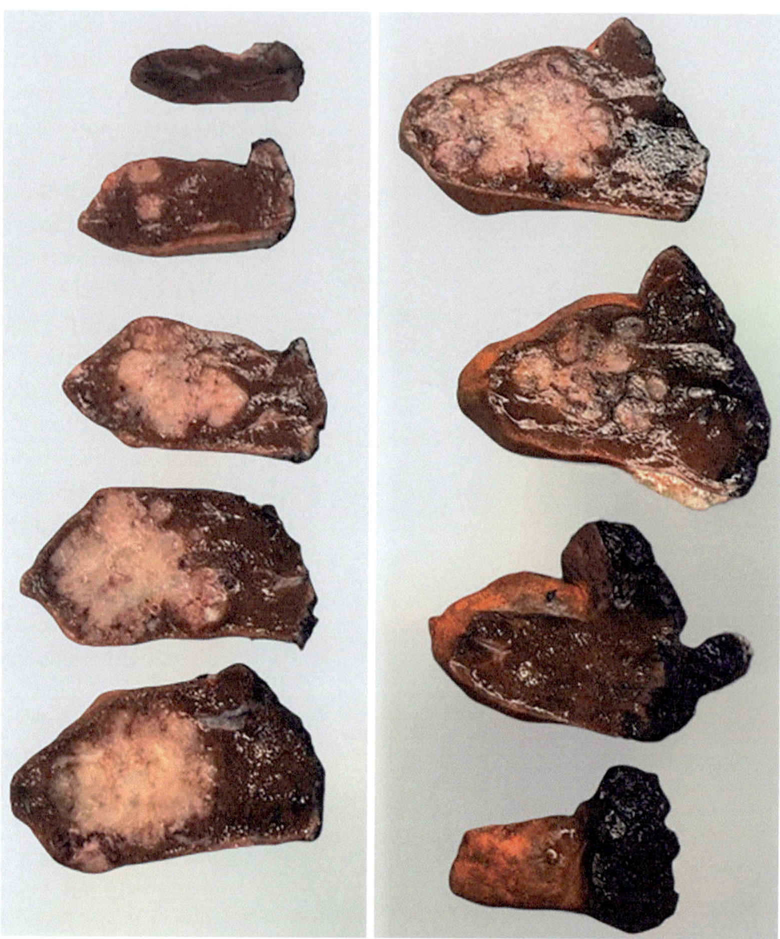

Fig. 10.11 Liver wedge with mass

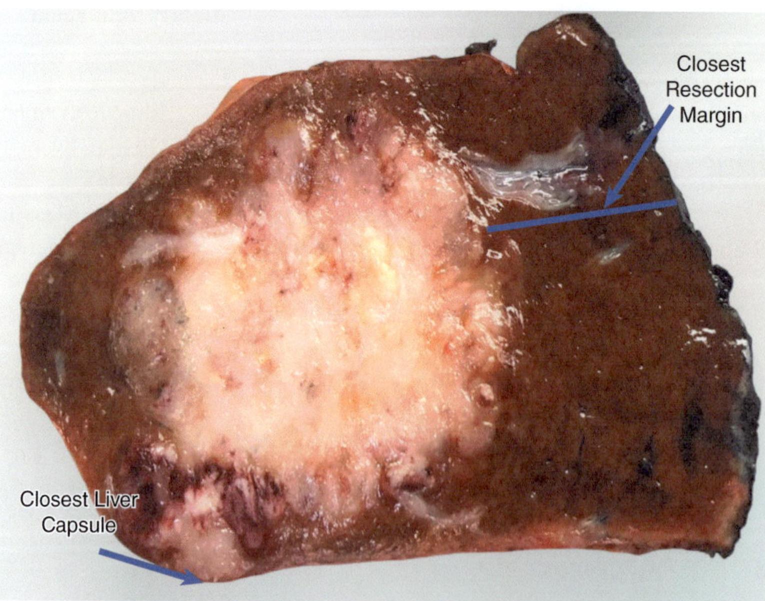

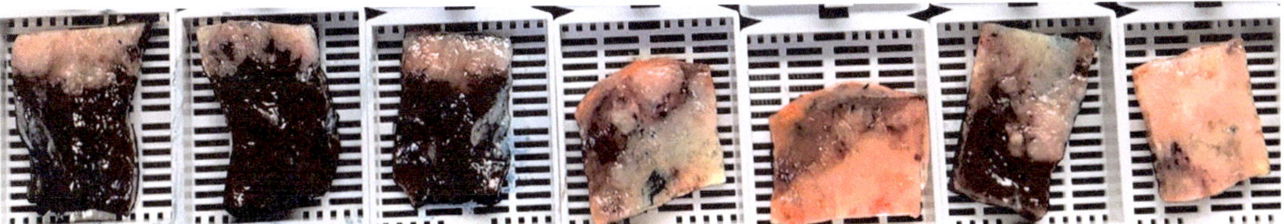

Fig. 10.12 Section submission

Fig. 10.13 Liver
segment orientation

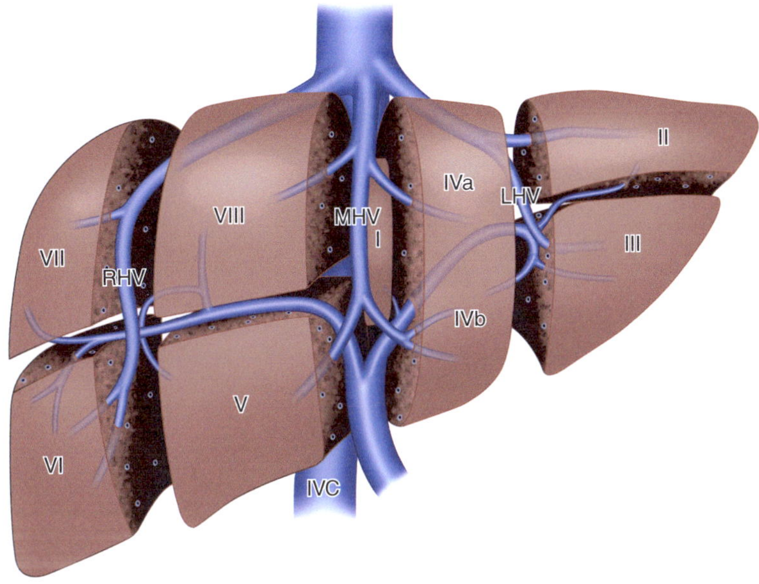

10.4 Liver Explant

Liver explant is the removal of the entire liver with attached gallbladder, if present. A healthy donor liver replaces the explanted recipient liver. Liver transplants are done for end-stage liver disease due to alcoholic liver disease, cirrhosis, or hepatitis. Before proceeding, check radiology for any lesion identified by imaging. Submit any nodule which is more than 1 cm or looks different from other nodules. Depending on pathologist's preference, orienting the liver by segments may be necessary. See Fig. 10.13 for an illustration of the liver oriented by segments.

Step 1: Before grossing, always look at the imaging studies of the patient. Note any lesions that were identified in the liver by imaging.

Step 2: Orient the liver. Figure 10.14a is the anterior surface, and Fig. 10.14b is the posterior surface.

Step 3: Measure, weigh, and describe the liver capsule.

Step 4: Measure the gallbladder, if present.

Step 5: Remove the gallbladder (Fig. 10.15) and gross as described in Sect. 10.2 Gallbladder.

Step 6: Shave and submit the hilar vessels, en face. The hepatic vein is noted with a blue arrow in Fig. 10.16.

Step 7: Serially section the liver from left to right lobe as seen in Fig. 10.17.

Step 8: Grossly assess the slices for macronodules that are greater than 5 mm. In Fig. 10.18, the slices are markedly variegated with numerous nodules but two macronodules are present. Right lobe 1.0 cm, segment 6 as noted by the blue arrow. The other nodule is 1.2 cm, present in the left lobe, segment 2 as noted by the red arrow.

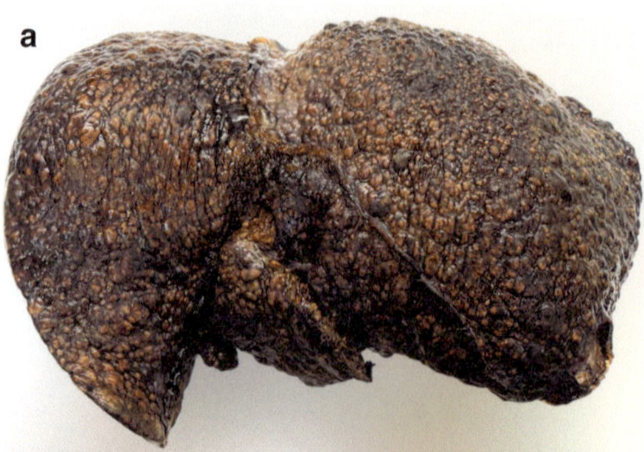

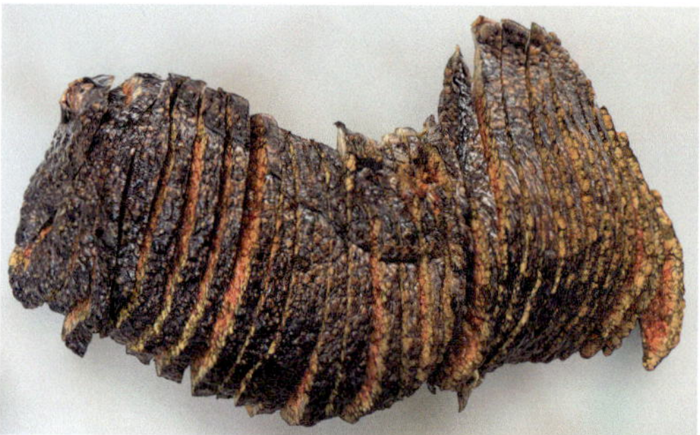

Fig. 10.14 (**a**) Liver anterior view; (**b**) liver posterior view

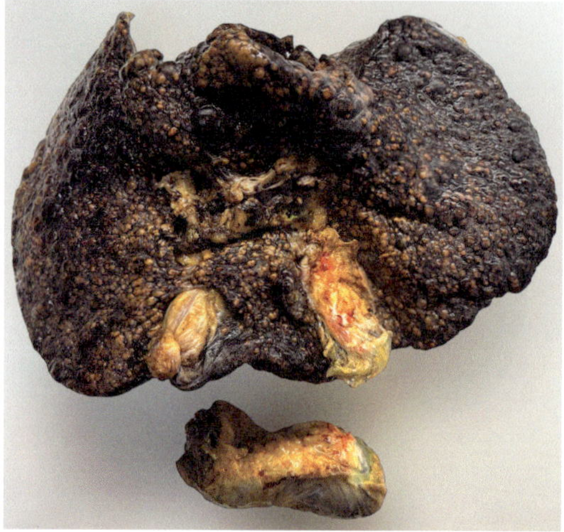

Fig. 10.15 Liver gallbladder removed

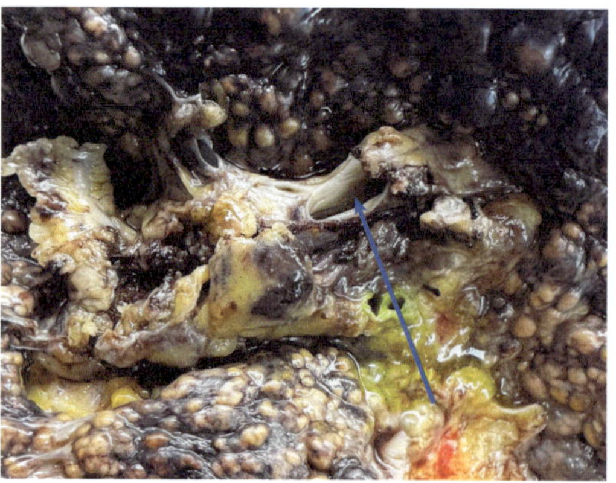

Fig. 10.16 Liver hilum

Fig. 10.17 Liver serially sectioned

Step 9: Measure the describe any macronodules and dictate where these nodules are located. Location can be designated by lobe or by liver segment. Communicate with the pathologists for instruction on how to designate location of any nodules.

Step 10: The gallbladder and hilar vessel margins are submitted. Representative sections of the designated nodules are submitted, and 1–2 sections of the right and left lobes are submitted as seen in Fig. 10.19.

Example Dictation

Specimen A is received in formalin labeled with patient's name, medical record number, "liver" and consists of a slightly dusky, tan-brown liver (25.6 × 15.9 × 6.6 cm, 1081 g) with attached

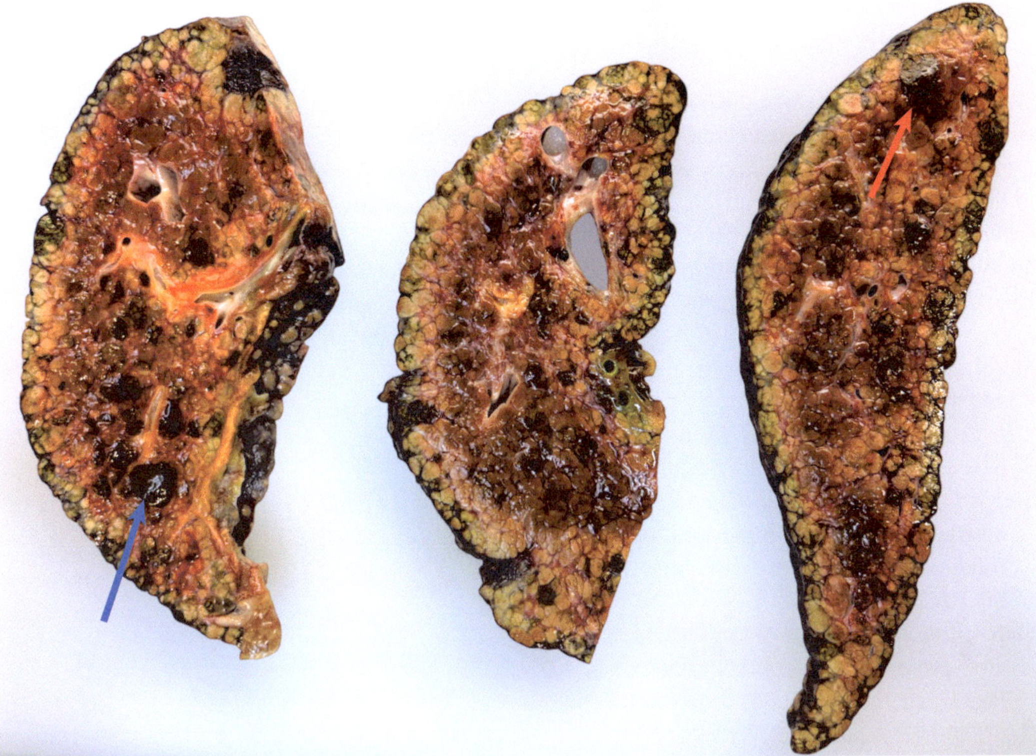

Fig. 10.18 Liver slices

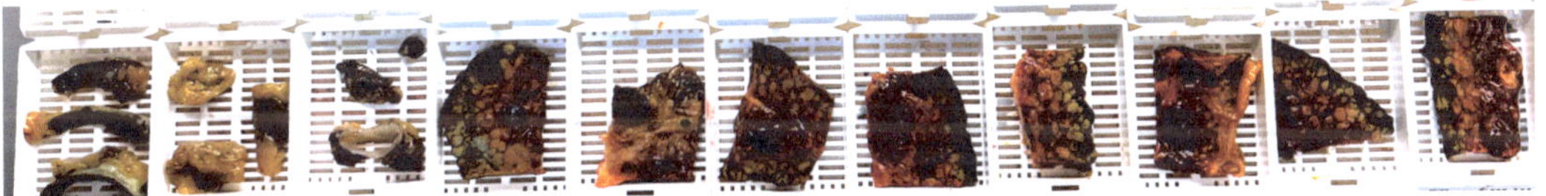

Fig. 10.19 Liver section submission

green gallbladder (8.5 × 3.4 × 3.3 cm) which is opened to reveal the wall thickness ranging from 0.2 to 0.3 cm, dark green velvety mucosa and markedly thickened dark green bile. A periductal lymph node (1.2 × 0.9 × 0.7 cm) is identified. The liver capsule is tan-brown and diffusely nodular with small nodules ranging from 0.3 to 0.5 cm and is serially sectioned to reveal diffusely nodular cut surfaces with small tan-brown, homogeneous nodules ranging from 0.1 to 0.4 cm, admixed with 2 tan-green, slightly variegated nodules, 1.0 and 1.2 cm present in the right segment 6 and left segment 2; respectively.

Section code

A 1: Cystic duct margin, en face and gallbladder, representative

A 2: Periductal lymph node, trisected

A 3: Liver hilum vasculature margin, en face

A 4: Segment 2 nodule, representative

A 5: Segment 6 nodule, representative

A 6: Left lobe, representative

A 7-A 8: Right lobe, representative

10.5 Pancreatic Tail: Level VI CPT 88309

When a lesion is present in the body or tail of the pancreas, a distal pancreatectomy can be performed. A distal pancreatectomy excises the mid to distal pancreas and the spleen. The spleen is removed with the pancreas because the splenic artery travels tightly along the majority of the pancreas and is difficult to separate.

Step 1: Describe and measure the pancreatic tail and the spleen (Fig. 10.20).

Step 2: Remove the staples from the proximal pancreatic margin (Fig. 10.21a).

Step 3: Orient the specimen. The splenic artery is positioned superior-posterior along the pancreas as shown by the blue arrow in Fig. 10.21b.

Step 4: Ink the pancreas. Inking is dependent of the preference of the pathologists. In Fig. 10.22, the ink code is as follows:

    Orange: superior
    Green: inferior
    Blue: anterior
    Black: posterior

Step 5: Shave the proximal pancreatic margin as shown in Fig. 10.23. Submit the margin en face.

Step 6: Serially section the remainder of the pancreas as shown in Fig. 10.24a.

Step 7: Identify and measure the lesion. Lesions of the pancreas can be very ill-defined as seen by the blue arrow in Fig. 10.24b.

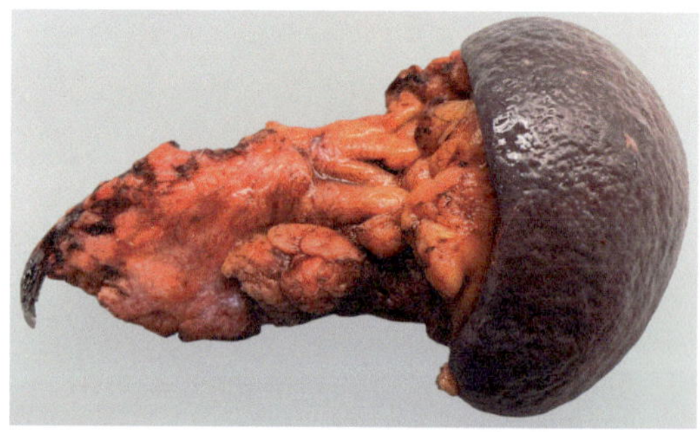

Fig. 10.20 Tail of pancreas and spleen

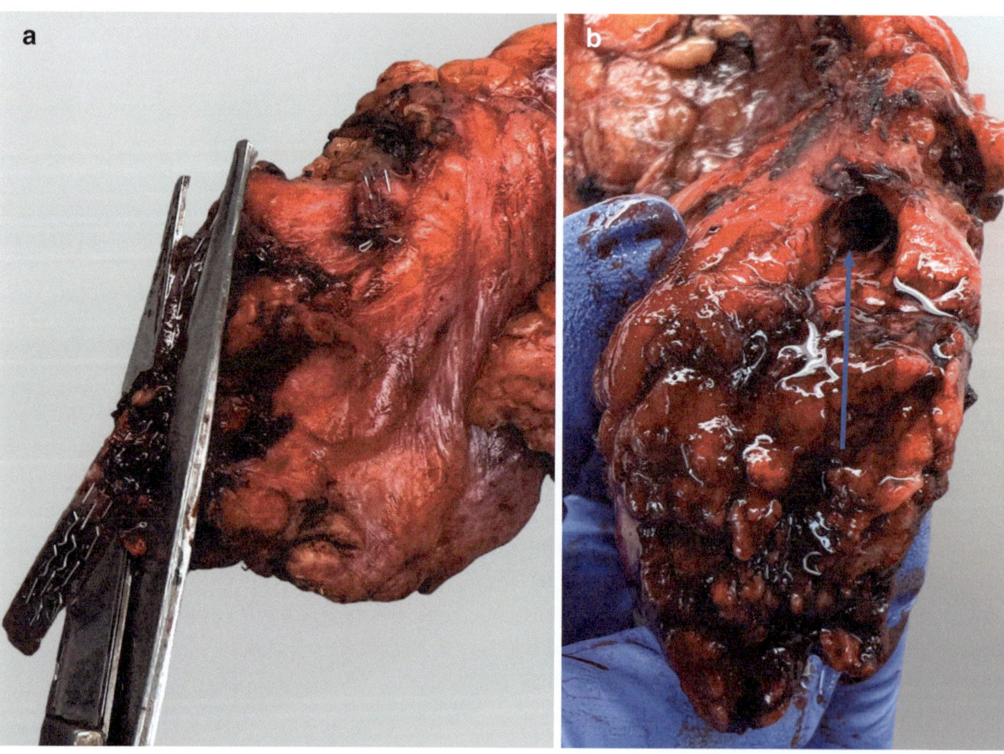

Fig. 10.21 (**a**) Proximal margin; (**b**) superior-posterior splenic artery

Step 8: Measure the lesion and measure the distance of the lesion to the proximal pancreatic margin and how close the lesion comes to the superior, inferior, anterior, and posterior aspects of the pancreas.

Step 9: Serially section the spleen and assess for any additional lesions present within the spleen (Fig. 10.25).

Step 10: Submit sections. Sections should include the proximal pancreatic margin, sections of the lesion in relation to the surrounding inks, and sections of the spleen as shown in Fig. 10.26.

Example Dictation

Specimen A is received in formalin labeled with patient's name, medical record number, "pancreas and spleen" and consists of a segment of tail pancreas (8.5 × 4.5 × 2.1 cm) with attached spleen (9.5 × 6.4 × 5.2 cm) which is serially sectioned to reveal tan-brown, lobular pancreatic parenchyma with a markedly ill-defined soft tan-yellow lesion (0.9 × 0.6 × 0.5 cm) coming within 7.3 cm of the proximal pancreatic resection margin and 2.1 cm from the distal pancreatic tail, coming within 0.8 cm of the anterior aspect, 0.8 cm from the posterior aspect, 0.2 cm from the inferior aspect, and 1.9 cm from the superior aspects of the pancreas. The spleen is serially sectioned to reveal homogeneous red-brown cut surfaces. (AI).

Ink code
    Blue: anterior
    Black: posterior
    Orange: superior
    Green: inferior
Section code
    A 1-A 2: Pancreatic margin, bisected, en face
    A3-A6: Two full-face sections of lesion, bisected
    A7-A8: Spleen, representative

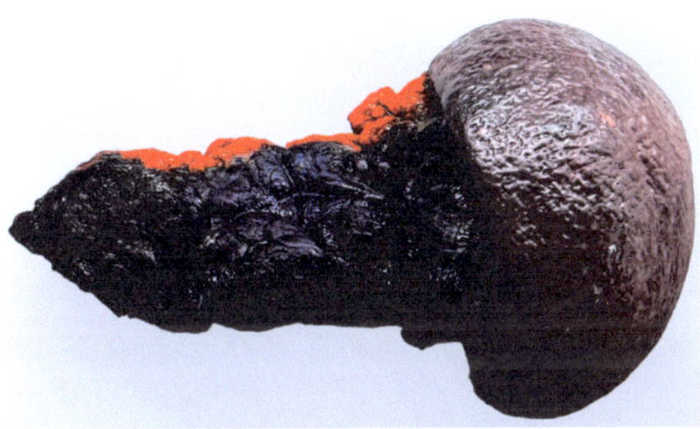

Fig. 10.22 Pancreas inked

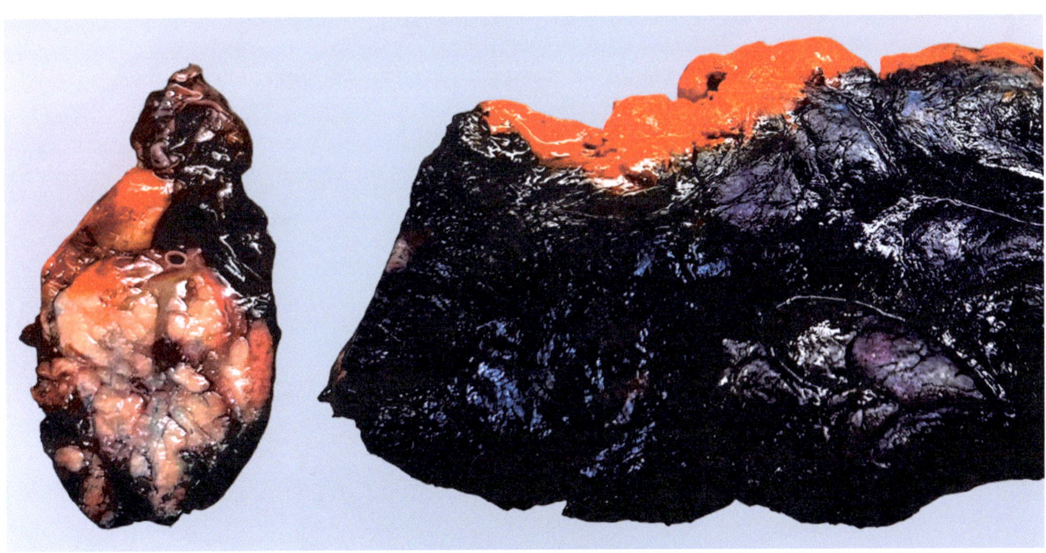

Fig. 10.23 Pancreatic margin

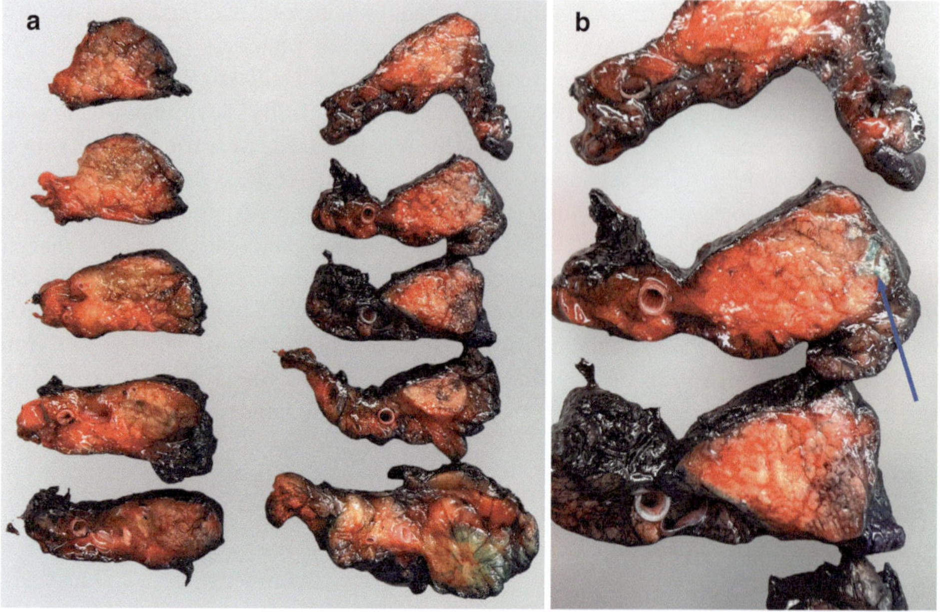

Fig. 10.24 (**a**) Pancreas serially sectioned; (**b**) pancreas lesion

Fig. 10.25 Spleen serially sectioned

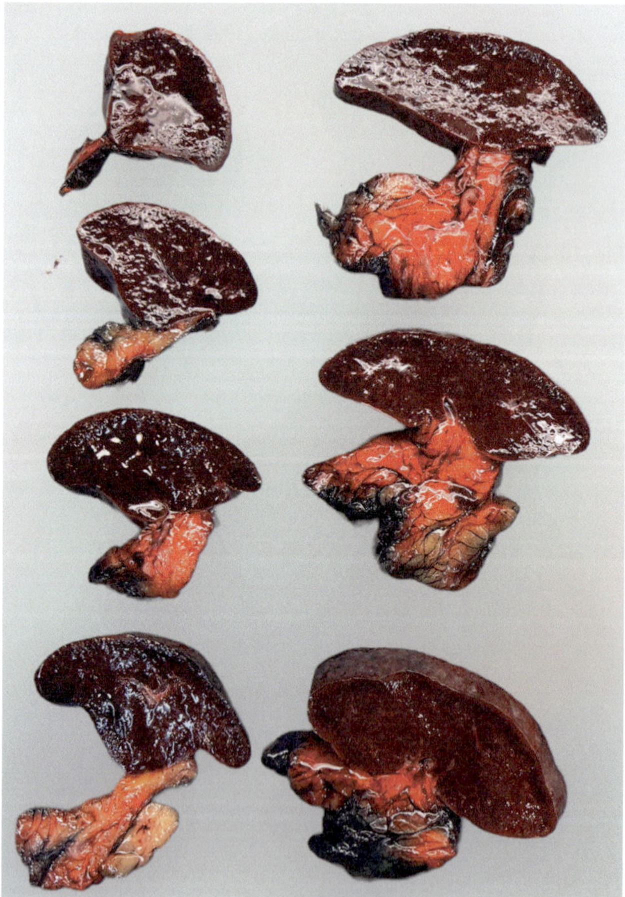

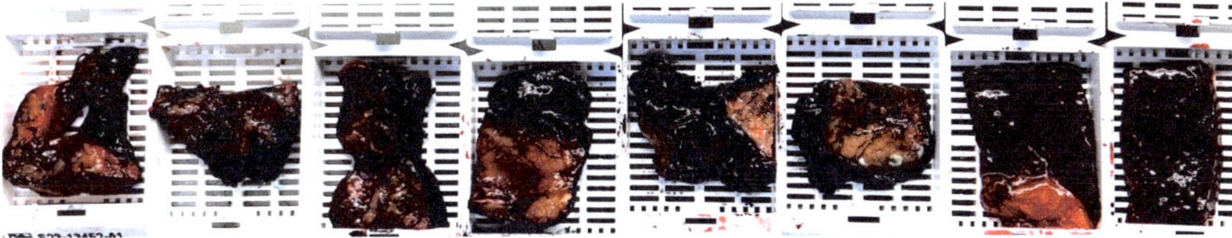

Fig. 10.26 Tail of pancreas and spleen section submission

10.6   Whipple with Pancreatic Primary: Level VI CPT 88309

A pancreaticoduodenectomy (Whipple) procedure is a complicated surgery consisting of the removal of the duodenum and pancreatic head. Additionally, the surgery includes stomach, common bile duct, hepatic duct, cystic duct, and gallbladder.

Cancer Protocol Breakdown Relative to Grossing Pancreas.

The cancer protocol for pancreaticoduodenectomy is for carcinomas of the pancreas only, not neuroendocrine tumors. See Table 10.3 for tumor descriptions.

Procedure: a pancreaticoduodenectomy is called a Whipple procedure and includes the duodenum and pancreatic head at minimum. Other procedures performed for carcinomas of the pancreas are excisional biopsies where the lesion is enucleated from the pancreas, total pancreatectomy where the entire pancreas is removed, or partial pancreatectomy which can include the body and/or the pancreatic tail.

Tumor site: This is where the mass is located such as the pancreatic head, uncinate process, pancreatic body, or pancreatic tail.

Tumor size: A three-dimensional measurement is stated in the gross description. The cancer protocol requires the greatest dimension. [2].

PT Category:

pT0: No evidence of primary tumor
pTis: Carcinoma in situ
pT1: Tumor less than or equal to 0.5 cm–2.0 cm in greatest dimension
pT2: Tumor greater than 2 cm and less than or equal to 4 cm in greatest dimension
pT3: Tumor greater than 4 cm in greatest dimension

Table 10.3 Tumor gross appearance of pancreas lesions

Pseudocysts	Unilocular cyst with turbid or hemorrhagic fluid
Pancreatitis	Acute: Enlarged pancreases with fat necrosis and hemorrhage Chronic: Small pancreases with fibrosis, dilated ducts and cysts
Intraductal papillary mucinous neoplasm	Main duct: Dilated ducts filled with mucin and papillary appearing areas Branch ducts: Multicystic ducts filled with mucin and papillary areas
Cystadenoma	Bosselated outer surface, multicystic spaces filled with watery or straw-colored fluid
Cystadenocarcinoma	Bosselated outer surface, multicystic spaces filled with watery or straw-colored fluid
Endocrine lesions	Solitary, well circumscribed, tan yellow/brown/red

pT4: Tumor involves the celiac axis or the superior mesenteric artery, and/or common hepatic artery, regardless of size [2]

Sites involved by direct tumor extension: These areas include the anterior and posterior surface, the vascular groove, the ampulla of Vater, duodenal wall, peripancreatic soft tissue, extrapancreatic common bile duct, stomach, superior mesenteric and portal vein, and artery and celiac axis.

Treatment effect: Analyze the patient's chart. If the patient received presurgery treatment such as chemotherapy, the entire lesion should be submitted to assess the effect that treatment had on the mass.

Margins: Dictate how close the mass comes to the margins or if the mass is directly extending to the margin. The areas to note are the pancreatic margin, the uncinate process, the bile duct margin, and the proximal and distal duodenal margins. See Fig. 10.27 for an illustration of Whipple anatomy.

Step 1: Orient the specimen. The pancreatic head inserts on the medial aspect of the duodenum with the pancreatic margin present medial to the remainder of the pancreas as shown in Fig. 10.28.

Step 2: Identify the margins and anatomical aspects of the pancreatic head. Figure 10.29a shows the pancreatic head margin (blue circle), the portal groove (SMA red arrow/SMV blue arrow), the retroperitoneal margin (black square), and the uncinate process (yellow arrow). Figure 10.29b shows the common bile duct margin (blue arrow) which is present superior-posterior to the pancreatic head.

Step 3: Shave and submit the proximal and distal margins of the duodenum and submit en face.

Step 4: Open the duodenum along the opposite aspect of the pancreatic head as shown in Fig. 10.30.

Step 5: Shave (Fig. 10.31) and submit the common bile duct and the pancreatic margin en face.

Step 6: Ink the margins and anatomical aspects of the pancreas. Figure 10.32a shows the uncinate process (yellow) and the anterior aspect of the pancreas (green). Figure 10.32b shows the pancreatic false margin (orange), the SMV (blue), and the SMA (red). Figure 10.32c shows the retroperitoneal margin (black).

Step 7: Place probes in the pancreatic duct and the common bile duct and extend the probes through the ampulla of Vater as shown in Fig. 10.33.

Step 8: Bivalve the pancreatic head through the ducts as shown in Fig. 10.34. This can be done

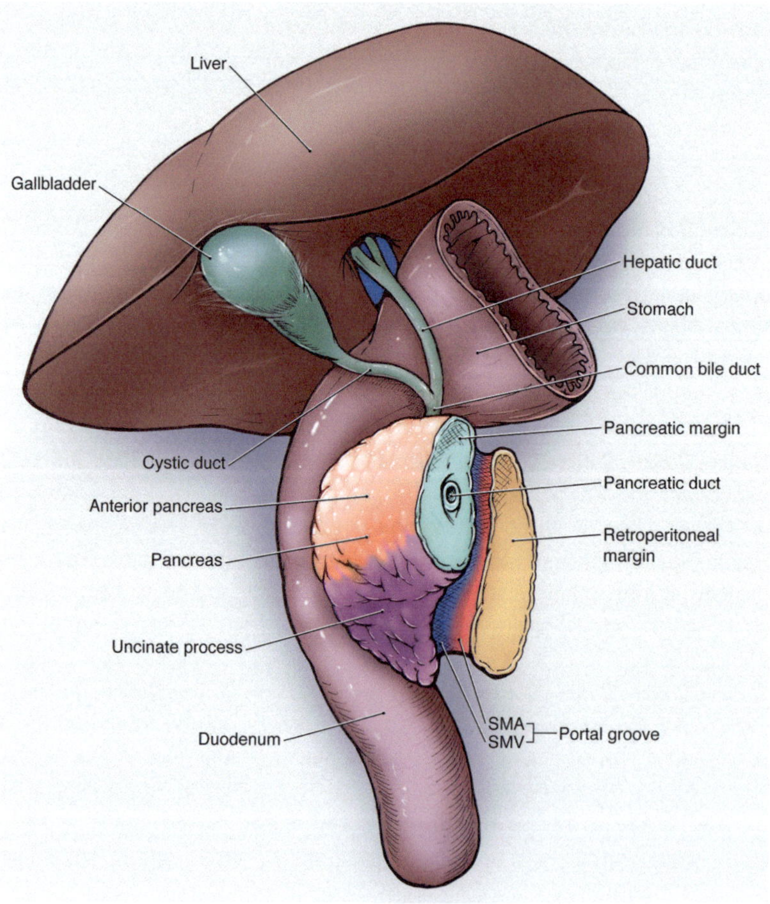

Fig. 10.27 Illustration of Whipple anatomy

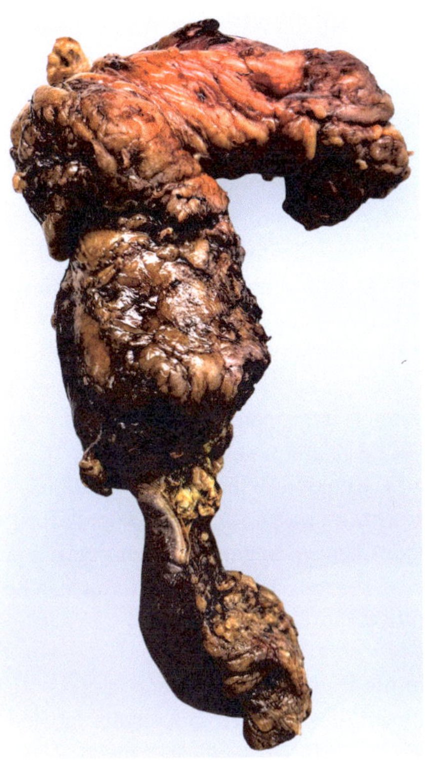

Fig. 10.28 Whipple specimen

by slicing down each probe separately or both probes together.

Step 9: Describe the common bile duct and the pancreatic duct. In Fig. 10.35, both ducts are slightly dilated.

Step 10: Shave the pancreatic margins and anatomical aspect. This step can also be done before bivalving the pancreatic head depending on the pathologists' preference and location of the lesion. The sections include anterior pancreas (green) and the uncinate process (yellow) in Fig. 10.36a. In Fig. 10.36b, the sections are the SMV (blue), the SMA (red), and the retroperitoneal margin (black). These sections are removed approximately 0.5–0.8 cm thick.

Step 10: Perpendicularly section the margins and submit on edge as seen in Fig. 10.37. Margins close to the lesion should be perpendicularly sectioned but margins far from the lesion can be submitted en face depending on the pathologist's preference. Perpendicularly sectioning allows for microscopic measurement of the lesion to the margin.

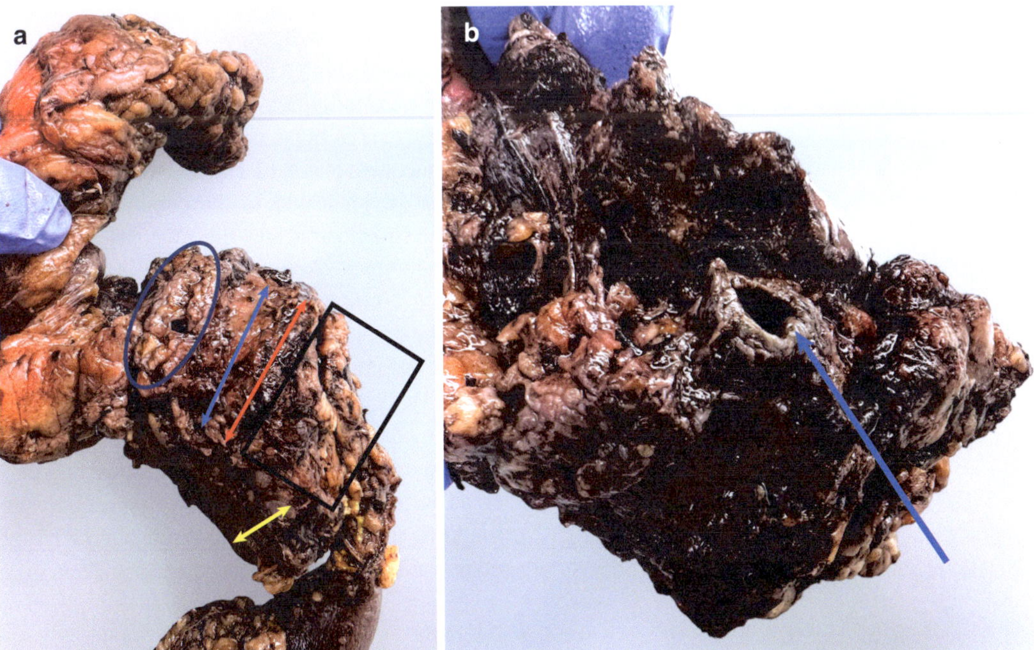

Fig. 10.29   (**a**) Pancreas aspect of Whipple; (**b**) common bile duct

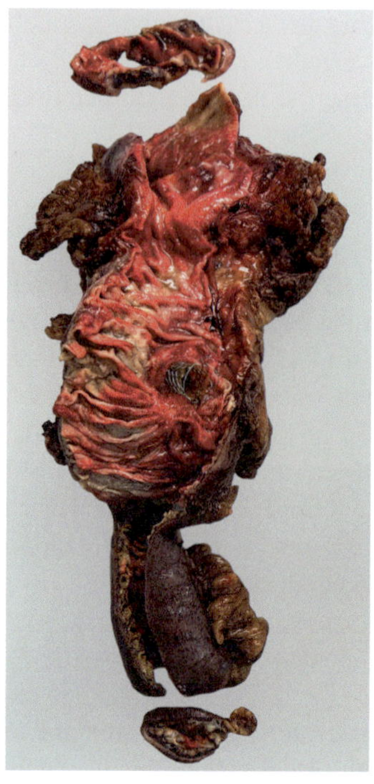

Fig. 10.30 Duodenum opened

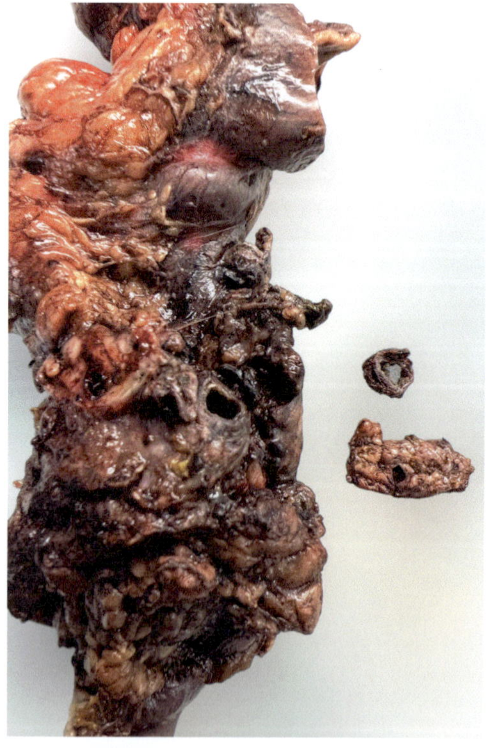

Fig. 10.31 Pancreatic margin and common bile duct margin

Step 11: Serially section the remainder of the pancreatic head. The lesion (blue arrow) in this example is posterior to the common bile duct as seen in Fig. 10.38. The lesion also minimally invades the posterior aspect of the common bile duct wall.

Step 12: Submit a fullface section of the lesion in relation to the common bile duct and pancreatic duct, if achievable. If not, submit representative sections of both ducts.

Step 13: Submit the remainder of the mass. Most often the entire lesion is submitted. If the lesion is large, communicate with the pathologist for instruction.

Step 14: Remove all the remaining adipose tissue as shown in Fig. 10.39 and palpate for lymph nodes. Depending on the pathologist's preference, the remaining adipose tissue can be submitted entirely.

Example Dictation

Specimen A is received in formalin labeled with patient's name, medical record number, "Whipple" and consists of a segment duodenum (21.2 cm in length by 2.0 cm in diameter) with attached head of pancreas (6.5 × 6.2 × 3.7 cm). The duodenum is opened to reveal tan-brown, folded mucosa with a stent placed in the common bile duct, extending through the ampulla of Vater. The pancreas is bivalved to reveal an ill-defined tan-white, firm lesion (2.1 × 1.9 × 1.5 cm) present at the posterior aspect of the common bile duct, with slight invasion into the mucosal surface of the duodenum. Additionally, the mass comes within 2.1 cm of the uncinate process, 1.1 cm from the anterior pancreas, 3.2 cm from the pancreatic resection margin, 2.1 cm from the SMA and SMV. Grossly the mass appears to extend into the retroperitoneal aspect, coming within 0.2 cm of the retroperitoneal margin. The remaining pancreas is lobulated and markedly pale. The surrounding adipose tissue is palpable for 15 lymph node candidates ranging from 0.1 to 1.7 cm.

Ink code

    Orange: pancreatic head false margin
    Blue: SMV
    Red: SMA

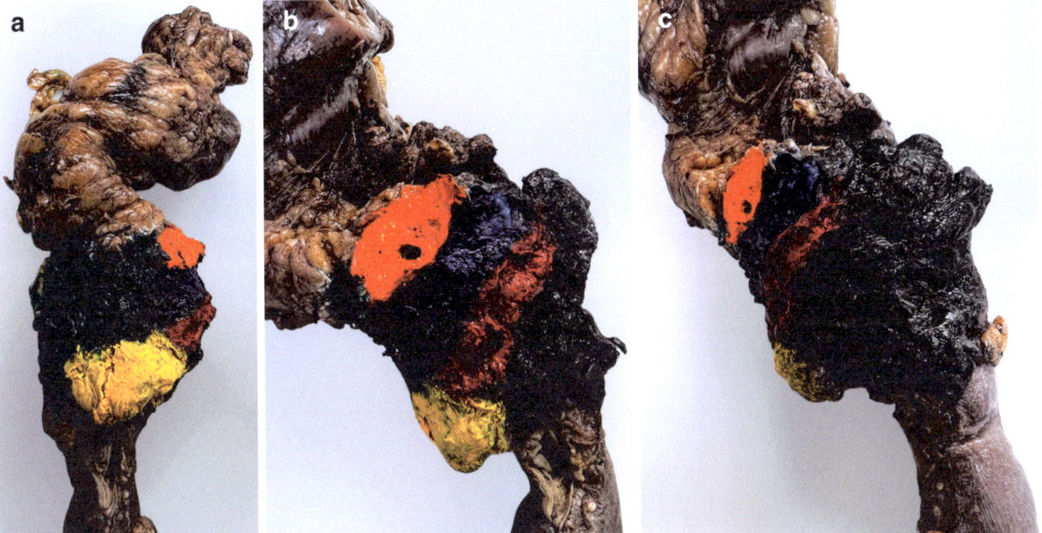

Fig. 10.32 (**a**) Anterior ink; (**b**) medial ink; (**c**) posterior ink

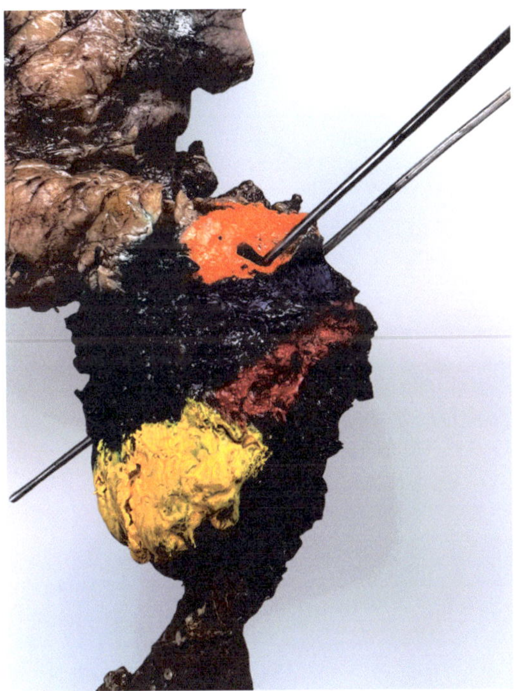

Fig. 10.33 Probes inserted

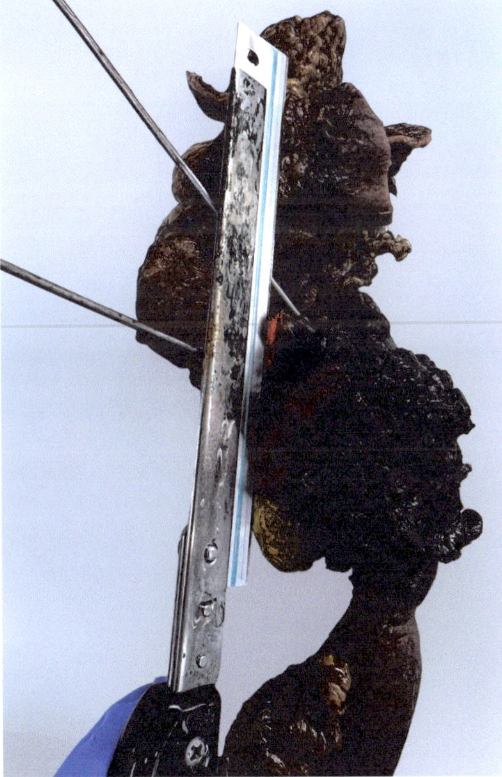

Fig. 10.34 Pancreatic head bivalved

Fig. 10.35 Pancreatic duct and common bile duct within pancreas

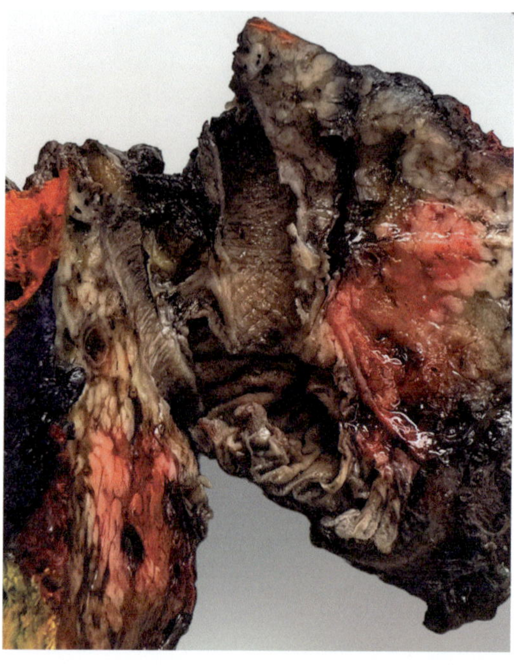

Fig. 10.36 (**a**) Anterior shave margins; (**b**) medial and posterior shave margins

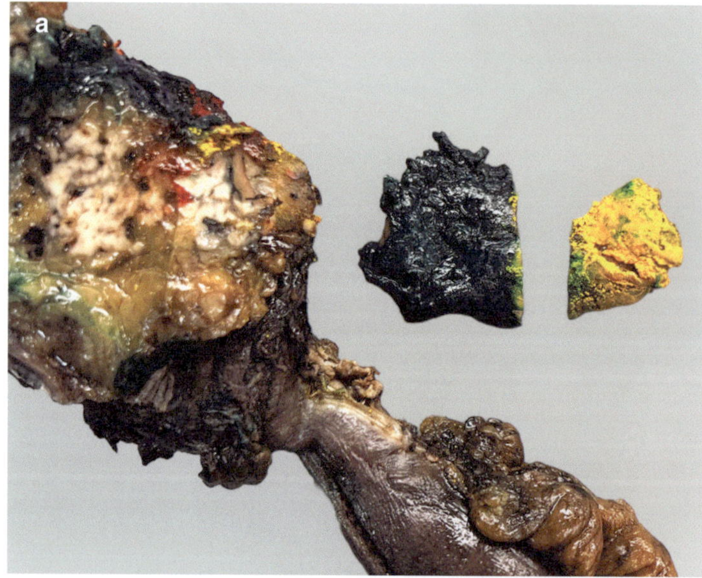

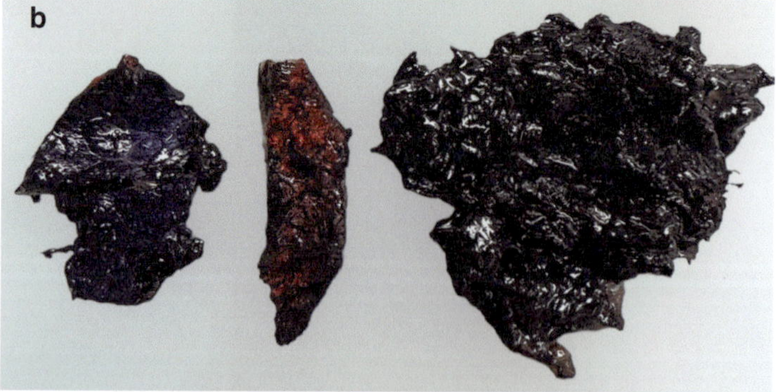

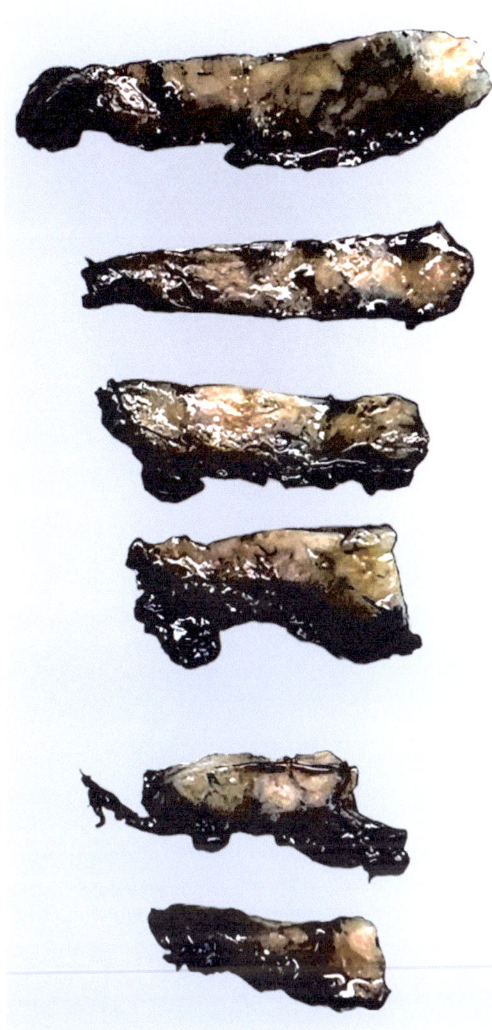

Fig. 10.37 Perpendicularly sectioned margins

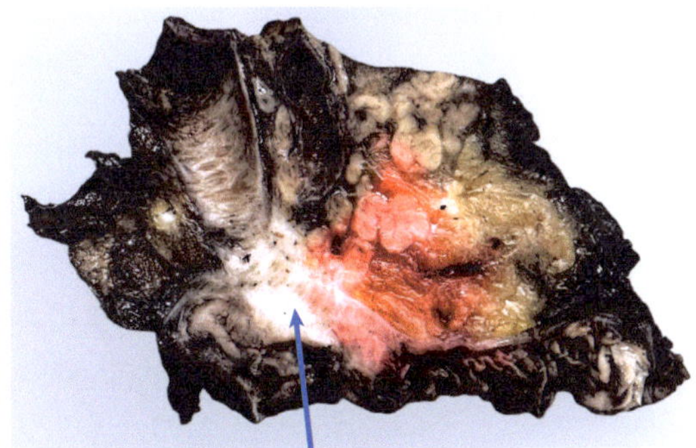

Fig. 10.38 lesion within pancreas.

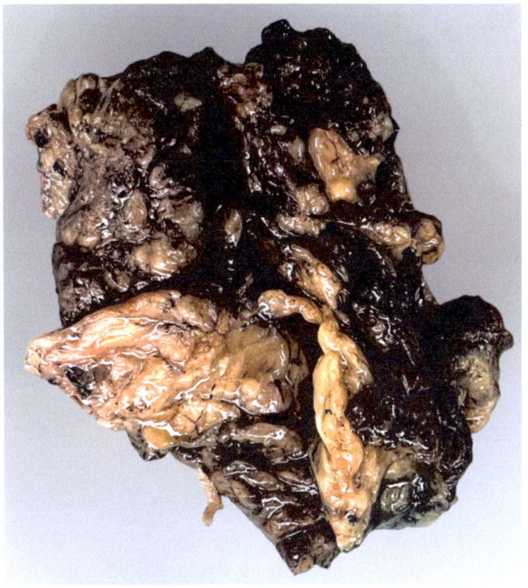

Fig. 10.39 Attached adipose tissue for lymph nodes

Black: retroperitoneal
Green: anterior pancreas
Yellow: uncinate process
Section code
A1-A2: Proximal stomach margin, bisected, en face
A3: Distal duodenal margin, en face
A4: Pancreatic head margin, en face
A5: Common bile duct margin, en face
A6-A7: Uncinate process, perpendicular
A8-A10: Anterior pancreas, perpendicular
A11-A12: SMV, representative
A13: SMA, representative
A14-A17: Retroperitoneal margin, perpendicular
A18-A21: Full-face section of mass surrounding and in relation to common bile duct and pancreatic duct
A22-A25: Remainder of mass surrounding ampulla (1 slice per 2 cassettes, bisected)
A26: Pancreas, representative
A27: Representative stomach and duodenum
A28-A30: Four lymph node candidates per cassette, whole
A31: One lymph node candidate, bisected
A32-A33: One lymph node candidate per cassette, whole

10.7   Whipple with Duodenal Primary: Level VI CPT 88309

Tumors present at or around the ampulla of Vater within the duodenum requires a Whipple procedure to remove the area. The duodenum and the head of the pancreas are directly connected and therefore are removed together.

Step 1: Describe and measure the specimen. This Whipple specimen example consists of the pancreatic head, a portion of duodenum, and often a small portion of the distal stomach (Fig. 10.40).

Step 2: Shave and submit the proximal and distal duodenal margins and submit en face as shown in Fig. 10.41.

Step 3: Identify the margins and anatomic aspects of the pancreas. This includes the pancreatic head margin, the portal groove where the superior mesenteric artery (SMA) and vein (SMV) were removed, the retroperitoneal margin, and the uncinate process as shown in Fig. 10.42.

Step 4: Identify and shave the common bile duct margin shown by the blue arrow in Fig. 10.43. This margin is submitted en face.

Step 5: Shave and submit the pancreatic head margin en face.

Step 6: Ink the margins and anatomical aspects of the pancreas. The pancreatic head margin has already been taken so the ink for the pancreatic head is now present on the false margin. It is optional to ink the pancreatic head false margin but it allows for easier orientation after the specimen is sectioned. In Fig. 10.44, the ink code is as follows:

    Red: pancreatic head false margin

    Blue: SMV

    Red: SMA

    Black: retroperitoneal

Step 7: Open the duodenum along the line opposite of the pancreas. In Fig. 10.45, the duodenum is open and the mass is exposed.

Step 8: Describe and measure the mass.

Step 9: Measure the distance of the mass to the proximal and distal duodenal margins.

Step 10: Shave all the pancreatic margins and aspects as seen in Fig. 10.46. These margins

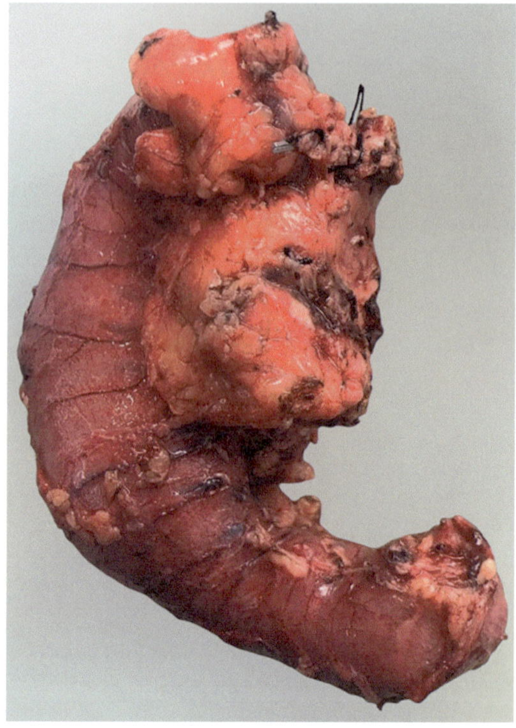

Fig. 10.40 Pancreaticoduodenectomy

can either be submitted enface or perpendicularly sectioned and submitted on edge.

Step 11: Bivalve the pancreatic head, exposing the pancreatic duct and common bile duct as shown in Fig. 10.47. This is best performed by placing probes in the pancreatic and common bile ducts and slicing along the probes from the duct margins toward the duodenum.

Step 12: Measure the greatest depth of invasion of the duodenal lesion into the pancreas. In Fig. 10.48, the extent of invasion is minimal. The lesion invades into the duodenal serosa without invasion into the pancreas as designated by the small blue arrow.

Step 13: Take sections of the duodenal lesion (blue arrow) in relation to the pancreas (green arrow), including the ampulla of Vater (red arrow) as shown in Fig. 10.49.

Step 14: Submit sections. Sections should include proximal/distal duodenum, common bile duct, pancreatic head, portal groove (SMA/SMV), retroperitoneal, uncinate process, duodenal lesion in relation to ampulla of Vater and pancreas (Fig. 10.50).

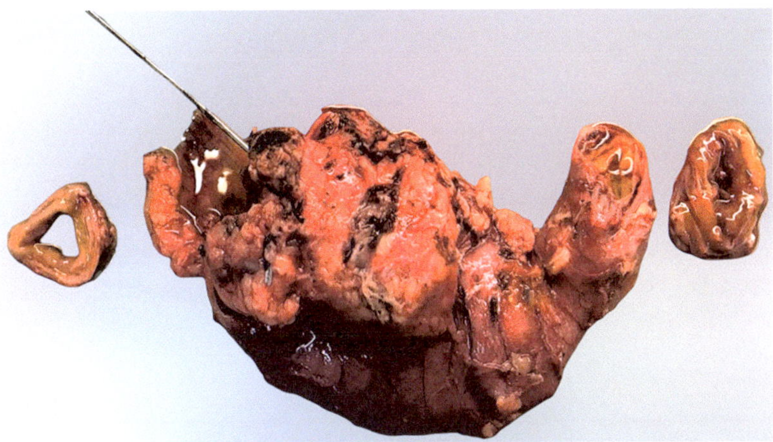

Fig. 10.41 Pancreaticoduodenectomy proximal and distal duodenal margins

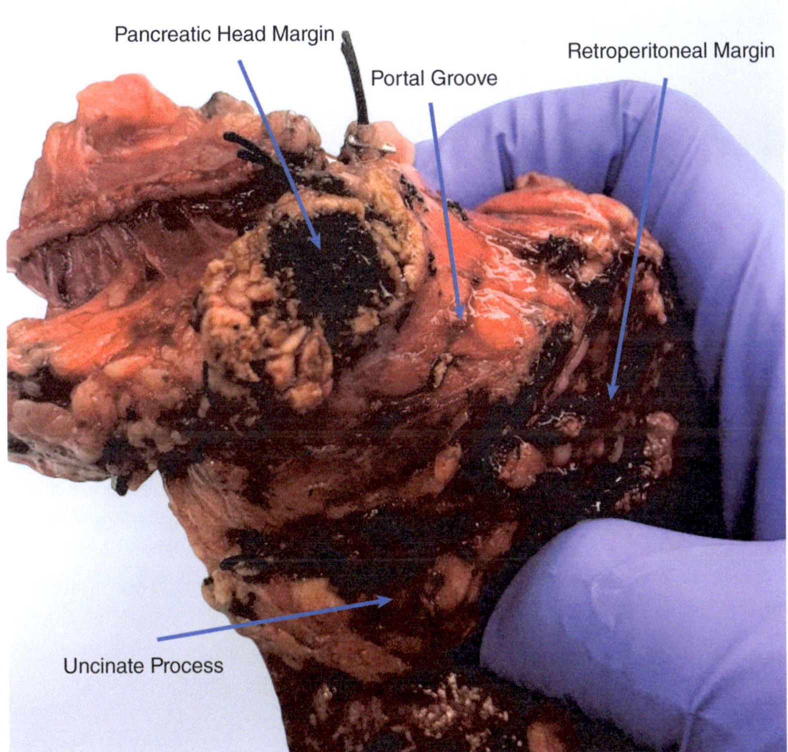

Fig. 10.42 Pancreaticoduodenectomy pancreatic margin

Example Dictation

Specimen A is received in formalin labeled with patient's name, medical record number, "Whipple" and consists of duodenum (19.2 cm in length by 2.2 cm in diameter) with attached head of pancreas (5.3 × 5.2 × 4.1 cm). The duodenum is opened to reveal a tan-brown, polypoid mass (2.6 × 1.9 × 0.7 cm) present at the ampulla of Vater. The mass comes within 9.1 cm of the proximal margin and 10.0 cm from the distal margin. The pancreas and duodenum are bivalved to reveal invasion of the mass into the duodenal serosal surface without invasion into the pancreas. The surrounding adipose tissue is palpable for 14 lymph node candidates ranging from 0.4 to 1.1 cm.

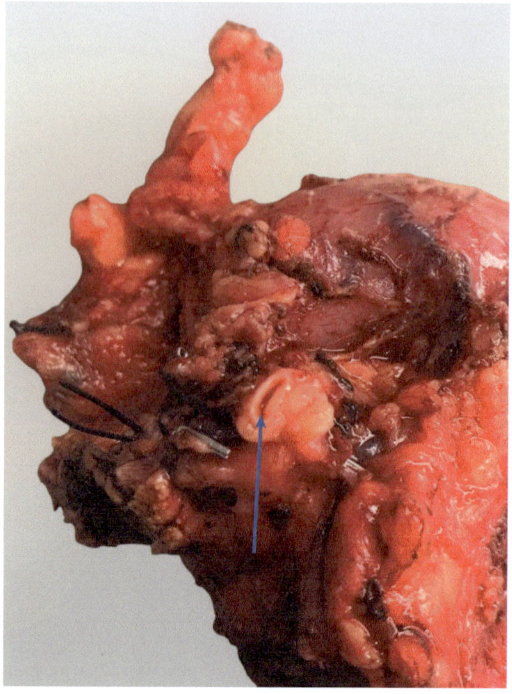

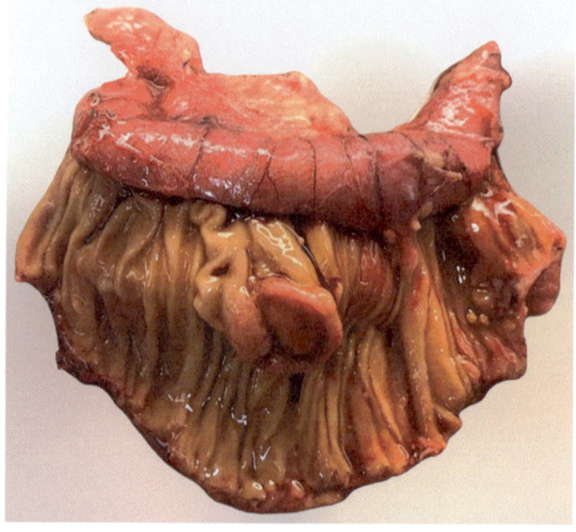

Fig. 10.45 Pancreaticoduodenectomy duodenum with mass

Fig. 10.43 Pancreaticoduodenectomy common bile duct margin

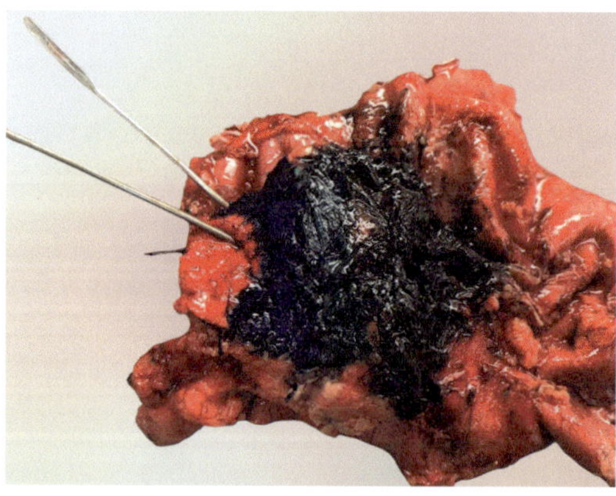

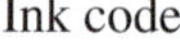

Fig. 10.44 Pancreaticoduodenectomy inked pancreatic, SMA, SMV, and retroperitoneal margins

Ink code

    Orange: pancreatic head false margin

    Blue: SMV

    Red: SMA

    Black: retroperitoneal

Section code

    A1-A2: Proximal duodenum margin, bisected, en face

A3: Distal duodenal margin, en face

A4: Pancreatic head margin, en face

A5: Common bile duct margin, en face

A6: Uncinate process, en face

A7: Anterior pancreas, en face

A8: SMV, en face

A9: SMA, en face

A10: Retroperitoneal margin, en face

A11-A12: Mass in relation to ampulla of Vater and pancreas, bisected

A13-A15:4 lymph node candidate per cassette, whole

A16-A17:1 lymph node candidate per cassette, bisected

Acknowledgments The author gratefully acknowledges Neha Varshney, MD, and Vamshi Vasantha Raya Gorantla, MBBS, for their contribution to this chapter.

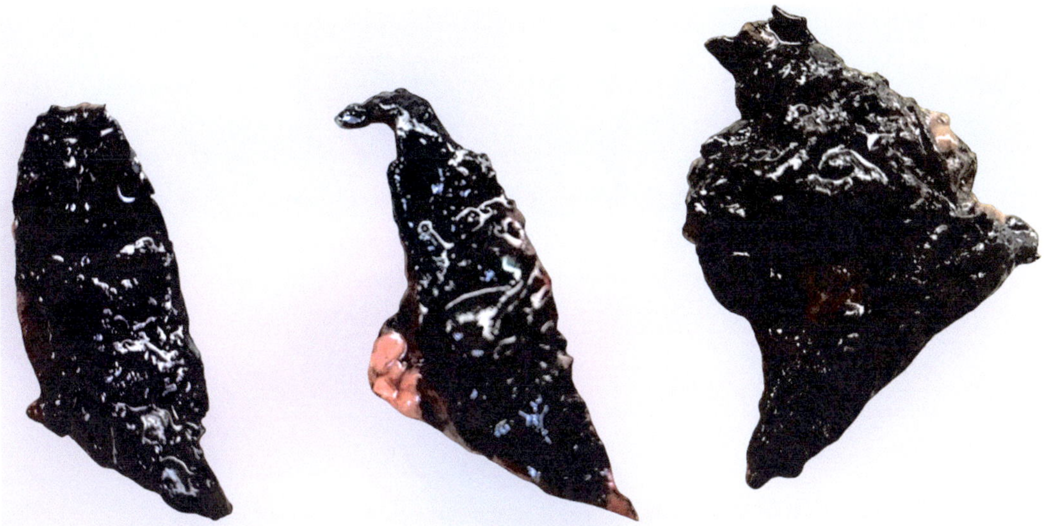

Fig. 10.46 Pancreaticoduodenectomy SMA, SMV, and retroperitoneal margins shaved

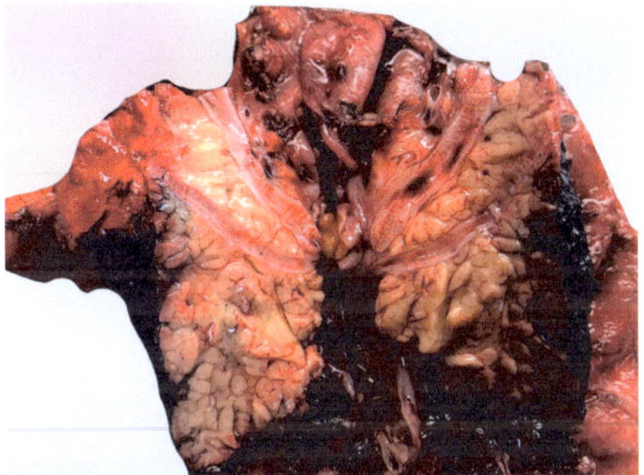

Fig. 10.47 Pancreaticoduodenectomy bivalve through CBD and pancreatic duct

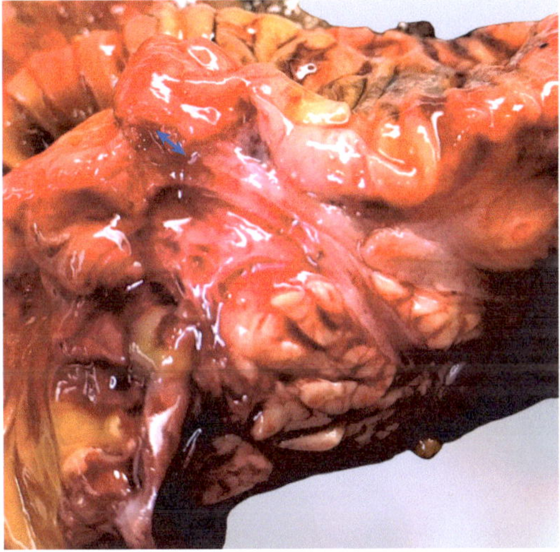

Fig. 10.48 Pancreaticoduodenectomy ampulla of Vater with mass

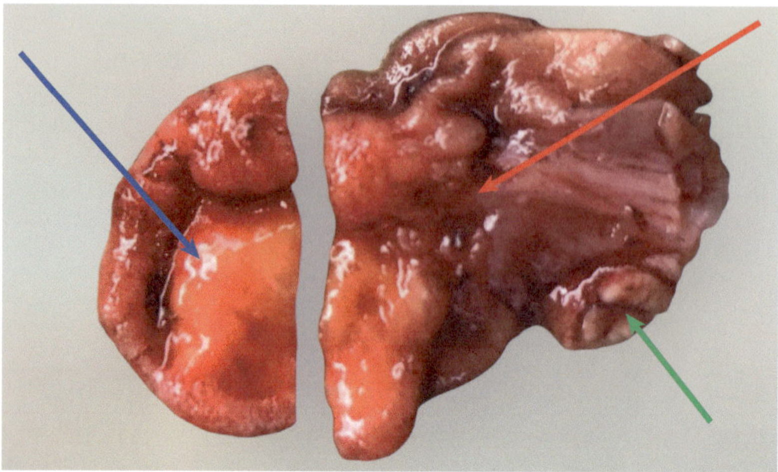

Fig. 10.49 Pancreaticoduodenectomy section of mass in relation to ampulla of Vater and pancreas

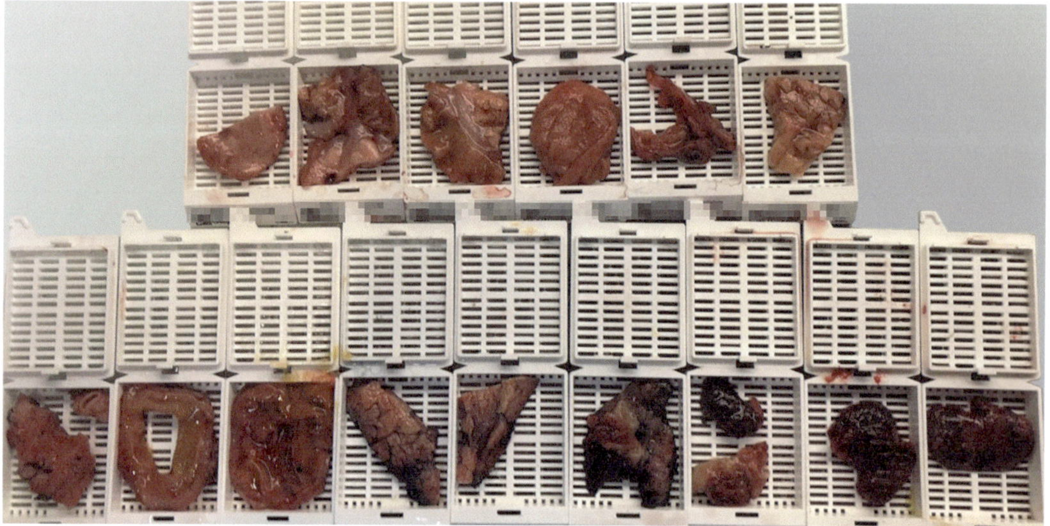

Fig. 10.50 Pancreaticoduodenectomy section submission

Quiz Questions

1. An intact cholecystectomy specimen is sent to pathology measuring 7.5 × 4.0 × 4.0 cm. Upon opening of the gallbladder, there are multiple tan green to yellow multifaceted stones and a small tan-yellow nodule measuring 0.9 × 0.8 × 0.3 cm. How should the nodule be grossed?
   (a) Submit 1 representative section of the nodule.
   (b) Submit nodule entirely.
   (c) Submit sections from the periphery of the nodule.
   (d) Describe the nodule but do not submit sections.

2. A 1.9 cm liver core biopsy is sent to the laboratory. The patient chart states a history of lymphoma but the current imaging indicated a possible adenoma. How should the responsible person proceed?
   (a) Place approximately 0.5 cm of the core in RPMI and submit the rest for normal processing
   (b) Place core in RPMI and wait for further instruction
   (c) Divide the core and submit in multiple cassettes
   (d) Submit core in 1 cassette

3. What is the structure designated by the black arrow in Fig. 10.51?
   (a) Quadrate lobe
   (b) Liver hilum
   (c) Caudate lobe
   (d) Gallbladder

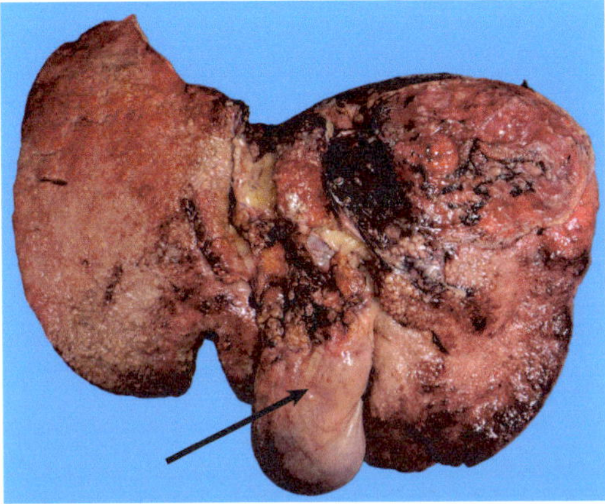

Fig. 10.51 Quiz question 3

4. A hepatectomy specimen was sent to pathology weighing 1200 gm, 12.9 × 7.9 × 7.2 cm. The outer surface of the liver capsule is smooth. Serial sectioning of the liver revealed 15 nodules ranging from 0.4 to 1.2 cm, surrounded by normal appearing liver parenchyma. What could be the most likely gross diagnosis?
   (e) Hepatocellular carcinoma
   (f) Hepatic cirrhosis
   (g) Metastatic carcinoma
   (h) Metastatic sarcoma

5. A hepatectomy specimen was sent to pathology weighing 1138 gm, 10.3 × 9.2 × 9.0 cm. The cut surface contains a tan mass with a central stellate scar. The patient had no previous history of liver diseases. What is the most likely gross diagnosis
   (a) Hepatic cirrhosis
   (b) Fibrolamellar variant of hepatocellular carcinoma
   (c) Hepatic adenoma
   (d) Metastatic carcinoma

6. A partial hepatectomy specimen was sent to pathology weighing 425 gm, 5.9 × 5.5 × 5.0 cm. The outer surface of the liver capsule is smooth and glistening. Serial sectioning of the liver revealed a tan red nodule (1.6 × 1.3 × 1.0 cm) surrounded by normal appearing liver. What could be the most likely gross diagnosis?
   (a) Hepatocellular carcinoma
   (b) Focal nodular hyperplasia
   (c) Hemangioma
   (d) Metastatic carcinoma

7. A 35-year female was found to have a nodule in the liver ultrasound. A partial hepatectomy specimen was sent to pathology weighing 155 gm, 4.1 × 3.4 × 3.1 cm. The outer surface of the liver capsule is smooth and glistening. Serial sectioning of the liver revealed a tan-brown nodule (1.2 × 1.2 × 1.1 cm) in a background of normal appearing liver. What could be the most likely differential?
   (a) Hepatocellular carcinoma
   (b) Focal nodular hyperplasia
   (c) Hemangioma
   (d) Hepatic adenoma

8. A 75-year female complaining of right upper quadrant pain, laboratory finding is suggestive of obstructive jaundice with ultrasound showing thickened gallbladder wall. On gross examination of the gallbladder, the wall is thickened ranging from 0. 3 to 0.8 cm and firm which lead to submission of the entire gallbladder wall for microscopic examination. What is the most important to rule out?
   (a) Cholecystitis
   (b) Cholelithiasis
   (c) Adenocarcinoma of the gallbladder
   (d) Cholecystitis with cholelithiasis

9. What margin is identified by the black arrow in Fig. 10.52?
   (a) Pancreatic margin
   (b) Retroperitoneal margin
   (c) Common bile duct margin
   (d) Cystic duct margin

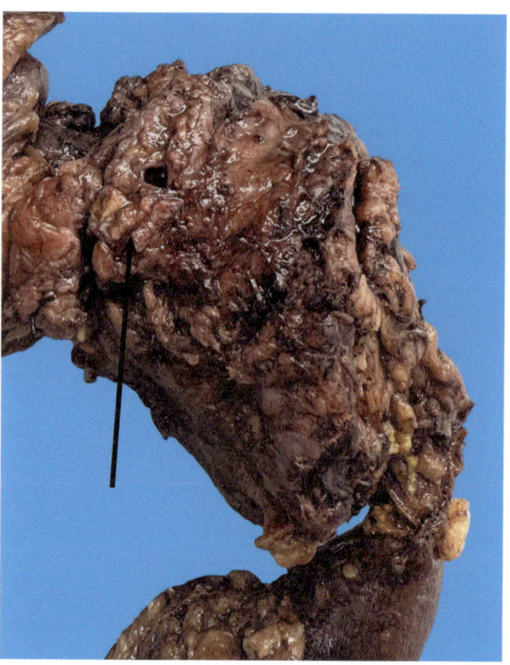

Fig. 10.52 Quiz question 9

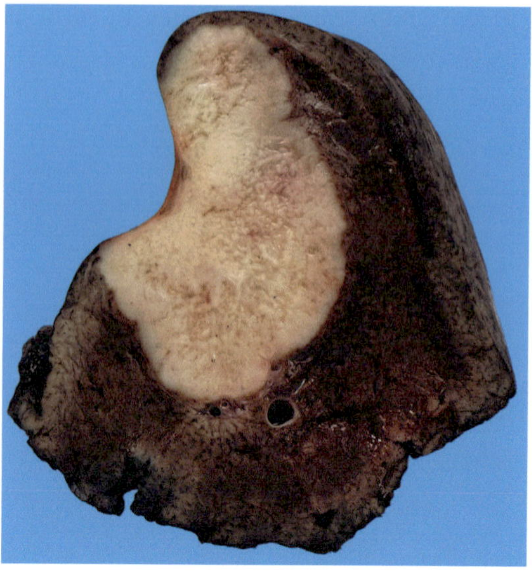

Fig. 10.53 Quiz question 10

10. A 65-year-old female complaining of mild abdominal pain. CT of the abdomen shows a solid mass measuring 3.0 × 3.6 × 2.6 cm in the liver. A partial liver resection is performed and the specimen was sent to pathology. Based on the gross appearance of the mass in Fig. 10.53, what is the gross diagnosis?

    (a) Liver scar
    (b) Cholangiocarcinoma
    (c) Liver abscess
    (d) Hepatocellular carcinoma

Answer Key

1. *(b) Submit nodule entirely*

    Explanation: Nodules of the gallbladder could be neoplastic. Since this nodule is small, it can be submitted entirely for microscopic assessment.

2. *(a)* Place approximately 0.5 cm of the core in RPMI and submit the rest for normal processing

    Explanation: In situations where a patient has a history of lymphoma in the past, always place a small amount of the tissue in RPMI. The remainder of the tissue can be processed as normal. If the biopsy is suggestive of lymphoma, then the tissue in RPMI can be used for flow cytometry.

3. (d) *Gallblatter*

   Explanation: The gallbladder is adhered to the liver between the quadrate lobe and the right lobe. The cystic duct extends from the gallbladder, converges with the hepatic duct to become the common bile duct as it enters the pancreas.

4. *(c) Metastatic carcinoma*

   Explanations: Most common malignancy of the liver is the hepatocellular carcinoma, which typically occurs in the background of hepatic cirrhosis. Hepatic cirrhosis has a nodular appearance on the outer and inner cut surfaces. Whereas metastasis to the liver is usually multiple, but the capsular outer surface is smooth, and sectioning of the liver reveals tan-brown normal appearing liver parenchyma with tan-white metastatic nodules. Sarcomas are by itself rare compared to carcinomas

5. *(b) Fibrolamellar variant of hepatocellular carcinoma.*

   Explanation: Fibrolamellar variant of hepatocellular carcinoma is the rare variant of hepatocellular carcinoma which arises in the background of normal liver. It has a characteristic central stellate scar radiating outwards. Focal nodular hyperplasia also show central stellate scar.

6. *(c) Hemangioma*

   Explanation: Cavernous hemangiomas are the most common benign neoplasm of the liver. They are mostly solitary tan red lesions present in a background of normal liver parenchyma.

7. *(d) Hepatic adenoma*

   Explanation: Hepatic adenoma is usually single or multiple, tan brown, circumscribed, unencapsulated nodules, so (d) is correct. Most other lesions have a white, solid appearance.

8. *(c) Adenocarcinoma of the gallbladder*

   Explanation: Thickened gallbladder in an elderly patient with obstructive symptoms should always be suspicious for cholangiocarcinoma. The entire gallbladder needs to be submitted for evaluation as this tumor is very subtle in gross appearance.

9. *(a) Pancreatic margin*

   Explanation: The pancreatic margin is where the surgeon transected the head of the pancreas from the remainder of the body and tail of the pancreas, so (a) is correct. It contains the pancreatic duct which runs along the middle of the pancreas to the ampulla of Vater. The retroperitoneal margin is the posterior aspect of the pancreas that is retroperitoneal in the abdomen. The cystic duct margin extends from the gallbladder and becomes the common bile duct margin as the cystic dust and hepatic duct margin converge and enter the pancreas. Chronic pancreatitis has shrunken small pancreases and a long-standing history of mild abdominal pain. In neoplasm like adenocarcinoma or other tumors, there will be a mass or cystic lesion.

10. *(b) Cholangiocarcinoma*

    Explanation: Cholangiocarcinoma grossly appears as a solid, firm, white-tan mass, so answer (b) is correct. Hepatocellular carcinomas are typically nodules that are tan-green and possibly encapsulated. An abscess area of the liver will be soft and friable while a scar will be fibrous and irregular.

References

1. "UMHS Department of Pathology Specimen To Charge Code Rapid Finder List," 2011.
2. "College of American Pathologists," June 2021. [Online]. Available: https://www.cap.org/protocols-and-guidelines/cancer-reporting-tools/cancer-protocol-templates. Accessed 21 Aug 2023.

Contents

The brain and the eye are often stressful specimens to handle. These specimens don't come across the gross bench very often so the lack of experience can be the biggest reason for stress. Taking photographs, knowing CPT codes (see Table 11.1) and consulting the pathologist can be the principal savior with these specimens.

Table 11.1 CPT codes [1]

Brain, meninges, other than tumor	88305
Brain, biopsy	88307
Brain/meninges, tumor resection	88307
Pterygium	88304
Endothelium	88304
Cornea	88304
Eye, enucleation	88307

11.1 Brain Biopsy: Level V CPT 88307

A brain biopsy is a procedure to remove a small amount of the identified lesion (abnormal tissue) found on imaging for examination under a microscope. Identification of malignant tumors, benign lesions, infections, and cysts can help dictate the appropriate surgery needed for complete resection/management.

Step 1: Describe and count the number of fragments present. Often 5+ fragments can be called an aggregate (Fig. 11.1)

Step 2: Measure the fragments in aggregate.

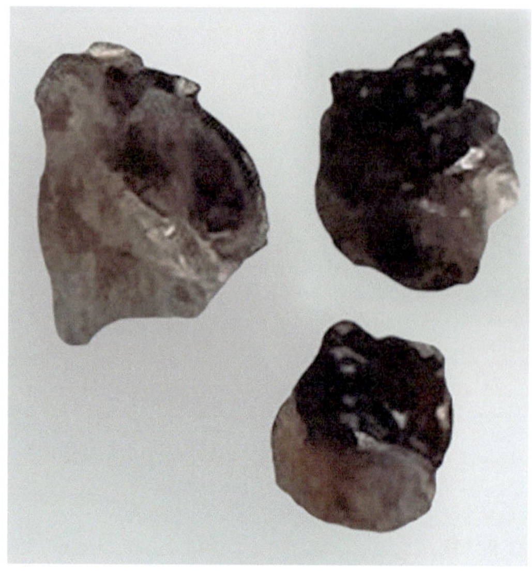

Fig. 11.1 Brain biopsy

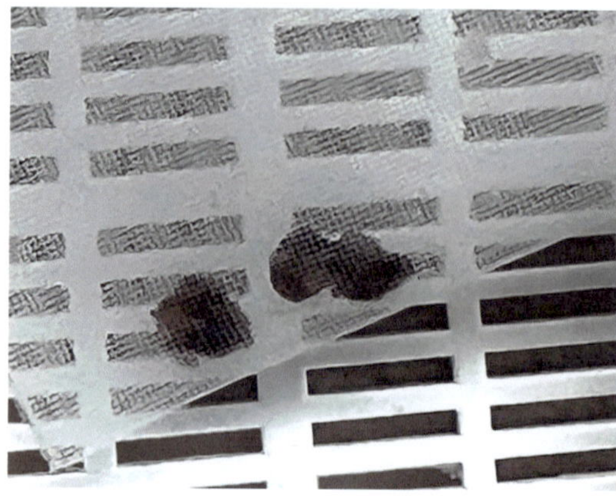

Fig. 11.2 Brain biopsy cassette submission

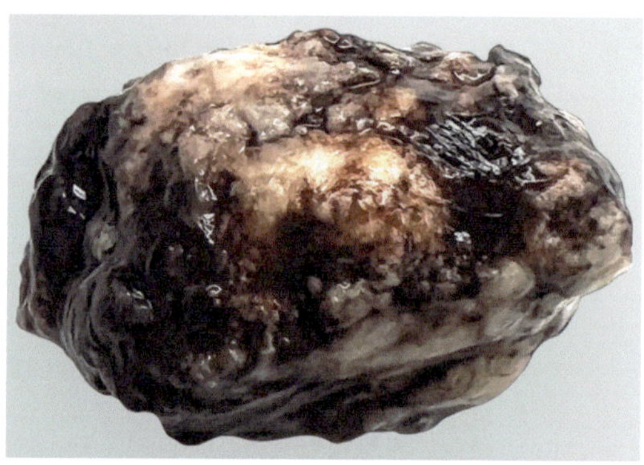

Fig. 11.3 Brain resection

Step 3: Submit the specimen entirely in a biopsy bag. If there is a large amount of tissue, it can be divided into multiple cassettes to be submitted (Fig. 11.2).

Example Dictation

Specimen A is received in formalin labeled with the patient's name, medical record number, "brain biopsy" and consists of 3 fragment of tan-brown, cauterized, and hemorrhagic tissue (0.8 × 0.7 × 0.3 cm) which is submitted entirely in a biopsy bag in A1.

11.2 Brain Resection for Tumor: Level V, CPT 88307

There are a multitude of benign and malignant brain tumors. These tumors must be resected as they can impinge on brain areas, causing a multitude of other symptoms.

Step 1: Measure and describe the specimen (Fig. 11.3).
Step 2: Serially section the specimen as seen in Fig. 11.4.
Step 3: Dictate the gross appearance of the cut surface of the specimen.

Step 4: Submit specimen entirely or representative sections.

In this example, the specimen is small and fits in only a few cassettes as seen in Fig. 11.5. However, if the specimen is large, then representative sections can be submitted. Often one section per centimeter of the overall size of the tissue, e.g., an 8-cm specimen will have 8 sections submitted.

Example Dictation

Specimen A is received in formalin labeled with the patient's name, medical record number, "brain resection" and consists of a single fragment of tan-brown, cauterized and hemorrhagic tissue (2.7 × 1.8 × 1.1 cm) which is serially sectioned to reveal solid tan, focally hemorrhagic cut

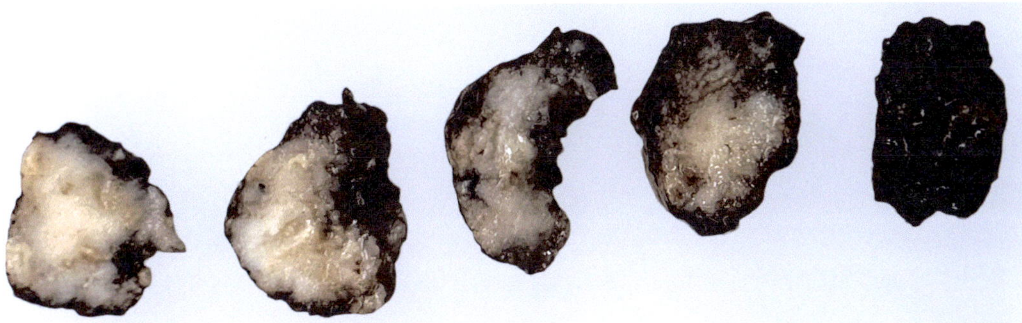

Fig. 11.4 Brain resection serially sectioned

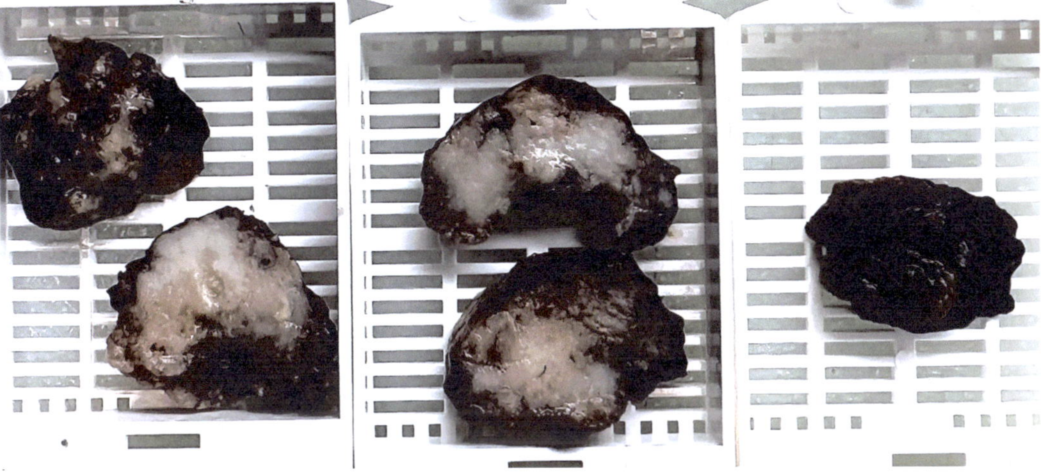

Fig. 11.5 Brain resection cassette submission

surfaces. The specimen is submitted entirely in A1-A3.

11.3 Cranial Bone: Level VI CPT 88309

Cranial bone can be removed for medical issues such as tumor invasion, blood clots, trauma, or swelling. Occasionally, the bone is kept sterile and frozen to be surgically inserted back into place, but often the bone is replaced with plates to cover the defect.

Step 1: Describe and measure the specimen.

Step 2: Orient the specimen. Figure 11.6a is the convex external surface of the cranium and Fig. 11.6b is the concave internal surface of the cranium.

In this example, a brain lesion has invaded into the internal surface of the cranium, through the bone and extended out the external side of the bone. Note the blue arrows in Fig. 11.6a, b designating the lesion.

Step 3: Ink the external, internal, and peripheral margin of the specimen as shown in Fig. 11.7a, b. This step is optional depending on the preference of the pathologist.

Step 4: Serially section the bone.

Step 5: Assess the cut surface of the bone for lesion involvement. In Fig. 11.8, the lesion is extending through the bone as noted by the blue line.

Step 6: Submit representative sections of the lesion with the greatest involvement and the lesion to the closest peripheral margin (Fig. 11.9).

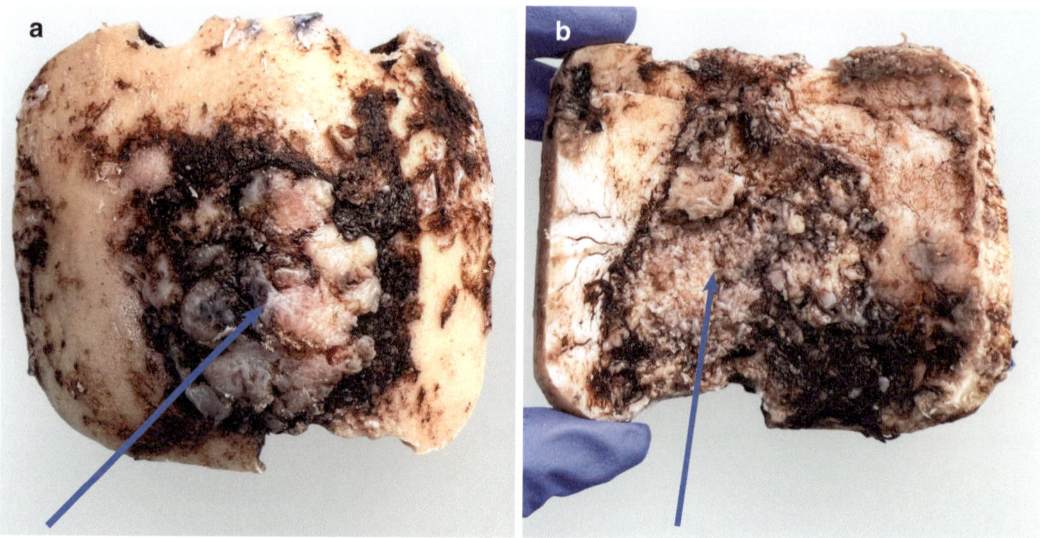

Fig. 11.6 (**a**) Cranial bone, external surface; (**b**) cranial bone, internal surface

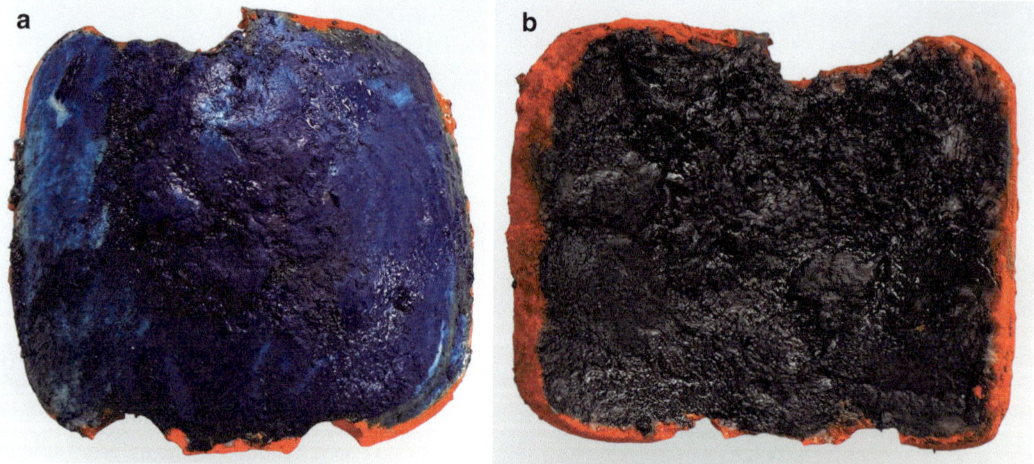

Fig. 11.7 (**a**) Cranial bone external ink; (**b**) cranial bone internal ink

Step 7: Bone will need to be decalcified before submitting to histology.

Example Dictation

Specimen A is received in formalin labeled with patient's name, medical record number, "partial cranium" and consists of a portion of unoriented cranial bone (8.6 × 7.4 × 0.9 cm) with identifiable area of erosion (4.5 × 4.2 cm) on the internal surface. The specimen is sectioned to reveal firm, tan bone with extension to the external surface, coming within 1.0 cm of the closest peripheral margin. Representative sections of the lesion in relation to the closest peripheral margin are submitted in A1-A2 (1 slice per 2 cassettes, bisected, post-decalcification).

Ink code

    Blue: External bone

    Black: Internal bone

    Orange: Peripheral margin

Fig. 11.8 Cranial bone serially sectioned

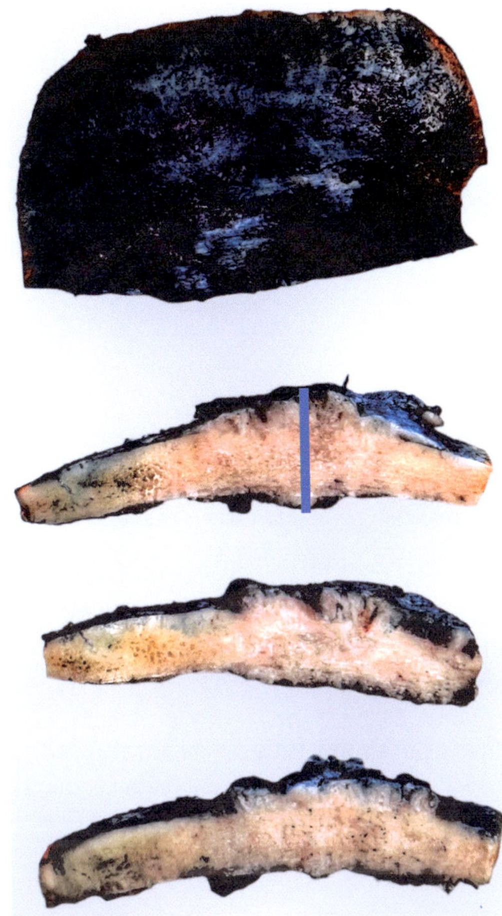

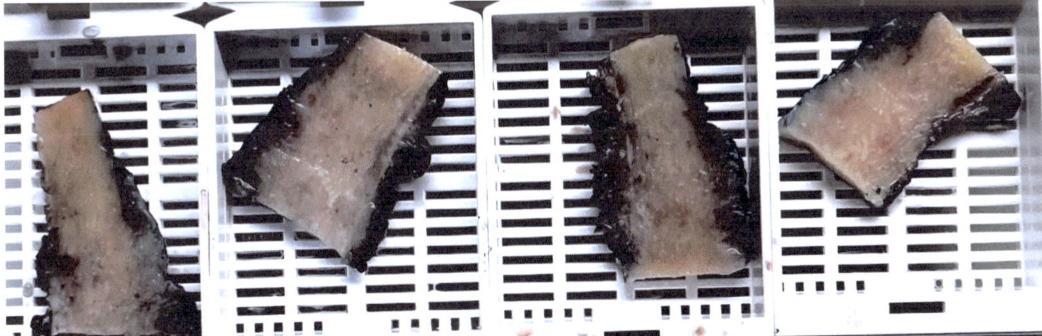

Fig. 11.9 Cranial bone section submission

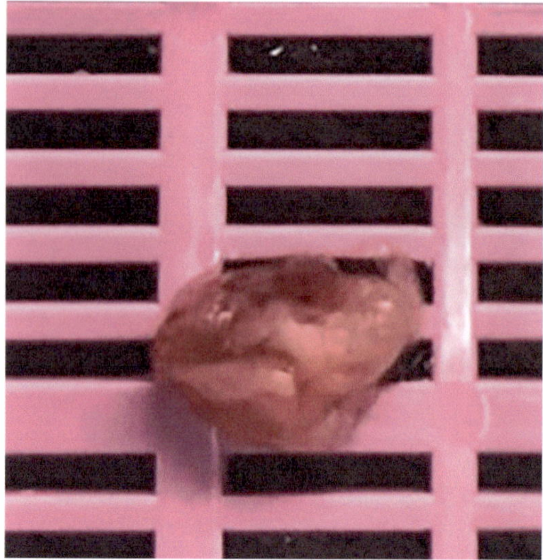

Fig. 11.10 Pterygium

11.4   Pterygium: Level III, CPT 88304

A pterygium is a raised area (abnormal growth of tissue) on the conjunctiva and adjacent cornea of the eye. These are benign lesions and can eventually obscure vision if left untreated.

Step 1: Measure and describe the specimen.
Step 2: Submit the specimen whole as seen in Fig. 11.10.

Example Dictation
Specimen A is received in formalin labeled with the patient's name, medical record number, "pterygium" and consists of a single fragment of tan-pink tissue ($0.9 \times 0.6 \times 0.5$ cm) which is submitted in toto in A1.

11.5   Endothelium: Level III, CPT 88304

Endothelium of the eye is translucent tissue that is present on the back of the corona. When received in the lab, it is incredibly hard to see in the container. Whether received fresh or in formalin, the tissue is very small and completely translucent. Once identified, do not take your

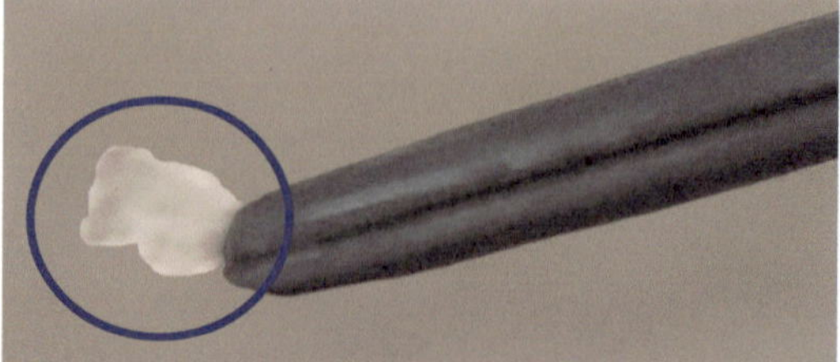

Fig. 11.11 Eye endothelium

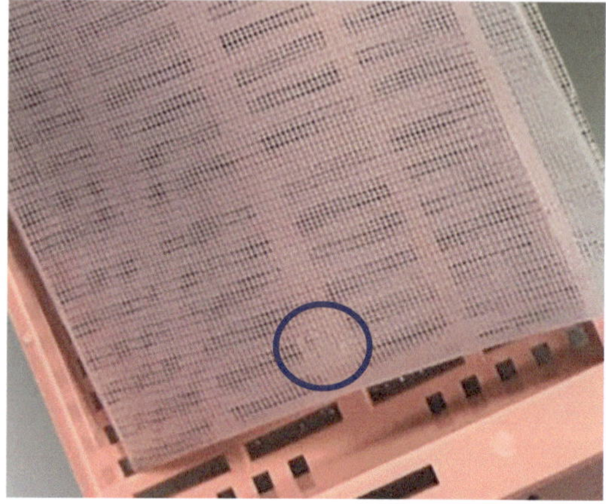

Fig. 11.12 Eye endothelium cassette submission

eyes off of it. Some labs chose to put ink or hematoxylin on these specimens so they can be seen in the biopsy bag.

Step 1: Identify the tissue in the container seen in Fig. 11.11 (blue circle).
Step 2: Describe and measure the specimen. Endothelium is almost completely translucent and difficult to identify in formalin.
Step 3: Place specimen in biopsy bag carefully as shown in Fig. 11.12 (blue circle).
Step 4: Submit the specimen entirely. It can be a common practice to dip the endothelium in hematoxylin to allow for better visualization of the tissue inside the biopsy bag.

Example Dictation
Specimen A is received in formalin labeled with patients' name, medical record number, "eye endothelium" and consists of a single translucent tissue fragment ($0.3 \times 0.3 \times 0.1$ cm) which is submitted in toto in a biopsy bag in A1.

11.6   Cornea: Level III, CPT 88304

When the cornea is damaged, it can lead to pain and cloudy vision. A corneal transplant can help these symptoms by removing and replacing the cornea with a donor cornea.

Step 1: Describe and measure (diameter) the cornea as seen in Fig. 11.13.
Step 2: Describe any areas of hemorrhage or lacerations on the cornea.
Step 3: The cornea is serially sectioned and submitted on edge shown with the blue lines in Fig. 11.14. However, it is common practice that the grossing person submits the cornea intact and the histotechnologist will serially section and embed the cornea after processing to ensure proper orientation.

Example Dictation
Specimen A is received in formalin labeled with patients' name, medical record number, "patients left cornea" and consists of an intact, semitranslucent cornea (0.7 cm in diameter) with a focal area of hemorrhage (0.3 cm in diameter) along one edge. The specimen is submitted in toto in A1.

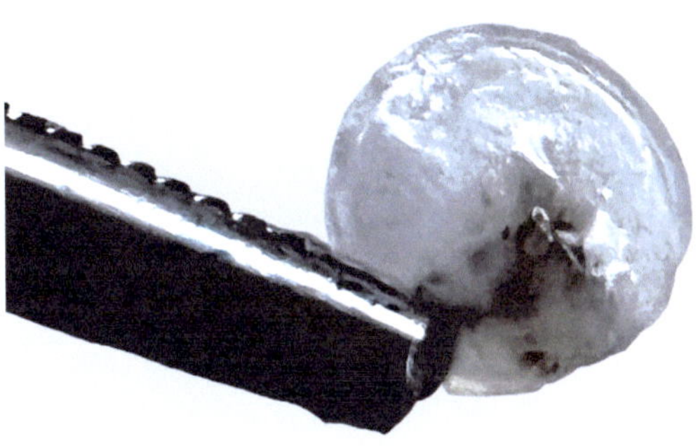

Fig. 11.13 Cornea

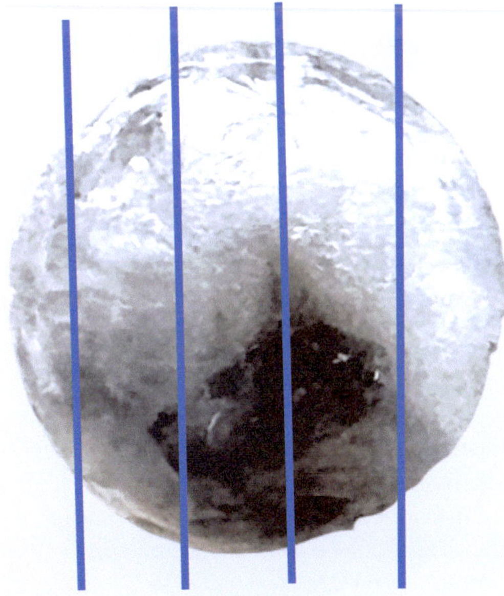

Fig. 11.14 Cornea serially sectioned

11.7   Eye Enucleation: Level V, CPT 88307

Eye enucleation specimens can occur for different reasons, such as trauma, blind painful eye, malignant lesion in orbit, or lesions surrounding the eye that are impinging on the eye (see Table 11.2 for the gross description of eye tumors). Fixing the eye in 10% buffered formalin for a few days before grossing is helpful. Always discuss eye enucleation specimens with the pathologist.

Enucleations for tumors rely heavily on the anatomic structures of the eye. Knowing the anatomy and grossing the eye based on anatomic structures will make signing out the case more streamlined.

Cancer Protocol Breakdown Relative to Grossing Eye

Procedure:

Local resection: Removing the tumor involved area only. This is often performed for melanomas of the uvea

Enucleation: Removal of the eye with no surrounding structures

Limited exenteration: A complete enucleation of the eye with only some of the surrounding structures such as conjunctiva or surrounding muscle

Complete exenteration: A complete enucleation of the eye including surrounding conjunctiva, soft tissue, and skin of the eyelids

Table 11.2 Gross description of eye tumor [2]

Eyelid tumors	They include a wide variety of skin and adnexal tumors
Melanocytic tumors	Well-defined tumors of variable color, ranging from amelanotic to dark brown and variegated
Retinoblastoma	The tumor has a white, encephaloid or brain-like appearance, with chalky areas of calcification and yellow necrotic areas
Vascular tumors Capillary hemangioma Cavernous hemangioma Malformations Hemangiopericytoma Angiosarcoma	• Deep lesions are well circumscribed and solid to cystic, with dilated vessels and with or without thrombus formation • May be polypoid with a stalk • Malignant lesions are ill defined
Germ cell tumors Dermoid cyst Teratoma	• Soft, round/oval solid to cystic lesion with thickened wall • Contain yellow, cheesy material (Dermoid) • Several tissue types like bone, tooth, cartilage (Teratoma)
Lacrimal gland tumors Pleomorphic adenoma Adenocarcinoma Adenoid cystic carcinoma Mucoepidermoid	Tumors of the lacrimal gland are similar to tumors of the salivary glands due to their shared embryologic origins Well-circumscribed, pseudoencapsulated, round to bosselated masses with a firm, whitish surface with occasional cysts, calcification, or cartilaginous areas. Can have infiltrative borders
Hematolymphoid tumors	Smooth distinct fleshy white to pink lesion that can be nodular ranging from a patch to a mass causing proptosis and displacement of the eyeball
Optic nerve tumors Astrocytoma (Juvenile) Malignant astrocytoma Meningioma	Most pilocytic astrocytoma's are soft, gray, and relatively discrete Optic nerve meningiomas are well circumscribed and surround the nerve, imparting a tubular appearance
Peripheral nerve tumors Neurofibroma Schwannoma Granular cell Malignant	Schwannomas are mainly solitary and globoid, with a smooth surface Neurofibroma has a variable gross presentation Granular cell tumors are uninodular and firm, homogeneous masses, tan to white in color MPNST shows a tan-white, fleshy cut surface, often with hemorrhage and necrosis
Bone and cartilage tumors	Variable; see relevant chapter
Adipose tissue tumors	*ALT/WDLS* may closely resemble normal fat or may appear whiter with a fibrous cut surface. Dedifferentiated areas can appear tan or gray and may have areas of necrosis. *Pleomorphic liposarcoma* usually appears white to yellow sometimes with myxoid areas and necrosis.
Muscle tumors Rhabdomyosarcoma	Most lesions present as poorly circumscribed, soft, fleshy, gelatinous masses with a pale-tan cut surface. Botryoid ERMS has a grape-like polypoid appearance
Histiocytic tumors	Soft tissue masses are usually firm, grayish to brownish in color, with smooth outer surface and yellowish cut surface
Fibrous tissue tumors (soft tissue)	Variable; see relevant chapter

Tumor site: The tumor site is broken down into quadrants (Fig. 11.15). First, trans-illuminate the eye to identify the quadrant and the tumor is located. Place a bright light behind the eye and allow the globe to illuminate. The dark area that does not illuminate should be the area of the tumor. A dissecting microscope works best.

Additionally, once the eye is opened, identifying the quadrant location of the tumor is necessary.

Tumor size: Measure the tumor in three dimensions with laterality (i.e., medial-lateral, anterior-posterior)

Distances: Measure the tumor distance to the limbus and to the posterior optic margin

Fig. 11.15 Eye
quadrant illustration

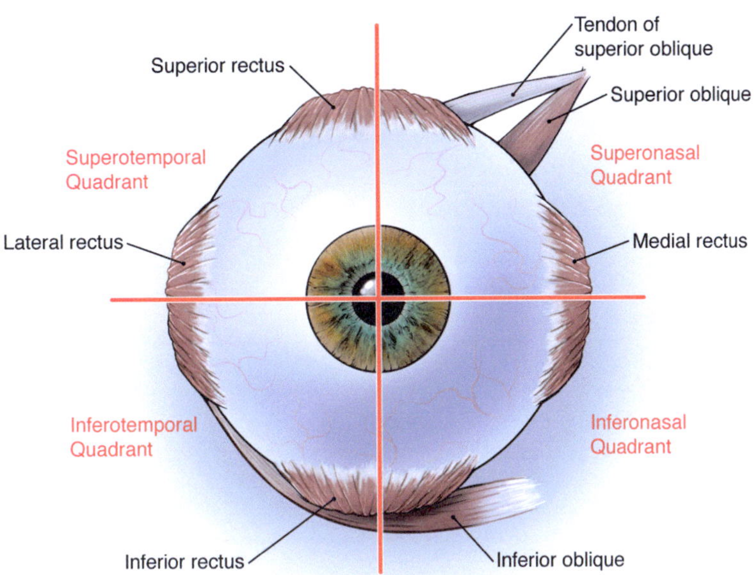

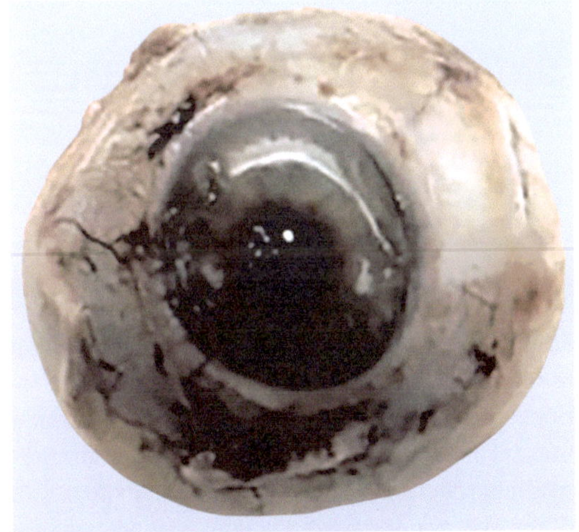

Fig. 11.16 Eye

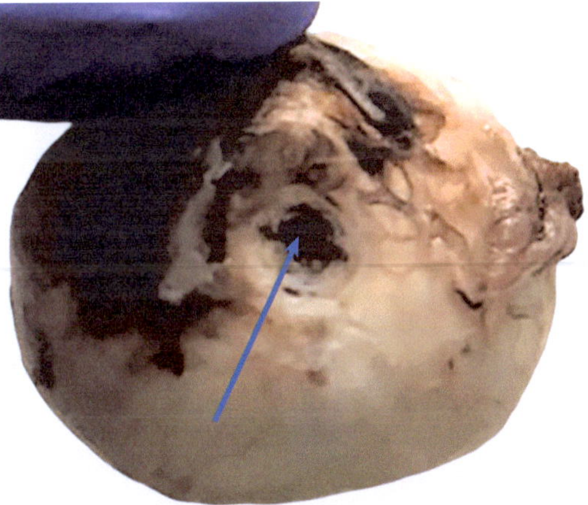

Fig. 11.17 Eye posterior view

Tumor growth pattern: Appropriately describe the tumor. (i.e., solid, cystic) [3]

Step 1: Measure the eye and describe the iris color and if there are ruptures in the globe shown in Fig. 11.16.

Step 2: Identify and measure the length of the optic nerve identified by the blue arrow in Fig. 11.17. In this example, the optic nerve is very short and has retracted into the eye post-surgical resection. If a length of the optic nerve is present, the margin of the optic nerve should be shaved and submitted en face.

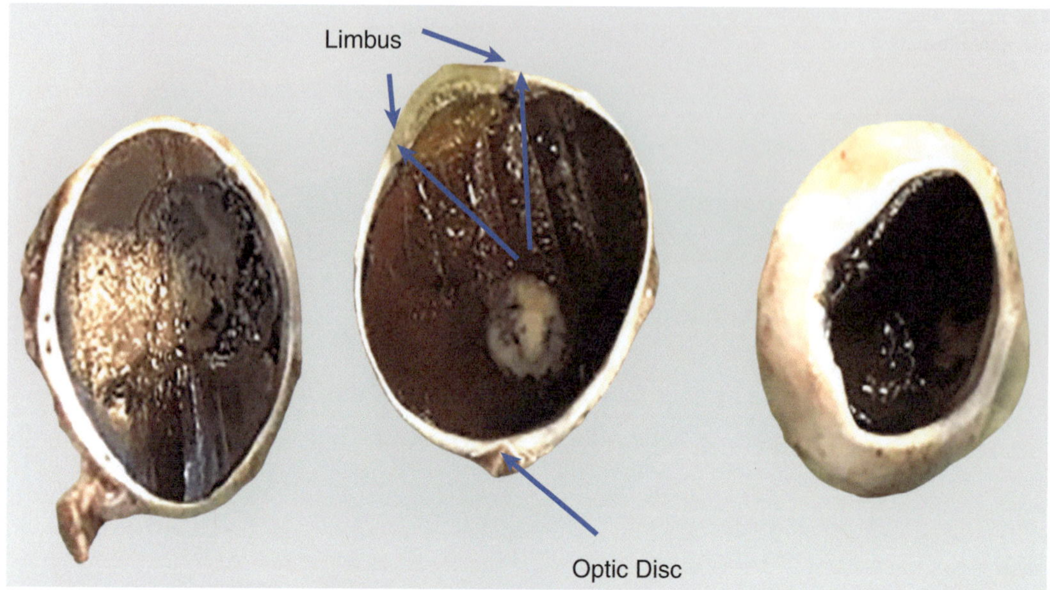

Fig. 11.18 Eye serially sectioned

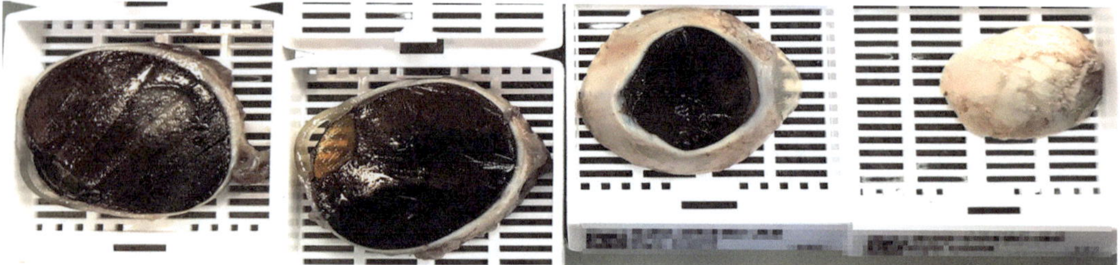

Fig. 11.19 Eye cassette submission

Step 3: Serially section the eye from medial to lateral as seen in Fig. 11.18. One slice should bivalve the optic nerve.

Step 4: Describe and measure the lesion and where it is present in the eye.

Step 5: Measure the lesion to the anterior limbus and posterior optic disc.

Step 6: Submit all sections as shown in Fig. 11.19. However, discuss the sections with the pathologist. It may only be necessary to submit the central slices that include the optic nerve.

Example Dictation

Specimen A is received in formalin labeled with patient's name, medical record number, "eye, left" and consists of an intact, slightly ragged eye enucleation (2.4 × 2.3 × 2.3 cm) with no identifiable length of ocular nerve present. The iris and pupil are markedly hazy. The specimen is serially sectioned to reveal a variegated white-black, irregular mass (1.6 × 0.8 × 0.8 cm) arising from the inferior-medial aspect of the eye, abutting the medial wall of the eye, coming within 1.2 cm from the anterior limbus and 0.9 cm from the posterior optic disc. The mass is diffusely surrounded by semitranslucent gelatinous material and hemorrhage.

Section code

    A1-A2: Mass in relation to optic nerve

    A3-A6: Remainder of medial and lateral eye

Acknowledgment The author gratefully acknowledges Youssef Al Hmada, MD, and Imran Ajmal, MBBS, for their contribution to this chapter.

Quiz Questions

1. Which is called the removal of the eye without surrounding structures or soft tissue?
   (a) Limited resection
   (b) Enucleation
   (c) Complete exenteration
   (d) Excision
2. What two structures are the limbus of the eye at the junction ?
   (a) Cornea and optic disc
   (b) Sclera and optic disc
   (c) Cornea and sclera
   (d) Cornea and pupil
3. Where is the corneal endothelium located in the eye?
   (a) Optic nerve margin
   (b) Exterior Sclera
   (c) Anterior Lens
   (d) Posterior cornea
4. For what reason pterygium is removed?
   (a) Causes blindness in the affected eye
   (b) Obscures vision of the affected eye
   (c) Can cause cancer of the affected eye
   (d) Causes cancer of the skin around the affected eye
5. What procedure is used to excise a very dark brown-black uveal lesion?
   (a) Corneal transplant
   (b) Complete exenteration including surrounding eyelid and surrounding muscle
   (c) Excision of the optic desc
   (d) Local resection

Answer Key

1. *(b) Enucleation*
   Explanation: An enucleation removes just the eye; therefore, "(b)" is correct. Limited resection of a portion of the eye. A limited exenteration removes the eye with minimal surrounding structures, and a complete exenteration includes the eye, all surrounding structures, and skin.
2. *(c) Cornea and sclera*
   Explanation: The limbus is the area of the junction of the sclera and cornea circumferentially around the cornea; therefore, "(c)" is correct. The remainder of the options does not form an actual junction. The optic disc is present on the posterior eye, and the pupil only forms a junction with the iris.
3. *(d) Posterior cornea*
   Explanation: The endothelium is only on the posterior cornea, so "(d)" is correct. The remaining options are incorrect as they are not part of the cornea. The optic nerve margin is the aspect of the optic nerve where the surgeon cuts to remove the eye. The lens functions with the cornea, but it is not part of the cornea, and the sclera is the white surrounding capsule of the eye.
4. *(b) Obscures vision of the affected eye*
   Explanation: A pterygium is a raised area on the conjunctiva of the eye. If left on the eye, these benign lesions can eventually obscure vision, so "(b)" is the correct answer. These lesions do not cause cancer of the eye or the skin surrounding the eye.
5. *(d) Local resection*
   Explanation: A local resection removes the tumor-involved area only. This is often performed for melanomas of the uvea, so "(d)" is the correct answer. An enucleation removes just the eye, whereas a limited exenteration removes the eye with some surrounding tissues, and a complete exenteration removes the eye, surrounding tissues, and skin.

References

1. "University of Michigan Health System Department of Pathology," 8 March 2011. [Online]. www.pathology.med.umch.edu/intra/templates/cribsheet.pdf. Accessed Tuesday August 2023.
2. Milman T, Grossniklaus H, Goldman-Levy G, Kivela TT, Coupland SE, White VA, Mudhar HS, Eberhart CG, Verdijk RM, Heegaard S, Gill AJ, Jager MJ, Rodrigues-Reyes AA, Esmaeli B, Hodge JC, Cree IA. The 5th edition of the world health organization classification of tumours of the eye and orbit. Ocular Oncol Pathol. 2023;
3. "College of American Pathologists," June 2021. [Online]. https://www.cap.org/protocols-and-guidelines/cancer-reporting-tools/cancer-protocol-templates. Accessed August 2023.

Grossing of Skin Specimens 12

Contents

Table 12.1 CPT codes [1]

Foreskin, newborn	88302
Foreskin, other than newborn	88304
Skin, plastics repair	88302
Skin, cyst/tag/debridement	88304
Skin, not cyst/tag/debridement	88305

Grossing skin specimens requires a highly consistent, almost obsessive-compulsive, approach to ensure that the pathologist can make an accurate diagnosis. Two essential elements that contribute to effective grossing are (1) understanding the lesion's nature and (2) preserving the specimens' proper orientation. Reference the CPT codes for charges pertaining to skin specimens (Table 12.1).

Acquiring clinical information regarding the lesion's location, size, color, and texture is crucial. This may be provided in the requisition or obtained by reviewing the patient chart. The clinical suspicion, whether it is benign, malignant, or inflammatory in nature, helps in the approach to microscopic examination and narrows the differential diagnoses. Preserving correct orientation is necessary to provide clinicians with valuable insights regarding the margin status of the specimen and guides future surgical planning and treatment decisions.

12.1 Skin Margins Explained

When submitting a skin specimen for histologic processing, careful consideration must be given to its proper orientation within the cassette. The correct positioning of the specimen is essential to ensure proper embedding, sectioning, and optimal visualization of appropriate tissue for the pathologist to make the correct interpretation from each tissue sample. In this regard, two common orientations are utilized: en face and perpendicular.

En face: The term "en face margins" refers to the positioning of the specimen in the cassette with the true margins facing down, as shown in Fig. 12.1. This is used for skin tips of serially sectioned excisional specimens and shave margins in some frozen sections and in Mohs surgery when it is important to examine the entire surgical margin, as shave margins have the advantage of sampling more quantity of tissue [2]. When the specimen is placed in the cassette with margins facing down, the histotechnologist cuts sections from the most superficial face, parallel to the skin surface. The true margin is in the first section placed on the glass slide. Thus, it is possible to determine if the tumor extends to the deep or lateral margins of the specimen.

Perpendicular section: These sections are cut perpendicular to the skin surface and margin, then placed in the cassette, with the cut surface facing down on edge. Thus, it is possible to visualize the entire skin thickness from the superficial epidermis to the dermis or subcutaneous fat (Fig. 12.1).

Shave section: This style of sectioning is removing a thin rim of the periphery of the skin that is full thickness to include superficial epidermis to the dermis or subcutaneous fat. These margins are submitted en face with the ink surface down in the cassette as shown in Fig. 12.1.

Tip section: Skin tips are the section where the ellipse of skin comes to a point on opposite sides. The tips are removed, and the true margin which is the most outer point of the tip is submitted en face in the cassette as shown in Fig. 12.1.

In the context of skin specimens, perpendicular sections are often used to evaluate the depth of tumor invasion, particularly in cases of melanoma (Breslow depth) or invasive squamous cell carcinoma. This information is crucial for determining the stage and, ultimately, the prognosis of the tumor, which guides treatment. The perpendicular sections can also visualize the relationship between the tumor and surrounding margins. For instance, the distance between the tumor and the closest margin can be specifically measured microscopically.

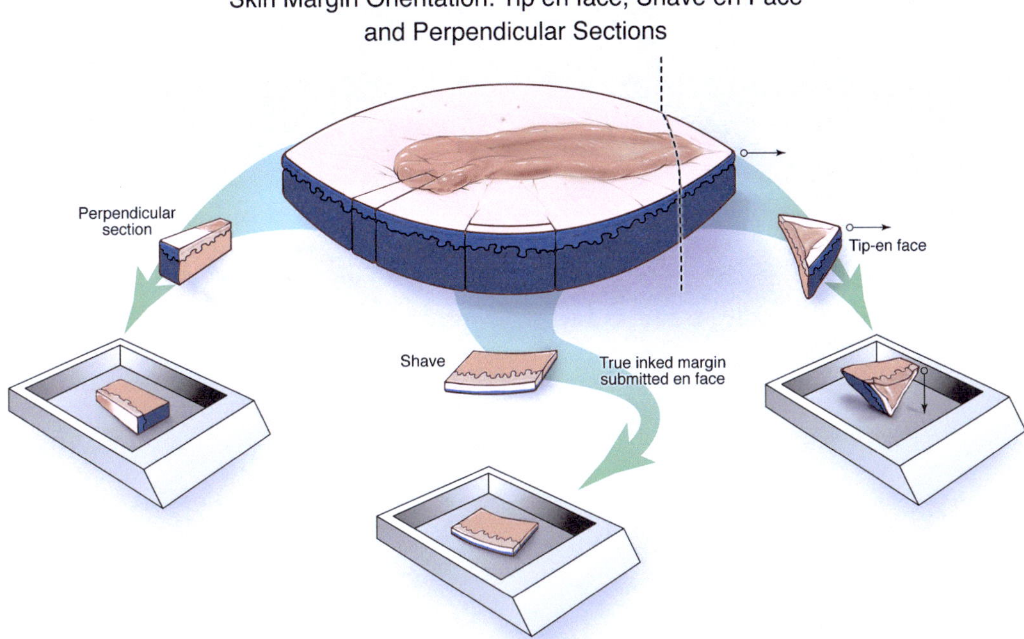

Fig. 12.1 Skin orientation: tips, shave, and perpendicular margins explained

12.2 Punch Biopsy: Level IV CPT 88305

A punch biopsy produces a skin sample with a full-thickness representation of the skin and subcutaneous tissue. A circular blade with a hollow center is used to punch out a small cylindrical piece of skin, much like a cookie cutter (Fig. 12.2). This enables the pathologist to make a detailed microscopic assessment of the epidermis, dermis, and often a portion of the underlying adipose tissue. Punch biopsies are valuable in cases where a lesion requires examination of the superficial and deep layers for an accurate diagnosis.

Step 1: Describe and measure the specimen (Fig. 12.2)

Step 2: Orient the tissue by finding the skin surface.

Step 3: Ink the margin, as shown in Fig. 12.3.

Step 4: If the skin surface's diameter is small (2–4 mm), the punch biopsy can be submitted in the cassette entirely on its side. If the punch diameter exceeds 5 mm, it is best to bisect the punch biopsy longitudinally/perpendicular to the skin surface.

Step 5: If the punch is bisected, place the cut surface facing down in the cassette.

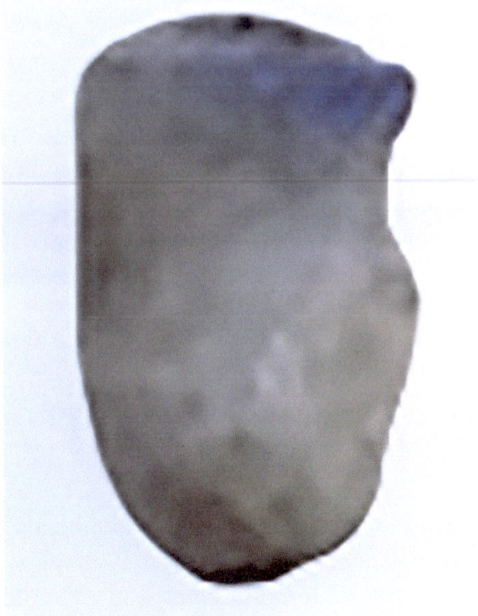

Fig. 12.2 Punch biopsy of the skin

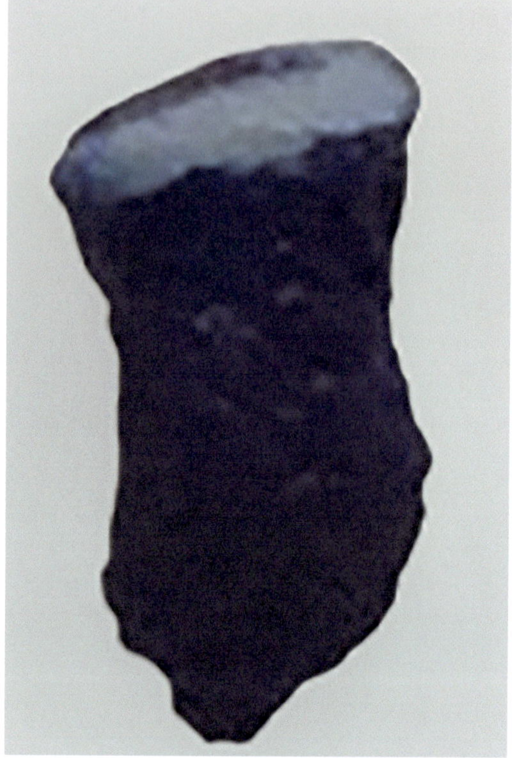

Fig. 12.3   Punch biopsy with inked resection margin

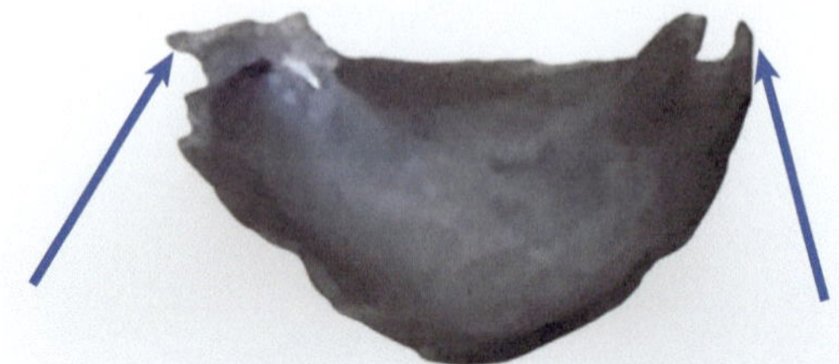

Fig. 12.4   Shave biopsy of the skin. The blue arrows indicate the biopsy edges curling in toward the deep margin

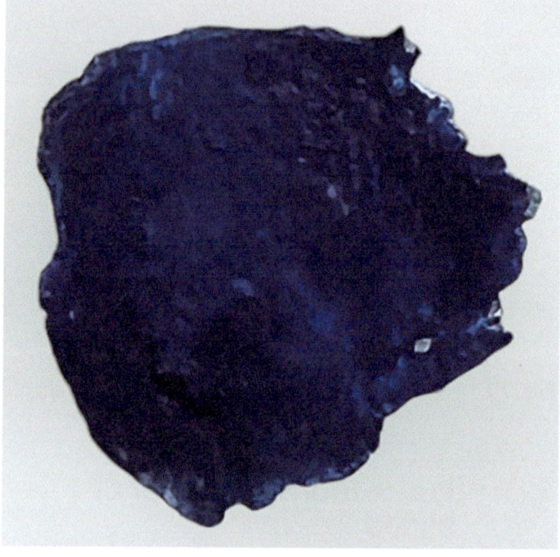

Fig. 12.5   Shave biopsy with inked deep margin

Example Dictation

Specimen A is received in formalin labeled with patient's name, medical record number, "Right thigh, punch biopsy" and consists of a single, tan-pink, punch biopsy (0.8 x 0.4 x 0.4 cm). The resection margin is inked blue, and the specimen is submitted entirely in A1.

12.3   Shave Biopsy: Level IV CPT 88305

A shave biopsy utilizes a flat blade, like a scalpel, to delicately remove a thin layer of skin. This technique allows for precise and controlled skin shaving, encompassing the epidermis to the level of the superficial or mid-dermis. This approach is commonly employed when a superficial or raised skin lesion needs to be assessed. This type of biopsy heals by second intention, typically not requiring sutures, and resulting in minimal scarring.

Step 1: Orient the specimen by identifying the skin surface and the deep margin. Sometimes differentiating between the two can be difficult. One trick: the skin surface of a shave biopsy specimen tends to curl toward the deep aspect. In Fig. 12.4, the edges curl (blue arrows) in toward the deep margin so the deep margin faces upward in this figure.

Step 2: Measure and describe the appearance of the skin surface.

Step 3: Ink the deep margin (Fig. 12.5).

Step 4: Small shave biopsies (0.2–0.3 cm) can be submitted entirely on edge [3]. Anything larger needs to be sectioned and placed on edge, as demonstrated in Fig. 12.6.

Step 5: Submit the shave biopsy entirely. Note that shave biopsies are submitted on edge in the cassette, mirroring the way they will be embedded, for appropriate evaluation.

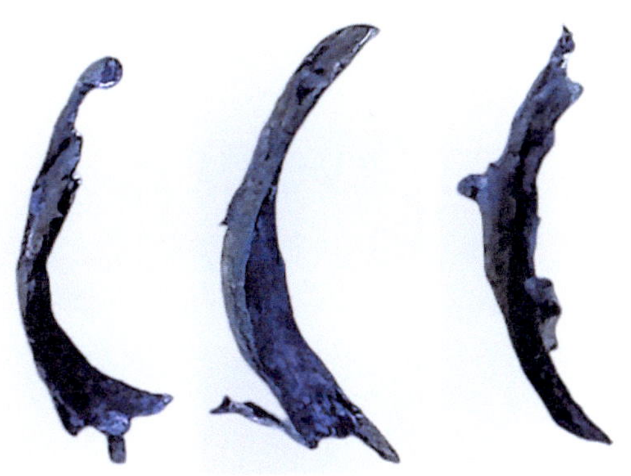

Fig. 12.6 Serially sectioned shave biopsy placed on the edge

Example Dictation

Specimen A is received in formalin labeled with patient's name, medical record number, "Right hand, shave biopsy" and consists of a single, tan-brown, variegated shave biopsy (1.2 x 1.0 x 0.2 cm). The resection margin is inked blue, and the specimen is trisected and submitted entirely in A1.

12.4 Skin, Plastics Scar Repair: Level II CPT 88302

A skin excision for cosmetic repair refers to skin removal during plastic surgery procedures. It encompasses abdominoplasty, facelift specimens, and scar revisions.

Step 1: Describe and measure the specimen (Fig. 12.7). If the specimen is large, weigh the specimen as well.

Step 2: Describe the skin surface and the presence of lesions or scars. Measure and detail the location of any lesions or scars that may be visible.

Step 3: Serially section the specimen, as seen in Fig. 12.8.

Step 4: Describe the cut surface of the specimen. In Fig. 12.9, fibrous scar tissue (blue arrow) is present under the skin surface, and an area of

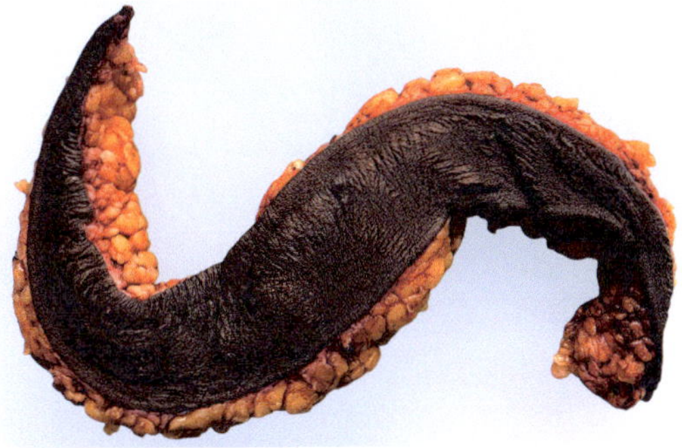

Fig. 12.7 Skin excision for scar, anterior view

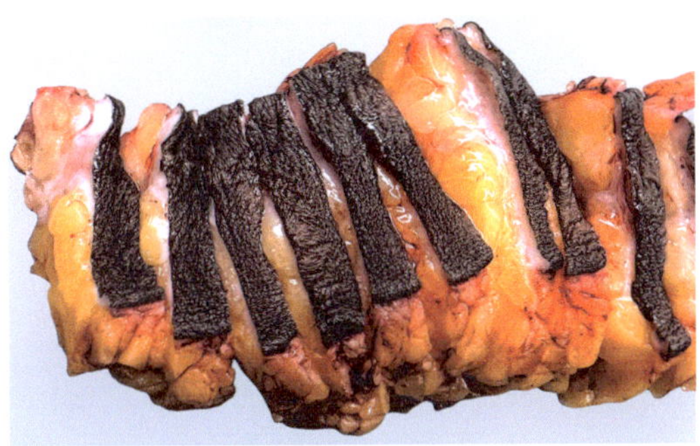

Fig. 12.8 Serially sectioned skin excision, superficial view

fat necrosis (blue circle) can be observed in the underlying adipose tissue. Measure the extent of fat necrosis with a percentage.

Step 5: Submit 1 or 2 specimen sections demonstrating scar and fat necrosis as seen in Fig. 12.10.

Example Dictation

Specimen A is received in formalin labeled with patient's name, medical record number, "abdominal scar repair" and consists of a single, unoriented skin excision (7.6 x 4.2 x 3.9 cm) with underlying adipose tissue. The skin surface contains a linear, well-healed scar (5.1 cm in length). The specimen is serially sectioned to reveal tan-yellow, lobulated cut surfaces with a focal area of fat necrosis (1.5 x 1.2 x 1.0 cm), which underlays the scar. A representative section is submitted in A1.

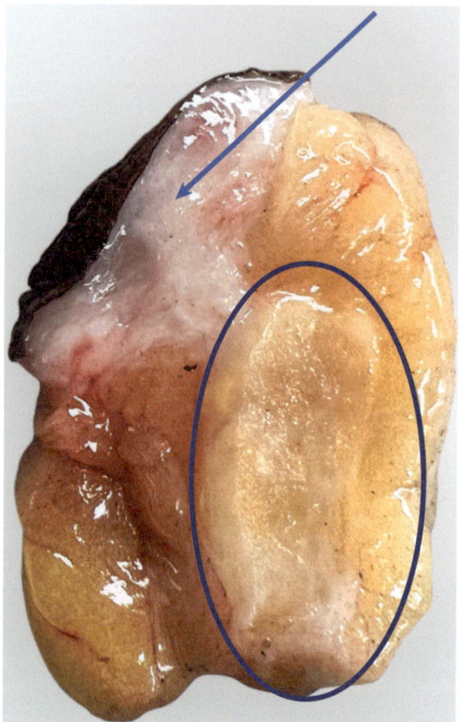

Fig. 12.9 Skin excision for scar, representative section. The blue arrow shows scar tissue under the skin. The blue circle indicates fat necrosis

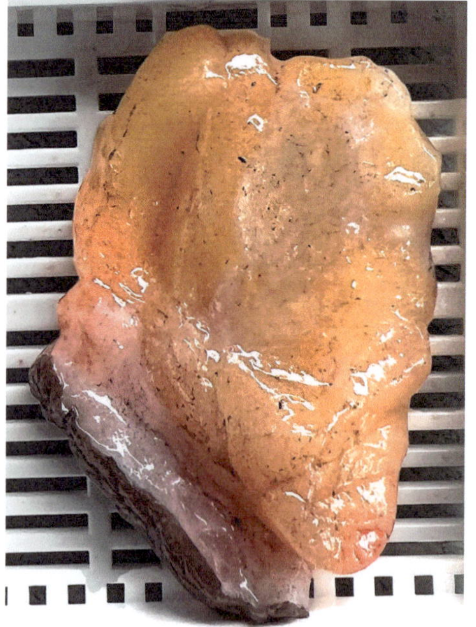

Fig. 12.10 Representative section submitted in the cassette

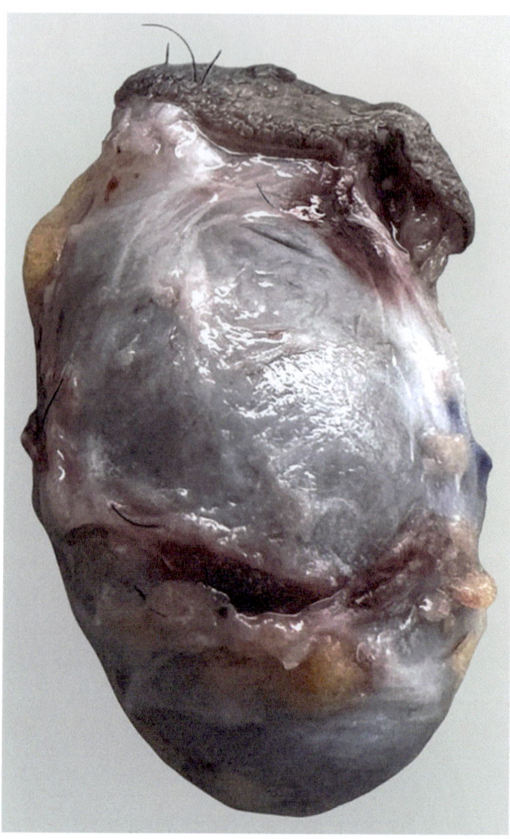

Fig. 12.11 Cyst with a segment of overlying skin

12.5 Cyst-Level III CPT 88304

Cysts encompass a heterogeneous spectrum of dermatological conditions characterized by a wall encompassing trapped material. The most common keratinous/epidermal cysts manifest a cell wall similar to the epidermis that is trapped within the dermis, producing keratinaceous, foul-smelling, caseous material which collects in the central cavity. The contents of other cysts may be liquid (steatocystoma multiplex) or semi-solid (pilar cysts).

Step 1: Describe and measure the cyst.

Step 2: Describe and measure the attached skin, if any. The skin on top of the cyst is depicted in Fig. 12.11.

Step 3: Describe whether the cyst is intact or ruptured.

Step 4: If the cyst wall is intact, ink the outer surface as seen in Fig. 12.12. If the cyst wall is already ruptured, then no ink is necessary.

Step 5: Serially section the specimen perpendicular to the skin so a little skin is attached to the cyst in each slice, if possible (Fig. 12.13).

Step 6: Describe the material present within the cyst.

Step 7: Submit 1 or 2 fullface sections of the cyst with attached skin, if any. Sections can be bisected if necessary. In some sections, like the one shown in Fig. 12.14, the cyst contents

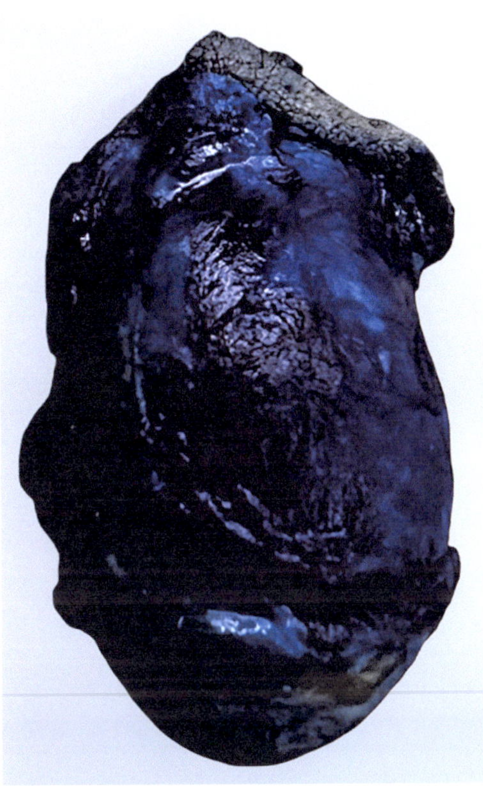

Fig. 12.12   Cyst with an inked outer surface

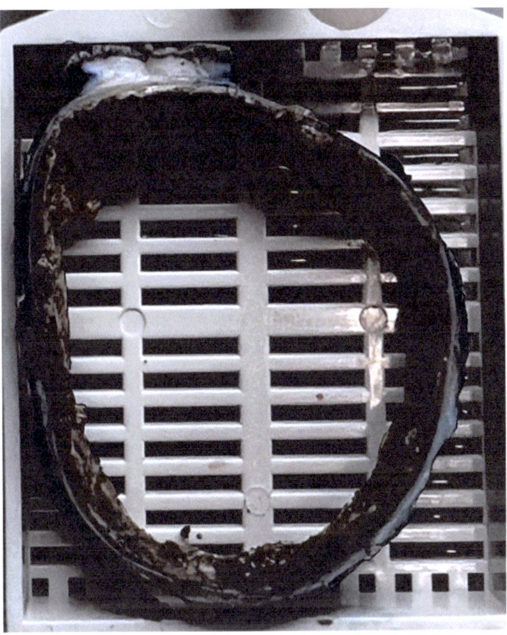

Fig. 12.14 Representative section of cyst submitted in the cassette. Specimen A is received in formalin labeled with patients name, medical record number, "Cyst" and consists of an intact cyst (2.1 x 1.9 x 1.5 cm) with overlying tan-brown skin (1.2 x 0.9 cm). The cyst capsule is inked blue and the specimen is serially sectioned to reveal brown, friable material within. Representative sections are submitted in A1-A2

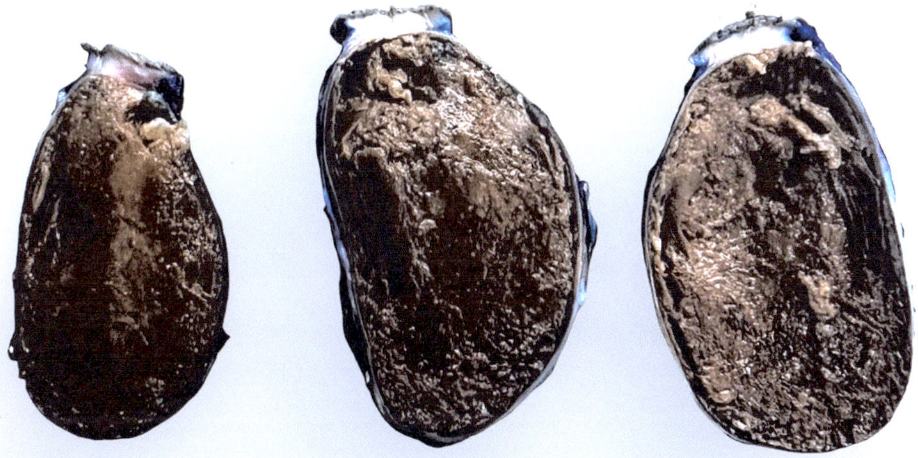

Fig. 12.13   Serially sectioned cyst with attached skin on each section

may be removed as the material can create sectioning difficulties for histology. If the cyst is ruptured, include a section with the rupture.

12.6   Keloid: Level III CPT 88304

A keloid is an aberrant proliferation of fibrous tissue within the dermis, often attributed to trauma or previous surgery in the affected region. These lesions exhibit a variable range in size, spanning from small papules to large nodules many centimeters in diameter, yet they are inherently benign.

Step 1: Describe and measure the specimen. Figure 12.15 shows a brown-gray, sessile skin excision.

Step 2: Identify the resection margin as seen in Fig. 12.16.

Step 3: Ink the resection margin (Fig. 12.17).

Step 4: Serially section the specimen and lay the sections flat, as demonstrated in Fig. 12.18.

Step 5: Describe the cut surfaces.

Step 6: Submit sections. If the specimen is small, it can be submitted entirely. Representative sections of a larger specimen are sufficient, approximately 1 section per 1 cm of the overall size.

Example Dictation

Specimen A is received in formalin labeled with patient's name, medical record number, "Right dorsal forearm" and consists of a brown-gray, sessile skin excision (4.9 x 2.3 x 1.9 cm). The resection margin is inked blue, and the specimen is serially sectioned to reveal tan-white, fibrous cut surfaces. Representative sections are submitted in A1–A5.

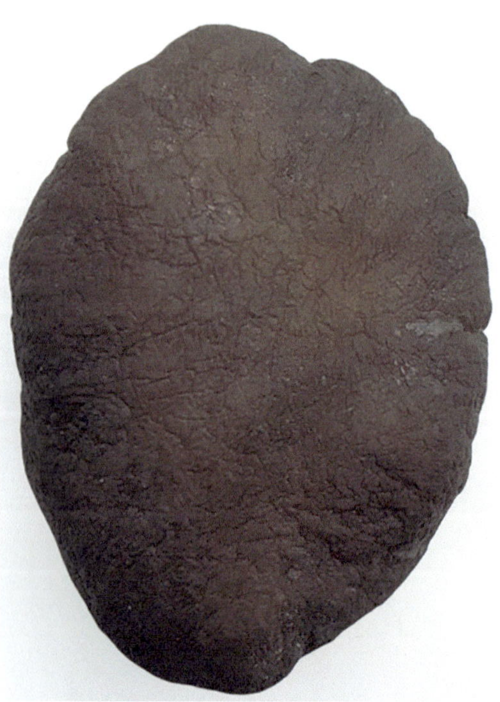

Fig. 12.15 Keloid resection specimen, superficial surface

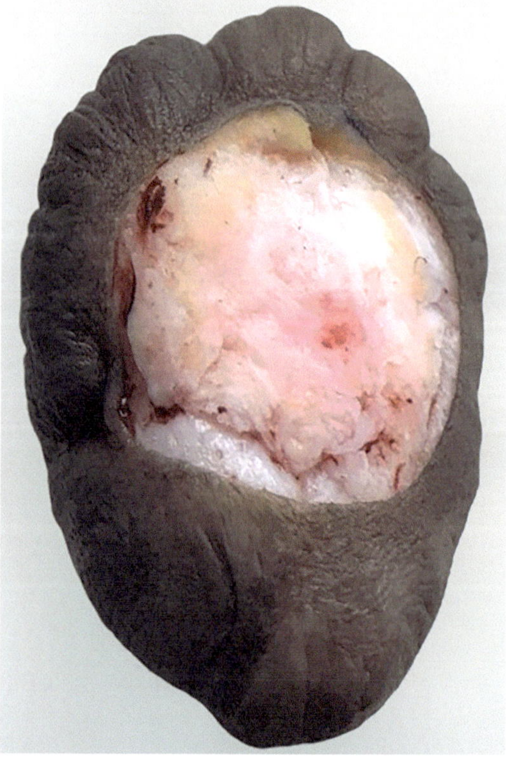

Fig. 12.16 Keloid resection specimen, deep surface, showing resection margin

Fig. 12.17 Keloid with inked resection margin

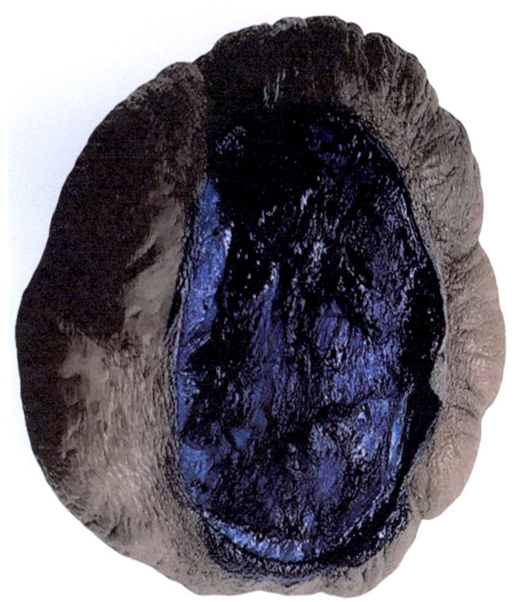

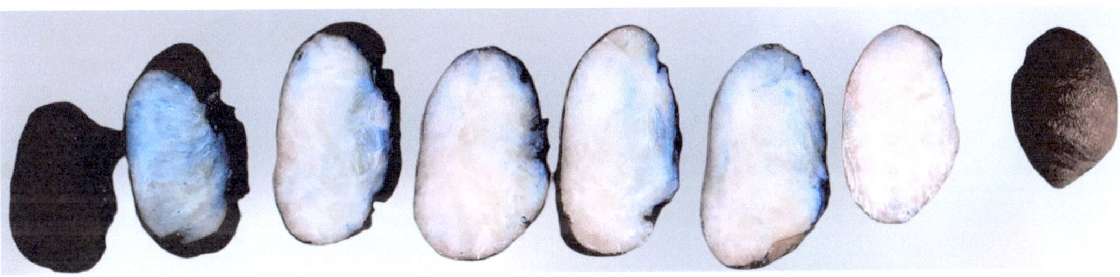

Fig. 12.18 Serially sectioned keloid excision

12.7 Foreskin, Other than Newborn: Level III CPT 88304

The foreskin of adult males is typically removed due to skin infection or phimosis. Often the foreskin does not retract. Foreskin of newborns and adults is grossed relatively the same way.

Step 1: Describe and measure the specimen. The skin surface of the foreskin is shown in Figure 12.19a, while Fig. 12.19b depicts the resection margin.

Step 2: Serially section the specimen and describe the cut surface as seen in Fig. 12.20.

Step 3: Submit representative sections. One or two representative sections are acceptable (Fig. 12.21).

Example Dictation

Specimen A is received in formalin labeled with patient's name, medical record number, "foreskin" and consists of an unoriented, wrinkled fragment of tan-brown skin (5.8 x 3.4 x 1.8 cm) which is serially sectioned to reveal tan-white, focally hemorrhagic cut surfaces. Representative sections are submitted in A1–A2.

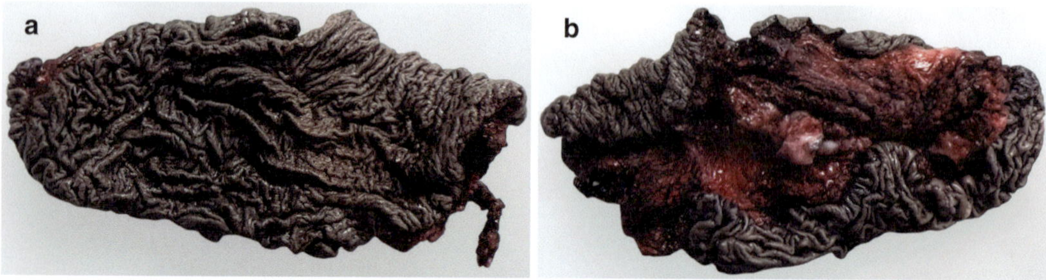

Fig. 12.19 (**a**) Foreskin, surface view; (**b**) foreskin, resection margin

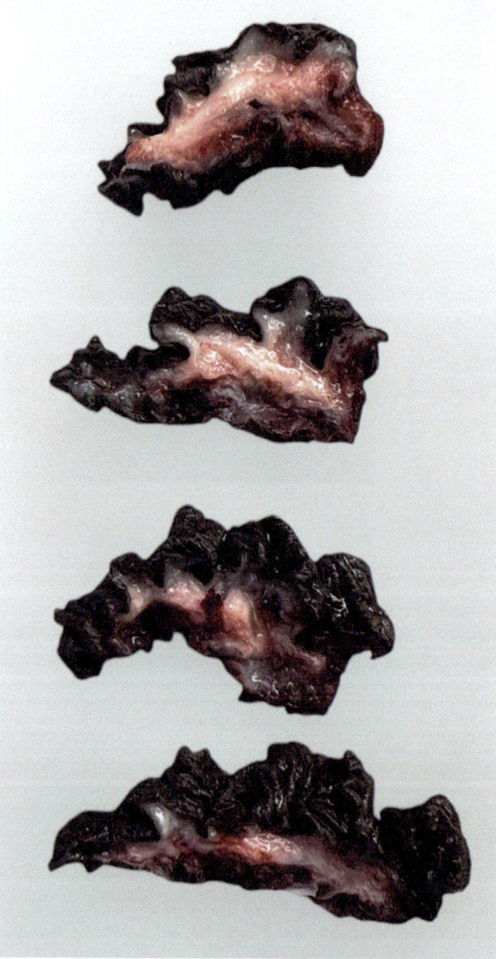

Fig. 12.20 Serially sectioned foreskin specimen

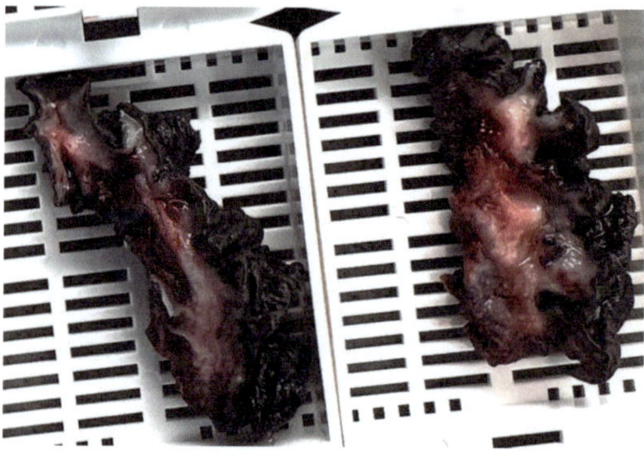

Fig. 12.21 Representative sections of foreskin submitted in the cassettes

12.8 Skin Excision, Other than Melanoma: Level IV CPT 88305

Skin excisions for cancers such as squamous cell carcinoma and basal cell carcinoma can range in size from very small to incredibly large, in all shapes and sizes. These cancers have the ability to metastasize, but the primary lesion is often localized, spreading outward or down into the dermis and soft tissue.

Spaghetti Excision Technique
The spaghetti procedure is performed for lentigo maligna and acral lentiginous melanoma, where

the margins are clinically ill-defined. The procedure excises a thin skin rim surrounding the lesion to assess the entire peripheral margin while initially leaving the lesion in place. The rim of skin is assessed microscopically for lesional cells. If the specimen is negative for tumor, the surgeon returns to the patient and excises the main lesion, already knowing the peripheral margins are free of tumor.

Step 1: Describe and measure the specimen. A ring of tissue can be challenging to measure. A length and thickness measurement of each spaghetti section is acceptable.

Step 2: Describe the orientation of the specimen. In Fig. 12.22, the surgeon oriented the specimen with a long stitch designating 12 o'clock and a short stitch designating 6 o'clock.

Step 3: Identify the true and false margins of the specimen. The outer edge of the specimen is the true margin. The inner edge is the false margin, and the open area inside the rim is where the lesion remains on the patient's skin.

Step 4: Submit margins en face. Inking the true margin is often helpful for the histology embedding person to identify the en face surface. In Fig. 12.23, the true margin is inked blue.

Step 5: Divide the specimen into quadrants. In Fig. 12.24, the specimen is divided into clock-face quadrants 12–3 o'clock, 3–6 o'clock, 6–9 o'clock, and 9–12 o'clock. A larger specimen may need to be sectioned more to fit into a cassette such as 12–2 o'clock, 2–4 o'clock, 4–6 o'clock, 6–8 o'clock, 8–10 o'clock, and 10–12 o'clock.

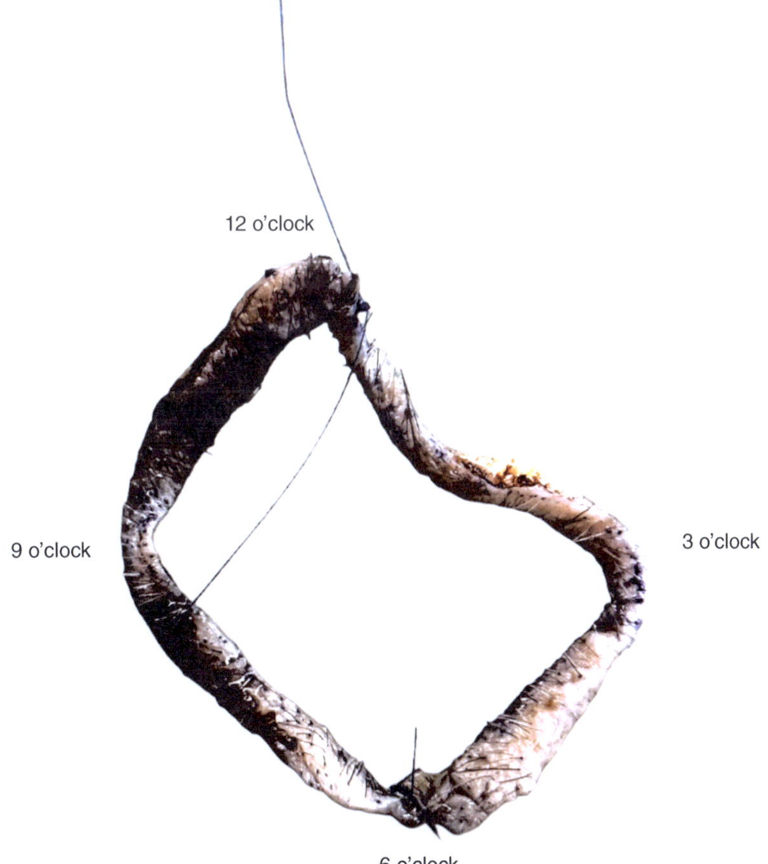

Fig. 12.22 An oriented specimen from spaghetti procedure

Step 6: Ink one end of the strip of skin to keep orientation. The red ink marks the proximal end of each strip in Fig. 12.25. When the sections are submitted, the red ink will orient the strip into the proximal and distal portions of each segment.

Step 7: The side of each strip that is inked blue is the true margin. All segments are submitted with the true margin (blue ink) en face (Fig. 12.26). Communicating with the histology technician to embed the blue ink en face is helpful. The histotechnologist can easily see the blue ink to assess the orientation of the tissue.

Example Dictation

Specimen A is received in formalin labeled with patient's name, medical record number, "spaghetti technique, right cheek" and consists of an annular excision of tan-pink skin (8.0 cm in length, 0.4 cm thick) which is oriented with a long stitch designating 12 o'clock and a short stitch designating 6 o'clock. The specimen is quadrisected, and the true margin is submitted en face.

Ink code
>   Blue: true margin
>   Red: proximal end of each segment

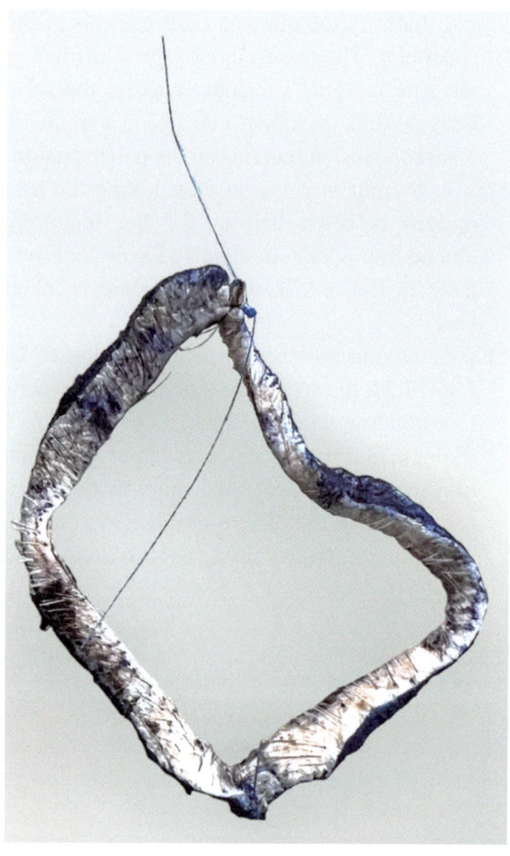

Fig. 12.23 The true margins are inked blue

Fig. 12.24 Specimen divided into clockface quadrants

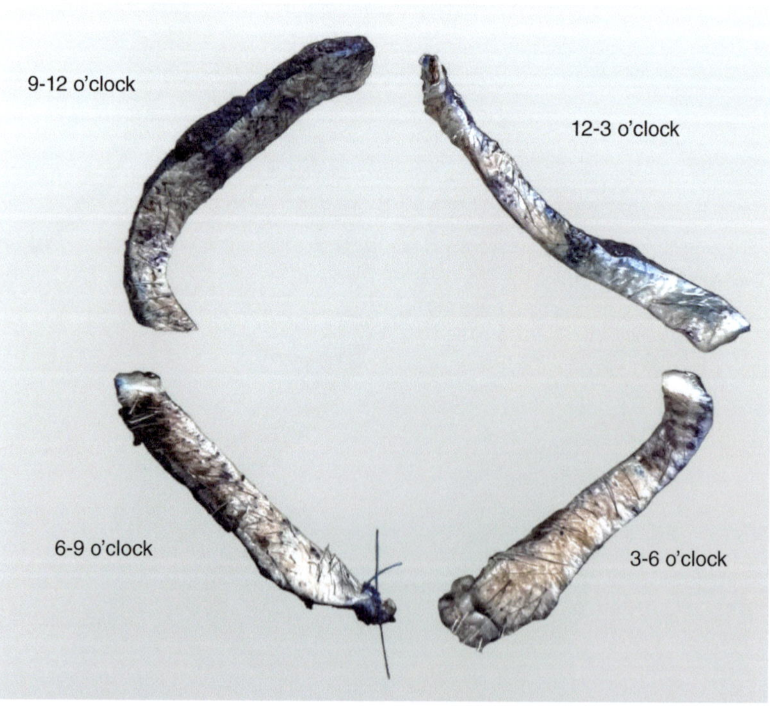

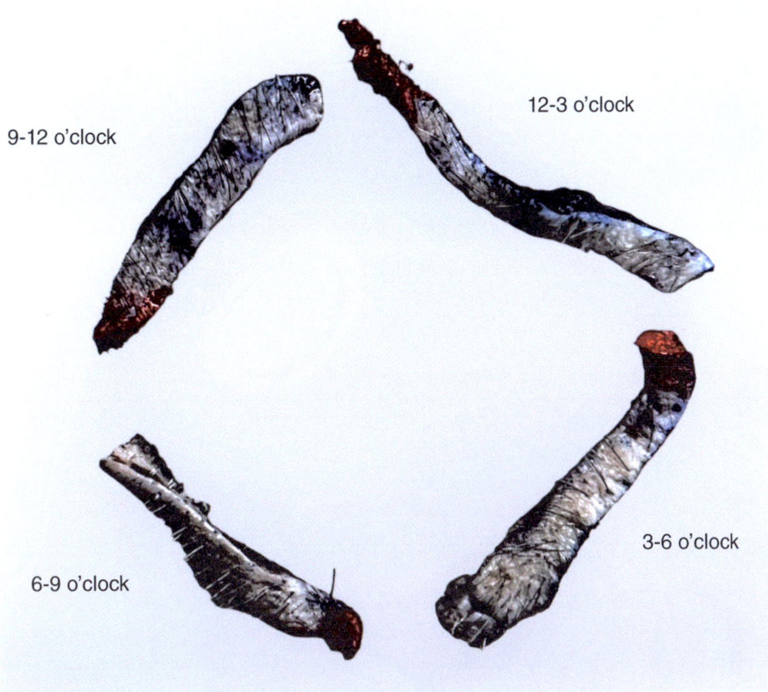

Fig. 12.25 Proximal end of each clockface quadrant strip is inked red

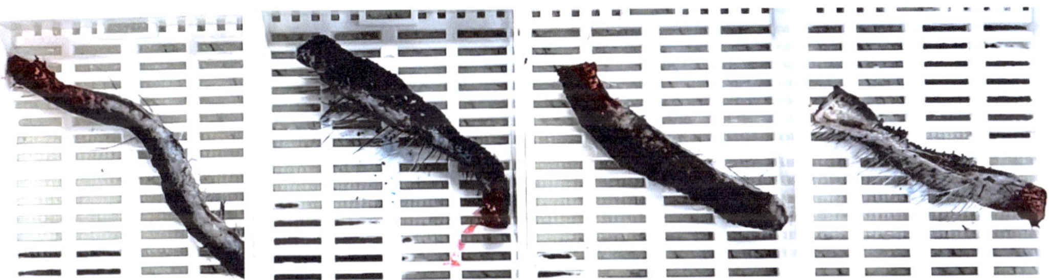

Fig. 12.26 True margins submitted en face in the cassettes

Section code
    A1: 12–3 o'clock, 2.0 x 0.4 cm section
    A2: 3–6 o'clock, 1.9 x 0.4 cm section
    A3: 6–9 o'clock, 2.1 x 0.4 cm section
    A4: 9–12 o'clock, 2.0 x 0.4 cm section

12.9   Unoriented Skin Ellipse: Level IV CPT 88305

Specimens are sometimes sent unoriented. In these cases, the grossing person cannot determine the orientation of the specimen relative to the patient.

Step 1: Describe and measure the specimen in three dimensions.

Step 2: Describe and measure the lesion. In Fig. 12.27, the area of concern was previously biopsied, leaving a well-healed scar (blue arrow) in place of the lesion, so the scar site area is measured.

Step 3: Measure the lesion or scar to the closest unoriented skin margin.

Step 4: Ink the resection margin. In Fig. 12.28, the margin is inked all one color because the specimen is unoriented. The grossing person cannot determine specific margins, so separate ink colors are not necessary.

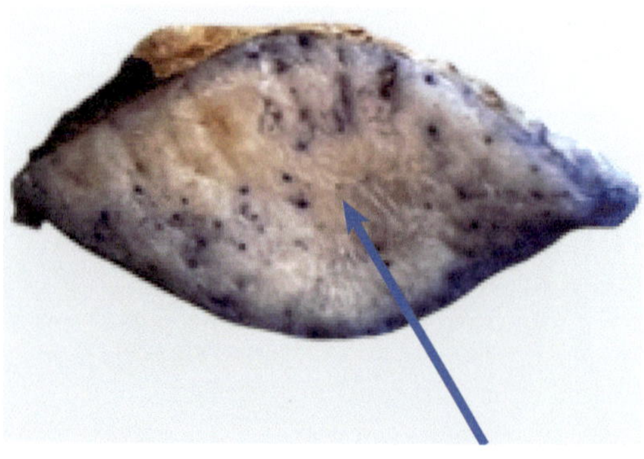

Fig. 12.27 Unoriented skin ellipse, anterior view. Blue arrow indicates lesion

Fig. 12.28 Unoriented skin ellipse, posterior view with inked resection margin

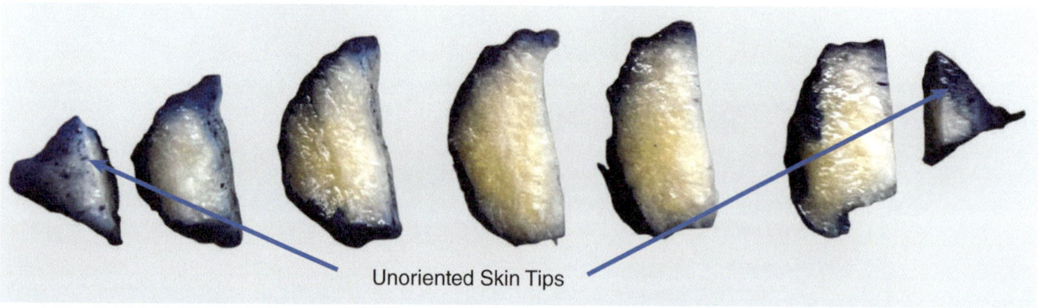

Fig. 12.29 Skin ellipse, serially sectioned. Tips shown by blue arrows

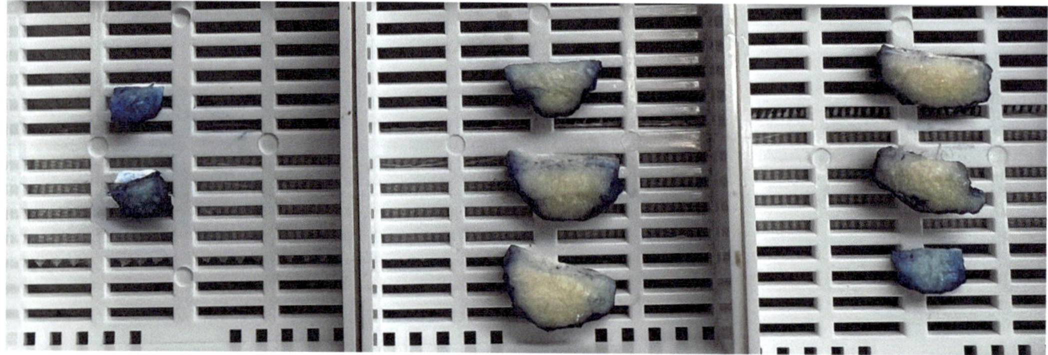

Fig. 12.30 Small unoriented ellipse submitted entirely in the cassettes

Step 5: Serially section the specimen perpendicular to the long axis. Sectioning in this plane will produce two unoriented tips, as shown by blue arrows in Fig. 12.29.

Step 6: Measure the depth of invasion of the lesion and determine the distance of the lesion from the deep margin, if possible.

Step 7: The specimen is submitted entirely because of its small size. Since the skin tips are unoriented, they can be submitted in the same cassette, as shown in Fig. 12.30.

Example Dictation

Specimen A is received in formalin labeled with the patient's name, medical record number, "Right back" and consists of an unoriented, tan-pink ellipse of skin (2.0 x 1.2 x 0.6 cm) with a well-healed previous biopsy scar (0.4 cm in diameter) on the skin surface coming within 0.2 cm from the closest unoriented margin. The resection margin is inked blue, and the specimen is serially sectioned to reveal tan, fibrous surfaces with underlying adipose tissue.

Cassette submission:
   A1: Unoriented tips, en face
   A2–A3: Body of specimen, entirely

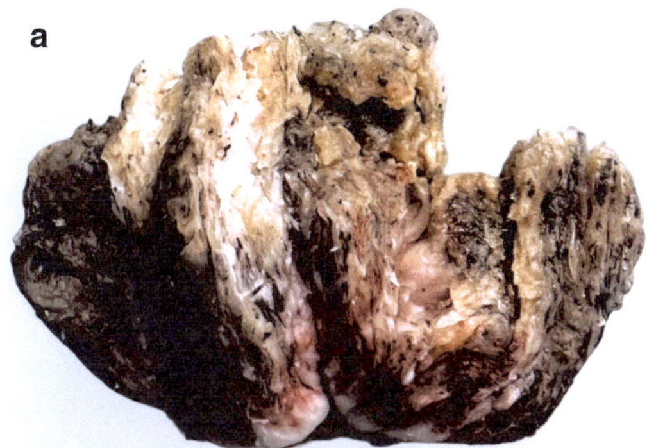

12.10 Unoriented Skin Ellipse with Oversized Lesion: Level IV CPT 88305

There may be clues as to the nature of the lesion that should be described at the grossing table. See Table 12.2 for common gross features of malignant skin tumors.

Table 12.2 Common gross features of malignant skin tumors that can be described

Squamous cell carcinoma	Thickened, ill-defined scaly plaque or ulceration on the skin surface; may form an exophytic mass Tan-white firm cut surfaces
Basal cell carcinoma (BCC)	*Nodular BCC*: Pearly pink or flesh-colored nodule. May have a central ulcer with a characteristic rolled border.
	Superficial BCC: Scaly erythematous lesion.
	Pigmented BCC: Similar to nodular and superficial BCC but has a pigmented surface.
	Infiltrative BCC: Tan-white (due to dense collagenous component), often shiny growths, may have visible blood vessels and ulcers.

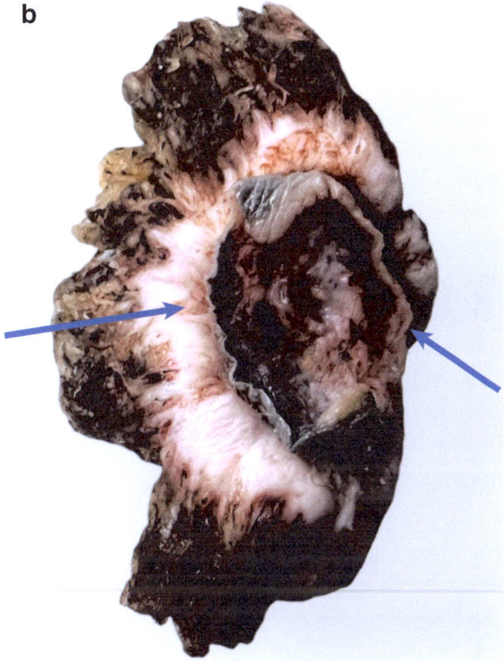

Fig. 12.31 (**a**) A tan-brown verrucoid skin lesion; (**b**) smaller skin ellipse with a larger overlying mass. Blue arrows outline skin excision margins

Step 1: Measure and describe the specimen (Fig. 12.31a). Reference Table 12.2 for gross identification.

Step 2: Identify the resection margin. In Fig. 12.31b, the ellipse of skin is considerably smaller than the large overlying mass and is unoriented. The blue arrows in Fig. 12.31b outline the periphery of the skin excision.

Step 3: Ink the resection margin of the skin, as seen in Fig. 12.32.

Step 4: Identify the unoriented tips of the skin ellipse. In Fig. 12.33, the tips are identified with blue arrows.

Step 5: Serially section the specimen. Note that some skin lesions are larger than the actual skin excision; the first few slices contain the lesion without attached skin. In Fig. 12.34, the blue arrows identify the skin tips, and the triangles identify the sections from the periphery, not having attached skin. These sections do not have a margin.

Step 6: Assess each section, identify the greatest depth of tumor invasion, and measure the distance between the lesion and the resection margin. Figure 12.35 contains an irregular line that demonstrates the tumor edge. The blue arrow in Fig. 12.35 shows the tumor in relation to the closest resection margin.

Step 7: Since the ellipse of skin is unoriented, the skin tips can be submitted in the same cassette. Representative sections of the lesion with the resection margin are submitted, including the section with the closest margin (Fig. 12.36).

Example Dictation

Specimen A is received in formalin labeled with patient's name, medical record number, "Right arm" and consists of an unoriented, tan-brown, verrucous, friable lesion (4.1 x 2.9 x 1.4 cm) with an underlying tan-brown, unoriented ellipse of skin (2.0 x 1.7 x 0.2 cm). The resection margin is inked blue, and the specimen is serially sectioned to reveal a tan-white, friable cut surface with a greatest lesion depth of invasion of less than 0.1 cm, coming within 0.6 cm of the resection margin.

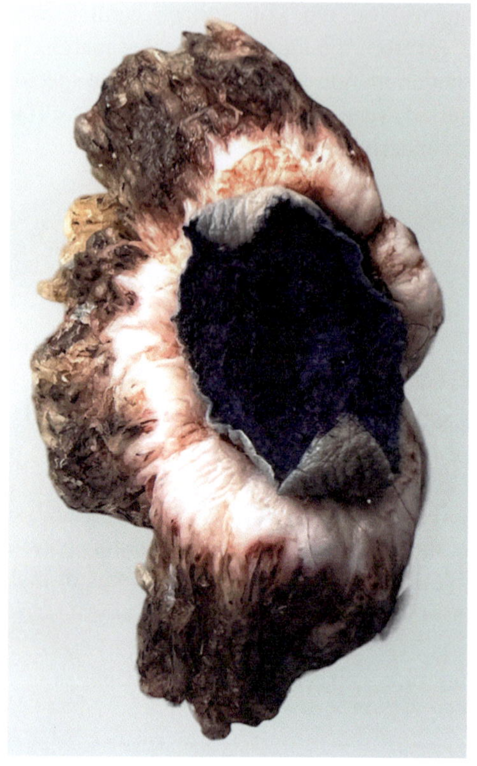

Fig. 12.32 Resection margin of skin inked blue

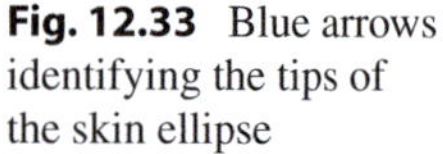

Fig. 12.33 Blue arrows identifying the tips of the skin ellipse

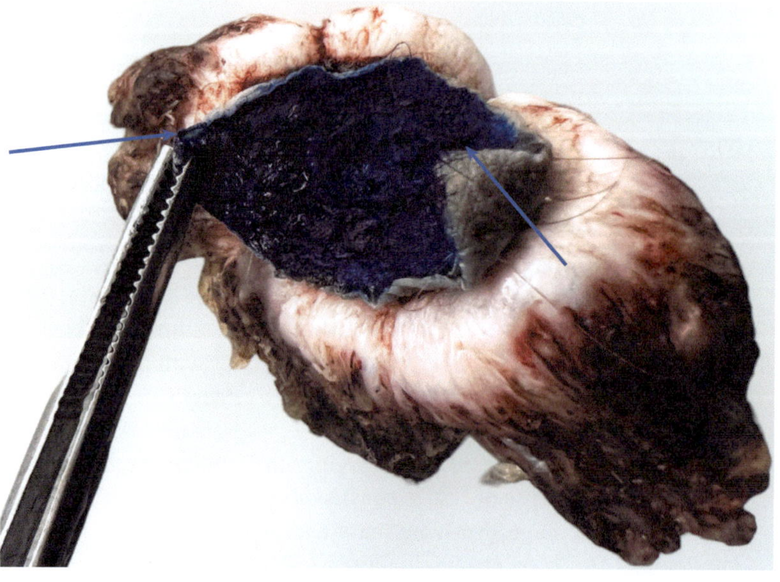

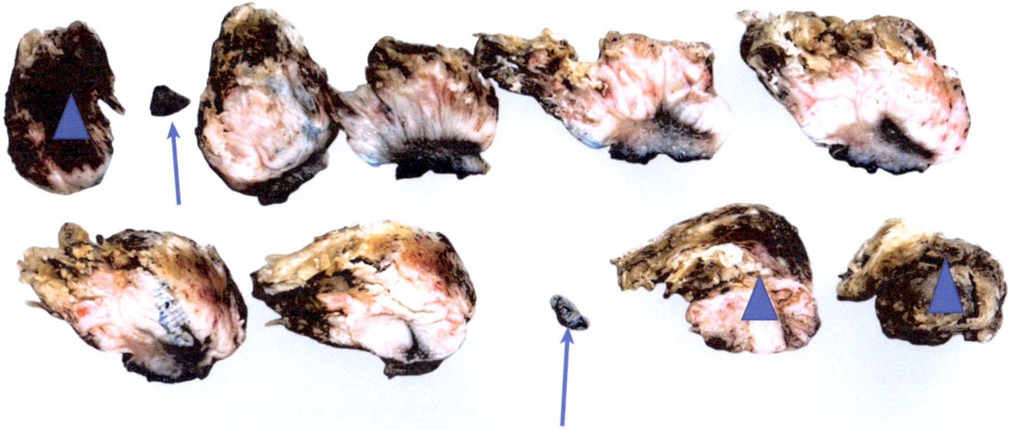

Fig. 12.34 Serially sectioned specimen. The blue arrows show skin tips, while triangles indicate sections without attached skin

Fig. 12.35 The tumor edge is shown with an irregular line with a blue arrow indicating its relation to the closest resection margin

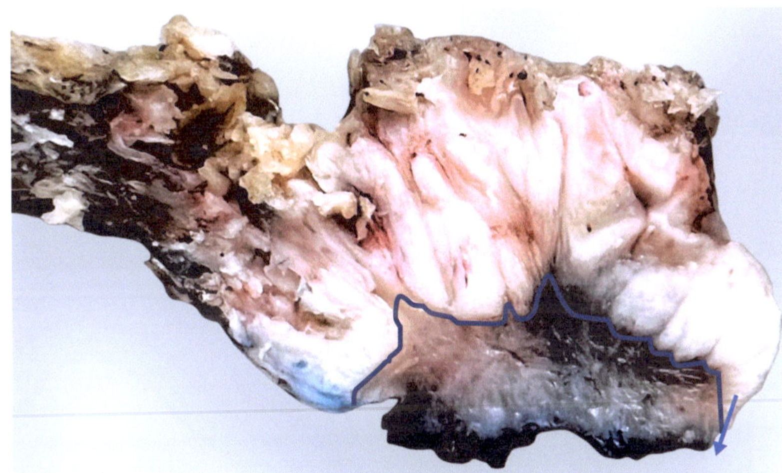

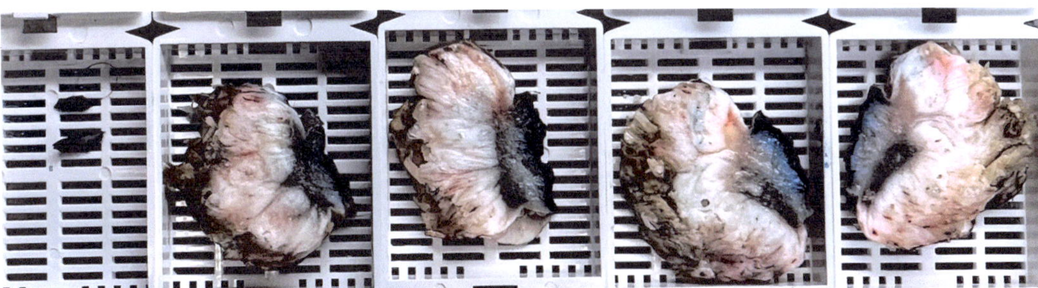

Fig. 12.36 Representative sections submitted in the cassettes

12.11 Oriented Ellipse of Skin: Level IV CPT 88305

An ellipse of skin that comes with orientation allows the grossing person to visualize the positioning of the specimen in vivo. The grossing person can also designate separate margins with ink so the closest margins can be identified microscopically.

Step 1: Orient the specimen. In Fig. 12.37, the specimen is oriented with a stitch at one tip designating 12 o'clock.

Step 2: Measure the specimen in three dimensions.

Step 3: Record the orientation of the specimen.

Step 4: Measure the lesion area (blue arrow in Fig. 12.37). Reference Table 12.2 for gross identification.

Step 5: Measure the distance between the lesion and the closest peripheral margin (12 o'clock tip, 3 o'clock margin, 6 o'clock tip, and 9 o'clock margin).

Step 6: Ink the margins. Pathologists may have different preferences with regard to inking an oriented specimen of this type. One method is using a variety of colored inks to establish orientation as follows in Fig. 12.38, the ink code is as follows:

    Orange: 3 o'clock margin

    Blue: 9 o'clock margin

    Black: Deep Margin

Step 7: Serially section the specimen from one tip to the other, laying each slice flat to allow for good visualization of the cut surfaces, as seen in Fig. 12.39.

Fig. 12.37 Oriented skin ellipse, anterior view, with a flesh-colored, well-circumscribed lesion indicated by the blue arrow

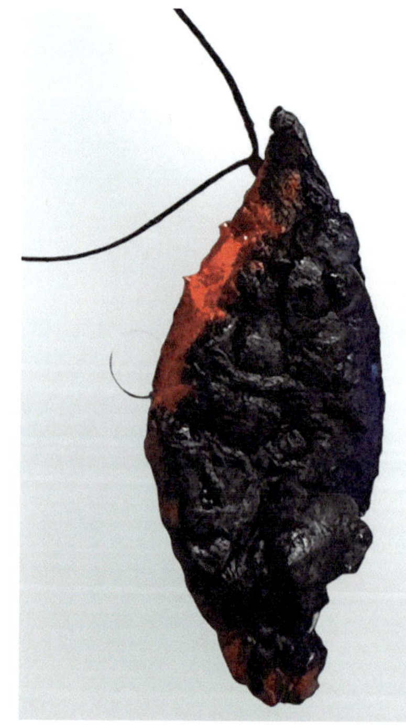

Fig. 12.38 Inked skin ellipse, posterior view

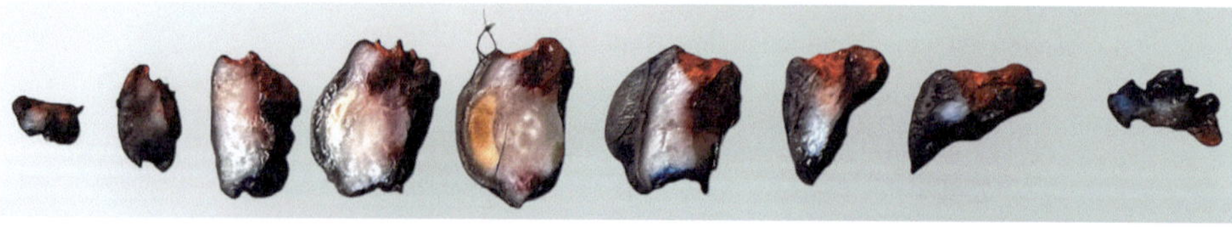

Fig. 12.39 Skin ellipse serially sectioned

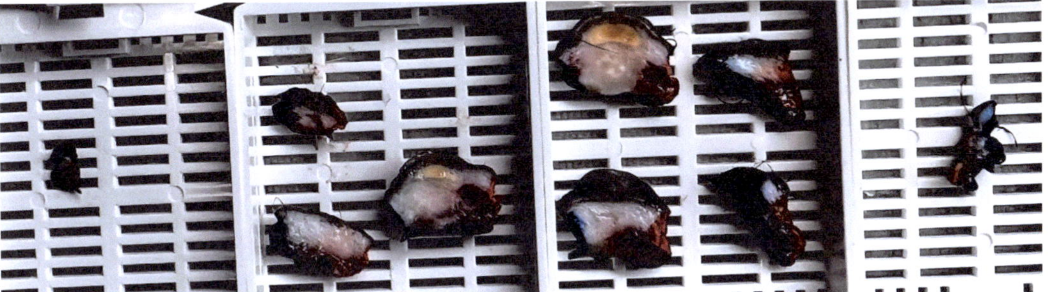

Fig. 12.41 Serially sectioned ellipse submitted entirely in the cassettes

Step 8: Measure the greatest depth of invasion and determine the measurement of the shortest distance between the lesion and the deep margin.

Step 9: Tips are submitted en face, which means the most outer point of the tip section is submitted down in the cassette (Fig. 12.40).

Step 10: The specimen is small and can be submitted in its entirety. Since the specimen is oriented, the tip orientation must be preserved, and the tips are submitted in separate cassettes as seen in Fig. 12.41. Another option is to place both tips in the same cassette, adding a different ink to one of the tips so the tips can be separately identified microscopically.

Example Dictation

Specimen A is received in formalin labeled with patient's name, medical record number, "left knee" and consists of a tan-brown ellipse of skin (2.5 x 1.5 x 1.0 cm) with a stitch at one tip designating 12 o'clock. The skin surface contains a tan-brown, flesh-colored, well-circumscribed lesion (0.5 x 0.4 x 0.2 cm), which comes within 1.0 cm from the 12 o'clock tip, 1.0 cm from the 6 o'clock tip, 0.2 cm from the 3 o'clock margin, and 0.2 cm from the 9 o'clock margin. The specimen is serially sectioned to reveal yellow cut surfaces of the lesion with no distinct invasion, coming closer than 0.6 cm of the deep margin.

Ink code
    Orange: 3 o'clock margin
    Blue: 9 o'clock margin
    Black: deep margin

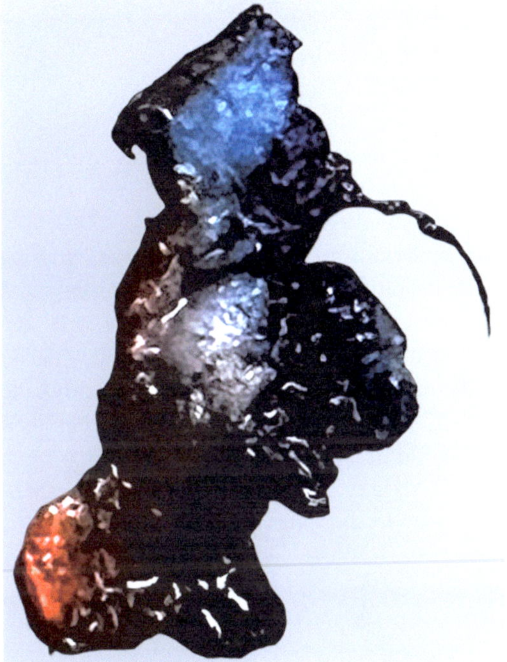

Fig. 12.40 One tip of the ellipse

Section code
    A1: 12 o'clock tip, en face
    A2–A6: Specimen entirely 12 o'clock to 6 o'clock
    A7: 6 o'clock, en face

12.12   Oriented Skin Excision: Level IV CPT 88305

Skin lesions can be excised producing a variety of tissue shapes and sizes. The margin edges are often irregular without clear tips. These specimens can be handled slightly different for ease at sign out.

Step 1: Describe and measure the specimen.

Step 2: Document the orientation of the specimen.

Step 3: Describe and measure the lesion. Reference Table 12.2 for gross identification.

Step 4: Measure the closest distance of the lesion to all peripheral margins (Fig. 12.42, blue arrows).

Step 5: Ink the specimen. In Fig. 12.43, five colors are used to designate the four peripheral and the deep margins.

> Blue: superior
> Green: inferior
> Red: medial
> Orange: lateral
> Black: deep

Step 6: Serially section the specimen and arrange the resulting slices on their edges as depicted in Fig. 12.44. Typically, the specimen is sectioned perpendicular to the long axis, which is medial to lateral in this example. Note that the two ends are sectioned slightly thicker than the middle.

Step 7: Serially section the end margins perpendicular to the long axis (Fig. 12.45). In this example, the margins are sectioned from superior to inferior. This allows microscopic measurement of the lesion to the medial and lateral margins.

Step 8: Measure the greatest depth of invasion and how close it comes to the deep margin.

Step 9: Submit the specimen with the appropriate orientation. In this example, the specimen is relatively small and submitted entirely from medial to lateral (Fig. 12.46). If the specimen is large, communicate with the attending for section submission.

Example Dictation

Specimen A is received in formalin labeled with patient's name, medical record number, "left forearm" and consists of a tan-pink skin excision (5.8 x 5.1 x 0.7 cm) with a short stitch designating superior and a long stitch designating lateral. The skin surface contains an ulcerated, tan-brown lesion (2.6 x 2.3 x 0.1 cm) which comes within 1.3 cm from the superior margin, 0.9 cm from the inferior margin, 1.6 cm from the medial margin, and 0.7 cm from the lateral margin. The specimen is serially sectioned to reveal tan-yellow cut surfaces with a greatest depth of invasion of 0.3 cm, coming within 0.2 cm of the deep margin.

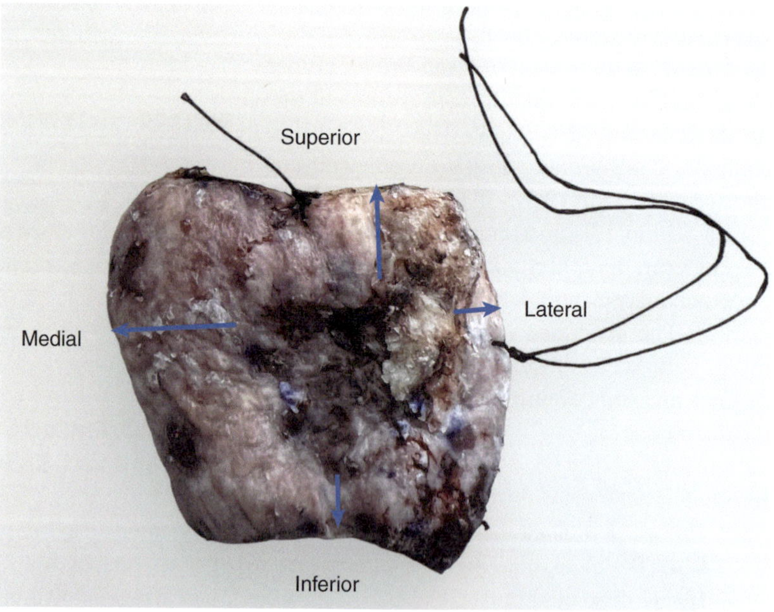

Fig. 12.42 Oriented skin excision, anterior view. The blue arrows indicate the distance of the lesion from the surrounding margins

Fig. 12.43 Inked skin excision, posterior view

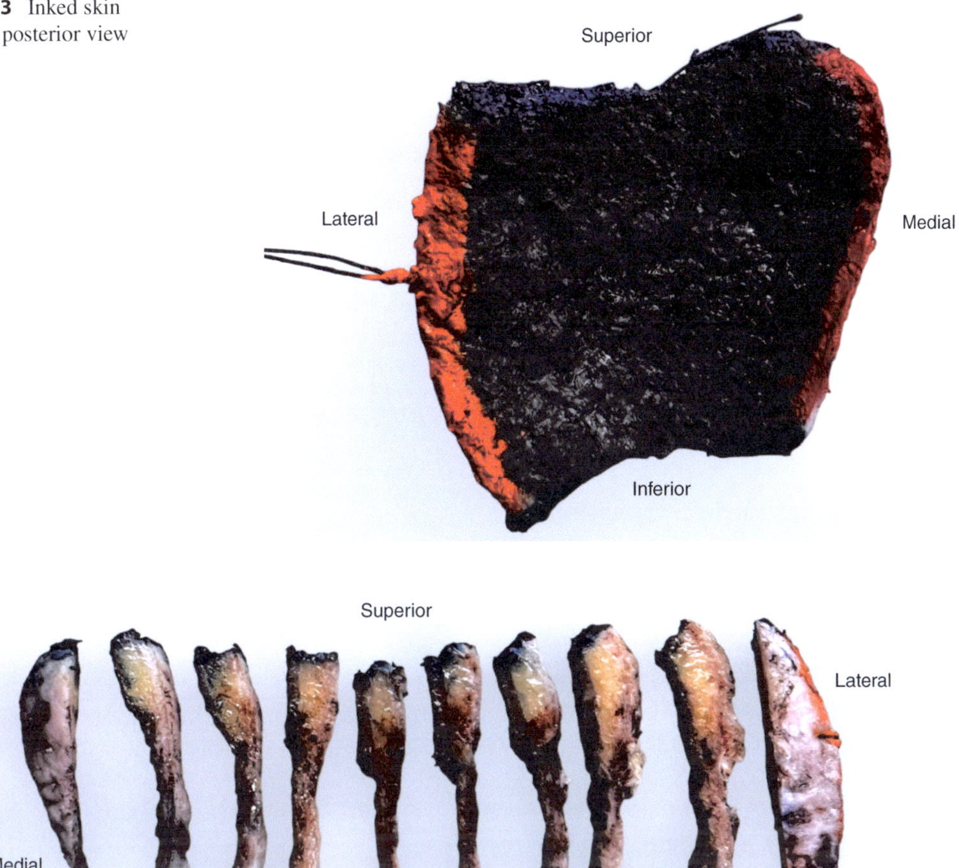

Fig. 12.44 Skin excision, serially sectioned

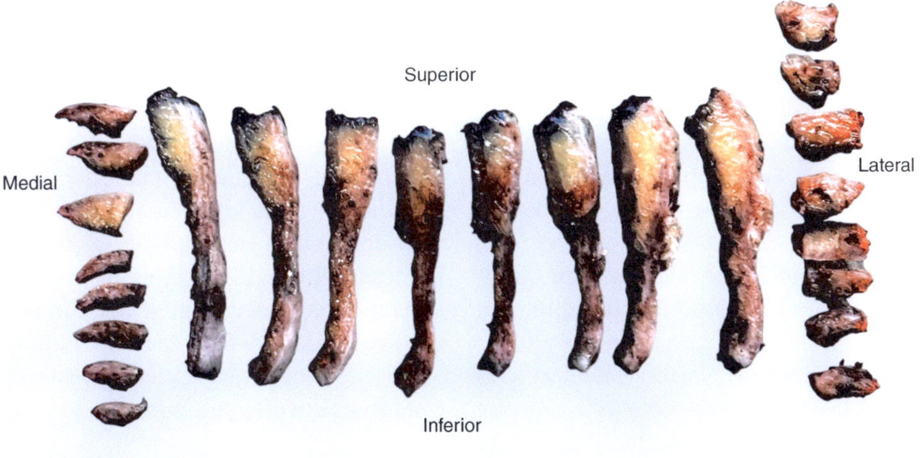

Fig. 12.45 Medial and lateral margins sectioned perpendicularly

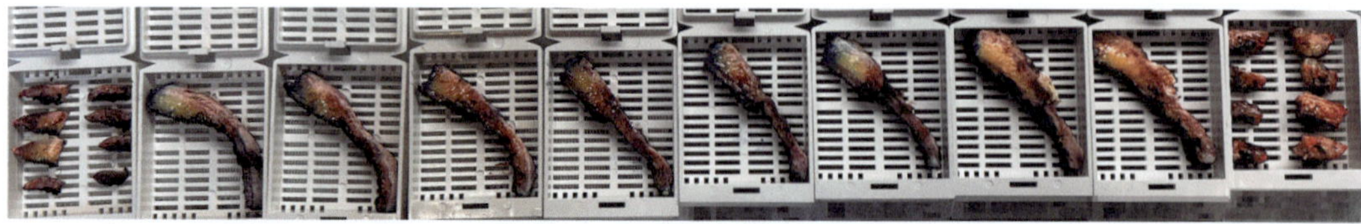

Fig. 12.46 Serially sectioned skin excision submitted entirely in the cassettes

Ink code

> Blue: superior
> Green: inferior
> Orange: lateral
> Red: medial
> Black: deep

Section code

> A1: Medial margin, perpendicular
> A2–A9: Specimen entirely from medial to lateral
> A10: Lateral margin, perpendicular

12.13 Skin Excision, Melanoma: Level IV CPT 88305

Although melanoma is not the most common type of skin cancer, it has the highest skin cancer mortality. This is because melanoma more commonly metastasizes to other organs, such as the lungs, liver, brain, or bones, when compared to basal and squamous cell carcinoma. This makes melanoma much more challenging to treat. The aim is to detect tumor early and completely remove the tumor before it spreads from the primary site.

Synoptic Breakdown Relative to Grossing (Table 12.3)

Procedure: Skin cancer specimens can range from punch, shave, or incisional biopsies to excision, re-excision with sentinel node(s) biopsy, and lymphadenectomy of regional nodes. Identify the procedure that was performed.

Laterality: Identify and mention if the specimen is from right, left, midline, or not specified.

Tumor Site: Identify which anatomical sites the lesion is located.

Tumor size, thickness, and the presence or absence of ulceration: Measure the lesion in three dimensions and also, measure the distance between the tumor and all surrounding skin margins. For melanoma, tumor thickness and the presence of ulceration are essential considerations for proper staging [4]. Reference Table 12.4 for tumor thickness and ulceration considerations. Once the specimen is sliced, identify and measure the greatest depth of tumor invasion and also, measure the distance between the tumor and the deep margin.

Table 12.4 pT classification.

Table 12.3 Synoptic breakdown relative to grossing

Synoptic breakdown relative to grossing
Procedure
Laterality
Tumor site
Multiple primary sites
Maximum tumor thickness
Macroscopic satellite nodules
Ulceration
Presence of perineural involvement
Presence of intravascular involvement
Distance from invasive melanoma to peripheral margin
Distance from invasive melanoma to deep margin

Table 12.4 pT classification

Important tumor size measurement considerations
pT0: No evidence of primary tumor
pT1a: Melanoma <0.8 mm in thickness, no ulceration
pT1b: Melanoma <0.8 mm in thickness with ulceration; or melanoma 0.8 to 1.0 mm in thickness with or without ulceration
pT2a: Melanoma >1.0 to 2.0 mm in thickness, no ulceration
pT2b: Melanoma >1.0 to 2.0 mm in thickness, with ulceration
pT3a: Melanoma >2.0 to 4.0 mm in thickness, no ulceration
pT3b: Melanoma >2.0 to 4.0 mm in thickness, with ulceration
pT4a: Melanoma >4.0 mm in thickness, no ulceration
pT4b: Melanoma >4.0 mm in thickness, with ulceration

12.14 Oriented Ellipse of Skin for Melanoma: Level IV CPT 88305

Excisions for melanoma can be a cumbersome task to gross because they often require a very wide margin producing a large specimen. It is best not to use black ink on these specimens as the ink pigment can resemble melanin pigment under the microscope. Melanomas sometimes demonstrate skip lesions/in transit metastases. These are separate areas of cancer in the skin adjacent to, but not connected to the primary lesion. See Table 12.5 for gross appearance of melanomas.

Step 1: Orient the specimen. In Fig. 12.47, the specimen is oriented with a notch placed by the surgeon (blue arrow) along the side designating superior and a stitch (red arrow) at one tip designating lateral.

Step 2: Measure the specimen in three dimensions.

Step 3: Determine and document the specimen's orientation.

Step 4: Measure the lesion area (Fig. 12.47, blue circle). Reference Table 12.5 for gross identification.

Step 5: Document the distance between the lesion and all peripheral margins (superior, inferior, medial, and lateral).

Step 6: Ink the peripheral and deep margins. Skin specimens can be inked in a variety of ways. The best approach is to ask the pathologist about their preference. In Fig. 12.48a and b, the superior, inferior, and deep margins are inked blue, green, and orange, respectively. When inking skin specimens for melanoma, it is best not to use black ink.

Step 7: Serially section the specimen with 1.5–2 mm sections, as seen in Fig. 12.49.

Step 8: Assess the cut surfaces to identify the greatest depth of invasion and distance between the lesion and the deep margin (Fig. 12.50).

Step 9: Unless the specimen for melanoma is very large, the specimen is typically submitted in its entirety, as seen in Fig. 12.51.

Step 10: Tips are submitted en face with the outer point of the tip facing down in the cassette, as seen in Fig. 12.52.

Example Dictation

Specimen A is received in formalin labeled with patient's name, medical record number, "left thigh" and consists of a tan-pink ellipse of

Table 12.5 Tumor gross appearance

Melanoma	Flat or slightly elevated surface, irregular margins. The color of these lesions ranges from tan, blue to black
Amelanotic melanoma	Flesh-colored or tan-red

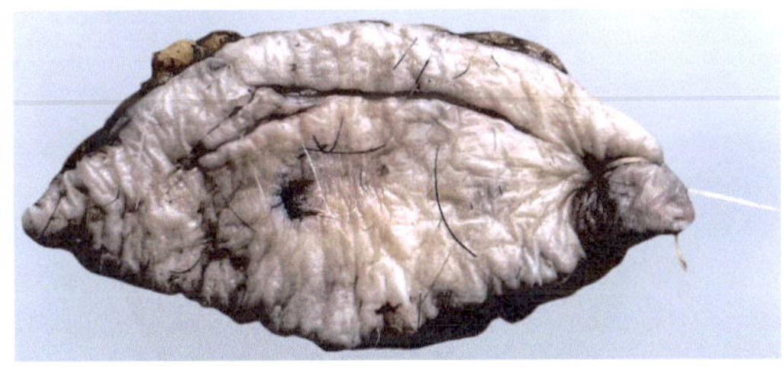

Fig. 12.47 Oriented skin ellipse, anterior view. A notch (blue arrow) indicates the superior side, and a stitch (red arrow) depicts the lateral tip

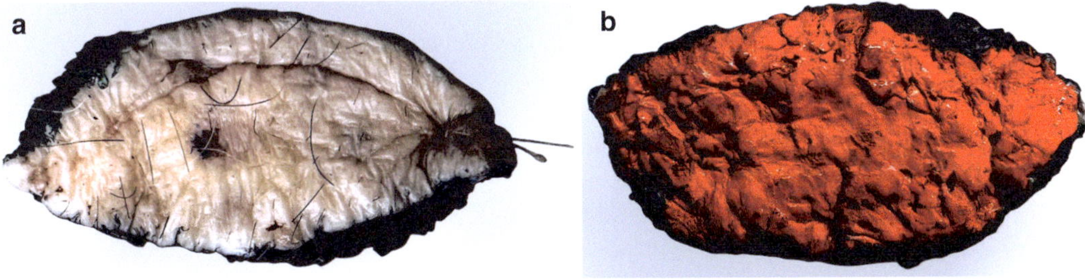

Fig. 12.48 (a) Inked skin ellipse, anterior view; (b) inked skin ellipse, posterior view

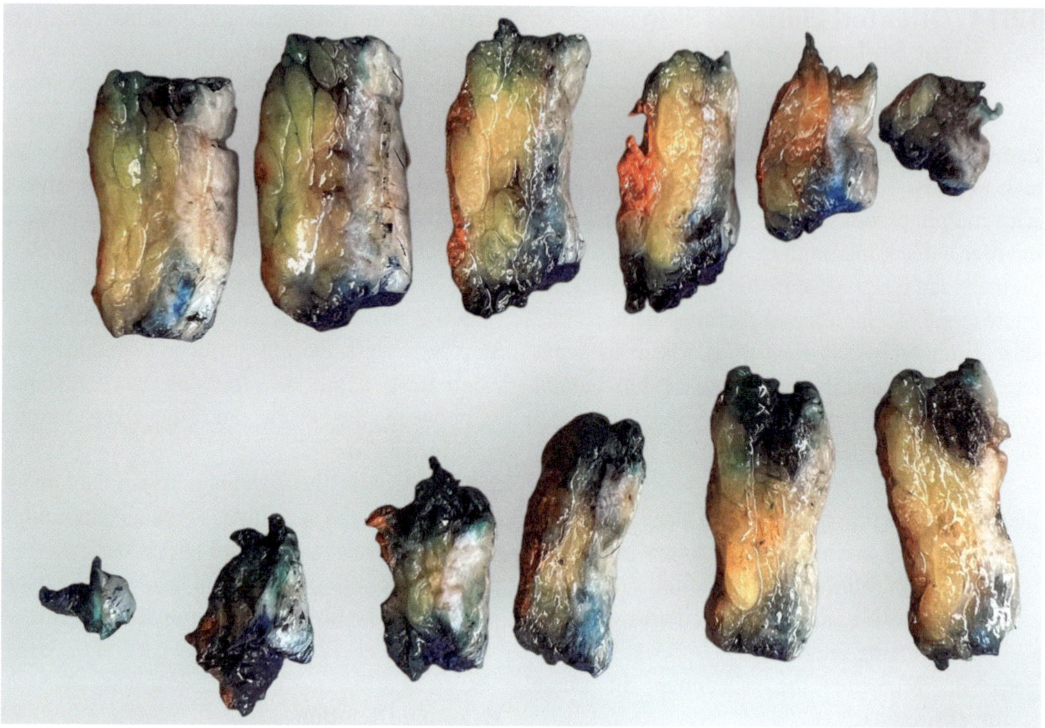

Fig. 12.49 Skin ellipse, serially sectioned

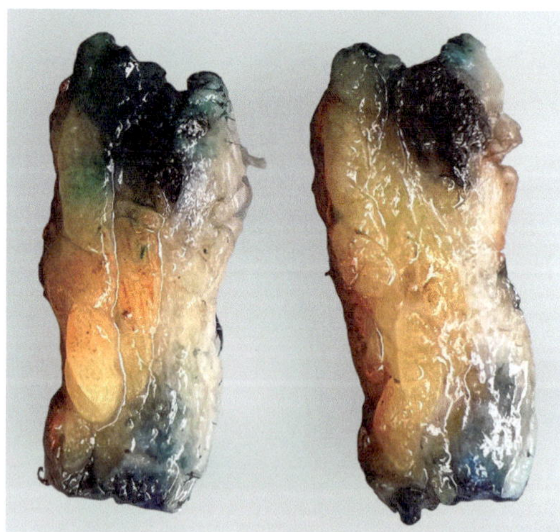

Fig. 12.50 The cut surfaces showing the lesion confined to the dermis

skin (3.8 x 1.9 x 1.0 cm) with a notch along one edge designating superior and a stitch at one tip designating lateral. The skin surface con-tains a scared, irregular tan-brown lesion (0.6 x 0.3 cm) which comes within 1.0 cm of the superior margin, within 0.8 cm of the inferior margin, within 2.2 cm of the medial margin, and within 2.4 cm of the lateral margin. The specimen is serially sectioned to reveal tan-yellow cut surfaces with invasion confined to the dermis and the lesion coming within 0.9 cm from the deep margin.

Ink code

    Blue: superior

    Green: inferior

    Orange: deep

Section code

    A1: medial tip, en face

    A2–A6: specimen entirely from medial to lateral

    A7: lateral tip, en face

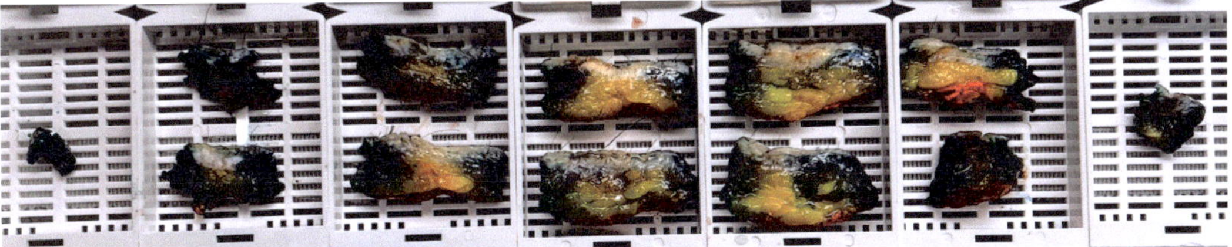

Fig. 12.51 Serially sectioned specimen submitted entirely in the cassettes

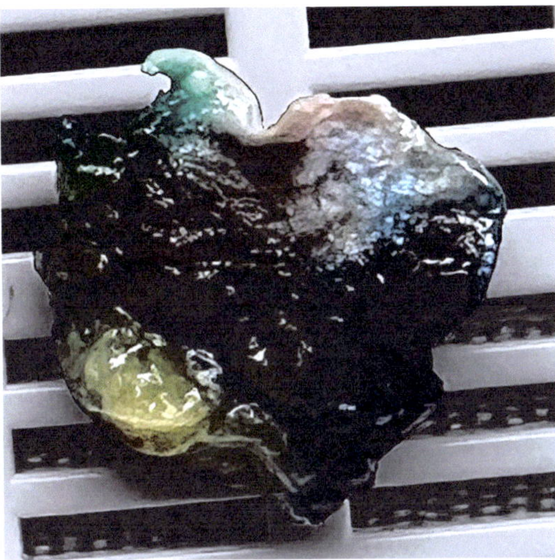

Fig. 12.52 The tip of the ellipse submitted en face in the cassette

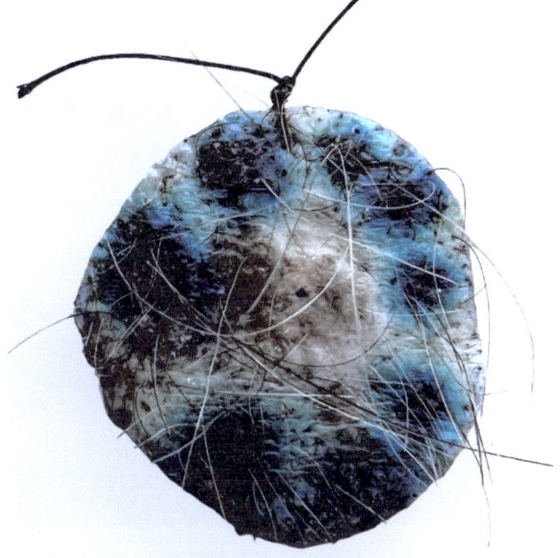

Fig. 12.53 An oriented circular skin excision. The skin surface contains an ill-defined, irregular tan-brown lesion

12.15 Oriented Circular Excision- Level IV CPT 88305

A circular-shaped skin excision does not have evident skin tips. If the pathologist wants skin tips, a thin shave of opposing margins can be taken and submitted en face. However, doing perpendicular margins allows for more surface area to be assessed, and microscopically the lesion distance can be measured from the margins.

Step 1: Describe and measure the specimen (Fig. 12.53).

Step 2: Measure the lesion. Reference Table 12.2 for gross identification.

Step 3: Measure the distance of the lesion to the peripheral margins.

Step 4: Document the orientation of the specimen.

Step 5: Ink the margins as seen in Fig. 12.54. Five colors are used to designate the four peripheral and deep margins as follows:

Red: 12 o'clock margin

Blue: 3 o'clock margin

Yellow: 6 o'clock margin

Green: 9 o'clock margin

Orange: Deep margin

Step 6: Serially section the specimen. Since the specimen is circular, sectioning in either of two directions is acceptable, either 12–6 o'clock or 3–9 o'clock. In Fig. 12.55, the specimen is sectioned from 12 to 6 o'clock.

Step 7: Assess the greatest depth of invasion and document the distance between the tumor and the deep margin. In Fig. 12.55, the lesion is superficial with minimal invasion.

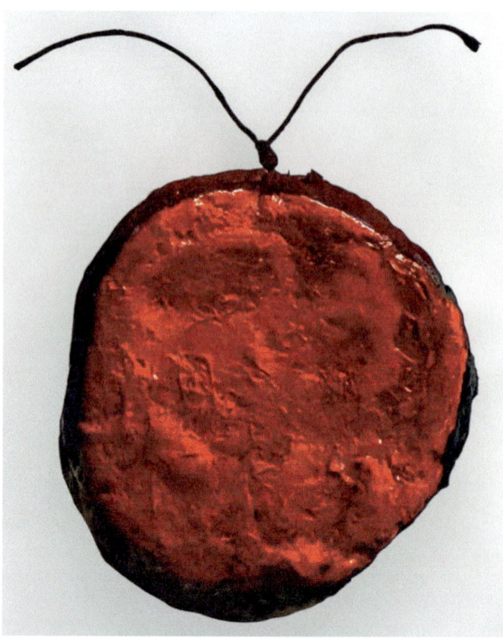

Fig. 12.54 Inked skin excision, posterior view

Step 8: Perpendicularly section the end margins. In Fig. 12.56, the 12 o'clock and 6 o'clock margins are perpendicularly sectioned.

Step 9: The specimen is submitted entirely from 12 o'clock to 6 o'clock, as seen in Fig. 12.57.

Example Dictation

Specimen A is received in formalin labeled with patient's name, medical record number, "Left Scalp" and consists of a tan-pink circular skin excision (4.2 x 4.1 x 1.0 cm) with a stitch designating 12 o'clock. The skin surface contains an ill-defined, irregular tan-brown lesion (1.2 x 1.0 cm) which comes within 1.0 cm from the 12 o'clock margin, 1.1 cm from the 3 o'clock margin, 1.2 cm from the 6 o'clock margin, and 1.0 cm from the 9 o'clock margin. The specimen is serially sectioned to reveal tan-yellow cut sur-

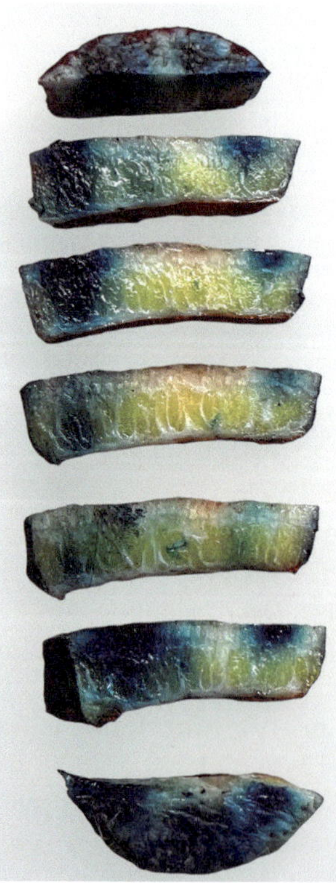

Fig. 12.55 Specimen serially sectioned from 12–6 o'clock

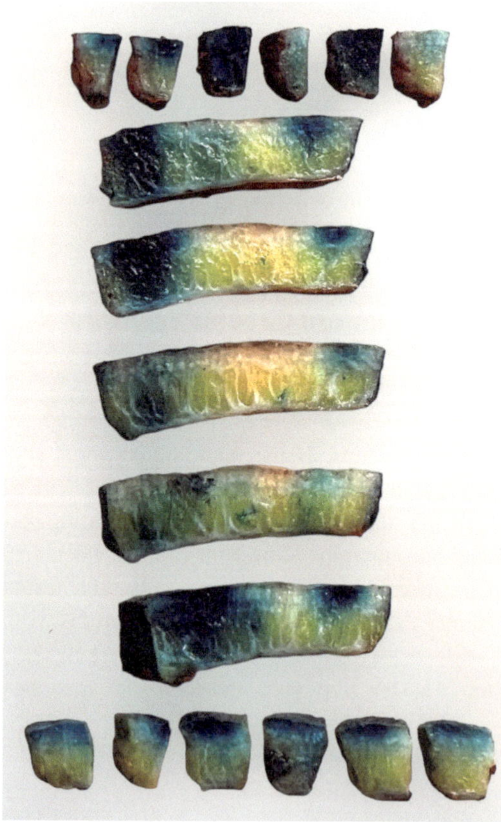

Fig. 12.56 12 o'clock and 6 o'clock margins perpendicularly sectioned

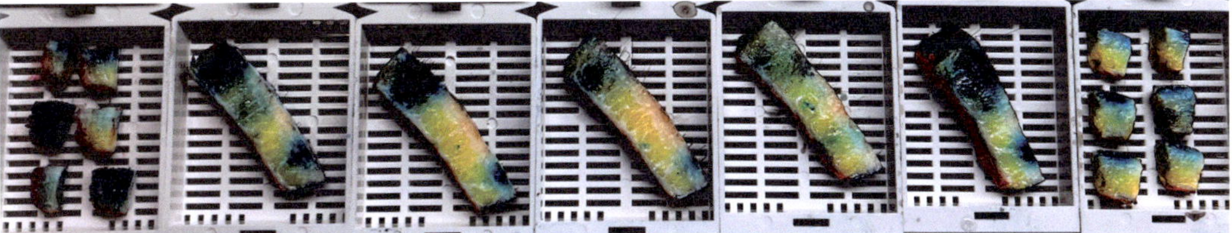

Fig. 12.57 Specimen submitted in its entirety in the cassettes

faces with a greatest depth of invasion of 0.1. The lesion comes within 0.9 cm from the deep margin, surrounded by blue dye.

Ink code
>   Red: 12 o'clock margin
>   Blue: 3 o'clock margin
>   Yellow: 6 o'clock margin
>   Green: 9 o'clock margin
>   Orange: deep margin

Section code
>   A1: 12 o'clock margin, perpendicular
>   A2–A6: Specimen entirely from 12 o'clock to 6 o'clock
>   A7: 6 o'clock margin, perpendicular

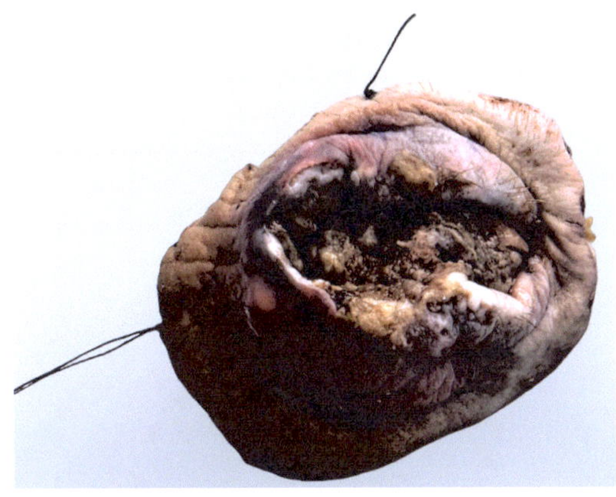

Fig. 12.58 Oriented resection specimen with upper and lower eyelid, peripheral skin, and the eye

12.16 Large Skin Excision with Multiple Anatomic Structures: Level IV CPT 88305

One of the most challenging considerations related to skin grossing is dealing with skin excision specimens that involve multiple anatomic structures. These specimens require careful attention to orientation and margins. Proper technique is necessary for sectioning and sampling. There should be a clear plan and rationale before sampling, based on anatomy and guidelines for each specimen type. This ensures quality and accuracy and avoids unnecessary errors. Involving the pathologist in grossing such specimens is never wrong since there is only one opportunity to gross the specimen correctly.

Following is an example of a complex specimen containing eyelid, orbit, optic nerve, and extraocular muscles.

Step 1: Identify all the anatomic structures present in the specimen. Figure 12.58 includes the upper eyelid, lower eyelid, peripheral skin, and the eye.

Step 2: Orient the specimen correlating with the anatomy.

Step 3: Describe and measure the specimen and dictate what anatomic structures are present.

Step 4: Measure the overall specimen.

Step 5: Measure individual anatomic structures.

Step 6: The skin excision has a set of margins, and the eye has its own separate set of margins. These margins include the optic nerve, superior rectus, inferior rectus, medial rectus, lateral rectus, superior oblique, and inferior oblique margins.

Step 7: Identify and shave the superior rectus and superior oblique margins (Fig. 12.59). These are submitted en face.

Step 8: Identify and shave the inferior rectus margin (Fig. 12.60). This margin is submitted en face.

Fig. 12.59 Superior
rectus and superior
oblique margins

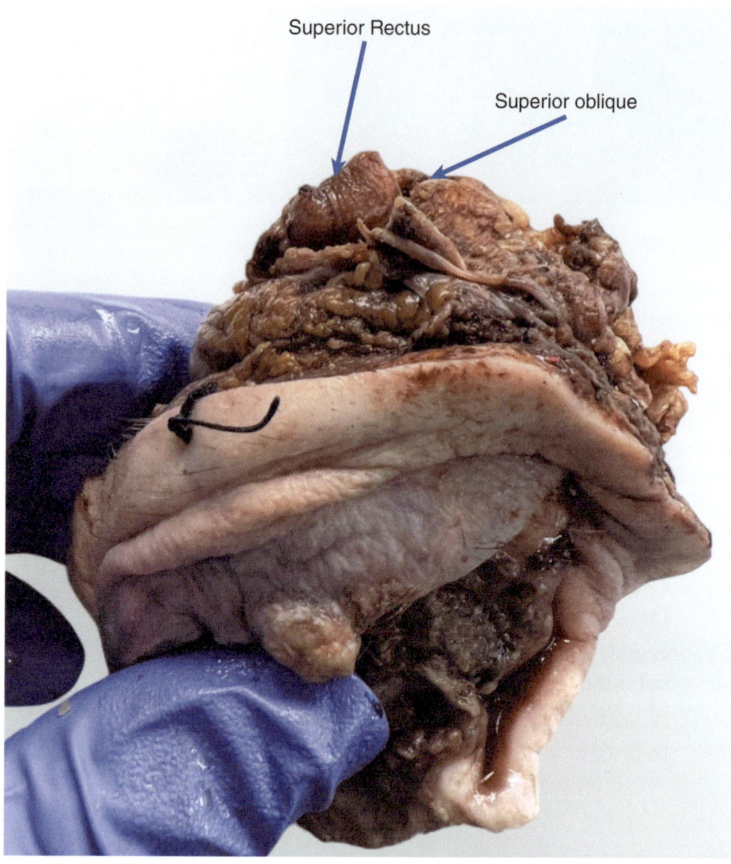

Fig. 12.60 Inferior
recuts margin

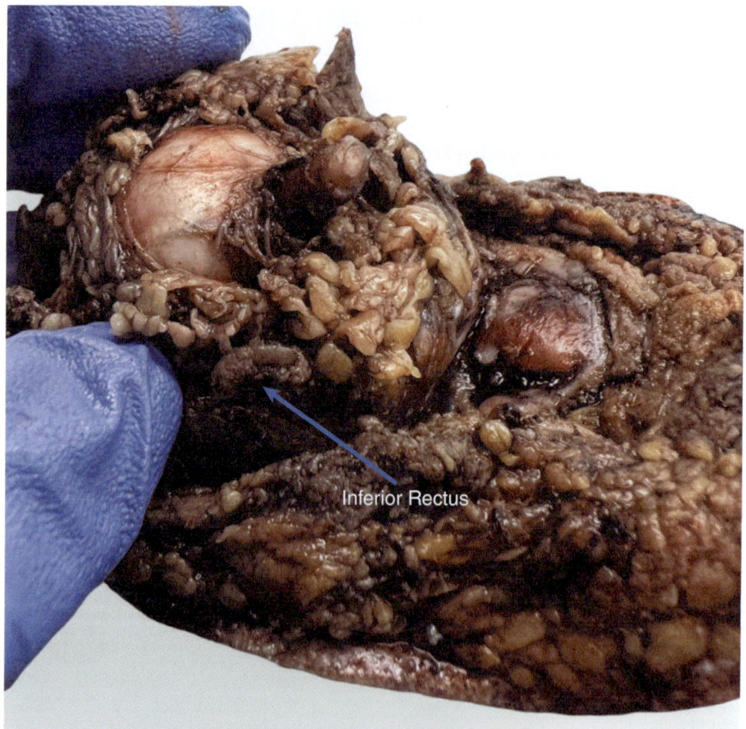

Step 9: Identify and shave the medial rectus and inferior oblique margins (Fig. 12.61). These margins are submitted en face.

Step 10: Identify and shave the lateral rectus margin (Fig. 12.62). This margin is submitted en face.

Step 11: Shave the optic nerve margin as seen in Fig. 12.63, and submitted en face.

At this point, the margins of the eye are complete, and attention can now be turned to the skin.

Step 12: Ink the specimen. It may be beneficial to discuss inking with the pathologists beforehand or at the bench with complicated specimens. In Fig. 12.64, the ink code is as follows:

> Blue: 12 o'clock margin
> Red: 3 o'clock margin
> Green: 6 o'clock margin
> Orange: 9 o'clock margin
> Black: Deep margin

It is important to discuss which margins are most important to the pathologist. One option is to shave the skin margin in a clockface fashion around the specimen and submit the margins en face. Another option is to submit the closest

margins perpendicularly, which is how this specimen was grossed.

Step 13: Serially section the specimen from 3 to 9 o'clock (which is medial to lateral) and lay each section flat to allow for the best assessment of the slices, as seen in Fig. 12.65.

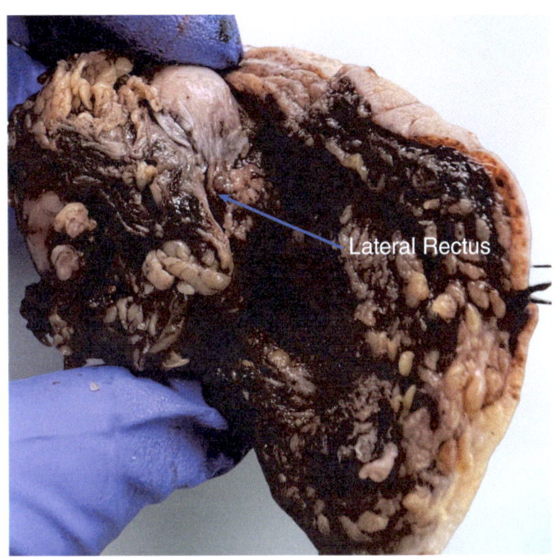

Fig. 12.62 Lateral recuts margin

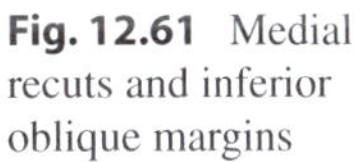

Fig. 12.61 Medial recuts and inferior oblique margins

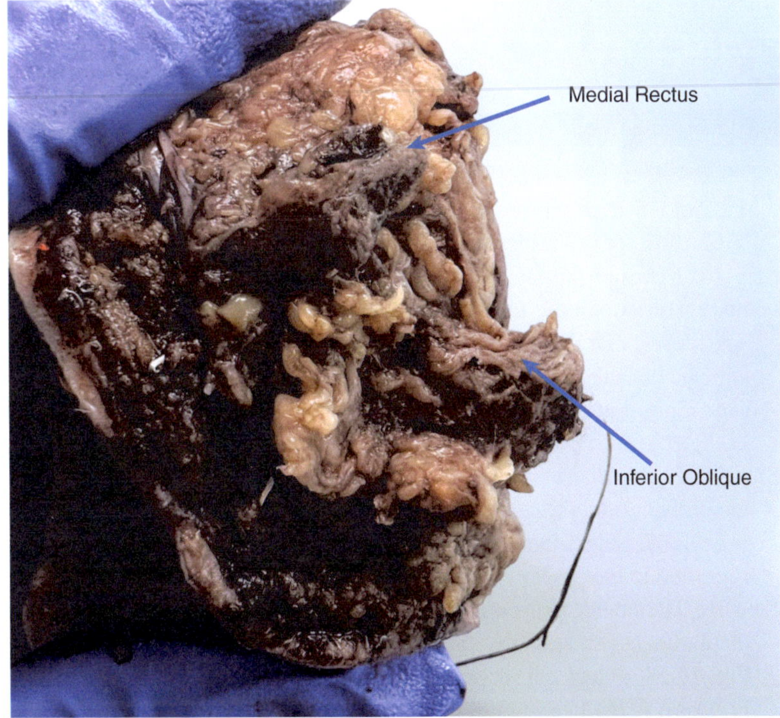

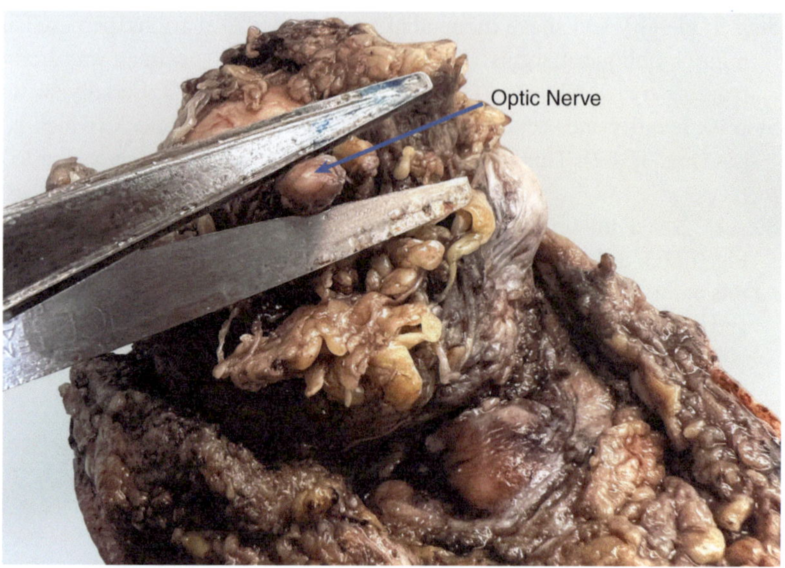

Fig. 12.63 Optic nerve margin being shaved

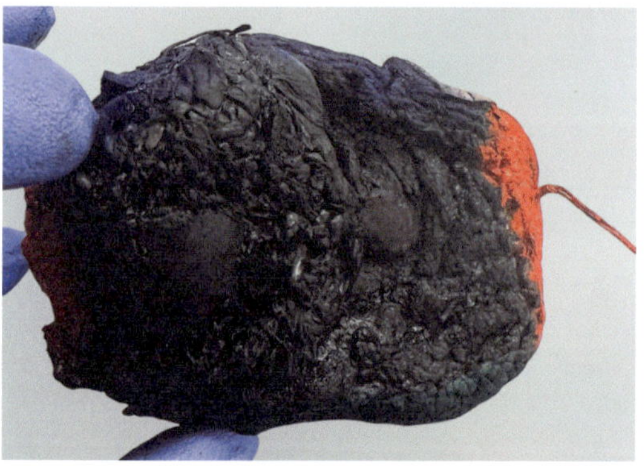

Fig. 12.64 Inked specimen, posterior view

Measure and describe the mass. Reference Table 12.2 for gross identification.

Step 14: Measure the smallest distance (closest margin) between the tumor and each margin. The closest margins can all be found in different slices. Take a perpendicular section of each margin in relation to the mass, as shown in Fig. 12.66.

Step 15: The medial margin is sectioned perpendicularly, as identified by the blue lines in Fig. 12.67. Select the section where the mass is closest to the medial margin.

Step 16: The lateral margin is sectioned perpendicularly as shown by the blue lines in Fig. 12.68. Select the section where the mass is closest to the lateral margin.

Step 17: Submit a fullface section of the mass. The fullface section does not need to include the closest margins because those margins have already been assessed and submitted. The purpose of these sections is to show what anatomic structures are involved by the mass. In Fig. 12.69, the section is quadrisected to fit the cassettes.

Step 18: With any complicated specimen, the sections submitted have no meaning unless the section code is specific. Ensure the section code explains exactly which section is present in each cassette (Fig. 12.70).

Example Dictation

Specimen A is received in formalin labeled with patient's name, medical record number, "right orbital lesion and orbital exenteration" and consists of an ellipse of tan-pink skin (7.6 x 5.9 x 4.4 cm) containing the upper lower eyelid and left orbital exenteration (3.2 x 2.5 x 2.5 cm) with attached length of optic nerve (0.9 cm in length). The specimen is oriented with a short stitch designating 12 o'clock and a long stitch designating 9 o'clock. At the lateral canthus, extending the entirety of the orbit to the medial canthus is an ulcerative, necrotic lesion encompassing the entirety of the antihelix and ulcerating through the lateral aspect of the helix (4.9 x 4.1 x 2.5 cm), obstructing the anterior skin aspect of the orbit. The mass comes within

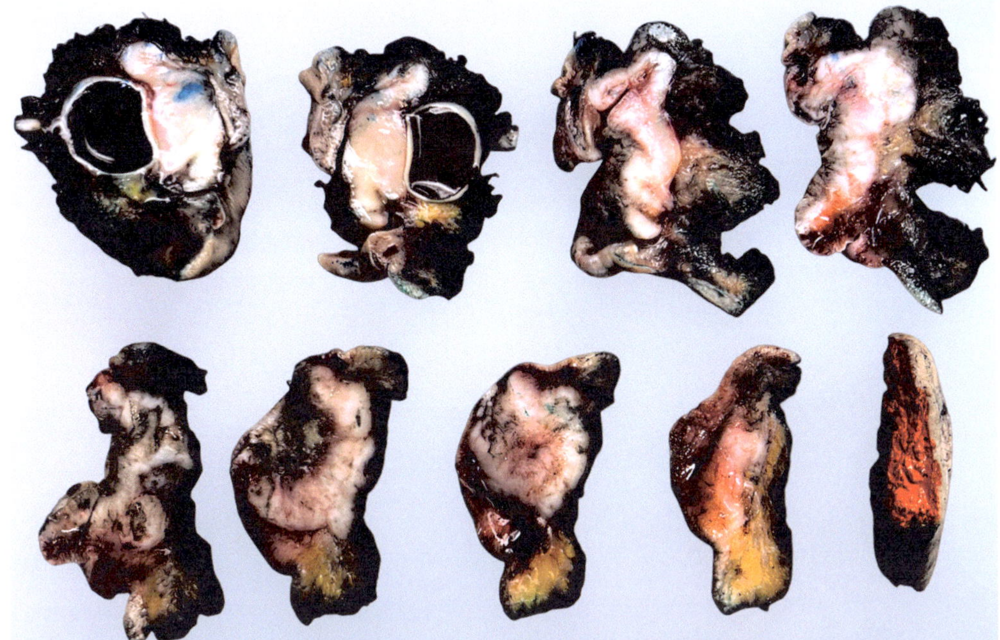

Fig. 12.65 Specimen serially sectioned from 3 to 9 o'clock (medial to lateral) and each section laid flat

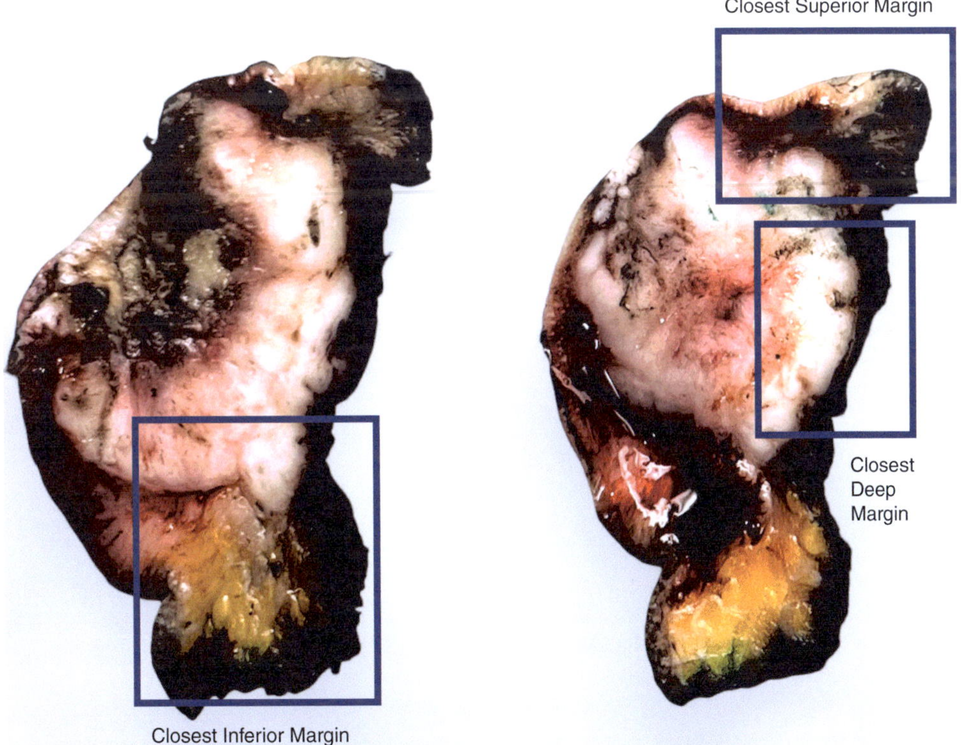

Fig. 12.66 Perpendicular sections showing the closest inferior margin and closest superior and deep margins

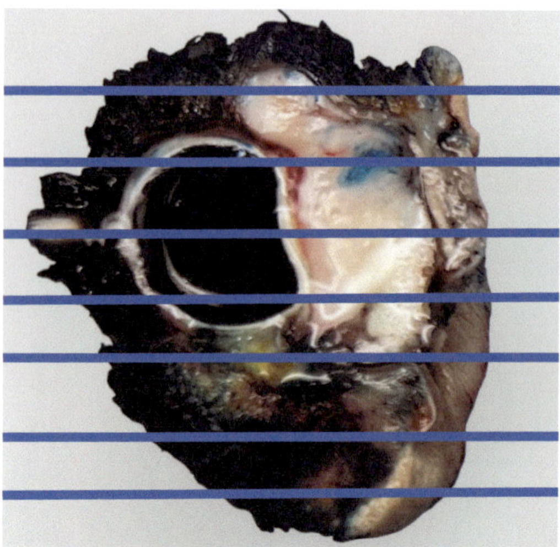

Fig. 12.67 The blue lines indicate how to cut the medial margin perpendicularly

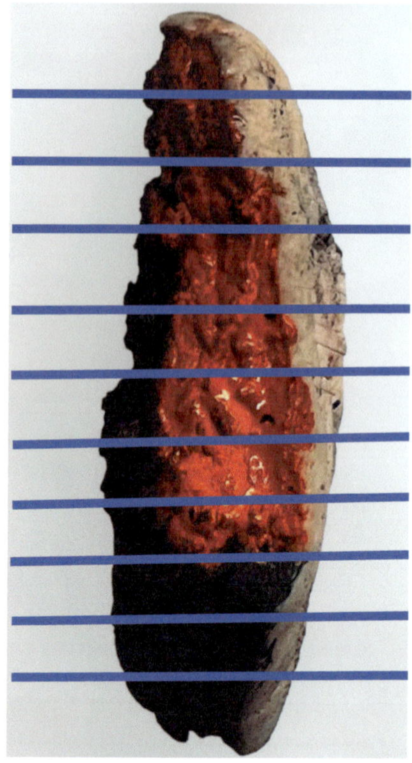

Fig. 12.68 The blue lines indicate how to cut the lateral margin perpendicularly

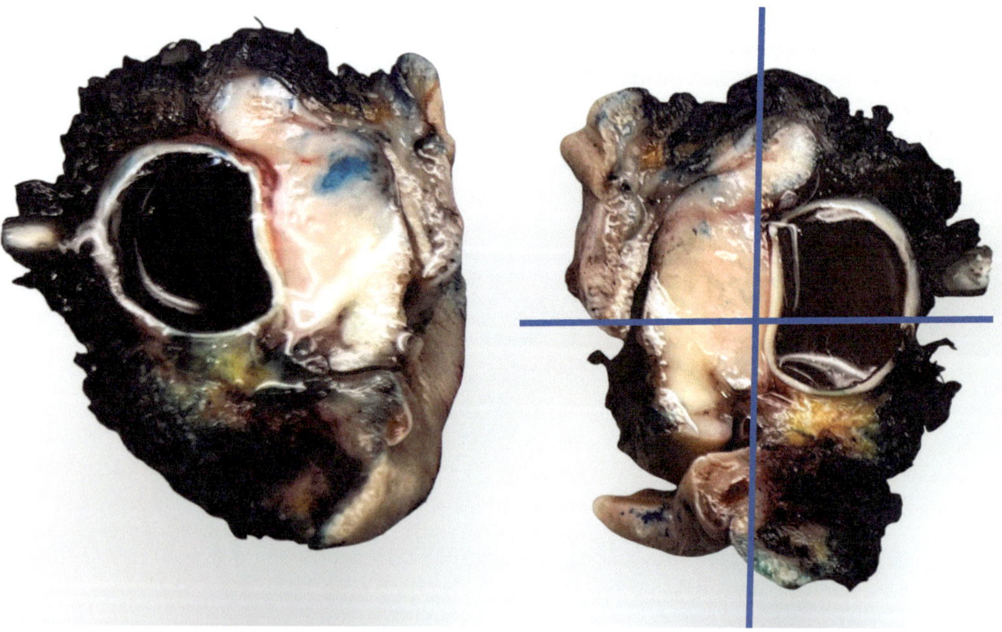

Fig. 12.69 Fullface section of the mass, quadrisected as indicated by the blue lines

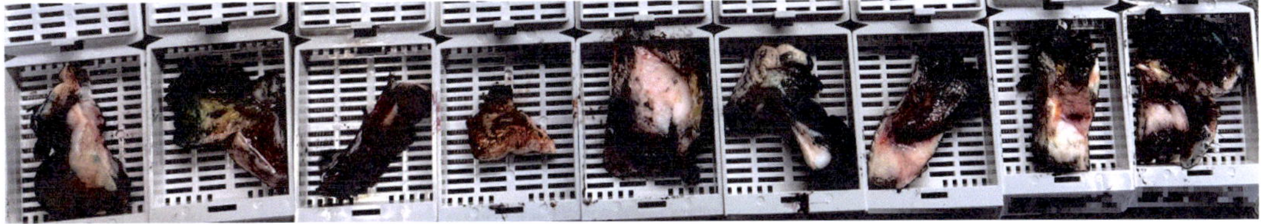

Fig. 12.70 Representative sections from the mass submitted in the cassettes

1.3 cm of the 12 o'clock margin, 0.7 cm from the 3 o'clock margin, 1.0 cm from the 6 o'clock margin, and 1.4 cm from the 9 o'clock margin. The specimen is serially sectioned to reveal an overall mass size of approximately 4.9 x 3.5 x 2.5 cm, coming within 1.0 cm of the 12 o'clock soft tissue margin, 1.5 cm from the 6 o'clock soft tissue margin, 2.2 cm from the 9 o'clock soft tissue margin, 1.1 cm from the 3 o'clock soft tissue margin, and less than 0.1 cm from the deep/posterior margin. Additionally, the mass abuts the orbit, pushing the orbit posteriorly without distinct invasion through the cornea or sclera.

Ink code

> Blue: 12 o'clock
> Green: 6 o'clock
> Red: 3 o'clock
> Orange: 9 o'clock
> Black: deep

Section code

> A 1: Superior rectus (inked blue) and superior oblique margins, en face
> A 2: Medial rectus (inked blue) and lateral rectus margins, en face
> A 3: Inferior rectus (inked blue) and inferior oblique margins, en face
> A 4: Optic nerve margin, en face
> A 5: Mass to closest 12 o'clock skin and soft tissue margin, perpendicular
> A 6: Mass in relation to closest 6 o'clock skin and soft tissue margin, perpendicular
> A 7: Closest medial skin and soft tissue margin, perpendicular (no mass present)
> A 9: Mass in relation to closest posterior/deep margin, perpendicular
> A 10–A13: Fullface section of mass in relation to eye
> A 14: Eye with cornea neck and lens

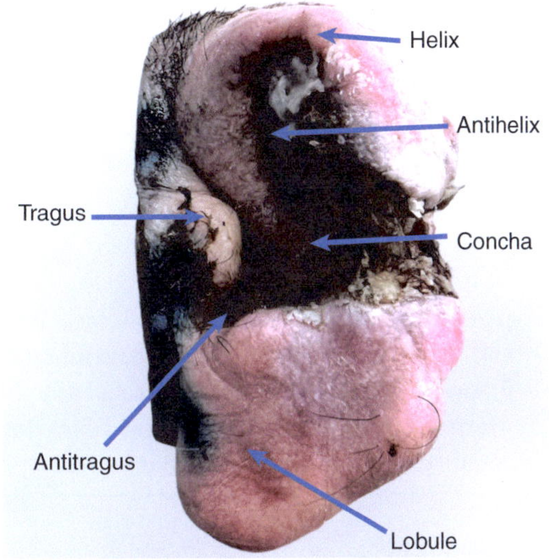

Fig. 12.71 Excision of the left ear

12.17 Large Skin Excision of One Large Anatomic Structure: Level IV CPT 88305

A skin excision, including a complete anatomic structure can be intimidating. With knowledge of basic anatomy, it is possible to determine the margins in the same manner as other skin excisions. No matter the structure, it is critical to determine the size of the mass and document the distance of the mass to the margins. As noted above, it is never wrong to involve the pathologist before the specimen is grossed. There is only one chance to get it right!

Step 1: Identify all the anatomic structures. In Fig. 12.71, the entirety of the left ear is present. Of course, the ear has multiple substructures which need to be identified.

Step 2: Describe and measure the specimen.

Step 3: Describe and measure the lesion in three dimensions. Reference Table 12.2 for gross identification.

Step 4: Describe all the structures involved by the lesion.

Step 5: Measure the lesions to the closest aspects of each peripheral margin. Figure 12.72a and b demonstrate the peripheral margins which are superior, inferior, anterior, and posterior.

Step 6: Identity the margins (Fig. 12.73a) and ink the resection margins. In Figure 12.73b, the ink code is as follows:

    Orange: superior
    Red: inferior
    Blue: anterior
    Green: posterior
    Black: deep/medial

Step 7: The auditory canal spans from the external ear to the tympanic membrane. Figure 12.74 shows the auditory canal margin which is present at the deep margin. Shave the auditory canal margin and submit en face.

Step 8: Serially section the specimen perpendicular to the long axis. In Fig. 12.75, the specimen is serially sectioned from superior to inferior.

Step 9: Measure the greatest depth of invasion.

Step 10: Measure the overall three dimensions of the lesion.

Step 11: Perpendicularly section the superior margin and submit sections of the lesion to the closest superior margin (Fig. 12.76).

Step 12: Perpendicularly section the inferior margin and submit sections of the lesion to the closest inferior margin (Fig. 12.77).

Step 13: Select representative sections. Figure 12.78a shows the selected slices, and Fig. 12.78b demonstrates the best method to transect the specimen (blue lines) so that they fit into the cassettes.

Step 14: Assess the sections including the auditory canal, to visualize if the lesion extends into the canal or to the auditory canal resection margin. In Fig. 12.79, the lesion does not extend into the auditory canal.

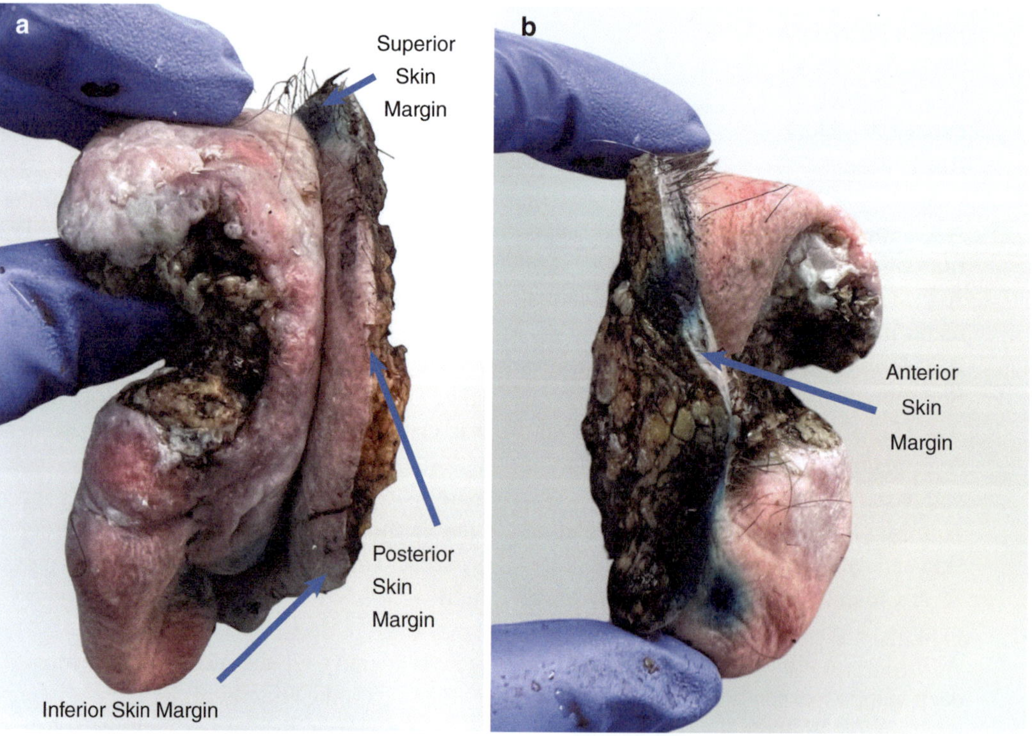

Fig. 12.72 (**a**) Left ear excision, posterior view; blue arrows indicate skin margins. (**b**) Left ear excision, anterior view; blue arrow indicates anterior skin margin

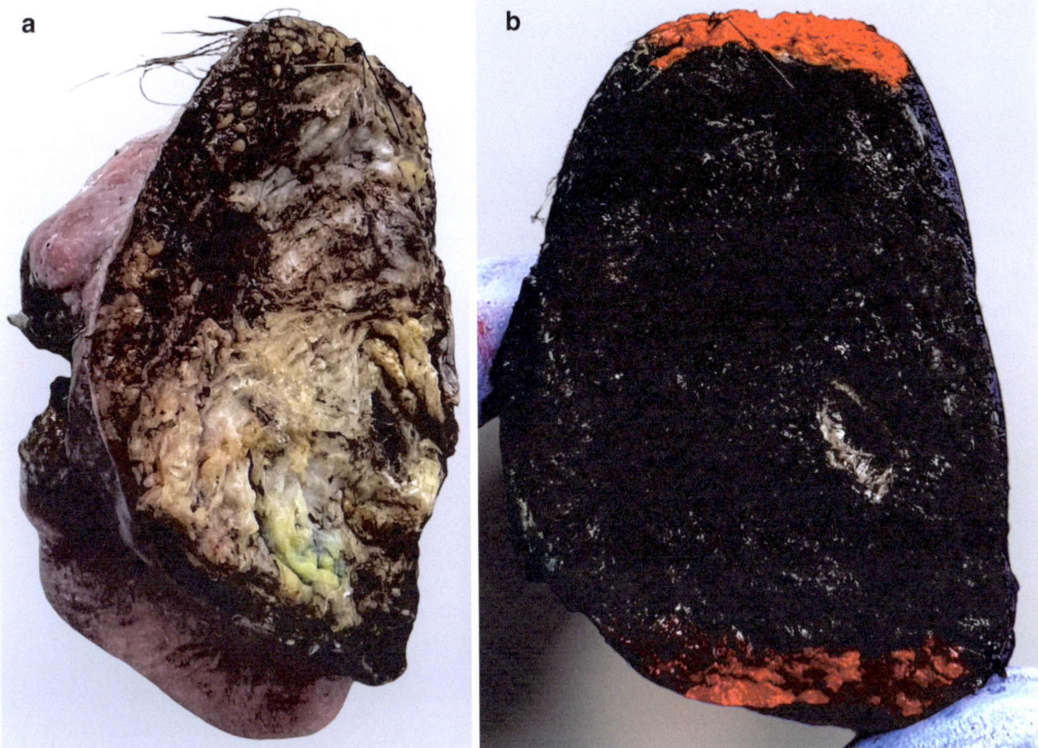

Fig. 12.73 (**a**) Resection margins; (**b**) resection margins, inked

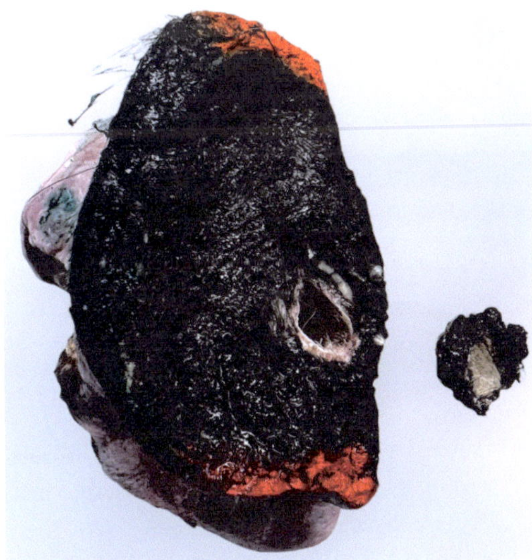

Fig. 12.74 Auditory canal margin, shaved

Step 15: The sections submitted are the auditory canal margin and representative sections that include the lesion to all peripheral margins and the deep margin (Fig. 12.80).

Example Dictation
Specimen A is received in formalin labeled with patient's name, medical record number, "left ear" and consists of a wide excision of the left ear (8.5 x 5.5 x 4.0 cm) with a stitch designating 12 o'clock and tan-pink skin. The ear is excised entirely and contains an ulcerative, necrotic lesion (4.2 x 2.5 cm) encompassing the entirety of the concha and antihelix and ulcerating through the lateral aspect of the helix. The lesion comes within 0.7 cm of the superior skin margin, 1.1 cm from the posterior skin margin, 0.7 cm from the inferior margin, and 2.1 cm from the anterior margin. The specimen is serially sectioned to reveal a greatest depth of invasion of approximately 2.2 cm, creating an overall mass of 5.2 x 4.9 x 2.2 cm, with the lesion invading through the cartilage of the helix and antihelix coming within 0.4 cm of the deep margin. Additionally, the mass does not appear to invade into the skin surface of the ear canal.

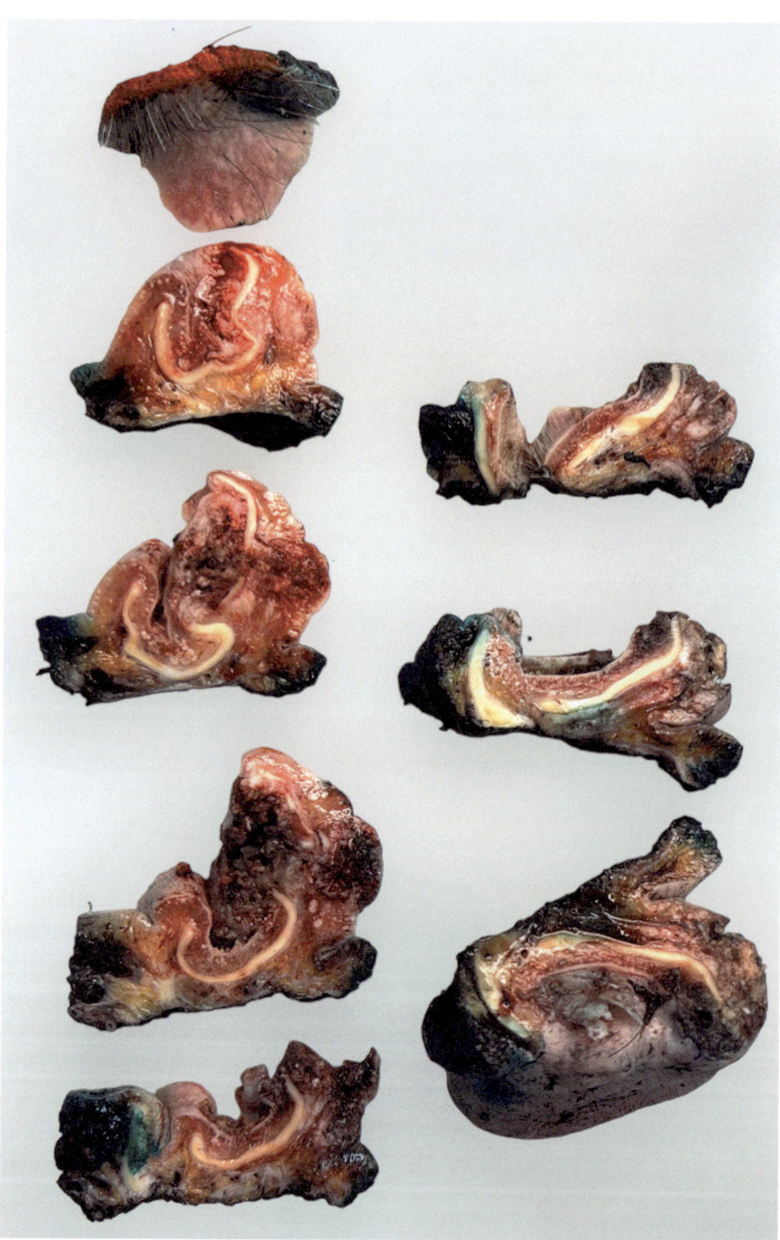

Fig. 12.75 Left ear resection specimen serially sectioned

Ink code

> Orange: superior margin
> Green: posterior margin
> Red: inferior margin
> Blue: anterior margin
> Black: deep/medial margin

Section code

> A1: Deep auditory canal margin, en face
> A2: Mass in relation to closest superior margin, perpendicular

A3–A5: Fullface section of mass in relation to anterior, deep, and posterior margins, trisected

A6–A7: Fullface section of mass in relation to anterior, deep, and posterior margins, bisected

A8: Mass in relation to the auditory canal, longitudinal, representative

A9–A10: Mass in relation to closest inferior margin, perpendicular.

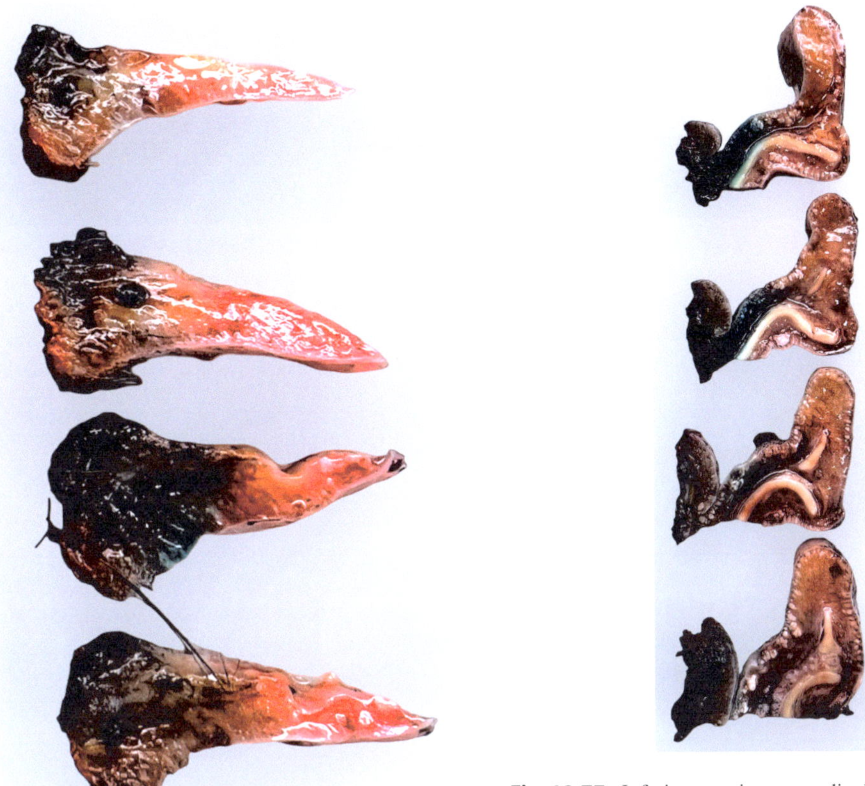

Fig. 12.76 Superior margin, perpendicularly sectioned

Fig. 12.77 Inferior margin, perpendicularly sectioned

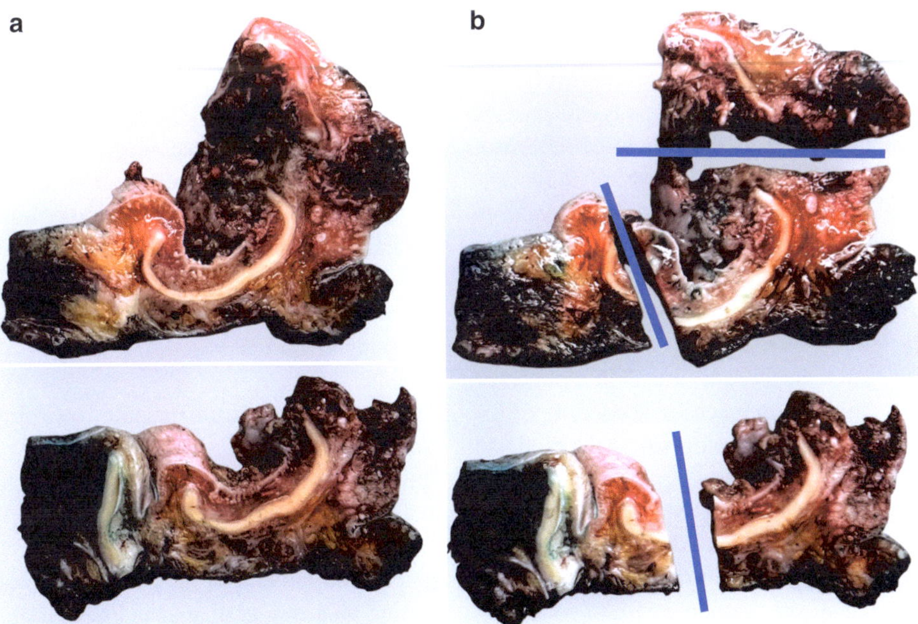

Fig. 12.78 (**a**) Representative sections with the lesion. (**b**) The blue lines indicate where the slices should be cut to fit into the cassettes

Fig. 12.79 Sections from the auditory canal

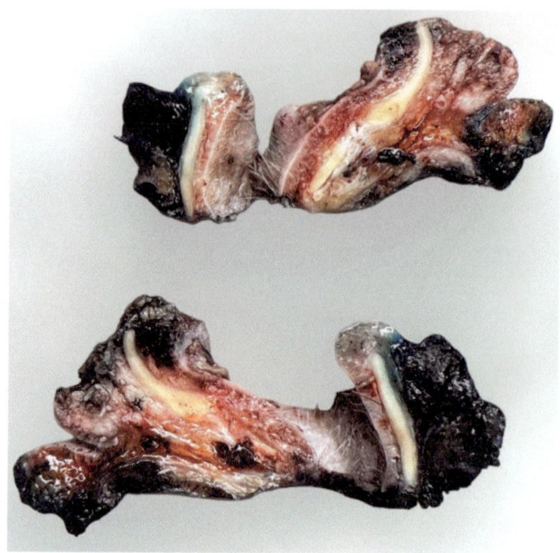

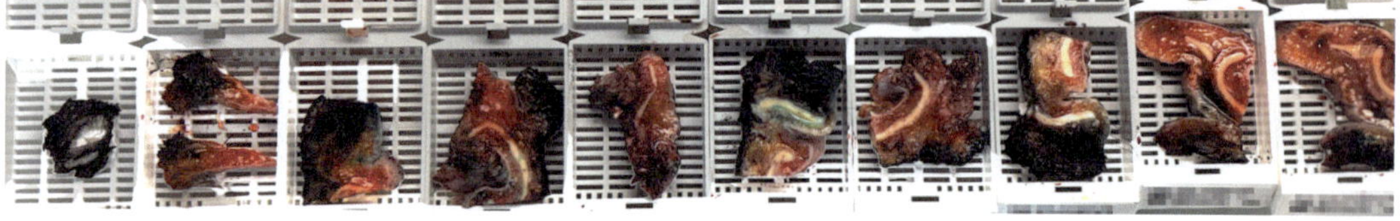

Fig. 12.80 Representative sections submitted in cassettes

12.18 A Special Consideration: Bedside Grossing by the Clinician

Some punch and shave specimens should be oriented and sectioned in specific ways to provide the pathologist with the best view of the histologic features needed to make a diagnosis. Unfortunately, the surface features needed to properly orient specimens before they are sectioned are difficult to detect at the pathology grossing table, for instance, the thread-like cornoid lamella in porokeratosis, a decompressed blister, or two adjacent specimens in a punch or shave specimen. In these cases, sectioning of the punch or shave can be performed by the clinician at the bedside. The grossing pathologist simply needs to embed the two halves of the punch or shave specimen with the cut edge down to provide the pathologist with the view of the tissue to make the requisite diagnosis. The following instructions can be shared with your dermatologists and surgeons!

The collaboration between clinicians and pathologists plays a crucial role in achieving accurate diagnoses in dermatopathology. For the clinician, the process of clinical-pathologic correlation begins even before the scalpel touches the skin. Several considerations need to be considered, such as the anatomic location for the biopsy, the type of biopsy, timing, depth, and breadth of the biopsy, and provision of important clinical information. This section, however, focuses on the benefits of grossing at the bedside. The value of bedside grossing is illustrated in the following scenarios.

Optimal Biopsy of and Bedside Grossing of Porokeratosis

The term porokeratosis describes lesions characterized by a cornoid lamella surrounding a central area with variable findings. Including the cornoid lamella in the biopsy is crucial for making an accurate diagnosis [5]. Sampling the center of the lesion will show only nonspecific findings. Improperly oriented biopsies, however, lead to the same nonspecific findings. To ensure proper orientation, a clinician can draw a line perpendicular to the cornoid lamella at the edge of the lesion. The punch biopsy is then centered at the intersection of the drawn line and the cornoid lamella. The punch specimen is bisected at the bedside along the previously drawn line, and the surgical pathology requisition should indicate that the specimen has been transected, and that the cut edges should be placed down in the block. (See Figs. 12.81a–c and 12.82) This ensures that the cornoid lamella will be present in cross-section on the slides which are produced. Thus, bedside grossing in coordination with the grossing person guarantees proper orientation, facilitating accurate histopathologic interpretation [7].

Draw a line perpendicular to the cornoid lamella at the edge of the porokeratosis patch using a skin marker as shown in Fig. 12.81a.

Before obtaining the specimen, center the punch on the intersection of the drawn line and cornoid lamella as seen in Fig. 12.81b.

A #15 scalpel blade is used to cut the punch specimen in half along the previously drawn line shown in Fig. 12.82c. The cut edges should be placed in the block facing downward to ensure that the cornoid lamella is present in the cross-section on the slides.

Shown in Fig. 12.82, bisecting along line A yields sections showing only normal skin, which lacks diagnostic significance. Similarly, bisecting along line B captures the center of the macule showing only nonspecific findings. While bisecting along path C and path D may seem promising, they provide views that can be confusing to the pathologist. Bisecting as directed above at the bedside produces the perfect sections for diagnosis.

Optimal Biopsy and Bedside Grossing of a Tense Blister

In cases of tense blisters like pemphigoid, capturing the "take off point" of the blister in the biopsy is essential to making a histopathologic diagnosis. It is recommended that punch biopsies include 70–75% perilesional skin and 25–30% blister so that the epidermis does not separate completely from the dermis during the procedure or processing. Random sections from punch biopsies that are performed in this manner miss the blister in 20–40% of cases. This requires multiple recuts and delays in diagnosis. Proper marking of the specimen before the procedure and bisection along the properly drawn line produces the proper view of the blister every time. (See Fig. 12.82) This approach also allows the clinician to put one-half in formalin for H&E sections

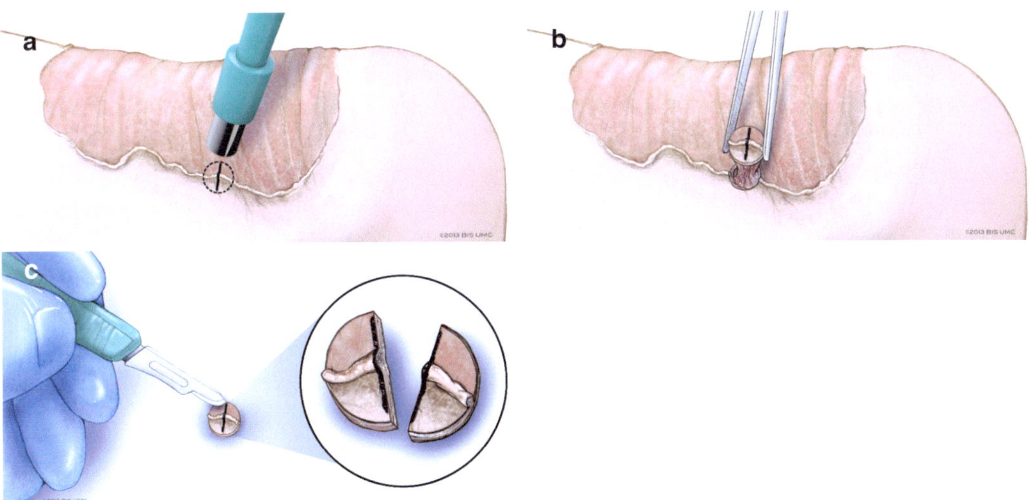

Fig. 12.81 (**a**) Excising a skin punch biopsy; (**b**) removing a skin punch biopsy; (**c**) bisecting a skin punch biopsy. (*From* Nobel et al. [6]; *with permission*)

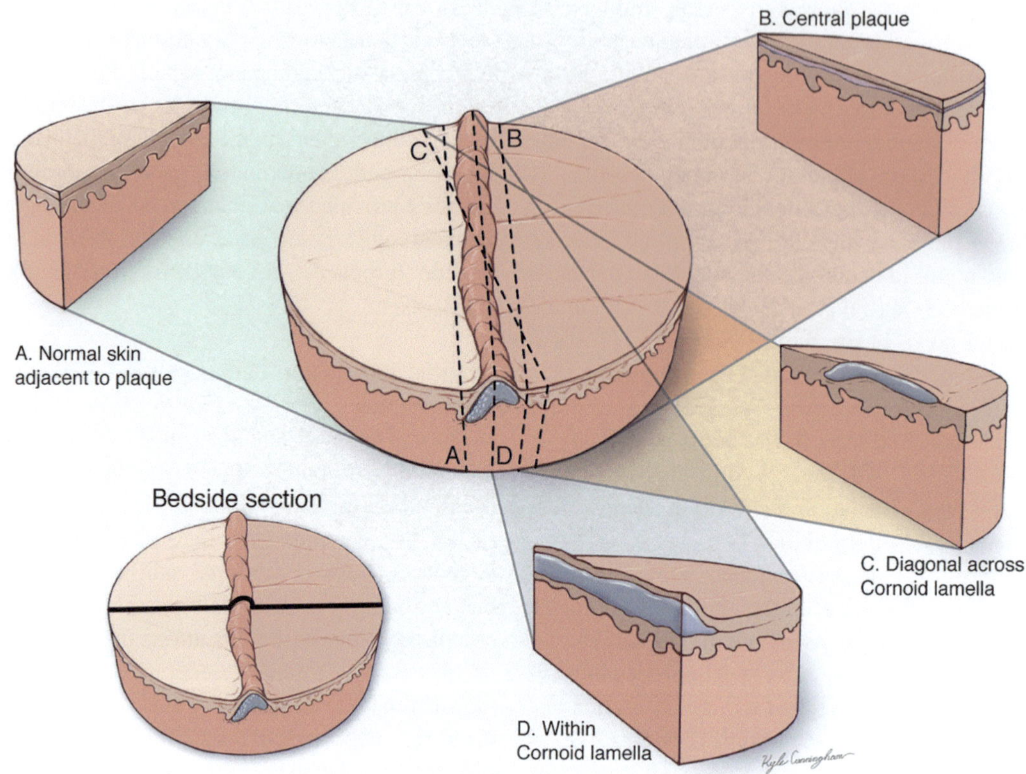

Fig. 12.82 Tissue planes for macules. (*From* Nobel et al. [6]; *with permission*)

and one-half in Zeus or Michelle's media for direct immunofluorescence processing.

Proper preparation of the lesion before the biopsy with a line drawn perpendicular to the edge of the blister (A) shown in Fig. 12.83 allows proper sectioning at the beside (B) and avoids the possibility of randomly bisecting the specimen at the grossing table which can lead to missing the blister completely (C).

Optimal Biopsy and Bedside Grossing of Vitiligo

For conditions like vitiligo, where comparing affected and normal pigmented skin provides the most information for the pathologist, correct punch sectioning at the bedside includes both lesional and perilesional skin in the same section (Fig. 12.83). This enables a direct comparison of the number of melanocytes using MART-1 or SOX-10 immunostains and aids in the interpretation of inflammatory changes at the margin of the vitiligo. Similar considerations apply to other

conditions, such as morphea, where subtle histopathology necessitates comparing the affected skin to normal skin.

Proper preparation of the lesion before the biopsy with a line drawn perpendicular to the junction of normal skin and vitiligo (A) allows proper sectioning at the beside (B), seen in Fig. 12.84. This avoids the risk of randomly bisecting the specimen at the grossing table, which can result in improper sections (C and D).

Optimal Biopsy and Bedside Grossing of Two Adjacent Lesions

Sometimes, a punch biopsy may contain two adjacent lesions within its circumference. By correctly sectioning the biopsy at the bedside, both lesions are visible in a single section. This approach allows for a comprehensive evaluation of each lesion without recuts. (See Fig. 12.84).

Clinicians choosing to bisect along line A at the bedside while visualizing both lesions

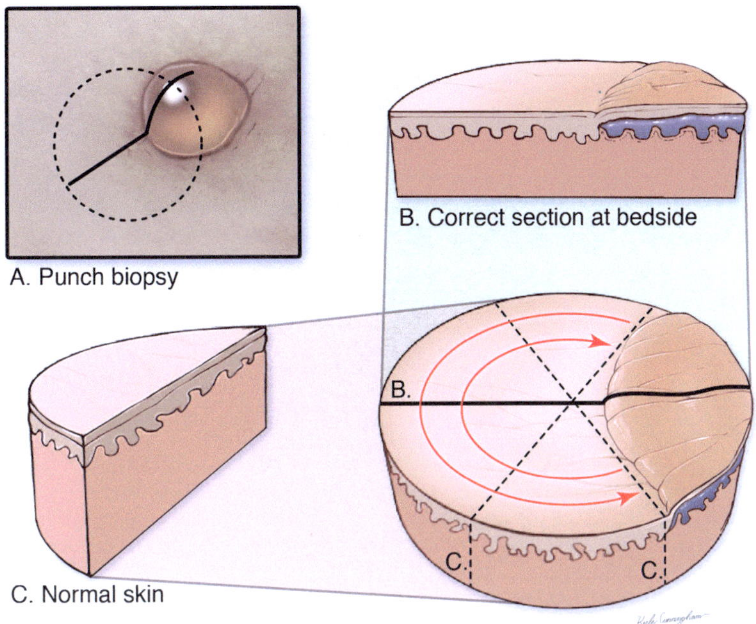

Fig. 12.83 Tissue planes for blisters. (*From* Nobel et al. [6]; *with permission*)

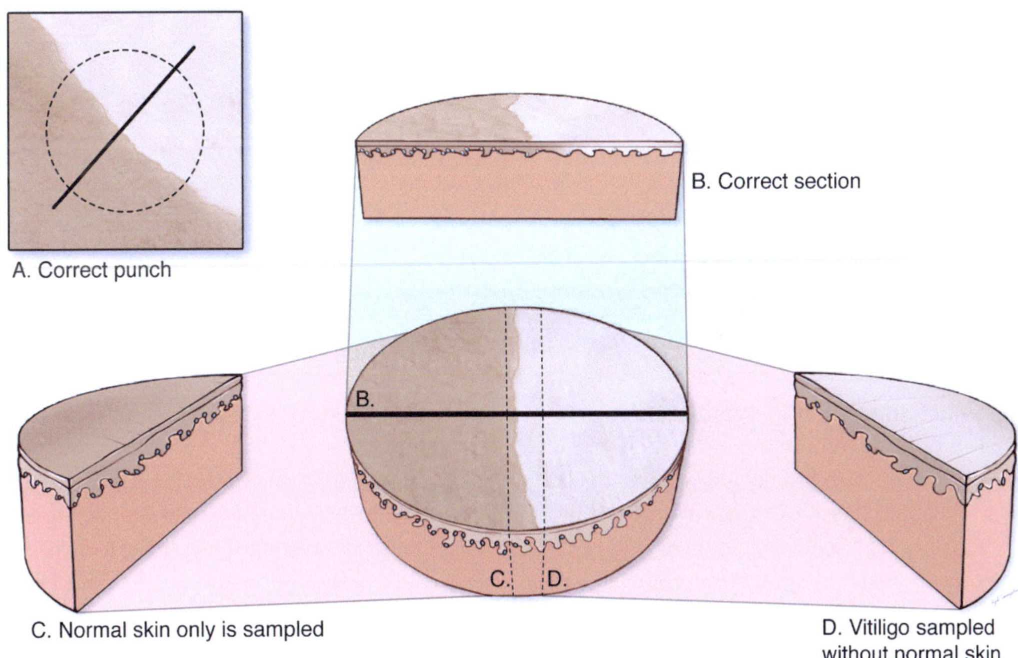

Fig. 12.84 Tissue planes of vitiligo. (*From* Nobel et al. [6]; *with permission*)

provides the specimen needed by the pathologist shown in Fig. 12.85. If the specimen is bisected randomly at the grossing table, suboptimal sections seen by the pathologist could be B, C, or D also shown in Fig. 12.85. Resectioning the tissue to identify lesions not present in the initial sections takes time and unnecessary effort.

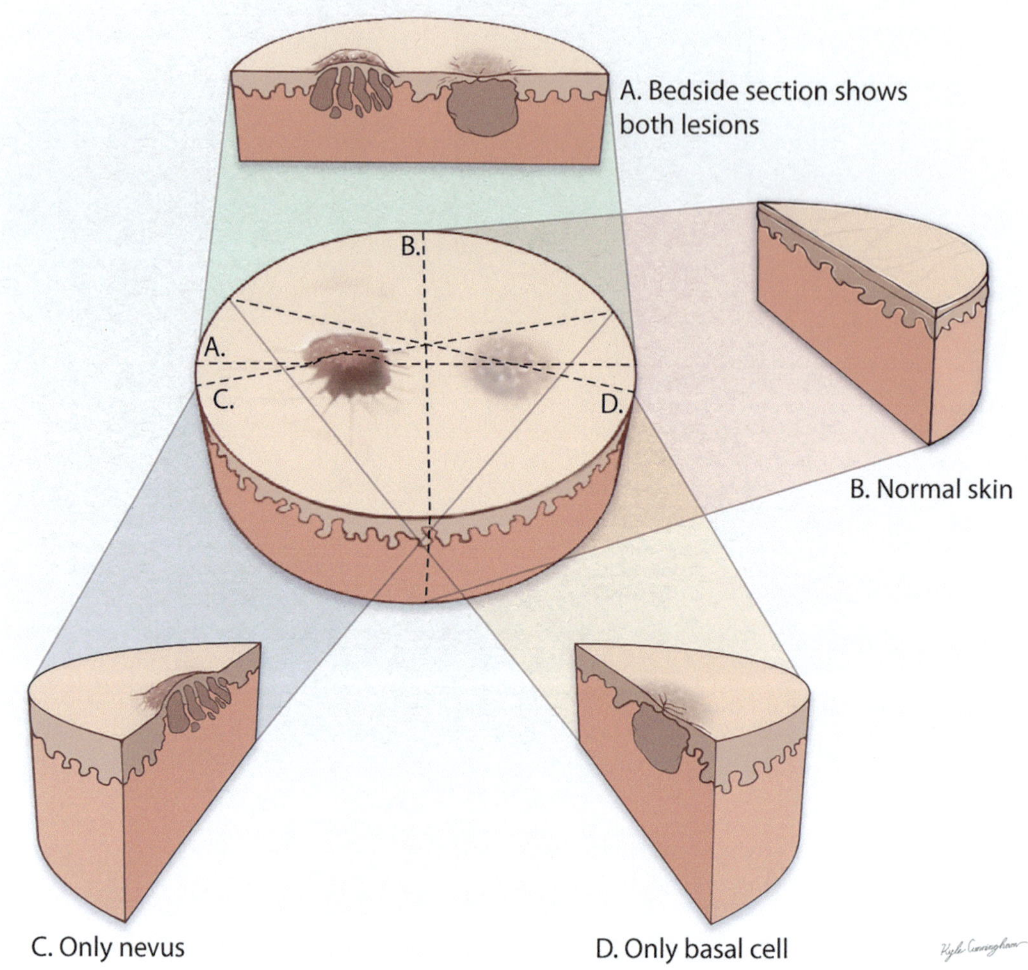

Fig. 12.85 Tissue planes of two lesions. (*From* Nobel et al. [6]; *with permission*)

Optimal Sampling of Pigmented Lesions Feared to be Melanoma.

When dealing with pigmented lesions, it is crucial to sample the thickest portion of the lesion and sample any visible ulceration (Fig. 12.85). This is optimally done by the clinician at the bedside. This approach ensures that the pathologist can determine the Breslow depth at the thickest portion of melanoma and allows the pathologist to see the ulceration which affects the AJCC staging of the melanoma to determine the patient's prognosis.

Bedside grossing ensures that the biopsy is bisected in a manner that positions the ulcerated and thickest portion of the melanoma are included in sections viewed by the pathologist shown in Fig. 12.86.

In conclusion, bedside grossing is a valuable tool that can be harnessed with proper collaboration and coordination between the pathologist and the clinician. It significantly improves the potential for obtaining the correct histopathologic diagnosis.

Disclosures Robert T. Brodell is a principal investigator for clinical trials (Novartis and Sanofi), the Corevitas psoriasis biologic registry, and owns stock in Veradermics, Inc. He has served on advisory boards for Amgen and Novan. Drs Illingworth and Awais have no conflicts of interest to disclose.

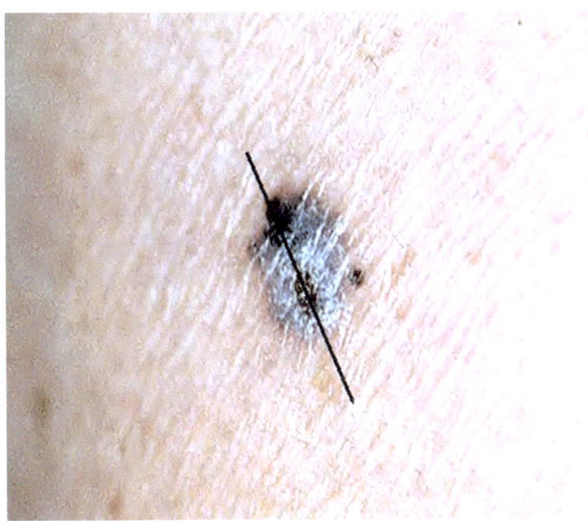

Fig. 12.86 Bisected plan of lesion

Acknowledgments The author gratefully acknowledges Robert T. Brodell, MD, FAAD, FRCP Edin, and Muhammad Awais, MBBS, for their contribution to this chapter.

Questions

1. A 67-year-old male presents with a lesion on the right cheek that has been growing for 6 months. He has a history of sun exposure and smoking. He denies any pain, itching, or bleeding. The lesion is 2 cm in diameter, raised, and firm with central ulceration. The excision specimen and cross-sections are shown in Fig. 12.87. After measuring the lesion and distance from margins, what is the most appropriate method of grossing this lesion?
   A. Ink, serially section the specimen and submit one representative section through the central lesion.
   B. Ink, serially section the specimen and submit one fullface section of the lesion.
   C. Ink, serially section the specimen and submit multiple sections perpendicular to the skin surface, including the margins.
   D. Serially section the specimen and submit multiple sections, excluding the margins.
   E. Breadloaf the specimen and submit every other section.

2. Which of the following statements is true regarding the orientation of skin specimens for histologic processing?
   A. En face margins are used to evaluate the depth of tumor invasion and the relationship with surrounding margins.
   B. Perpendicular sections are used for tips of a skin ellipse.
   C. En face margins and perpendicular sections are interchangeable and can be used for any skin specimen.
   D. Perpendicular sections are used to assess the tumor thickness and the distance between the tumor and the closest margin.
   E. En face margins are used to visualize the entire lesion thickness.

3. What is the CPT code for skin cyst removal?
   A. 88,300
   B. 88,302
   C. 88,304
   D. 88,305
   E. None of the above

4. A 45-year-old male presents with a suspicious mole on his back enlarging over the past few months. An excision is performed,

Fig. 12.87 Quiz question

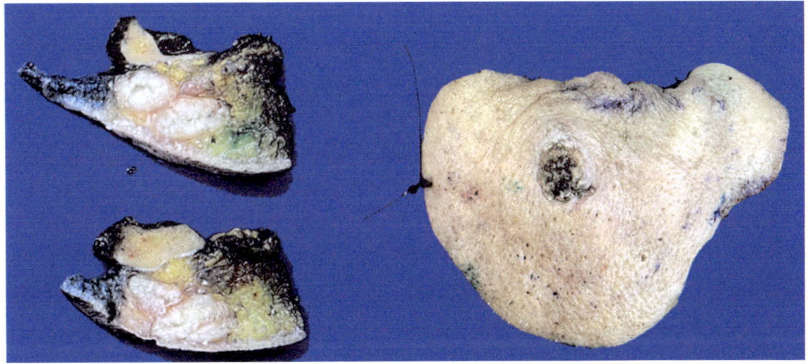

and the specimen shows a melanoma with a thickness of 1.5 mm and ulceration. What is the pT stage for this melanoma?

A. pT1a
B. pT1b
C. pT2a
D. pT2b
E. None of the above

5. Which of the following is the correct color scheme for inking skin specimens for melanoma?

A. Superior: blue, Inferior: green, Medial: red, Lateral: yellow, Deep: orange
B. Superior: green, Inferior: blue, Medial: red, Lateral: yellow, Deep: black
C. Superior: blue, Inferior: green, Medial: yellow, Lateral: red, Deep: black
D. Superior: yellow, Inferior: blue, Medial: red, Lateral: green, Deep: black
E. Superior: red, Inferior: yellow, Medial: blue, Lateral: green, Deep: black

6. What should be the ratio of perilesional skin to blister in punch biopsies of large tense blisters like pemphigoid?

A. 70–75% perilesional skin and 25–30% blister
B. 50% perilesional skin and 50% blister
C. 60% perilesional skin and 40% blister
D. 40% perilesional skin and 60% blister
E. None of the above

7. At approximately what measurement in diameter will the grossing person bisect a punch biopsy?

A. 1 mm
B. 2 mm
C. 4 mm
D. 5 mm

8. A perpendicular section of the mass in relation to the true margin allows for what information that a shave or tip submitted en face?

A. Microscopic measurement of the mass to the margin
B. Diagnosis of a positive or negative margin
C. Histology of the mass
D. All of the above

9. A 2.5 unoriented skin ellipse is received in the gross room. How should this specimen be inked?

A. No ink necessary
B. Ink each half of the resection margin in separate colors dividing the specimen down the middle
C. Ink the entire resection margin 1 color
D. Ink the resection margin in 3 colors, separate colors on each long edge and a third color on the deep surface

10. Shave biopsies are submitted in what orientation?

A. Skin surface en face
B. On edge
C. Deep margin en face
D. None of the above

Answer Key

1. C. Ink, serially section the specimen and submit multiple sections perpendicular to the skin surface, including the margins.

   Explanation: The image shows an irregular ulcerated lesion. The sections show a mass with a tan-white cut surface that invades into subcutaneous adipose tissue. This is a potentially malignant lesion, and it should be serially sectioned after inking the margins, and multiple sections need to be submitted, including the margins. This method allows for assessing tumor depth, size, and margin status, which are important prognostic factors for cutaneous malignancies. Submitting one random section or one fullface section may not be representative of the entire lesion and may miss areas of invasion or maximum tumor depth. Breadloafing the specimen and submitting every other section may also miss areas of invasion.

2. **D. Perpendicular sections are used to assess the tumor thickness and the distance between the tumor and the closest margin.**

   Explanation: In the context of skin specimens, perpendicular sections are used to assess the depth of tumor invasion and the distance between the tumor and the closest margin. En face margins and perpendicular sections are not interchangeable and have different purposes. En face orientation is used for tips and shave margins, while perpendicular sections are used for evaluating tumor thickness and margin distance.

3. **C. 88,304.**

   Explanation: CPT code 88304 is used for skin specimens that require gross and microscopic examination, such as skin cysts or tags that are removed and sent to pathology for evaluation. CPT codes 88,300 and 88,302 are used for gross examination only or gross and microscopic examination of less complex specimens, respectively. CPT code 88305 is used for skin specimens that require special stains or additional work beyond gross and microscopic examination. Therefore, the correct answer is CPT code 88304.

4. **D. pT2b.**

   Explanation: According to the American Joint Committee on Cancer (AJCC) staging system for melanoma, a melanoma that is >1.0 to 2.0 mm in thickness with ulceration is classified as pT2b. Therefore, the correct answer is D.

5. **A. Superior: blue, Inferior: green, Medial: Red, Lateral: Yellow, Deep: Orange**

   Explanation: When inking skin specimens for melanoma, it is best not to use black ink because it can interfere with the pathologist's ability to assess the specimen's margins accurately.

6. **A. 70–75% perilesional skin and 25–30% blister**

   Explanation: To make a histopathologic diagnosis in cases of tense blisters like pemphigoid, capturing the "take-off point" of the blister in the biopsy is crucial. Punch biopsies should include 70–75% perilesional skin and 25–30% blister so that the epidermis does not separate completely from the dermis during the procedure or processing.

7. **D. 5 mm**

   Explanation: At approximately 5 mm the punch biopsy can be bisected, so D is correct. Bisecting a punch biopsy smaller than 5 mm is diameter may resort is tangential or poor sectioning. When a punch biopsy is bisected, the bisected/cut surface is submitted down in the cassette.

8. **D. All of the above**

   Explanation- A perpendicular section that includes mass is submitted on edge and allow for microscopic measurement of the mass to the true margin. If the mass is present at the margin, then the margin is positive for tumor; and if the mass is not present at the margin, then it is negative for tumor. Also, if the perpendicular section includes the mass, then histology of the mass can also be assessed making D the correct answer.

9. **C. Ink resection margin one color**

   Explanation- When an ellipse of skin is received unoriented by the surgeon, there is no way to decipher each margins orientation. The margin should always be inked but in this case different ink colors will not designate specific margins so one ink color covering the entire resection margin is acceptable, so answer C is correct. This allows to visibility of the margin even though the margin is not specifically designated.

10. **B. On edge**

    Explanation- Submitting skin shave biopsies on edge allows for microscopic visualization of the full thickness of the specimen (epidermis and dermis) to assess the lesion and extent of the lesion; therefore, B is correct. Submitting the skin shave biopsy with the epidermis en face will only allow for microscopic visualization of epidermal cells and the deep margin en face will only visualize the dermis. On edge is the only way to visualize both structures.

References

1. FirstPath. 2009–2023. [Online]. Available: https://www.firstpathlab.com/cpt-codes/. Accessed 2 Jun 2023.
2. Ranjan R, Singh L, Arava S, Singh M. Margins in skin excision biopsies: principles and guidelines. Indian J Dermatol. 2012;6(59):567–70.
3. Dimenstein I. Grossing biopsies: an introduction to general principles and techniques. Ann Diagn Pathol. 2009;2(13):106–13.

4. Protocol for the examination of biopsy specimens from patients with melanoma of the skin. College of American Pathologists; 2021.

5. Reed C, Reddy R, Brodell R. Diagnosing porokeratosis of mibelli every time: a novel biopsy technique to maximize histologic confirmation. Cutis. 2016;3(97):188–90.

6. Noble CA, Bhate C, Duong BT, Cruse AR, Brodell RT, Hanus RC. Clinical-pathologic correlation: the impact of grossing at the bedside. Semin Diagn Pathol. 2024;S0740–2570(24):00006. https://doi.org/10.1053/j.semdp.2024.01.007. Epub ahead of print. PMID: 38336505.

7. Tumminello K, Cochran C, Brodell R. The appearance or disappearance of the cornoid lamella due to the level and direction of sectioning in porokeratosis. J Am Acad Dermatol. 2022;4(86):145–6.

Index